Advanced Laboratory Methods in Haematology

Advanced Laboratory Methods in Haematology

Edited by

R. Martin Rowan FRCP(G) FRCP(E) FRCPath
Formerly Department of Haematology, Western Infirmary,
Glasgow, UK

Onno W. van Assendelft MD PhD
Centers for Disease Control and Prevention, Atlanta,
Georgia, USA

F. Eric Preston MD FRCP FRCPath
UK National External Quality Assessment Scheme for
Blood Coagulation, University of Sheffield, Sheffield, UK

A member of the Hodder Headline Group
LONDON • NEW YORK • NEW DELHI

First published in Great Britain in 2002 by
Arnold, a member of the Hodder Headline Group,
338 Euston Road, London NW1 3BH

http://www.arnoldpublishers.com

Distributed in the United States of America by
Oxford University Press Inc.,
198 Madison Avenue, New York, NY10016
Oxford is a registered trademark of Oxford University Press

Whilst the advice and information in this book are believed to be true and accurate at the date of going to press,
neither the authors nor the publisher can accept any legal responsibility or liability for any errors or omissions that
may be made. In particular (but without limiting the generality of the preceding disclaimer) every effort has been
made to check drug dosages; however it is still possible that errors have been missed. Furthermore, dosage
schedules are constantly being revised and new side-effects recognized. For these reasons the reader is strongly
urged to consult the drug companies' printed instructions before administering any of the drugs recommended in
this book.

British Library Cataloguing in Publication Data
A catalogue record for this book is available from the British Library

Library of Congress Cataloging-in-Publication Data
A catalog record for this book is available from the Library of Congress

ISBN 0 340 80617 6 (hb)

1 2 3 4 5 6 7 8 9 10

Commissioning Editor: Georgina Bentliff
Production Editor: Anke Ueberberg
Production Controller: Martin Kerans
Cover design: Terry Griffiths
Typeset in 10 on 12 pt Minion by Phoenix Photosetting, Chatham, Kent
Printed and bound in Italy by Giunti

Contents

Contributors

David Barnett DipMS PhD
Department of Haematology, Royal Hallamshire Hospital, Sheffield, UK

Giuseppe d'Onofrio MD
Research Centre for Automated Methods in Haematology, Department of Haematology, Università Cattolica, Roma, Italy

Elena M. Faioni MD
Angelo Bianchi Bonomi Haemophilia and Thrombosis Centre, University of Milan, Milan, Italy

Berend Houwen MD PhD
Department of Pathology and Human Anatomy, Loma Linda University Medical School, Loma Linda, California, USA

Steve Kitchen PhD
Sheffield Haemophilia and Thrombosis Centre, Royal Hallamshire Hospital, Sheffield, UK

George G. Klee MD PhD
Department of Laboratory Medicine and Pathology, Mayo Clinic and Mayo Foundation, Rochester, Minnesota, USA

John A. Koepke BS MS MD FCAP
Formerly Duke University Medical Center, Durham, North Carolina, USA

Pier M. Mannucci MD
Angelo Bianchi Bonomi Haemophilia and Thrombosis Centre, University of Milan, Milan, Italy

John D. Olson MD PhD
Department of Pathology, University of Texas Health Science Center, San Antonio, Texas, USA

F. Eric Preston MD
University of Sheffield, Sheffield, UK

John T. Reilly MD FRCP FRCPath
Department of Haematology, Royal Hallamshire Hospital, Sheffield, UK

Katayoun Rezvani BSc MBBS MRCP DipRCPath
Department of Haematology, Imperial College School of Medicine, London, UK

R. Martin Rowan FRCP(G) FRCP(E) FRCPath
Formerly Department of Haematology, Western Infirmary, Glasgow, UK

Annette Schlueter MD PhD
Department of Pathology, The University of Iowa, Iowa City, Iowa, USA

Patricia Schryver BS
Department of Laboratory Medicine and Pathology, Mayo Clinic and Mayo Foundation, Minnesota, USA

Douglas A. Triplett MD
Department of Pathology, Ball Memorial Hospital, Muncie, Indiana, USA

Onno W. van Assendelft MD PhD
Centers for Disease Control and Prevention, Atlanta, Georgia, USA

Anton M.H.P. van den Besselaar MD
Department of Haematology, University Hospital, Leiden, The Netherlands

Isobel D. Walker MD FRCPath
Department of Haematology, The Royal Infirmary, Glasgow, UK

Sunitha N. Wickramasinghe PhD MB FIBiol FRCP FRCPath
Department of Haematology, Imperial College School of Medicine, London, UK

Mark Worwood BSc PhD FRCPath F Med Sci
Department of Haematology, University of Wales College of Medicine, Cardiff, UK

Gina Zini MD
Research Centre for Automated Methods in Haematology, Department of Haematology, Università Cattolica, Roma, Italy

Preface

The International Council (formerly Committee) for Standardization in Haematology (ICSH) was established to promote and encourage the improvement of methods, to promote the development of standards needed to achieve international comparability of results of haematological analyses, and to provide a forum for communication on these topics by the professions concerned with haematology laboratory functions. Towards these goals, the work of ICSH includes (i) the development of international reference standards of haematological importance, (ii) collaboration with appropriate bodies in various countries to establish comparable national and secondary reference standards, (iii) standardization of analytical methods used in haematology, (iv) selection of appropriate tests to support the different requirements of clinical medicine, research and epidemiology within the limits of resources and facilities available to laboratories, and (v) development of quality assurance programmes.

Biological sciences depend extensively on measurement, defined by the International Organization for Standardization (ISO) as that set of operations whose object it is to determine the values of a quantity. This requires the application of the scientific principles of a measurement process: the measurement must be traceable, directly or indirectly, to an international metrological standard. All diagnostic laboratory equipment and methods must be standardized for relevant measurements and users need to be assured of the control of precision and accuracy of these measurements. ICSH is thus especially concerned with guidelines, recommendations, standards, standard materials and their application for the calibration of all equipment and apparatus used in the haematology laboratory, from simple haemocytometer chambers and pipettes to the most complex automated multiparameter analytical systems.

ICSH is the standardizing authority of the International Society of Hematology and is in official relations with the WHO as a non-government organization (NGO). ICSH has associations with allied professional societies and with industry on various aspects of laboratory practice. There are established collaborative links with other international organizations, such as the International Society of Laboratory Haematology (ISLH), the International Society of Blood Transfusion (ISBT), the International Society on Thrombosis and Haemostasis (ISTH), the International Federation of Clinical Chemistry and Laboratory Medicine (IFCC), the World Association of Societies of Pathology (WASP), and close liaison with a number of national organizations, notably the National Committee for Clinical Standards (NCCLS) in the United States of America.

In addition to creating written and material standards and guideline documents, ICSH fulfils a major educational role by presenting symposia and workshops in association with meetings of professional societies, particularly the International Society of Hematology. Over the years, ICSH has published a series of books on diverse haematological topics including red cell counting methods, standardization, modern concepts in haematology, abnormal haemoglobins and thalassaemia, quality control, advances in haematology laboratory methods, quality assurance and management and practice.

Laboratory practice evolves rapidly with greater diversity of testing and increasing automation but against a need for cost containment and increasing accountability. This latest volume reflects these advances and the necessary reactions to them with each chapter written by acknowledged international experts in their particular field. The aim has been to produce a balanced, topical but at the same time readable volume reflecting the latest best laboratory haematology practice.

This book is intended primarily for haematologists and technical staff working in haematology laboratories, but it will also be of value to students and their teachers. The book will also be of interest to laboratory workers in disciplines other than haematology, to healthcare administrators and to public health authorities.

R.M. Rowan, Glasgow, UK
O.W. van Assendelft, Atlanta, GA, USA
F.E. Preston, Sheffield, UK

Introduction

At the IXth Congress of the European Society of Haematology, a symposium on *Erythrocytic Methods and their Standardization* was held on 31 August 1963. Papers were presented and discussed on the red blood cell count, the packed cell volume and trapped plasma, the mean red cell diameter, the measurement of haemoglobin concentration, and results of national and international haematological trials. At this symposium a Standardising Committee of the European Society of Haematology was also founded:

> '1. In order to bring about the international comparability of results of haematological analysis, the persons present, representatives of the European Society of Haematology, of national haematological societies, of clinical pathology societies as well as other national, international and supranational societies and corporations, have decided to found a Standardising Committee of the European Society of Haematology.'

This newly founded Standardising Committee immediately proceeded to make recommendations for the standardization of the determination of haemoglobin concentration in human blood. The symposium proceedings, edited by Ch. G. de Boroviczeny, were published by S. Karger, Basel/New York in 1964 (Bibl. Haemat., Fasc. 18).

In 1964, at the Xth Congress of the International Society of Haematology, a second symposium, *Standardization, Documentation and Normal Values in Haematology*, was held. At this time it was proposed to enlarge the Standardising Committee of the European Society of Haematology to include members from outside the European Society and to create an international standardizing committee of haematology. Again, symposium proceedings edited by Ch. G. de Boroviczeny were published by S. Karger, Basel/New York (Bibl. Haemat., Fasc. 21, 1965).

At the Xth Congress of the European Society of Haematology a third symposium, *Standardization in Haematology III*, was held. The name of the standardizing committee was changed to the International Committee for Standardization in Haematology of the European Society of Haematology and the symposium proceedings, again edited by Ch. G. de Boroviczeny, were published by S. Karger, Basel/New York (Bibl. Haemat., Fasc. 24, 1966).

The standardizing committee finally became the International Committee (now Council) for Standardization in Haematology (ICSH) at the XIth Congress of the International Society of Haematology in 1966.

ICSH continued to organize or sponsor free-standing symposia, and symposia or educational sessions at international or regional meetings. A number of these resulted in further publication of proceedings and other publications.

New York, September 1968/Milan, November 1968:
Astaldi, G., Sirtori, C. and Vanzetti, G. (eds) (1970) *Standardization in Hematology*. Milan: Franco Angeli Editore.

Munich, 1970:
Izak, G. and Lewis, S.M. (eds) (1972) *Modern Concepts in Hematology*. New York: Academic Press.
S. Giovanni Rotondo, 1971:
Astaldi, G., Gusso, G., Tentori, L. and Torlontano, G. (eds) (1972) *Standardization in Haematology and Clinical Pathology*. Fogia: Archivio Casa Sollievo della Sofferenza.

Jerusalem, 1974:
Lewis, S.M. and Coster, J.F. (eds) (1975) *Quality Control in Haematology*. London: Academic Press.
R.M. Schmidt (ed.) (1975) *Abnormal Haemoglobins and Thalassaemia*. New York: Academic Press.

Berlin, 1979/Montebello, 1980:
Lewis, S.M. and Verwilghen, R.L. (eds) (1988) *Quality Assurance in Haematology*. London: Baillière Tindall.
van Assendelft, O.W. and England, J.M. (eds) (1982) *Advances in Hematological Methods: the Blood Count*. Boca Raton, FL: CRC Press.

Amsterdam, 1994:
Huefner Memorial Symposium: Analytical and Physiological Aspects of 100 Years of Hemoglobin Research. *Lab. Hemat.* (1995) **1**: 30–36; 143–169.
S.M. Lewis, S.M. and Koepke, J.A. (eds) (1995) *Hematology Laboratory Management and Practice*. Oxford: Butterworth-Heinemann.

Laboratory practice has changed in recent years. Instrumentation has become more complex and automated; labour, instrumentation and reagent costs have increased; clinicians look forward to increased accuracy and decreased turn-around times; laboratories are held more accountable to hospital management, auditors, health authorities and regulators, and, of course, to its customers. The present volume, with sections on blood cell counting, haemoglobinometry, abnormal haemoglobin detection, erythrocyte sedimentation, haematopoietic factors and coagulation, discusses some of the methodological advances and some of the newer measurable parameters in the haematology laboratory.

1

The blood count

1

Quality assurance for basic haematology cell counts

GEORGE G. KLEE AND PATRICIA SCHRYVER

INTRODUCTION

The production of valid analytical test results is dependent on many factors, including robust procedures for collection of specimens, pre-analytical processing, measurement of each of the parameters, validation of the test information, and timely reporting of both test values and reference data. To assure that each of these procedures is functioning properly, the system needs statistically valid monitoring programmes for each of these functions. There is generally a trade-off between the robustness of the procedure and the intensity of the control system required to maintain the performance. A robust procedure which is stable and reproducible requires less monitoring than one that is less reliable or unstable. The design of both the laboratory procedures and their accompanying quality control systems are critically dependent on the existence of well-defined performance criteria. Unfortunately, even though haematology cell counts are frequently ordered, there is no consensus for performance criteria for most of these procedures.

This chapter discusses seven important areas to be included in a quality assurance programme for laboratory testing of haematological cell counts:

- specimen identification
- specimen integrity
- analytical imprecision
- analytical bias
- medical review criteria
- quality control monitors
- assay turnaround time.

1.1 SPECIMEN IDENTIFICATION

Specimen identification is an important factor that is difficult to control and even more difficult to monitor. The 'right' result on the wrong patient can often be more dangerous than the other sources of error, because two patients may be inappropriately treated (both the patient initially found to have the wrong report and the second patient whose specimen was involved in the mix-up). Zero tolerance for misidentification errors is the goal for specimen identification; however, this is impossible. For fully automated systems, a working target could be less than one error in 100 000 specimen collections. Experimental studies have shown that most manual processes have an identification error rate of 1–20/10 000, which is far greater than this target (Houwen, 1990). Therefore, automated identification systems are highly recommended.

Closed-loop systems utilizing bar codes and bar code readers are an effective way of reducing identification errors. The term 'closed loop' designates that all the information transfer steps from the initial identification of the patient, which include the collection of the specimen, processing of the specimen, measurement of the analytes, generation of the reports and archiving of the information, are performed by systems that electronically link the elements together. These closed-loop systems require a positive patient linkage for each step in the process, often through the use of bar code labels and direct interface of the analytical instruments to the laboratory and/or medical information system. Many of the current haematology cell counters and laboratory computer systems have bar code readers and computer interfaces to facilitate this process. Using bar code readers and duplicate entry of keyboard data, error rates as low as 3/100 000 have been reported (Houwen, 1990).

1.1.1 Use of delta checks for confirmation of identification

Effective monitoring systems for detection of error rates of less than 1/100 000 are difficult to construct. Delta checking, in which a patient's test values are compared with previous test values, has been proposed as a mechanism to detect specimen misidentification (Houwen and Duffin, 1989). The differences between two consecutive test values on a patient are dependent on multiple factors, such as the time between the collections, the biological variability of the analyte, and medical condition of the patient, receipt of blood transfusions as well as the laboratory processes for collection, transport, processing and measurement. Each of these processes adds variation to the test values. Overall, the difference between two reported values in the same patient is often as large as the differences in test values between two randomly selected patients.

The limits used for delta checking need to be carefully defined. If the check limits are set too small, there will be numerous false-positive signals, whereas if the limits are too large, the system will not be able to detect real errors. Table 1.1 shows selected percentile limits for the distribution of the absolute value of the difference between measurements of repeat specimens from 2247 patients having a second specimen collected within 72 hours of their first specimen while at the Mayo Clinic hospitals and outpatient services. These data are from an integrated practice that has about 350 000 patient registrations per year and about 2000 hospital beds. These distributions represent the absolute value of the differences of measurements performed in a centralized laboratory using three Coulter STKS instruments which are calibrated to provide similar results. The distribution of these differences reflects the pre-analytical, analytical, and post-analytical changes.

Table 1.2 shows how the distributions of the delta values between serial measurements on a patient broaden as a function of the time interval between the measurements. The table is derived using data from 3500 to 8100 pairs of specimens which were collected between 1 and

Table 1.1 *Distribution limits for the absolute value of the delta between repeat specimens collected within 72 hours*

Measurement	Units	70%	80%	90%	95%	98%	99%	99.5%	99.9%
Haemoglobin	g/dL	1.0	1.3	2.1	2.8	3.6	4.2	4.9	6.0
Haematocrit	%	3.1	4.2	6.3	8.1	10.6	12.6	14.8	19.2
Erythrocytes	$\times\ 10^{12}$/L	0.35	0.47	0.72	0.94	1.22	1.43	1.63	2.05
MCV	fL	0.8	1.1	1.5	1.9	2.8	3.6	5.3	7.6
Leucocytes	$\times\ 10^{9}$/L	2.6	3.7	5.5	7.4	9.8	12.8	19.1	45.6
Platelets	$\times\ 10^{9}$/L	35	50	78	109	150	179	224	280
MPV	fL	0.4	0.5	0.8	1.0	1.3	1.7	2.3	3.0
RDW	%	0.3	0.4	0.6	0.8	1.2	1.6	2.0	4.0
Neutrophils	$\times\ 10^{9}$/L	2.69	3.66	5.46	7.18	8.76	10.9	12.67	16.91
Lymphocytes	$\times\ 10^{9}$/L	0.46	0.61	0.9	1.18	1.56	2.03	2.36	3.91
Monocytes	$\times\ 10^{9}$/L	0.21	0.3	0.45	0.6	0.8	0.9	1.05	2.18
Eosinophils	$\times\ 10^{9}$/L	0.08	0.11	0.19	0.29	0.42	0.54	0.76	1.25
Basophils	$\times 10^{9}$/L	0.03	0.06	0.12	0.19	0.28	0.36	0.4	0.5

MCV, mean cell volume; MPV, mean platelet volume; RDW, red cell distribution width.

7 days apart (the values for ≤ 3 days are slightly different from Table 1.1 because this data file contains multiple specimens per patient, whereas the first file is based on the subset with only two specimens per patient). Some measurements, such as mean cell volume (MCV), mean platelet volume (MPV), red cell distribution width (RDW) and basophil granulocytes, are relatively stable with time, while others, such as haemoglobin, haematocrit, leucocytes and platelets, can change quite dramatically. Delta checks that span longer time intervals would include a larger number of patients, but the wider ranges further diminish the probability of detection of sample mix-ups. Potential improvements in error detection could occur if longer time intervals were used for the stable measurements and shorter time intervals for the more volatile measurements.

Table 1.2 *Effect of time interval between collections on 95% limits of absolute value of delta between measurements*

Measurement	Units	≤ 1 day	≤ 2 days	≤ 3 days	≤ 4 days	≤ 7 days
Haemoglobin	g/dL	2.3	2.4	2.6	2.7	2.8
Haematocrit	%	6.7	7.3	7.7	7.8	8.0
Erythrocytes	$\times\ 10^{12}$/L	0.77	0.83	0.89	0.90	0.93
MCV	fL	1.9	1.9	2.0	2.0	2.1
Leucocytes	$\times\ 10^{9}$/L	6.4	6.5	6.8	6.9	7.0
Platelets	$\times\ 10^{9}$/L	75	81	90	99	113
MPV	fL	0.9	0.9	1.0	1.0	1.0
RDW	%	0.8	0.8	0.9	0.9	1.0
Neutrophils	$\times\ 10^{9}$/L	6.01	6.31	6.55	6.61	6.71
Lymphocytes	$\times\ 10^{9}$/L	1.01	1.05	1.09	1.09	1.12
Monocytes	$\times\ 10^{9}$/L	0.57	0.59	0.59	0.60	0.61
Eosinophils	$\times\ 10^{9}$/L	0.21	0.24	0.25	0.26	0.28
Basophils	$\times\ 10^{9}$/L	0.20	0.20	0.20	0.20	0.20

MCV, mean cell volume; MPV, mean platelet volume; RDW, red cell distribution width.

The statistical power of delta checking systems for detection of specimen identification errors is relatively low. The percentage distribution limits for delta checks listed in Table 1.1 are quite large. When wide ranges (such as 99.9th percentile) are used as delta check limits, the utility of this procedure for detection of sample identification errors is quite low, because a large percentage of randomly selected patients would have values matching within these limits. If tighter check limits are used (such as the 70th percentile), fewer randomly selected patients have values within these limits, but many (30%) repeat values from the same patient would be triggered as sample mix-ups.

The performance characteristics of eight delta check rules were evaluated for their utility in identifying specimen misidentification. The rules evaluated were:

- Rule A – any of the 13 tests outside delta limits;
- Rule B – all of the 13 tests outside delta limits;
- Rule C – haemoglobin, leucocyte, erythrocyte *or* platelet count outside delta limits;
- Rule D – haemoglobin, leucocyte, erythrocyte *and* platelet count outside delta limits;
- Rule E – neutrophil, lymphocyte, monocyte, eosinophil *or* basophil outside delta limits;
- Rule F – neutrophil, lymphocyte, monocyte, eosinophil *and* basophil outside delta limits;
- Rule G – MCV, MPV *or* RDW outside delta limits;
- Rule H – MCV, MPV *and* RDW outside delta limits.

The limits used in the evaluation were the 70, 80, 90, 95, 98 and 99% limits shown in Table 1.1. The control group was composed of the 2247 patients whose paired test values were used to generate Table 1.1. The test group was computer-generated by pairing the initial value from the control group with the value randomly selected from the remaining 2246 initial values. Sensitivity was calculated as the percentage of the mismatched paired data which violated the control rules, while specificity was calculated from the number of matched pairs which violated the rules. Table 1.3 and Figure 1.1 show the receiver operating characteristics (ROCs) for these rules.

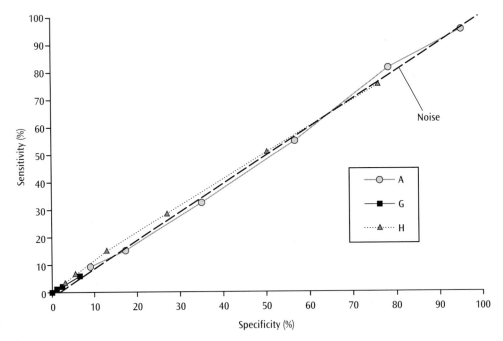

Fig. 1.1 *Receiver operating characteristics for delta check rules A, G and H (see text for details).*

Table 1.3 *Receiver operating characteristics for the power of delta check rules to detect specimen misidentifications*

Measurements	Limits	'And-ing' together Sensitivity	100 – specificity	'Or-ing' together Sensitivity	100 – specificity
All 13 haem tests	99%	0	0	9	9
	98%	0	0	15.1	17
	95%	0	0	32.5	34.9
	90%	0	0	54.9	56.6
	80%	0	0	81.4	78.2
	70%	0	0	94.8	94.8
Haemoglobin,	99%	0	0	2.54	3.0
leucocytes, RBCs,	98%	0.04	0.04	4.6	6.0
platelets	95%	0.09	0.09	12.4	14.6
	90%	0.4	0.53	22.7	25.5
	80%	1.16	2.45	43.2	45.6
	70%	4.54	6.9	58.3	60.0
Neutrophils,	99%	0	0	3.87	4.0
lymphocytes,	98%	0	0	6.85	8.14
monocytes,	95%	0	0	16.55	18.69
eosinophils,	90%	0	0.04	30.7	33.51
basophils	80%	0.40	0.09	53.18	50.86
	70%	1.64	1.96	68.55	71.16
MCV, MPV, RDW	99%	0	0	3.64	3.0
	98%	0.18	0.13	6.76	5.52
	95%	0.4	0.31	15.09	12.86
	90%	1.27	1.07	28.57	27.01
	80%	2.4	2.31	51.13	50.33
	70%	6.05	6.45	75.57	75.79

RBCs, red blood cells; MCV, mean cell volume; MPV, mean platelet volume; RDW, red cell distribution width.

An ideal discriminator (100% sensitivity and 100% specificity) would be represented by the left vertical axis and the upper horizontal axis. The diagonal line represents random noise. All the delta check rules are close to random noise in terms of their power to detect specimen misidentification. Three of the 'better' rules (A, G and H), as shown in Figure 1.1, also are close to random noise. Two other rules (B and F) had very low sensitivity for error detection; in fact, no patients from either the control or the test group had all 13 parameters outside any of the limits tested.

Houwen and Duffin (1989) have advocated the use of delta checks for the detection of random errors. By setting limits at about 99.5% and also making their check limits a function of the initial test value, they were able to identify 'suspicious' cases, which were subjected to further investigation. Since these extreme delta values seldom occur naturally, it is probably appropriate to investigate the clinical status of these cases. On the other hand, one should not assume that these delta check systems detect most of the sample mix-ups. A recent Q-Probe study of 703 laboratories by the College of American Pathologists showed that flags for test values exceeding delta check limits were the third most frequent cause for CBC specimen rejection (Jones *et al.*, 1995). These 'suspicious' cases probably warrant further investigation, but the inherent lack of sensitivity and specificity of delta check rules does not justify using these rules for specimen rejection based on suspected specimen identification errors.

1.2 SPECIMEN INTEGRITY

For haematology specimens, three major problems in specimen integrity are clumps (aggregations and clots), haemolysis and cellular degeneration. Most current instruments have flags to detect erythrocyte agglutination and platelet clumps. In addition, most laboratories have their personnel check the specimens for visible clots in the EDTA tubes. Clot formation is generally caused by improper mixing and/or improper collection technique. The usual corrective action for clotted specimens is to redraw the specimen, which is both inconvenient and expensive.

Haemolysis has a direct effect on the erythrocyte count and the red cell parameters. Some analysers have a check for haemolysis and most have checks for red blood cell (RBC) fragments. Cellular degradation is generally a function of storage time and temperature. Leucocytes and platelets are most susceptible to degradation. Most analyser manufacturers have recommendations for specimen storage conditions and maximum allowable storage times.

A College of American Pathologists Q-Probe study analysed specimen acceptability issues from 703 laboratories processing an aggregate of about eight million complete blood counts (Jones et al., 1995). About 35 000 specimens were rejected (0.45%). Specimen integrity issues accounted for 88% of the rejections as listed below:

- clotted specimen (64.8%)
- insufficient quantity (10.1%)
- improperly labelled (5.1%)
- clumped platelets (2.2%)
- haemolysis (2.0%)
- contamination with intravenous solution (1.6%)
- improper container (1.4%)
- delayed delivery (0.9%).

The relative frequency of specimen problems was over fourfold greater for complete blood count specimens collected in microtube containers. Clotted specimens and insufficient quantity accounted for 89% of the microtube specimen problems. These authors recommend that laboratories establish quality improvement programmes which monitor rejected specimens and focus corrective action plans on the most frequent causes of rejection.

1.3 ANALYTICAL IMPRECISION

Several systems have been used to propose tolerance limits for the analytical precision of laboratory measurements: previous performance records of the instruments, ratio of analytical to biological variation, clinical perceptions without significant changes, and the effects of laboratory tests on clinical outcomes (Barnett, 1968; Statland et al., 1978; Elion-Gerritzen, 1980; Fraser, 1987).

The standard practice in most laboratories is to document the imprecision of the instrument by calculating the mean (x), standard deviation (SD) and coefficient of variation (CV) of approximately 20 measurements of three levels of control. The precision goals for that instrument are set at $x \pm 2SD$ for each level of control. The less reproducible instruments are assigned wider performance controls. This method of setting imprecision performance limits is quite arbitrary, but serves to assure that the laboratory is functioning 'as good as it was yesterday'. Unfortunately, it does not have any relationship to the clinical use of the tests.

Much of the literature on precision goal setting focuses on clinical chemistry analytes; however, the principles are the same for haematology tests. Tonks (1963) empirically suggested that total allowable analytical error should not exceed one-quarter of the normal reference interval. Since reference intervals typically are set at $x \pm 2SD$ (biological across-population), this recommendation implies that the analytical SD should be less than the biological SD. Mathematically, it can be shown that if the analytical SD is less that one-quarter of the biological SD then the total SD of the combination of the two variances is only increased by < 3%. Assuming that the analytical and biological variances are independent, then:

$$SD^2_{total} = SD^2_{biological} + SD^2_{analytical}$$

If $SD_{analytical} < \frac{1}{4} SD_{biological}$, then:

$$SD^2_{total} < (1 + 1/16) SD^2_{biological}$$
$$SD_{total} < 1.03 \, SD_{biological}$$

This concept is illustrated in Figure 1.2 for biological CVs varying from 1 to 15% and analytical CVs of 1–5%.

The choice of how the biological variation is defined depends on the clinical use of the laboratory test. If the test is used for diagnosis (separation of individual from a population at risk) then the across-population biological SD is used. If the test is used to monitor progression of an analyte within a specific person over time, then the within-person biological variation would be used (Fraser *et al.*, 1990). The choice of the time interval (short-term versus long-term) and the conditions of specimen collection (time of day, position, fasting state, etc)

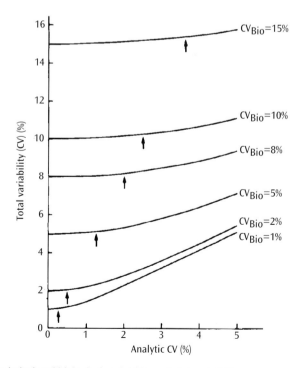

Fig. 1.2 *Effect of analytical and biological variability on total variability.*

used for the biological reference study depends on the conditions used for monitoring (Statland *et al.*, 1978).

Another method proposed for estimating imprecision tolerance goals is to ask practising clinicians to determine what degree of test change would alter their medical decision (Barnett, 1968; Elion-Gerritzen, 1980). Some elaborate case scenarios have been designed to collect this information. Following this approach, Thure and Sandberg (1993) used 11 case histories to estimate the imprecision goal for haemoglobin and recommended 2.8% (range of 0–7.8%). One of the problems of this approach is that it generally focuses on individual patients and may not take into account the aggregate influence of these laboratory parameters on large numbers of patients.

A fourth approach to defining laboratory performance goals is to analyse the impact of the laboratory test on medical outcomes. Most of this work has focused on simulation studies, because it is difficult to carry out randomized, blinded, controlled clinical studies (Klee 1990, 1993).

Data from some of these studies are summarized in Table 1.4. Current precision performance based on measurement of pools appears to be acceptable for the precision goals; however, tight instrument precision is important for assuring instrument accuracy and the bias goals are more difficult to achieve if precision is low.

Table 1.4 *Imprecision goals (for normals) as determined by various approaches*

Analyte	Coefficient of variation (CV)			
	Pools[a]	Biological/analytical[b]	Clinician[c]	Cases[d]
WBCs	1.7–2.1 %	2.83, 7.8 %	16.4 %	–
RBCs	0.5–1.8 %	0.87 %	–	–
HGB	0.4–1.3 %	0.70, 1.2 %	3.6, 2.8 %	4.8, 13.4%
MCV	0.5–1.3 %	0.77 %	3.2 %	–
Platelet	0.8–2.1 %	3.5, 3.3 %	–	–

WBCs, white blood cells; RBCs, red blood cells; HGB, haemoglobin; MCV, mean cell volume.
[a]Tatsumi *et al.* (1996).
[b]Klee (1990), Statland *et al.* (1978), Fraser (1987).
[c]Barnett (1968), Fraser (1987).
[d]Thure and Sandberg (1993), Elion-Gerritzen (1980).

1.4 ANALYTICAL BIAS

Shifts in analytical measurements due to analyser drift, calibration changes and/or reagent lot changes are major laboratory performance issues (Klee, 1997). When an analyser has a shift in the set point of calibration, there can be dramatic changes in the percentage of patients having test values exceeding critical decision thresholds. In an era of managed care and critical pathways, these shifts can create major downstream costs. Table 1.5 shows that very small shifts in the set point of a haematology analyser can cause major changes in the number of patients having test values outside the normal reference range. Shifts in haemoglobin of ±0.5 g/dL cause changes of +34% to –28% in the number of patients having haemoglobin concentrations below 10 g/dL. In the leucocyte channel, shifts of ±0.2 × 10⁹/L can cause changes of –15.0% to +17% in the number of patients flagged as 'leucopenic'. Similarly, shifts of ±2.0 fL in the MCV changes the percentage of patients classified as 'macrocytic' by +69% to –45%.

Variations in patient populations can be used to calculate performance target limits for analytical bias (Tatsumi *et al.*, 1996). Using this algorithm, analytical bias performance goals

Table 1.5   *Effect of analytical bias on distribution of patient values outside decision level*

Haemoglobin (female)

Bias (g/dL)	Decision level % ABN	6.0 g/L change	Decision level % ABN	10.0 g/dL change
−0.5	1.1%	−50%	10.8%	−28%
−0.2	1.7%	−23%	13.1%	−13%
0	2.2%	0%	15.1%	0%
+0.2	3.0%	+35%	16.9%	+12%
+0.5	4.2%	+91%	20.2%	+34%

Leucocyte count

Bias (cells/µL)	Decision level % ABN	3500/µL change	Decision level % ABN	10 500/µL change
−200	5.1%	−15%	17.9%	+5.3%
−100	5.6%	−7%	17.5%	+2.9%
0	6.0%	0	17.0%	0%
+100	6.5%	+8%	16.6%	−2.4%
+200	7.0%	+17%	16.2%	−4.7%

MCV

Bias (fL)	Decision level % ABN	80 fL change	Decision level % ABN	100 fL change
−2	2.7%	−44%	4.9	+69
−1	3.6%	−25%	3.8	+31
0	4.8%	0%	2.9	0
+1	6.4%	+33%	2.2	−24
+2	8.7%	+81%	1.6	−45

Platelet count

Bias (cells/µL)	Decision level % ABN	100 000/µL change	Decision level % ABN	400 000/µL change
−25 000	4.2%	−35%	6.8	+33%
−10 000	5.4%	−17%	5.7	+12%
0	6.5%	0%	6.1	0%
+10 000	7.6%	+17%	4.6	−10%
+25 000	9.8%	+51%	3.9	−24%

ABN, abnormal; MCV, mean cell volume.

were calculated for the lower and upper ranges of the haematology test parameters. These data were based on 20 consecutive distributions, with over 1000 patient values in each. The variation of the percentage of the distribution having values outside the reference range was calculated for each group and the analyte range corresponding to ±1SD of the distribution was selected as the bias goal. The rationale for using the variation of patient distribution to set control limits for analytical bias is that the percentages of the patients exceeding decision thresholds are generally fairly constant from day to day, and clinicians generally know these ranges of variation, at least intuitively. When there is an unusual change in the test value distribution, specialist clinicians become suspicious of analytical shifts and may call the laboratory to check if the assay has shifted. By linking analytical bias goals to the usual changes in the test distributions, the laboratory should be alerted to changes that are large enough to cause clinical concerns prior to the notification (angry calls) from clinicians.

The numbers in Table 1.6 show that the bias performance goals are tightest (< 1%) for the red cell and platelet indices and widest (5–14%) for the leucocyte count. Most of the other parameters have bias performance goals in the 1–5% range.

Table 1.6 *Bias performance goals from patient distributions*

Analyte	Units	Level I	Goal	CV (%)	Level II	Goal	CV (%)
Haemoglobin	g/dL	11.9	0.26	2.2%	15.5	0.18	1.2%
Haematocrit	%	35	0.70	2.0%	45	0.61	1.4%
Erythrocytes	$\times 10^{12}$/L	2.9	0.07	2.5%	4	0.05	1.2%
MCV	fL	81.5	0.7	0.8%	98.3	0.7	0.7%
Leucocytes	$\times 10^{9}$/L	3.5	0.2	4.9%	10.5	0.5	5.1%
Platelets	$\times 10^{9}$/L	150	4.0	2.7%	450	17.3	3.8%
MPV	fL	7.3	0.04	0.6%	11	0.22	2.0%
Neutrophils	$\times 10^{9}$/L	1.7	0.11	6.5%	7	0.5	7.5%
Lymphocytes	$\times 10^{9}$/L	1	0.05	4.7%	3	0.09	3.0%
Monocytes	$\times 10^{9}$/L	0.03	0.01	3.5%	1.00	0.05	5.3%
Eosinophils	$\times 10^{9}$/L	0.04	0.005	13.9%	0.35	0.03	7.1%
Basophils	$\times 10^{9}$/L	–	–	–	0.1	0.001	8.8%

CV, coefficient of variation; MCV, mean cell volume; MPV, mean platelet volume.

1.5 MEDICAL REVIEW CRITERIA

Automated cell counters can rapidly and efficiently process haematology profile tests when all measurements are normal. Unfortunately, in most complex medical centres, 40–50% of the specimens have at least one abnormality flag which requires further verification (Davis, 1994; MacDonald *et al.*, 1996). Each further verification step requires additional resources and delays the reporting of test results. A key step in most of these review processes is examination of the blood smear morphology, which is labour-intensive and time-consuming (especially if the slide is not already made). Therefore, it is important to clearly define the flagging criteria to identify medically relevant problems while maximizing the number of specimens that can be 'autoverified' (Koepke, 1994; Lacombe *et al.*, 1995; Chapman, 1997). Various expert systems are being developed to assist with this autoverification process. The basic elements in these systems are:

- instrument flags
- limit checks
- delta checks
- quality controls
- moving averages of patient values.

Additional information which helps these decisions is as follows:

- age and gender of patient
- diagnosis of patient
- medical speciality/physician
- prior test values
- prior verification of same flag.

Currently there is no consensus about the various verification parameters or the review limits. Some of the items typically flagged are (Davis, 1994; MacDonald *et al.*, 1996; Chapman, 1997):

- blasts (review limit ≥ 1)
- immature granulocytes (review limits > 2 to > 5%)
- atypical lymphocytes (review limits > 1 to 5%)
- left shift
- nucleated RBC
- RBC anisocytosis
- RBC fragments
- RBC agglutination
- platelet anisocytosis
- platelet clumps.

In addition, there often are limit checks for quantitative measurements requiring further review (Davis, 1994; MacDonald *et al.*, 1996; Chapman, 1997):

- leucocytosis (review limits > 20 to > 99.9×10^9/L)
- leucopenia (review limits < 1.0 to < 3.4×10^9/L)
- neutrophilia (review limits > 5.2 to > 13.0×10^9/L)
- neutropenia (review limits < 1.0 to < 2.2×10^9/L)
- lymphocytosis (review limits > 2.6 to > 5.5×10^9/L)
- lymphopenia (review limits < 0.8 to < 1.6×10^9/L)
- monocytosis (review limits > 0.5 to > 2.0×10^9/L)
- eosinophilia (review limits > 0.4 to > 1.5×10^9/L)
- basophilia (review limits > 0.2 to > 0.5×10^9/L)
- anaemia (review limits < 5.0 to < 11.0 g/dL)
- erythrocytosis (review limits > 6.0 to > 8.0×10^{12}/L)
- thrombocytopenia (review limits < 40 to < 125×10^9/L)
- thrombocytosis (review limits > 600 to > 999×10^9/L)
- macrocytosis (review limits > 100 to > 105 fL)
- microcytosis (review limits < 60 to < 70 fL)
- anisocytosis (review limits RDW > 16 to > 17.5 %)
- pancytopenia (review limits WBC < 3.0×10^9/L, RBC < 3.5 to < 4.0×10^{12}/L, platelets < 100 to < 125×10^9/L).

The lack of consensus, indeed the wide variance in review limits, may be due to multiple factors. First, there is no reference document endorsed by expert panels such as ICSH and NCCLS for these medical review limits (Koepke, 1994; Lacombe *et al.*, 1995). Secondly, there are variations in the performance of cell counters, although most instruments are capable of performing well within the relatively narrow limits used for medical review. Thirdly, the practices and expertise of the medical centres as well as the mix of patients seen at these centres vary markedly.

The goals of computerized 'expert' system use for review are to assure consistency of review and increase the number of test results which can be released without film review and/or retesting (Davis, 1994). Several mechanisms have been used to advance these goals: (i) subsetting specimens into patient categories so that specific review rules can be used for each category; (ii) retaining a file of those patients whose test results have already been reviewed to expedite the review of future specimens; and (iii) implementing reflex testing algorithms to further characterize those specimens with measurements exceeding the first level review criteria.

The subsetting of patient categories can be performed using information obtained from electronic medical record systems (such as specific disease diagnosis or therapy programmes) and/or simple demographics from the laboratory information system (such as age, gender and medical discipline of the physician seeing the patient). Examples of how this information could be used are to set lower anaemia review limits for patients on renal dialysis, who often have lower haemoglobin concentrations, or to alter the review limits for neonatal infants. For centres without electronic medical record linkages, the use of special order codes could help to expedite test review. For example, if different test numbers are used for blood test requests for oncology patients or post-bone marrow transplant patients, then different review criteria could be applied to these alternate test numbers. In essence, many different 'tests' are mapped to be the same measurement procedures on the haematology analyser, the differences in the test codes being predominately the review criteria.

1.6 QUALITY CONTROL MONITORS

The objectives of analytical quality control monitors for haematology cell counters are to assure that the instruments are performing within the expected standards while generating few false positive alarm situations. A recent review of quality control practices in 505 US hospital laboratories indicated that most out-of-control events were false positives that were resolved simply by retesting the controls (Steindel and Tetrault, 1998). Unfortunately, this study did not address the issue of false negatives nor the power of the QC system to detect real errors when they occur. This question of error detection is directly tied to the performance criteria discussed in previous sections, because the detection rates are dependent on the magnitude of the changes considered unacceptable.

Two major techniques are used to monitor the analytical performance of cell counters: moving-window averages of test values (especially RBC indices, e.g. the 'Bull' algorithm) and measurement of stabilized reference materials (Koepke, 1994; Lacombe et al., 1995). Each of these programmes has both advantages and deficiencies. The power of any of these techniques to detect true assay changes is related to the relative size of the variance of the control parameter compared with the size of the change allowed by the performance limits.

The variation of the red cell indices is relatively small compared with the variation of the other cell parameters, and therefore these indices are widely used in moving-average QC systems. The variation of the moving averages of the red cell indices depends on the size of the window used, the statistical weighting functions and the heterogeneity of the patient population. The technique developed by Bull et al. (1974) works well for laboratories performing screening studies for relatively healthy outpatients, but may have numerous false positives in laboratories serving multiple subspeciality clinics, especially oncology treatment programmes and burns units (Cembrowski and Westgard, 1985). The major advantages of this procedure are its low cost (no reagents or control material) and its long-term stability (assuming the patient mix does not change). The major disadvantages of this system are that it monitors only the red cell parameters and that the system can detect only systematic errors but not random errors. The other test parameters, such as counts of platelets, leucocytes and leucocyte subsets, have large population variations, and therefore moving-window averages of small numbers of patient values ($n < 20$) also have large variations. This causes the system to have little statistical power to detect real assay changes. Even for red cell parameters, the moving-window averages fail to detect concurrent changes of red cell counts and haemoglobin concentrations due to the ratioing of these parameters in the calculation of the indices (Tramacere et al., 1991). Random test errors are 'averaged' out of these moving-window averages and therefore are not detected. Replicate testing of a subset of patients could be used to detect random errors (Cembrowski et al., 1988).

The mainstay of most analytical monitoring programmes for red cell counts is the measurement of stable reference controls. The advantage of these programmes is that they directly monitor each of the parameters being reported on patient samples. In addition, these controls can detect both systematic errors (bias) and random errors (imprecision). The disadvantages are the cost (of both the controls and the reagents), the lack of stability of some of the materials, the variable reliability of the target values assigned to the control materials, and the necessity to measure the controls frequently in order to have adequate power for early detection of analytical errors.

In addition to the moving averages of red cell indices and stable reference controls, valuable quality control information can be obtained by monitoring patient test results. The distribution of the test values from large numbers of patients is generally quite stable over time (Table 1.6). Therefore, changes of the test distribution can be used as a supplementary method for detecting analytical bias (Klee, 1997; Smith and Croft, 1997). In addition, cross-indexing the patient test values with International Classification of Disease (ICD) codes and/or the diagnostic-related groups (DRGs) used for billing can provide valuable insights into the relationship between laboratory errors and patient outcomes (Winkelman and Mennemeyer, 1996).

1.7 ASSAY TURNAROUND TIME

Along with analytical accuracy and precision, timeliness is an important parameter for quality laboratory performance (Steindel, 1995). There are no national or international standards for turnaround time (TAT), but delayed reports (those exceeding the expectations of the clinicians) are a source of frustration in most medical practices. Therefore monitors of TAT have become an important part of most laboratory quality control programmes (Hilborne *et al.*, 1989).

The College of American Pathologists (CAP) has surveyed laboratory TAT through their Q-probes studies (Steindel, 1995). The median time between collection and reporting for haemoglobin measurements in US hospital emergency departments was 25 minutes in 1990 and 23 minutes in 1993. The fastest 10% returned results within 15 minutes. The slowest 10% had a median response time of 40 minutes.

Multiple factors influence TAT. Standardization and monitoring of the collection processes and transport processes are two factors that have been shown to reduce TAT (Steindel and Howanitz, 1997). Interestingly, dedicated 'STAT' laboratories and laboratories with computer systems did not have improved TAT. Laboratories with well-defined transportation processes with effective monitoring programmes had better TAT.

A 1997 CAP Q-probe study of routine outpatient test TAT showed that the median collection-to-report time for a complete blood count was 59 minutes, with 90% completion rate of 165 minutes during weekdays and 123 minutes on weekends (Steindal and Jones, 1997). The within-laboratory processing time had a median TAT of 32 minutes and a 90th percentile of 77 minutes. In this study, laboratories with computer systems incorporating electronic reporting had faster TAT, whereas centres with computer-generated labels versus handwritten labels had comparable TATs. Delivery times from external collection sites were important factors for those laboratories performing community outreach services.

1.8 CONCLUSIONS AND RECOMMENDATIONS

Quality assurance programmes for haematology cell counts involve multiple parameters that do not have well defined performance specifications. This chapter has attempted to discuss the issues involved in establishing quality control programmes for these parameters and to provide illustrative examples of the quality control programmes that are used by some medical centres and/or instrument manufacturers. Each medical laboratory should carefully analyse the needs of its practice and design a quality assurance programme to meet these needs.

Managed care programmes and the implementation of practice care guidelines are beginning to standardize medical practice. With this standardization, there is an increased need for across-laboratory consistency of test results. To achieve this goal, further standardization in assay performance and assay calibration will be necessary. Hopefully this standardization movement will lead to an overall improvement in haematology laboratory performance rather than a consensus towards mediocre performance.

REFERENCES

Barnett, R.N. (1968) Significance of laboratory results. *Am. J. Clin. Pathol.* **69**, 671–6.

Bull, B.S., Elashoff, R.M., Hilbron, D.C. *et al.* (1974) A study of various estimators for the deviation of quality control procedures from patient erythrocyte indices. *Am. J. Clin. Pathol.* **61**, 473–81.

Cembrowski, G.S., Lunetzky, E.S., Patrick, C.C. and Wilson, M.K. (1988) An optimized quality control procedure for hematology analyzers with use of retained patient specimens. *Am. J. Clin. Pathol.* **89**, 203–10.

Cembrowski, G.S. and Westgard, J.O. (1985) Quality control of multichannel hematology analyzers: evaluation of Bull's algorithm. *Am. J. Clin. Pathol.* **83**, 337–45.

Chapman, M. (1997) Hematology review criteria and its impact on workflow and productivity. *Lab. Hematol.* **3**, 48–52.

Davis, G.M. (1994) Autoverification of the peripheral blood count. *Lab. Med.* **25**, 528–31.

Elion-Gerritzen, W.E. (1980) Analytical precision in clinical chemistry and medical decisions. *Am. J. Clin. Pathol.* **73**, 183–95.

Fraser, C.G. (1987) Desirable standards for hematology tests: a proposal. *Am. J. Clin. Pathol.* **88**, 667–9.

Fraser, C.G., Petersen, O.H. and Larsen, M.L. (1990) Setting analytical goals for random analytical error in specific monitoring situations. *Clin. Chem.* **36**, 1625–8.

Hilborne, L.H., Oye, R.K., McArdle, J.E. *et al.* (1989) Evaluation of stat and routine turnaround time as a component of laboratory quality. *Am. J. Clin. Pathol.* **91**, 331–5.

Houwen, B. (1990) Random errors in hematology tests: a process control approach. *Clin. Lab. Haematol.* **12**, 157–68.

Houwen, B. and Duffin, D. (1989) Delta checks for random error detection in hematology tests. *Lab. Med.* **June**, 410–7.

Jones, B.A., Meier, F. and Howanitz, P.J. (1995) Complete blood count specimen acceptability: a College of American Pathologists Q-Probe study of 703 laboratories. *Arch. Pathol. Lab. Med.* **119**, 203–8.

Klee, G.G. (1990) Performance goals for internal quality control of multichannel haematology analyzers. *Clin. Lab. Haematol.* **12**, 65–74.

Klee, G.G. (1993) Tolerance limits for short-term analytical bias and analytical imprecision derived from clinical assay specificity. *Clin. Chem.* **39**, 1514–8.

Klee, G.G. (1997) A conceptual model for establishing tolerance limits for analytic bias and imprecision based on variations in population test distributions. *Clin. Chim. Acta* **160**, 175–80.

Koepke, J.A. (1994) Let's improve the flagging of abnormal hematology specimens. *Med Lab Observ* **22**, 6.

Lacombe, F., Cazaux, N., Briais, A. *et al.* (1995) Evaluation of the leukocyte differential flags on an hematologic analyzer. *Am. J. Clin. Pathol.* **104**, 495–502.

MacDonald, A.J., Bradshaw, A.E., Holmes, W.A. and Lewis S.M. (1996) The impact of an integrated haematology screening system on laboratory practice. *Clin. Lab. Haematol.* **18**, 271–6.

Smith, F.A. and Kroft, S.H. (1997) Optimal procedures for detecting analytic bias using patient samples. *Am. J. Clin. Pathol.* **108**, 254–68.

Statland, B.E., Winkel, P., Harris, S.C. *et al.* (1978) Evaluation of biologic sources of variation of leukocyte counts and other hematologic quantities using very precise automated analyzers. *Am. J. Clin. Pathol.* **69**, 48–54.

Steindel, S.J. (1995) Timeliness of clinical laboratory tests: a discussion based on five College of American Pathologists Q-probe studies. *Arch. Pathol. Lab. Med.* **119**, 918–23.

Steindel, S.J. and Howanitz, P.J. (1997) Changes in emergency department turnaround time performance from 1990 to 1993: a comparison of two College of American Pathologists Q-probe studies. *Arch. Pathol. Lab. Med.* **121**, 1031–41.

Steindel, S.J. and Jones, B.A. (1997) Routine outpatient test turnaround time 97-03: data analysis and critique. Northfield, IL: College of American Pathologists.

Steindel, S.J. and Tetrault, G. (1998) Quality control practices for calcium, cholesterol, digoxin, and hemoglobin. *Arch. Pathol. Lab. Med.* **122**, 401–8.

Tatsumi, N., Tsuda, I., Shimizu, A. *et al.* (1996) Basic performance evaluation of the new hematology analyzer, CELL-DYN®4000: Japanese hematology analyzer study group. *Lab. Hematol.* **2**, 157–61.

Thure, D.B. and Sandberg, S. (1993) Clinical goals for measurement of hemoglobin in primary care as assessed by paper vignettes. *Upsala J. Med. Sci.* **98**, 331–4.

Tonks, D.B. (1963) A study of accuracy and precision of clinical chemistry determinations in 170 Canadian laboratories. *Clin. Chem.* **9**, 217–33.

Tramacere, P., Marocchi, M.D., Gerthoux, P. *et al.* (1991) Inefficiency of moving average algorithm as principal quality control procedure on Technicon System H6000. *Am. J. Clin. Pathol.* **95**, 218–21.

Winkelman, J.W. and Mennemeyer, S.T. (1996) Using patient outcomes to screen for clinical laboratory errors. *Clin. Lab. Man. Rev.* **10**, 134–42.

2

The blood cell count

BEREND HOUWEN

INTRODUCTION

The blood cell count is one of the key components of haematology testing and differs fundamentally from clinical chemistry tests of soluble blood components. While the latter are based on enzymatic, physical, chemical or immunochemical analysis of the coagulated blood's serum, often by colorimetric or densitometric assays, the blood cell count is dependent on the enumeration of individual particles (cells) suspended in anticoagulated, whole blood. However, the blood count also measures various attributes of the cells counted, such as cell volume, cytoplasmic complexity, staining capability, etc., adding entirely new dimensions to simple enumeration of suspended blood cells. Ideally, the cells should not have changed by blood collection, anticoagulation or manipulation and storage. Unfortunately this is not so: handling cells outside the body may result in blood cell activation, as with platelets, while anticoagulation and storage may result in other secondary changes. The currently widely used anticoagulant ethylene diamine tetra-acetic acid (potassium or sodium salts of EDTA) affects the cell membrane of many cell types and contributes to cell volume increases over time. These changes influence some of the cell analysis procedures, particularly those in which measurement of cell attributes is involved. Newer anticoagulants, not yet released for general use, may alleviate some of these problems.

The methodologies used for electronic measurements, such as cell count, cell volume, cell type, RNA content, etc., often call for compensating algorithms in order to match analyser results with those obtained by reference methods. While it is not possible to discuss in this chapter all methods used for electronic blood cell analysis in detail, the most commonly used methods and their 'reference' method-based counterparts will be included.

2.1 BASIC BLOOD CELL COUNTING PRINCIPLES AND METHODOLOGIES

The primary method for blood cell counting has been the microscope-based 'chamber' or haemocytometer count. The basic principles include pretreatment of whole blood in such a way that the cells of interest – white blood cells (WBCs), red blood cells (RBCs) or platelets – may be made visible for a microscopy optical count. The treated blood is dispensed in a haemocytometer, which is a thick glass slide with three parallel platforms in the middle. The platforms are separated by grooves and differ slightly in height: the outside platforms are exactly 0.1 mm higher than the central platform. This allows a special, thick, perfectly plane coverglass to create a space defined by the chamber height (0.1 mm) and the surface area of the central platforms. The counting chambers have a grating that divides the surface into squares, typically 1 mm apart and subdivided into 16 smaller squares of 0.25 × 0.25 mm. With the coverglass in place, a capillary tube filled with the diluted blood is made to touch the groove at the edge of the coverglass. The fluid will fill the space under the coverglass by capillary action but care must be taken to fill only the space below the coverglass without air bubbles or overflowing. After letting the cells settle for a few minutes, those that are of interest, e.g. WBCs, present in a minimum of four large squares (1 mm × 1 mm), are counted by microscopy (different rules apply for RBC and platelet counts). For a WBC count of 5×10^9/L, the chamber count per four squares will be 100, assuming that the depth of the counting chamber is exactly 0.1 mm. Unfortunately, the tolerances for counting chambers in themselves can account for errors as large as ±7% (Dacie and Lewis, 1975). Dilution errors and uneven distribution of cells in the counting chamber are other contributing factors, resulting in a 95% confidence limit of 18.5% when 200 cells are counted (using two chambers and one pipette). Using four chambers and two pipettes, counting 400 cells reduces the confidence limit to 12.8% (Henry, 1991).

The haemocytometer method applies to all three basic blood cell types – red cells, white cells and platelets – and as well as having problems with accuracy, it is also time-consuming and rather imprecise (Table 2.1). Imprecision is a particularly serious problem at clinical decision levels for low white cell and platelet counts, where the method essentially fails because of poor reproducibility. The problems with imprecision are not just methodological; many basic haematology parameters have very wide dynamic ranges, often starting at zero or near-zero values and vastly exceeding the normal reference intervals for those parameters. This is another difference between haematology parameters such as the WBC and platelet count and most clinical chemistry measurements. While zero or near-zero values as well as extremely high values for WBC and platelet counts are associated with serious clinical conditions, similar outlying values would not be compatible with life for most chemistry parameters, and will therefore mostly be encountered in haematology testing. Obviously this poses significant challenges for performance and quality control for haematology analysers that are quite different from those in clinical chemistry.

A prime reason for imprecision of the particle count is that the distribution of particles (cells) suspended in solution (blood) is random and their count is therefore affected by sampling error or Poisson distribution. The Poisson distribution, like the binomial distri-

Table 2.1   *Imprecision (CV%) for different haematological parameters for manual and electronic methods*

	Manual/haemocytometer		Electronic methods	
	Literature[a]	Actual[b]	Literature[a]	Actual[b]
Haemoglobin (N)	2	0.75	< 1.5	≤ 0.65
Haematocrit (N)	2	1.27[c]	< 1.5	≤ 0.65
WBC count (N)	6.5	6.0	< 3.0	≤ 2.0
WBC count (L)	15	ND		
RBC count (N)	4.3	ND	< 1.5	≤ 0.65
Platelet count (N)	11	10–15	1–3	≤ 1.7
Reticulocyte count (N)	40[d]	15[e]	< 10	5–7

N, a value for the parameter tested within the reference interval for normal adult individuals; L, values tested below the reference interval; CV, coefficient of variation; Hgb, haemoglobin; Hct, haematocrit; PLT, platelet; RBC, red blood cell; WBC, white blood cell; ND, no data.
[a]Literature data were obtained from: Henry (1991) – Hgb, Hct, WBC, RBC, PLT; Dacie and Lewis (1975) – PLT; Miale (1982) – reticulocyte.
[b]All of the test results listed were performed in the authors' laboratory.
[c]Performed by skilled technologists, using microscope-based readings of spun haematocrit tubes from fresh, normal samples obtained by venepuncture.
[d]Data for normal counts on 1000 RBCs counted on a single blood film.
[e]Performed by skilled technologists on normal and patient samples with reticulocyte counts <2.0% with 2 × 2000 RBCs counted on two different blood films.

bution, describes the probability of discrete events occurring within a given time or number of repetitions. In our case, this means that the fewer the particles counted, the wider the dispersion of an individual counting result around a 'perfect' mean value. The Poisson distribution is described by a single parameter, λ, and will approach normal (Gaussian) distribution even with low values for λ (Diem, 1962). We may therefore assume that the variation in the count is given by the standard deviation:

$$SD = \sqrt{[\Sigma \ (x - \mu)^2/(n - 1)]}$$

where x is the individual count from observations 1 to n; μ is the mean number of particles counted per test; and n is the number of tests performed. However, unlike the standard deviation, the Poisson error is expressed in integers. Therefore, if the count is based on a specific volume of blood analysed, and not on a fixed number of cells counted, then imprecision of the cell count will be greatly influenced by the actual particle/cell concentration in any given blood sample. Other formulas for Poisson distribution assume a correction factor primarily based on λ, e.g. $1.84 \times \sqrt{\mu}$, for calculating 95% confidence intervals (Schumacher, 1997).

Even though modern haematology analysers count many more cells than the chamber count procedure, their results still remain affected by Poisson distribution. This is because of the wide dynamic range for WBC and platelet counts, and the limit to the maximum volume of blood that can be analysed in these instruments. Thus, WBC and platelet counts will show more imprecision at lower than normal levels. This is extremely unfortunate since many clinical decisions are based on low counts, and incorrect interpretation of a patient's clinical condition during suppressed blood counts may have severe implications. To overcome this problem, many automated haematology analysers have built-in algorithms to create 'prolonged' counts in samples with low numbers of WBCs and/or platelets. In fact, such 'prolonged' counts involve the analysis of a greater than normal volume of blood, resulting in more cells counted and reduced imprecision. For an example of the effects on imprecision of the number of cells counted, see Table 2.2. As indicated in this table, sampling error is not dependent on the concentration of particles in suspension, but on the actual number of particles counted. This means that an error rate of 1% or more will always occur if less than 8000 particles are counted, regardless of the type of instrument or technology used. It also means that in order to achieve error rates consistently below 1%, it is necessary to count 25 000 particles or more. While this may be possible for some cell types at normal concentrations, it is generally not feasible at low cell counts. This is because of the fixed dilution rate of whole blood used by all blood cell counters, often ±1:500, which brings the final cell concentration in specimens with an already suppressed WBC or platelet count down even further. While it would be desirable to count greater numbers of cells in such situations, this is not possible with current technology because of whole blood viscosity. In patients with suppressed WBC and platelet counts, the RBC count may be normal, and lowering the dilution ratio for the blood sample would result in increased viscosity and red cell coincidence. The only solution currently available is a prolonged counting period, when the analyser senses a low WBC and/or platelet count.

Table 2.2 *Effects on imprecision of the number of cells counted*

Particles counted	SD	95% confidence interval (± 2SD)	CV (%)	Poisson error
10	±3.2	4–16	32	±4
25	±5.0	15–35	20	±5
50	±7.1	36–64	14.2	±8
100	±10.0	80–120	10	±10
500	±22.36	455–545	4.5	±23
1 000	±31.62	937–1 063	3.2	±32
2 500	±50.0	2 400–2 600	2.0	±50
8 000	±89.44	7 801–8 199	1.1	±90
25 000	±158.11	24 684–25 316	0.6	±159

An additional difficulty with automated blood cell counting can be discrimination of the cells of interest, e.g. platelets from debris or small red cells, etc. This is one of the reasons why, for cell types such as platelets, the use of two or more parameters allows a more accurate definition of platelets as the targeted cell type. Typically, such multi-parameter analyses cannot be obtained by the counting technique most commonly used, i.e. aperture impedance flow. The principle of this basic cell counting method is simple (Fig. 2.1) and is based on blood cells suspended in an electrolyte solution passing an aperture between two differently charged compartments (Coulter, 1956). The passage of a blood cell through the narrow aperture causes resistance or 'impedance' of the direct current (DC) between the two electrodes, measured as a change in voltage. For cells passing through the centre of the aperture, the change in voltage is proportional to cell volume as long as the cells are spherical, such as white cells. For red cell and platelet volume measurements, correction factors have to be used to calculate the volume, because of their non-spherical shape. While most voltage changes (pulses) relate to cells passing the aperture, and therefore to a cell 'count', some considerations apply.

It is assumed that cells pass the aperture in single file, and that coincidence is absent or minimal, or at least that the rate of coincidence is known and can be corrected. A low coincidence rate requires the blood sample to be diluted, usually at a ratio of 1:500. Even at this dilution not all cells pass in single file. Cells can pass the sensing aperture (or sensing zone) in different ways: as single objects; by passing too close together, one cell behind another, to be

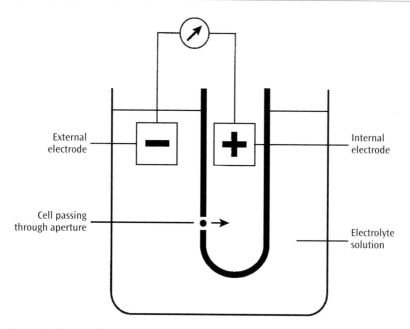

Fig. 2.1 *Schematic diagram of a particle counter based on electrical resistance (impedance). To allow electrical conductivity, cells are suspended in an electrolyte solution that is moved from its reservoir through the aperture into the 'counting tube', and then into a waste container. The flow of cells through the aperture causes a voltage change ('pulse') that (i) enumerates and (ii) sizes the cells passing through.*

fully separated as individual objects; or by passing simultaneously through the sensing zone (Fig. 2.2). While two red cells or a red cell passing simultaneously with a white cell will be recognized as an abnormal signal, this is not the case for a platelet coinciding with a red cell. This has been one of the major obstacles to developing a platelet reference counting method (an immunoflow-based method is currently being evaluated; see Section 2.8). Coincidence effects can seriously affect the accuracy of the cell count and although haemodilution prevents it to some degree, it would take a very narrow sensing zone and much higher blood dilution than are currently used to prevent coincidence effects completely. All haematology analysers currently on the market therefore use coincidence correction algorithms, which in the main work satisfactorily, as judged by acceptable linearity for RBC, WBC and platelet counts.

2.2 OTHER PROBLEMS/ISSUES

The direct current itself causes the development of small bubbles in the electrolyte solution, often below the detection limit, but potentially capable of causing falsely elevated cell counts. Recirculation of blood cells through the aperture may cause a similar problem.

Larger than appropriate and abnormal pulses are caused by cells passing, not through, but away from the axial flow through the centre of the aperture (Thom, 1969). Systems equipped with hydrodynamic focusing use sheathed flow surrounding the sample flow containing the blood cells (Thom and Kachel, 1970). This improves results in two ways: it is easier to maintain the cells in single file, reducing coincidence effects; and at the same time the sheath flow keeps the sample flow well centred and avoids those inappropriately large pulses. In analysers without focused flow, such large pulses have to be eliminated from volumetric analysis (but not from the cell count). This is achieved by truncation of the histogram so that

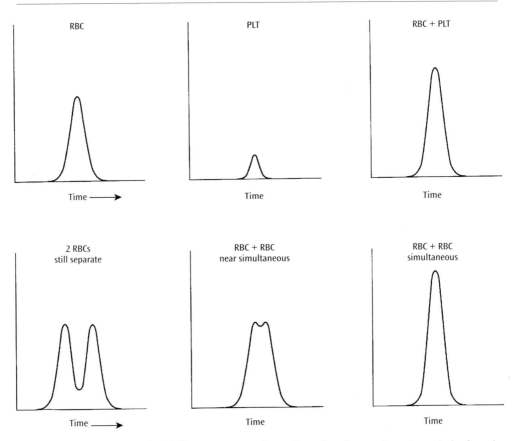

Fig. 2.2 *The different panels in this figure represent pulse configurations from an impedance device for red blood cells (RBCs) and platelets (PLTs) in different relations. The much smaller PLT pulse, while perfectly recognizable by itself, becomes easily obscured by the much larger pulse from a RBC when both cells travel through the measuring orifice at the same time (coincidence). RBC coincidence pulses can occur in different types, depending on the proximity of two RBCs when passing the measuring orifice.*

only cells falling within certain cell volume-related criteria are included in volumetric analysis (Fig. 2.3). This process is often called 'pulse editing' and may influence the cell count itself, as well as causing some loss of information for cell volume-related measurements.

To create circumstances whereby only targeted cell types are detectable by the analytical system for a count, the anticoagulated and diluted blood sample is often exposed to some form of chemical treatment. This may result in lysis of certain cell types (RBCs, platelets) and/or in changes in other cell types (WBCs, WBC subsets, reticulocytes). Lysing cells results in debris, ghosts, stroma, etc., and to ensure that these, as well as electrical noise and small bubbles, are excluded from analysis, a volumetric threshold is set and only signals above the threshold are analysed. This threshold is set individually by different manufacturers, mostly around the equivalent of 2 fL.

The limitations of impedance flow (DC system) for white cell differential counting have generated developments either to enhance it or to replace it altogether. These include a radio frequency (RF) sensor that is able to measure cellular 'complexity' or content. For cells with a complex content, i.e. neutrophils or eosinophils containing a segmented nucleus plus large numbers of granules, RF measurements result in a signal different from that for lymphocytes without granules or other nuclear and cytoplasmic complexities. Addition of a laser

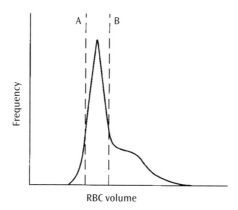

Fig. 2.3 *This histogram represents the frequency of cells with a given (red blood cell, RBC) volume in a particular blood sample. The cells to the right of the discriminator 'B' are considered doublets, caused by coincidence counts, and their cell volume is therefore artificially inflated. By truncating the histogram and eliminating smaller RBCs (left of discriminator 'A'), as well as doublets, a central population remains for which a mean cell volume can be calculated.*

detection unit has also been used and has resulted in further resolution of white cell sub-populations. Other developments have included cytochemical treatment and special channels for some cell types, including immature cells. All of this has resulted in further refinements in blood cell classification and has been applied in leucocyte differential counting in the clinical laboratory.

Other major approaches for leucocyte differential counting have started from entirely optical, often laser-based, focused flow platforms. Here again, as in impedance flow, cells are sent in single file through a sensing zone, but instead of changes in direct current or radio frequency, a variety of light-based properties of blood cells are used. These include forward light scatter (FSc), side scatter (SSc), light absorption and fluorescence (if fluorescence-based cell probes or labels are used) (Fig. 2.4). Light sources vary from multi-wavelength 'white' light to laser sources with different wavelengths (often in the red or blue visible light range) and either gas (helium–neon or argon ion) or diode. The angles of light scatter signal analysis often differ between manufacturers, and other techniques such as polarized laser light may be used, but the basic principles remain the same for all platforms.

Because of the versatility of the optical focused flow platform, many current haematology analysers have an optical flow system either integrated with impedance flow or entirely optically based (Crosland-Taylor, 1953). The reason for the combination of technologies is not caused by problems in counting efficiency or accuracy by the flow-based platforms. Instead, the narrow sensing zone of the flow platform and signal speed generally allow higher flow rates than in most impedance-based systems. The primary problem is with cell sizing of non-spherical cells (red cells and platelets) by a FSc signal. These cells give irregular signals, depending on the way they project themselves to the (laser) light, resulting in very different signals for essentially the same cell volume. One manufacturer has solved this problem by isovolumetric sphering of the red cells and shows results generally equivalent to cell sizing by hydrodynamically focused impedance flow (Paterakis *et al.*, 1994). Optical flow systems offer a variety of elegant solutions to distinguish different white cell types. Methods include the use of fluorescent and non-fluorescent probes, and also (enzyme) cytochemistry. While it is certainly possible to include monoclonal antibodies for cell identification, as is done in

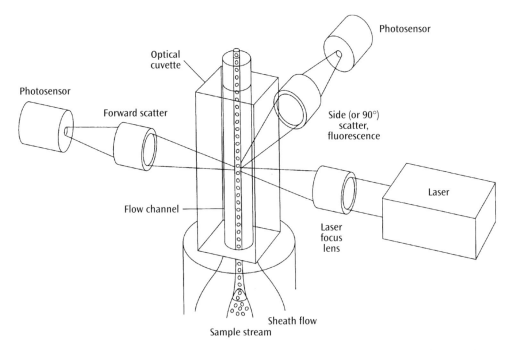

Fig. 2.4 *Schematic drawing of a flow cytometer with detection capability of forward scatter (representing cell volume; laser wavelength), side scatter (representing cellular contents; laser wavelength) and/or side fluorescence (light emitted by a fluorescent probe; longer than laser wavelength). Depending on the use of beam splitters (dichroic mirrors) and band filters, emitted light of different wavelengths can be measured separately. Light sources for flow cytometers are usually lasers, mostly emitting light at 488 nm. Semiconductor lasers, emitting at 633 nm, have recently become used in routine clinical instruments.*

leukaemia/lymphoma phenotyping (*US-Canadian Consensus Recommendations*, 1997; Orfao *et al.*, 1999) and in reference flow cytometric WBC differential counting (Lebeck *et al.*, 1993; Hubl *et al.*, 1997), this is too laborious and far too expensive to be used in a routine clinical setting.

The enumeration of various white cell populations has become much better over time, because of improved biosensor systems and because of vastly increased computing power, allowing for more complex software algorithms. Together, these result in ever-improving electronic leucocyte differential counts. The results in terms of laboratory practice have been impressive. In less than 20 years, these systems have replaced manual differential counting in about half of all patient samples (Houwen and Koepke, 1990; Kickler, 2000).

2.3 PERFORMANCE GOALS FOR THE BLOOD CELL COUNT

The criteria for reference counting as set forth by the International Council for Standardization in Haematology (Lewis, 1990) in general also apply to routine, clinical counting as performed by electronic analysers. These criteria state that:

- the method must be suitable for all specimens in health and disease;
- the cells of interest must be discriminated from all other cell types and particles;

- the cells should be counted only once (and one at a time);
- the count should be made from a representative sample of the blood specimen;
- the counts should be made from an accurately known volume of (diluted) blood.

The last requirement may not always apply, e.g. not when ratio counts are being used as in the candidate reference immunoflow method for platelet enumeration (see also p. 32).

Overall, the setting of performance goals for analytical processes is not an easy task. As discussed above, the wide dynamic range for many haematology parameters creates significant issues with accuracy and reproducibility at low values (Poisson error). Additionally, it can make an enormous difference to performance requirements whether the test is used for screening purposes, case finding, diagnosis or monitoring (see also Table 8.5, p. 188). Of the several attempts that have been made to set performance goals for haematology analysers, only one is listed (NCCLS, 1996), while recognizing that currently similar efforts are being made to develop such goals for the International Organization for Standardization (ISO) document covering *in vitro* diagnostic devices.

2.4 CALIBRATION AND QUALITY CONTROL APPROACHES

Calibration materials should be available for all analysers, for all parameters that can be calibrated. These materials should not be the same as the quality control (QC) materials, and in fact may differ substantially since their use is to provide a set point for a particular parameter not a day-to-day monitoring of a parameter at different levels. The provider of the calibrator material is responsible for the 'assignment of values' of the calibrator. This involves a process where an analyser is first carefully calibrated against whole blood reference methods (NCCLS, 1998). Then calibrator material is run on the analyser and test results are recorded for the parameter(s) for which the calibrator is intended. These are typically the mean values of multiple measurements, usually in more than one laboratory. After validation of the results obtained in these reference laboratories, the mean of all recorded values is 'assigned' to the calibrator material. The calibrator should be stable for its shelf-life, and its manufacturer should ensure that such stability is monitored. Subsequent use of the calibrator 'in the field' will now enable a user to check and, if necessary, adjust the analyser to the 'assigned' value of the calibrator. This procedure ensures that results for blood specimens analysed on all instruments of a given model will show worldwide homology.

All manufacturers have to supply QC materials, in many situations mandated to monitor test performance at three levels: normal, below normal and above normal. These materials should have prolonged stability, often beyond 60 days. Typically, results are expressed in QC charts (Levy-Jennings type), and are also compared with the results obtained using the same materials on the same analyser type in other laboratories (peer comparison). Sometimes such analyses are offered in real time through electronic (modem-based) submission of QC data, but mostly such results are analysed after the laboratory has submitted its QC results from a defined period (usually 1 month).

Proficiency testing, by testing one or more unknown samples at set intervals, is also often mandated by regulatory bodies, and in some countries is required for laboratory certification.

A powerful QC mechanism is provided by analysis of the moving average of certain parameters of the blood cell count, particularly those that show limited dynamic range for normal and patient data (Levy *et al.*, 1986; Smith and Kroft, 1997). Algorithms for such analysis exist in most of the high-end instruments and are available in most laboratory computer information systems.

2.5 PERFORMANCE OF THE BASIC CELL COUNT: RBCS, WBCS AND PLATELETS

Blood specimens obtained for the cell count will require adequate anticoagulation, and directions for suitable collection procedures and anticoagulants must be followed (NCCLS, 1991a,b). The following aspects of electronic cell counting performance should always be provided by the manufacturer in the instrument specifications: inaccuracy, imprecision (including the level at which this was tested), dynamic range, linearity and carry-over. Potential interferences and remedies, where available, should be listed. In addition, manufacturers should provide data on long-term stability of specific analyser counts (and other measurements) and on specific storage conditions for patient specimens. Protocols and testing procedures can be found in the literature (NCCLS, 1992; ICSH, 1994a; Weber et al., 1995), and it is recommended (and often mandatory) that the user confirms the instrument manufacturer's specifications prior to instrument installation for clinical use.

2.6 RED BLOOD CELL COUNTING

The RBC count itself has limited clinical use but is needed to calculate the following RBC indices: mean cell volume (MCV), mean cell haemoglobin (MCH) and mean corpuscular haemoglobin concentration (MCHC). These, combined with the red cell distribution width (RDW) and, in some analysers, with cellular mean haemoglobin concentration (CMHC) and cellular haemoglobin (Hgb) distribution width, can provide valuable information in patients with anaemia, thalassaemia trait, etc. (Bessman et al., 1983).

Because red cells are the most frequent cell type in blood, their count is also most severely affected by coincidence effects. A check for RBC linearity by diluting a blood sample with a high RBC count (naturally or artificially elevated) will reveal whether the coincidence algorithm installed by the manufacturer functions properly.

The reference method for RBC counting is based on single channel electronic counts, by impedance, using highly diluted blood samples, while correcting for the known coincidence characteristics of the counting device at the blood dilution used. By using specific aperture sizes, white cells can be excluded from the count (ICSH, 1994b).

For red cells, not only is the count important, but so also are their volumes and volume distribution. Because normal and most patients' red cells are non-spherical, volume measurements can pose some intricate problems. Red cell volume measured by impedance technology may suffer from inaccuracy due to shape change in cells passing the measuring aperture. This so-called 'shape factor' is a result of shear force applied to the deformable red blood cell while exposed to the vacuum forces needed to create the high flow rates through a narrow orifice. Typically, instruments not using focused flow show more shape change than those equipped with sheath flow. Shape change causes microcytic, hypochromic red cells to appear smaller than they really are. This results in a compensation for a low MCHC, thus more or less 'normalizing' such values for anaemias with hypochromic RBCs and reducing the dynamic range of the MCHC parameter (Thom and Kachel, 1970; Bull et al., 1996).

Red cells can sometimes be found as two or more populations in the same patient, as indicated by differences in MCV and/or CMHC. This potentially valuable observation has yet to be generally incorporated in haematology analysers. Situations where it could be useful include monitoring patients treated for microcytic or megaloblastic anaemia where the abnormal cells can readily be distinguished from the emerging normal red cell population. It would thus be possible to track the progress and the efficacy of treatment in terms of actual change and improvement in red cell populations, rather than by more indirect measurements such as RDW, haemoglobin concentration, serum iron or ferritin, etc. Measurement of red cell (and reticulocyte) cellular haemoglobin content has been used in situations of emerging iron deficiency or iron mobilization, and in the treatment of iron deficiency anaemia (Mohandas *et al.*, 1992; Brugnara *et al.*, 1999).

Interferences of the RBC count include cold agglutinins as well as haemolytic anaemia associated (cold) autoantibodies against red cells (see Table 2.3). Because most clinical cell

Table 2.3 *Possible interferents with the blood count*

Parameter	Interferent	Effect on parameter
WBC	Unlysed RBC	False >
	NRBC	False >
	Cryoglobulin/fibrinogen	False >
	Platelet clumps	False >
	Monoclonal proteins	False >
	Microclots or partial clotting of specimen	False <
	Fragile WBC (e.g. CLL)	False <
	Storage (cell decay)	False <
RBC	Microclots or partial clotting of specimen	False <
	Severe microcytosis	False < (inappropriate RBC discriminator settings)
	Cryoglobulins	False <
	Autoagglutination	False <
	(*in vitro*) Haemolysis	False <
Hematocrit[a]	Sickling	False >
	Prolonged storage	False >
	Microclots or partial clotting of specimen	False <
	Cryoglobulins	False <
	(in vitro) Haemolysis	False <
	Severe hyperglycaemia	False <
	Short sample (excess EDTA)	False <
Platelets	Severe microcytosis	False >
	RBC fragments	False >
	WBC fragments	False >
	Giant platelets	False <
	EDTA-induced platelet clumping	False <
	Heparin-induced platelet clumping	False <
	Platelet satellitosis	False <
Reticulocytes	RBC inclusions	False >
	RBC parasites (malaria)	False >
	WBC fragments	False >
	Platelet clumps and giant platelets	False >
	Prolonged storage	False <

CLL, chronic lymphocytic leukaemia; NRBC, nucleated red blood cell; RBC, red blood cell; WBC, white blood cell.
[a]Most of these apply to mean cell volume measurements as well.

counting methods are performed at room temperature, this may cause the red cells to agglutinate *in vitro*, even when the specimen container was warmed up prior to analysis. It is also relevant to note that, *in vitro*, over time, red cells start to take up water, more so when stored at room temperature than at 4°C. This is in part the result of deoxygenation and the resulting uptake of CO_2. The carbonates formed by CO_2 bind water and the result is an increase in MCV, partially reversible upon oxygenation of the blood sample (Bryner *et al.*, 1997). Reagent systems in some instruments alter the water content of RBCs and may thus mask this time-dependent *in vitro* storage effect. Manufacturers should state long-term stability data for MCV at different temperatures.

2.7 WHITE BLOOD CELL COUNTING

The WBC count is an important part of haematology testing since reliable, and relatively narrow, normal reference intervals have been established in the USA for various age and ethnic groups for both sexes (van Assendelft, 1991). Therefore, a low or elevated WBC count carries clinical significance and should lead to further investigation if the count is used as a screening test. Very low WBC counts are particularly important, because at levels $<0.5 \times 10^9$/L severe risk of infection exists for the patient. WBC counts are also used to monitor treatment of patients with infections, solid tumours, leukaemia and other forms of haematological malignancy. The reference method for the WBC count is the electronic, single channel count similar to the RBC count described above (ICSH, 1994b). The blood sample will have undergone red cell lysis and an aperture size appropriate for WBC measurements will be used.

In haematology analysers, the WBC count is also obtained after red cell lysis, but a white cell volume distribution histogram is relatively uninformative without further processing. Coincidence rarely causes WBC counting problems except when very high levels are encountered. Fragile white cells generally do not pose as much of a problem in the count as in blood film preparations, mainly because the shear forces of electronic blood cell analysis are smaller than in wedge blood film preparation. In chronic lymphocytic leukaemia (CLL), a typical example of fragile cells, the electronic white cell and lymphocyte counts will therefore most likely reflect the true count.

Apoptotic white cells and white cell fragments can be present in blood samples from patients with myelodysplastic syndromes, and are sometimes induced *in vitro* even in normal specimens. This is particularly the case when samples have been stored under inappropriate conditions (temperature too high, storage time too long). However, in most situations there will be limited presence of apoptotic cells or cell fragments, and hence limited or minimal interference. In patients with bone marrow suppression and low WBC counts due to cytotoxic chemotherapy or with fragile white cells (apoptotic), white cell fragments may cause interference with the platelet count.

White cell count interference can occur from lyse-resistant red cells (most often in thalassaemia and sickle cell disease patients) and from nucleated red blood cells (NRBCs). (For possible interferences see Table 2.3.) Although clinically relevant interference from NRBCs is rarely seen at or below 5 NRBC/100 white cells, it can be important to correct the WBC count in samples with appreciable numbers of NRBCs (>10/100 WBCs). Even in those cases, the importance is relative: at 10 NRBCs/100 WBCs, a count of 6.5×10^9/L (which is normal) after correction changes to 5.85×10^9/L (which is still normal). Therefore, the clinical importance of some of these corrections is limited, and the laboratory should weigh the effort of manually correcting the WBC count against the improvement in clinical information thus obtained.[1] Since low WBC counts hold significant clinical information, it is important that such counts are accurate. Absence of carryover from previous analyses is therefore crucial in obtaining accurate results. Instrument specifications should include data on carryover of white cells. Manufacturers should also state long-term stability and recommended storage conditions for WBC counts on their analysers.

2.8 PLATELET COUNTING

With the advent of multi-channel automated haematology analysers, platelet counts have become an integral part of routine testing since the 1980s. Platelet count reference intervals have been established for various ethnic and age groups, for both sexes (van Assendelft, 1991).

Platelet counts are especially useful for patients with malignancies, in whom thrombopoiesis is adversely affected either directly by the disease or indirectly by cytotoxic chemotherapy. Low platelet counts may expose patients to severe bleeding complications that are, for the most part, preventable by prophylactic platelet transfusions. There is thus a growing emphasis on accurate ultra-low platelet counts, so that transfusions can be given at the appropriate time and for appropriately low counts.

High platelet counts are generally a smaller problem, at least in terms of a diagnosis of thrombocytosis or thrombocythaemia. However, when platelets are present in high numbers they are often activated, leading (i) to variable attachment to monocytes, and (ii) to micro-aggregate formation, making it difficult to obtain stable, accurate and reproducible counts in these patients.

In virtually all haematology analysers, platelets are counted in unlysed whole blood. Using single-parameter mode, e.g. in impedance flow counting, platelets are separated from red cells by a linear discriminator. Often this discriminator is not fixed in one position, but can float to make the best possible distinction between platelets and red cells. There are several reasons why this is not always successful. When the red cells are small, as in microcytosis, or when red cell fragments are present, the distinction between red cells and platelets becomes tenuous. This leads to significant inaccuracies in the platelet count, especially when it is low, because of admixture of small red cells or fragments into the platelet count. A similar situation exists when the platelet count is low, even when the MCV is normal. Again, in these situations the automatic placement of the discriminator is variable, often inaccurate, resulting in imprecise and inaccurate counts. This is all the more significant because patients with very low platelet counts are prone to bleeding, and accurate counts are deemed necessary to determine the correct timing for transfusion to prevent bleeding. So far a clinical policy based on transfusing platelets prophylactically when the counts drop to certain levels has been successful in that currently very few patients with low platelet counts due to cytotoxic chemotherapy or after bone marrow/stem cell transplantation develop severe bleeding complications. However, the relative scarcity of platelets for transfusion has caused a demand for lowering the count threshold still further. This, in turn, has created a need for greater accuracy and precision at low counts.

Technological progress in platelet counting has mainly come from optical platforms using dual-parameter measurement, e.g. platelet volume determined by FSc and platelet

---

[1]The manual WBC count correction for NRBCs is performed as follows: NRBCs are identified on a Wright-Giemsa or similarly stained blood film, and expressed as NRBCs/100 WBCs. The instrument WBC count is then corrected for the excess NRBCs, assuming that all NRBCs are identified by the analyser as WBCs, using the following equation: [(100 − no. of NRBCs per 100 WBCs) × (uncorrected WBCs)] ÷ 100.

fluorescence or light absorbance (either based on platelet content or derived from monoclonal antibody labelling). This two-parameter approach separates platelets more effectively from non-fluorescent red cells and red cell fragments and cell debris (Fig. 2.5). While most analysers still use single-parameter analysis as the main mode for platelet counting, it appears that in future, for low counts and for interference by small red cells and red cell fragments, the optical method will be preferred.

Similar to RBCs, several 'indices' have been derived for platelets, with the most commonly used being the mean platelet volume (MPV) and platelet distribution width (PDW). Contrary to the RBC indices, the clinical value of MPV and PDW is limited. A high MPV has been used as an indicator for emerging young platelets (Bessman, 1982). However, the specificity of MPV is restricted and is likely to be replaced by the platelet RNA content ('reticulated platelets') at some time in the future (Kienast and Schmitz, 1990; Ault and Knowles, 1995; Dale et al., 1995). Currently, reticulated platelets remain a research parameter without a commonly accepted definition, and, although promising as a new tool for measuring platelet production and turnover, must await further development before introduction as a general, clinical laboratory parameter.

The absence of a viable reference count method remains a problem with clinical platelet counting: the haemocytometer method is too imprecise. Recently, a task force of the International Society for Laboratory Hematology (ISLH) and ICSH has developed a monoclonal antibody and flow cytometry (immunoflow) based protocol that has been tested as a candidate reference method. It is expected that this method can establish reference values, even at very low platelet counts, for the evaluation and validation of automated clinical analyser results. A robust and transferable platelet reference count should also improve the homology between counts on different analyser platforms and between different manufacturers.

Interference with platelet counting includes EDTA-induced clumping, platelet rosetting of neutrophils, very high levels of Intralipid® intravenous (i.v.) feeding and rare forms of

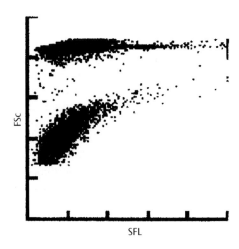

Fig. 2.5 *The scatterplot represents two cell populations: the upper population consists of red blood cells (RBCs) and reticulocytes, and the lower cell population of platelets. Overlap between large platelets and smaller RBCs often occurs in single-parameter measurements based on cell volume alone. In the method represented here, the fluorescent content of platelets moves the larger and more fluorescent platelets away from the RBC and reticulocyte population, creating an effective enumeration of platelets without interference from small RBCs or red cell debris.*

hyperlipaemia (for other possible interferences see Table 2.3). As indicated above, apoptotic white cell fragments and fragile white cells (CLL) may also interfere with platelet counting. EDTA-induced clumping is caused by IgG and/or IgM anti-platelet antibodies active in the presence of EDTA and is usually entirely an *in vitro* phenomenon (Pegels *et al.*, 1982; Casonata *et al.*, 1994). Repeat collection of the patient's blood in a different anticoagulant such as sodium citrate may eliminate EDTA-induced platelet clumping and allow an electronic count. The solution for the other problems is far from simple, and one may have to rely on an estimate of the platelet count from microscopy of the stained blood film.

2.9 PACKED CELL VOLUME

Strictly speaking, the packed cell volume or, as it is more commonly termed, the haematocrit (Hct), like the haemoglobin (Hgb) determination, is not part of the blood count proper, although an electronically determined Hct is entirely derived from blood counting parameters, namely red cell count and volume. For interferences, please refer to Table 2.3.

The reference method for packed cell volume by centrifugation has been the subject of many years of scrutiny and evaluation. The Cytometry Panel of ICSH and others have published several papers on the topic and the issue may finally be laid to rest by accepting an indirect method (ICSH, 1980; Bull and Rittenbach, 1990; Bull, 2000). One of the problems with the earlier method was that it required the incorporation of radiolabelled albumin to measure plasma trapped between the packed RBCs. This was not only cumbersome to carry out, but the labelled albumin became unavailable. The indirect method uses the haemoglobin concentration of the cells in the red cell column of a spun blood sample (Bull and Rittenbach, 1990; Bull, 2000). The assumption is that this represents a direct measurement of the actual MCHC and that the Hct can therefore be calculated by dividing this measurement by the sample's direct Hgb concentration before centrifugation since

$$MCHC = Hgb/Hct.$$

In the final analysis, it appears that the borosilicate glass of the microhaematocrit tubes used for this 'reference method' dehydrates those red cells that have the most contact with the glass walls of the tubes just to the extent that this water loss compensates for the amount of trapped plasma.

For practical purposes the spun haematocrit is applied for instrument calibration, using low-power microscopy for backlit and parallax-free readings and the Vernier scale of the microscope stage for calculating the proportion of the red cell column relative to the total column of RBCs and plasma combined (NCCLS, 1993a). However, care must be taken that blood is aerated before any Hct measurements are made, manually or electronically, because of water shifts into the RBC as a result of deoxygenation and the subsequent formation of carbonates (Bryner *et al.*, 1997).

Haematology analysers measure Hct either by summing all the pulses in the RBC channel (direct Hct measurement) or, in case of instruments with pulse editing, by multiplying the MCV calculated from a truncated red cell volume distribution histogram by the RBC count. Pulse editing excludes large (and very small) red cells from the calculation and instead bases the Hct on the cells in the central part of the red cell volume distribution. This causes some loss of information as it creates a Hct based on the cell volumes of a selected population of red cells close to the MCV, but not on the individual cell volume of all red cells. This results in a somewhat dynamically challenged Hct, which becomes apparent when MCHC calculations from different instruments (with direct Hct measurement and with Hct based on truncated red cell populations) are compared with a reference MCHC based on reference Hgb measurement and spun Hct (Bull *et al.* 1996). Reproducibility of the electronically obtained haematocrit is generally excellent (Table 2.1).

The clinical usefulness of a Hct obtained from a haematology analyser is limited, and for determining a patient's red cell mass, the use of Hgb rather than Hct measurements should be encouraged. However, in many clinical environments, as well as in some leading medical journals, the Hct has remained popular. This does not always serve diagnostic efforts to the best extent. When the spun Hct is obtained from venous blood, and if read by experienced staff under appropriate conditions, accuracy and precision can be quite good (Table 2.1). However when blood is obtained by microcollection and read by non-technologist staff using hand-held 'haematocrit reading devices', the Hct becomes more of an estimate than an accurate test. This microcollection-based technique is commonly used in many emergency rooms, operating rooms, intensive care units and neonatal environments. It is unlikely that under such circumstances a reading can be obtained which is reliable enough to document a 10% blood loss. It might be more appropriate to replace this test with near-patient haemoglobin determination.

2.10 COMBINING PARAMETERS: THE 'HAEMOGRAM' AND THE 'COMPLETE BLOOD CELL' COUNT

The combination of red cell, white cell and platelet counts with haemoglobin and haematocrit determination constitutes a basic 'haemogram' without a leucocyte differential count. The amount of information from the haemogram, especially in regard to flagging abnormalities, may appear limited, but this does not affect many of its clinical applications for monitoring, screening or case finding. Combined with the RBC indices – MCV, MCH, MCHC and RDW – and especially when combined with a reticulocyte count, a haemogram provides powerful information in anaemia patients (Fourcade *et al.* 1999). Several efforts have been made to use such information in rule-based systems in order to separate iron deficiency anaemia from other types of microcytic anemia such as thalassaemia trait (England, 1989; Green and King, 1989; Houwen, 1989). Overall, the success of such rule-based systems has been limited.

An extension of the haemogram became available when this basic count was combined with an electronic differential analysis of the WBC population. While initially the focus was to develop automated microscopes, the cost and relatively low throughput of this technology have led to other forms of electronic cell analysis, based on flow systems. The earliest systems were based on enzyme-cytochemistry and light-scattering properties of leucocytes (Mansberg *et al.*, 1974). In the 1980s, a new, partial differentiation of WBCs became available, based on volumetric distribution of WBCs (Bain *et al.*, 1984). With further improvements this became known as a three-part WBC differential (Johnston, 1985; Richardson-Jones *et al.*, 1985; Payne *et al.*, 1987) and to this date probably remains the most commonly used electronic method for a partial 'screening' differential WBC count. Lymphocytes and granulocytes, in particular, can be identified by this method, with a middle or mixed cell population including monocytes separating the two. However, it became clear that a WBC count combined with a volumetric three-part differential would not yield information beyond a limited number of blood cell types, and although useful for screening purposes, it lacked definition and finesse for definitive answers in complex situations.

The haemogram combined with a five-cell type WBC differential count and flagging system for abnormalities is often called a 'complete blood cell count' (CBC; also called a 'full blood count', FBC). Instrument flagging by the five-cell type WBC differential may trigger the requirement for a blood film review, and sometimes for a WBC differential by visual microscopy. Numerical results (counts, volume measurements, cell distributions) from the analyser's basic 'haemogram' parameters may also be used as flagging criteria and can be incorporated into quite elaborate algorithms that can signal the presence of qualitative abnormalities above a certain trigger level (Thalhammer-Scherrer *et al.*, 1997). The decision levels for abnormal cell types are outlined in NCCLS (1992), based on common experience in clinical laboratories, using the 100 WBC microscopy differential count. Using newer data, based on flow cytometric analysis, it is likely that some of these decision levels will undergo some adjustment in the near future. Manufacturers should state instrument flagging performance in their specifications, including a general description of the normal and patient populations studied.

The CBC plus its flagging system can complete the haematological analysis in about 45% of patient specimens in most tertiary care hospitals and in greater proportions in most other hospitals and outpatient services, depending on specific case loads. Given the economic constraints within laboratories, there is a strong desire to reduce manual blood film reviews even further without affecting the quality of the laboratory output. This has led to the concept of the electronic 'extended differential' count.

2.11 EXTENDED DIFFERENTIAL COUNTING

With improved technology in terms of instrument fluidics, reagent systems, electronics and computing, instrument users and manufacturers have started looking at broader analytical capabilities and applications for haematology analysers. Such increased capability is now being offered on some analysers as 'full' leucocyte differential counting, including enumeration of cell types normally not found in the blood, or present at very low levels only (the 'extended differential' count, EDC). In addition, many analysers now include optical platelet counting and integrated reticulocyte counting often with measurement of reticulocyte maturity. Other new applications for automated haematology cell counters include cell counting of bone marrow, body fluids and automated urinalysis. These broader applications became possible because of concerted efforts between manufacturers, experts and regulators, and have been instrumental in opening up new fields for automated electronic cell analysis. It has also stimulated the development of new 'reference' methods for the evaluation of emerging new technology and its applications. Reference methods were originally based on visual microscopy methods only, but increasingly have begun to include alternate methodologies such as flow cytometry (Table 2.4).

Table 2.5 presents an overview of cell types included in the EDC. One specific cell type, identified in some countries as a 'band' or 'stab' cell, and in other countries not counted but indicated by an equally difficult to standardize 'left shift' flag, will currently not be included in the EDC. The reason for this is the lack of international agreement on how to define and/or express 'band' cells or 'left shift' by light microscopy. Faced with this lack of agreement, even among experts (Bentley *et al.*, 1994; Cornbleet and Novak, 1995), it will be virtually impossible for manufacturers to standardize and calibrate an electronic method for enumerating such cells. Even more problematic might be the rather vague descriptive term 'left shift', which is based on an overall morphological impression (not count) of morphology parameters including toxic changes in neutrophils, Döhle bodies and the possible presence of more

Table 2.4 *Reference methods for blood cell counting*

Cell type	Manual (current/extinct)	Other (current/experimental)
Red blood cells (RBCs)	Counting chamber (E)	Single channel impedance count (C)
White blood cells (WBCs)	Counting chamber (E)	Single channel impedance count (C)
Platelets	Counting chamber ($\pm$ E)	Immunoflow (C)
Reticulocytes	Manual count (C) -2×2000 RBCs	Flow cytometry (exp)
Five-cell differential (neutrophils + lymphocytyes + monoctyes + eosinophils + basophils)	Manual count (C) $-$ blood film 2×200 WBCs	Flow cytometry (CD45, PI) (C)
Nucleated red blood cells	Manual count (C) $-$ NRBCs per 1000 WBCs	Flow cytometry (PI and antibody-based) (exp) $-$ CD45, CD14 (CD13)
Immature granulocytes (promyelocytes + myelocytes + metamyelocytes)	Manual count (C) $-$ blood film 2×200 WBCs	Flow cytometry (antibody-based) (exp) $-$ CD45, CD11b, CD16
Variant/atypical lymphocytes	Manual count (C) $-$ blood film 2×200 WBCs	
Blasts	Manual count (C) $-$ blood film 2×200 WBC	Flow cytometry (antibody-based) (exp)
Haemopoietic progenitor cells	Flow cytometry (C) $-$ CD34	

C, currently used; E, extinct (no longer in use); exp, experimental; NRBCs, nucleated red blood cells.

immature granulocytes such as metamyelocytes and myelocytes. Monoclonal antibody-based flow cytometry might offer a better solution than the highly subjective interpretation of what constitutes a mature segmented neutrophil and what determines a slightly more immature 'band' cell (Fujimoto *et al.*, 2000).

Other cell types such as NRBCs and immature granulocytes[2] can be defined by morphology, antibody-based flow cytometry (Tsuji *et al.*, 1999) or both (Table 2.4). Improved electronic cell identification has opened up the possibility for automated enumeration of all or most white cells, even in blood specimens with significant pathology. This could have significant consequences for further automating leucocyte differential counting in a much greater proportion of specimens. A recently published survey (Konno and Kanda, 1996) of hospitalized patients lists the frequency of abnormalities encountered (Table 2.5). It is obvious from these data that reliable identification of just the two most frequently

[2]It has been generally agreed within the Extended Differential Task Force of the International Society for Laboratory Hematology (ISLH) to group metamyelocytes, myelocytes and promyelocytes as immature granulocytes. Band neutrophils are included in the neutrophil group.

Table 2.5 *Cell types included in the traditional and the extended electronic differential count (proportional) and absolute (n × 10⁹/L)*

Traditional	Reference interval[a]		Extended	Limit	Frequency[b]
	n	**%**			
Neutrophils	1.89–5.32	38–68	Left shift	Varies	NA[c]
Lymphocytes	1.39–3.19	22–50	Immature granulocytes	> 1%	11%
Monocytes	0.30–0.76	5–11.4	NRBCs	> 1%	2%
Eosinophils	0.05–0.35	0.8–5.3	Blasts	> 1%	0.7%
Basophils	0.01–0.06	0.2–1.0	Atypical lymphocytes	> 10%	0.3%
			Haematopoietic progenitor cells	NA	
			Other	0.2%	

[a]Based on 328 medical students (male = 195 and female = 133). Analysed in the author's laboratory by Sysmex XE-2100 haematology analyser (Sysmex Corp., Kobe, Japan).
[b]Clinical frequency in patient specimens (*n* = 24 579) (Konno and Kanda, 1996).
[c]Neither 'band' (or 'stab') cells nor left shifted cells are currently included in the extended differential count, but they are included in the neutrophil group.
NA, not available; NRBCs, nucleated red blood cells.

occurring abnormal cell types, i.e. immature granulocytes and NRBCs, will significantly reduce manual (or automated) microscopy. Microscopy will thus be pertinent only to those samples selected either by the laboratory's management decisions and/or by the inability of the analyser to deal with a specific abnormality. An example of a management-based decision would be microscopy review (not differential count) of a blood film on every newly admitted patient. Other examples are blood specimens from selected patient categories or with results outside set limits for white cell counts, red cell indices, a first time abnormal platelet count, etc.

The methods by which different analysers achieve a leucocyte differential count of the five normally present cell types (neutrophils, lymphocytes, monocytes, eosinophils, basophils) and of the EDC all differ and are based on the inherent (often proprietary) technologies used. None so far uses monoclonal antibodies routinely, mainly because of inconvenience and cost. The time required for incubation with a monoclonal antibody would increase the turnaround time significantly, and reimbursement requirements for a major cost increase are adverse factors for the routine use of fluorescent or otherwise labelled monoclonal antibodies. One of the purposes of the electronic CBC and EDC is to reduce (expensive) manual microscopy, not to increase the costs per test further.

2.12 ANALYSER FLAGGING PERFORMANCE

The clinically important issue with any electronic CBC and EDC is the false-negative (FN) rate for flagging abnormalities: ideally it should be very low if not zero. From the laboratory perspective this is, of course, also important, but on the other hand a low false-positive (FP) rate is essential to keep the laboratory costs of operating a particular technology or instrument reasonable. Typically, operating costs in the haematology laboratory are more than 50% generated by personnel/staffing and a high microscopy review rate adversely affects the now almost universal intent to reduce laboratory expenditure. Most haematology analysers show a balance between FN and FP rates so as to create reasonable, although perhaps not ideal, end results.

Representing flagging results in terms of overall sensitivity and specificity is often misleading, and it can be more informative to present data separately for normal specimens (all or nearly all should be unflagged) and patient specimens with qualitative, quantitative abnormalities and mixed abnormalities (all specimens with morphological abnormalities should be flagged). Although guidelines for analyser performance are available (NCCLS, 1992; ICSH, 1994a; Weber *et al.*, 1995), these are no longer sufficient even for routine testing conditions, especially for cells occurring as rare events, and efforts are underway within ICSH and ISLH to improve existing testing protocols.

Several analysers are now equipped with user-adjustable levels for morphology flags, allowing clinical laboratories to adjust flagging results to their specific caseloads. Ultimately, though, it is expected that most flagging will be replaced by definitive analyser results, obviating secondary testing (by manual or automated microscopy). This will move electronic analysers from screening devices to a definitive and mature technology.

2.13 RETICULOCYTE COUNTING

Electronic reticulocyte counting has caused a revolution as well as an evolution for this cell type. The reticulocyte count is indicative of the RBC production rate and is, therefore, useful in conditions such as anaemia, haemolysis, etc. However, the count imprecision of the manual microscopic method renders it almost useless (Table 2.1).

Improvements in the electronic reticulocyte count are largely based on the counting of larger numbers of reticulocytes (reduction of Poisson error) and on the consistent application of reticulocyte properties (mainly stainable RNA) as criteria for identification of a cell as a reticulocyte. Currently, coefficients of variation (CVs) for reticulocyte counts at normal, adult levels by electronic cell counters are in the order of 5–7%, compared with 40% for routine manual counts (Table 2.1). Electronic counting has also led to the more general use of the 'absolute' reticulocyte count, expressed as the number of cells per unit volume ($\times 10^6/L$) rather than as a proportion (%) of RBCs. Using an absolute reticulocyte count no longer requires correction for anaemia and should lead to a more appropriate use of reticulocyte enumeration (NCCLS, 1993b).

An important issue concerns the definition of the reticulocyte population, or more specifically, whether 'bone marrow' or 'shift' reticulocytes should be included in the count. Shift reticulocytes have been considered an expression of erythropoietic stress and therefore their exclusion from the reticulocyte count has been advocated (Hillman, 1969). However, most electronic reticulocyte counts include these cells. This is still somewhat controversial, since the reticulocyte count is considered to reflect the actual rate of RBC production and shift reticulocytes are considered a spillover of red cell precursors from a hypercellular, stressed bone marrow that are not representative of the RBC production rate.

What has created additional excitement about electronic reticulocyte analysis is the availability of two entirely different new aspects of this cell type: reticulocyte Hgb and RNA content. Measurement of haemoglobin content in individual cells, including reticulocytes, has stimulated the idea that iron deficiency may possibly be diagnosed at an early stage of red cell development. This has been investigated for clinical usefulness in a series of different conditions, with somewhat variable results and less favorable predictive values of a positive test for more complex conditions. By far the best results were obtained in patients with uncomplicated iron deficiency anemia (Brugnara *et al.*, 1999), but in patients with end-stage renal disease positive tests yielded low predictive values (Fishbane *et al.*, 1997; Mittman *et al.*, 1997).

The second reticulocyte parameter that has been developed is called immature reticulocyte fraction (IRF) and is based on the RNA content of reticulocytes (Davis *et al.*, 1989; Houwen, 1992). Reticulocytes gradually lose their RNA and ultimately become RNA-free red cells, while RNA-rich, more immature reticulocytes are found in a relatively narrow reference interval in normal, healthy adults. Immature reticulocytes appear in larger than normal proportion when the red cell production increases. This is the case when erythropoiesis is stimulated by haematins such as oral or parenteral Fe supplements in iron deficiency anaemia, vitamin B_{12} in pernicious anaemia, and erythropoietin in end-stage renal disease. Somewhat surprisingly, IRF has also shown usefulness in patients recovering from cytotoxic chemotherapy and in the early phases of engraftment of bone marrow or stem cell transplants (Davis *et al.*, 1989). In fact, these patients show upward changes in IRF prior to changes in reticulocyte count and, in the case of transplanted patients, often prior to upward changes in white cell and platelet counts, as the first indicator of stem cell engraftment. There is now a large body of data in the literature, based on different methodologies to measure IRF, which supports these observations (Davis, 1996). Thus it appears that IRF changes are an indication of the rate of change in red cell production rates: in other words IRF reflects the second derivative of the red cell production process and the reticulocyte count the first derivative, i.e. the production rate itself.

Electronic counting of reticulocytes has created a major change in the evaluation of red cell production and bone marrow erythropoiesis. Unfortunately, this change is mostly limited to the laboratory environment and has yet to be incorporated, on a large scale, into clinical decision-making.

2.14 DATA PRESENTATION

Analysis (and presentation of data) varies from manufacturer to manufacturer, and often even by type of analyser from the same manufacturer. This lack of standardization may give 'character' to a specific line of products but it is counterproductive in an environment where a product mix is present. It also makes interfacing and data handling by laboratory information systems (LIS) much more complex and therefore carries a high cost. It would be preferable to have some standardization in data format and presentation. This is becoming more and more important with an ever-increasing number of cell types and their attributes being analysed electronically.

Most commonly used multi-parameter instruments display results as a mixture of graphical and numerical data. The graphical display combines single-parameter histograms with bivariate scatterplots. Only the more basic analysers show just histogram displays (or none at all) with numerical data. When more than two parameters are used, multiple scatterplots are often available with individual cell populations labelled by different colours. While this is certainly helpful, it would be even more helpful if industry could decide on uniform colour coding for at least the major leucocyte subsets.

Cell populations can be identified by discriminators of various kinds (straight lines, gates of different sizes and shapes, sometimes automatically adjusted, sometimes manually); sometimes the discriminators, analysis gates and analysis grids are visible to the user, and sometimes they are not. Cell populations can also be identified by various derivatives of cluster analysis instead of discriminators. Of these methods, automatically adaptable cluster analysis (by a process of optimization called 'bootstrapping') is probably the most versatile. It requires computing power now readily available on most modern small computer systems and can be carried out in real time.

2.15 DATA INTERPRETATION: CAN DATA BE TRANSFORMED INTO INFORMATION?

Regardless of the complexity of data and number of parameters generated by automated haematology analysers, there remain basically two levels of interpretation: the first is within the laboratory and may be carried out by different individuals with differing levels of expertise, often sequentially; and the second is at the clinical user site. The two levels do not necessarily require the same data. In fact, even information derived from the same data will still be different for the two sites. The clinical site operates with the knowledge of the patient's clinical condition; the laboratory focus is whether the data are reliable or not, without much clinical interpretation.

While the basic parameters of the haemogram, the CBC, and even the EDC, have remained the same, whether done manually or electronically, the addition of many numerical parameters such as red cell indices, red cell distribution width, cellular haemoglobin content, IRF, MPV, PDW, etc., are often beyond the grasp of most clinicians. Frequently these parameters disappear from view among the 25–40 measurements that are contained in a CBC/EDC report and constitute data overload for the clinician. It will be necessary to apply a new focus to the many parameters produced by current haematology analysers. It is important that electronic blood cell analysis has become increasingly reliable, but it is also necessary to recognize that the data are becoming too complex and cumbersome for general clinical usefulness. For new and potentially very useful parameters, such as IRF, it will be necessary, for successful clinical implementation, to look beyond 'the box' and to consider ways to transform IRF data into useful information.

Data should not always be looked at in isolation; often it can be more useful to review data as part of a string in a patient's course rather than as a single measurement 'snapshot', and to compare the behaviour of different parameters over a given time-frame. Graphical as well as numerical displays may be helpful, as may be the use of some form of interpretative software. Such changes should take data from where it has been since the inception of clinical laboratories: a mass of numbers as the laboratory's output rather than a set of well organized data, ultimately transformed into clinically useful information.

2.16 CONCLUSIONS

Since the introduction of the electronic cell count into the clinical laboratory in 1956, dramatic changes in clinical laboratory practice have occurred. Increasingly we see a move away from manual, microscopy methods towards electronic technology. The advantages of this shift are several. Analytical speed has much improved with enormous reductions in 'turnaround time' from test requisition to validated, chartable results in the hands of the clinician. The quality of electronic test results, in terms of both accuracy and precision, has improved for virtually all haematology tests. This improvement has been seen both in specimens with normal results and, even more so, in patient samples with significant abnormalities. Modern haemato-oncology practice would be unthinkable without electronic cell analysis. Extended differential counting and electronic analysis of bone marrow and body fluids are now being clinically applied, although not yet on the same scale as the CBC for blood specimens.

However, the management of data obtained by these electronic devices is lagging behind considerably. Essentially the data are presented in a format that has not changed since the inception of clinical laboratory testing in the early 1900s: a series of numbers, occasionally accompanied by a brief commentary, often formalized. There is a clear need for innovative approaches to stem the current trend of increasing numbers of parameters, resulting in data overload for clinicians. There is an equal need for algorithms that turn those data into information. This information could become extremely powerful if trends in sequential patient data were taken into account and were somehow related to treatment intervention schemes. That would take the practice of laboratory haematology out of its current stagnant backwater and could create new ways of diagnosing and monitoring health and disease.

REFERENCES

Ault, K.A. and Knowles, C. (1995) In vivo biotynilation demonstrates that reticulated platelets are the youngest platelets in circulation. *Exp. Hematol.* **23**, 996–1001.

Bain, B., Dean, A. and Broom, G. (1984) The estimation of lymphocyte percentage by the Coulter Counter Model S-Plus III. *Clin. Lab. Haematol.* **6**, 273–85.

Bentley, S.A., Johnson, T.S., Sohier, C.H. and Bishop, C. (1994) Flow-cytochemical differential leukocyte analysis with quantitation of neutrophil left shift. An evaluation of the Cobas-Helios analyzer. *Am. J. Clin. Pathol.* **102**, 223–30.

Bessman, D. (1982) Prediction of platelet production during chemotherapy of acute leukemia . *Am. J. Hematol.* **13**, 219–27.

Bessman, J.D., Gilmer, P.R. and Gardner, F.H. (1983) Improved classification of anemias through MCV and RDW. *Am. J. Clin. Pathol.* **80**, 322–6.

Brugnara, C., Zurakowski, D., DiCanzio, J. *et al.* (1999) Reticulocyte hemoglobin content to diagnose iron deficiency in children. *J. Am. Med. Assoc.* **281**, 2225–30.

Bryner, M., Westengard, J., Klein, O. and Houwen. B. (1997) The relationship of red blood cell volume to oxygenation and deoxygenation. *Clin. Lab. Haematol.* **19**, 99–103.

Bull, B.S. (2000) Is the packed cell volume reliable? *XIIIth International Symposium on Technological Innovations in Laboratory Hematology*, Banff, Canada.

Bull, B.S., Aller, R. and Houwen, B. (1996) MCHC: red cell index or quality control parameter? *Proceedings of the XXVI International Society of Haematology Meeting*, Singapore, 40–43.

Bull, B.S. and Rittenbach, J.D. (1990) A proposed reference haematocrit derived from multiple MCHC determinations via haemoglobin measurements. *Clin. Lab. Haematol.* **12**(Suppl.), 43–53.

Casonato, A., Bertomoro, A., Pontara, E. *et al.* (1994) EDTA dependent pseudothrombocytopenia caused by antibodies against the cytoadhesive receptor of platelet GpIIB-IIIA. *J. Clin. Pathol.* **47**, 625–30.

Cornbleet, P.J. and Novak, R.W. (1995) Lack of reproducibility of band neutrophil identification despite the use of uniform criteria. *Lab. Hematol.* **1**, 89–96.

Coulter,W.H. (1956) High speed automatic blood cell counter and cell size analyzer. *Proc. Nat. Electronics Conf.* **12**, 1034–40.

Crosland-Taylor, P.J. (1953) A device for counting small particles suspended in fluid through a tube. *Nature* **171**, 37–8.

Dacie, J.V. and Lewis, S.M. (1975) In: *Practical Haematology*, 5th edn. Edinburgh: Churchill Livingstone, 27.

Dale, G.L., Friese, P., Hynes, L.A. and Burstein, S.A. (1995) Demonstration that thiazole-orange-positive platelets in the dog are less than 24 hours old. *Blood* **85,** 1822–5.

Davis, B.H. (1996) Immature reticulocyte fraction: by any name, a useful clinical parameter of erythropoietic activity. *Lab. Hematol.* **1**, 2–8.

Davis, B.H., Bigelow, N.C., Ball, E.D. *et al.* (1989) Utility of flow cytometric quantification of reticulocyte maturity as a predictor of engraftment in autologous bone marrow transplantation. *Am. J. Hematol.* **32**, 81–7.

Diem, K., ed. (1962) *Documenta Geigy Scientific Tables,* 6th edn. Basle: Ciba-Geigy, 184.

England, J.M. (1989) Discriminant functions. *Blood Cells* **15**, 463–71.

Fishbane, S., Calgano, C., Langley, R.C. Jr. *et al.* (1997) Reticulocyte hemoglobin content in the evaluation of iron status of hemodialysis patients. *Kidney Int.* **52**, 217–22.

Fourcade, C., Jary, L. and Belanoui, H. (1999) Reticulocyte analysis provided by the Coulter GEN.S: Significance and interpretation in regenerative and nonregenerative hematologic conditions. *Lab. Hematol.* **5**, 153–8.

Fujimoto, H., Sakata, T., Hamaguchi, Y. *et al.* (2000) Flow cytometric method for enumeration and classification of reactive immature granulocyte populations. *Cytometry*, in press.

Green, R. and King, R. (1989) A new red cell discriminant incorporating volume dispersion for differentiating iron deficiency anemia from thalassemia minor. *Blood Cells* **15**, 481–91.

Henry, J.B. (1991) In: *Clinical Diagnosis and Management by Laboratory Methods*, 18th edn. Philadelphia: WB Saunders, 566.

Hillman, R.S. (1969) Characteristics of marrow production and reticulocyte maturation in normal man in response to anemia. *J. Clin. Invest.* **48**, 443–53.

Houwen, B. (1989) The use of inference strategies in the differential diagnosis of microcytic anemia. *Blood Cells* **15**, 509–32.

Houwen, B. (1992) Reticulocyte maturation. *Blood Cells* **18**, 167–86.

Houwen, B. and Koepke, J.A. (1990) The classic manual differential count and current multiparameter electronic cell analysis: the end of an era? *Sysmex J.* **13**, 47–57.

Hubl, W., Wolfbauer, G., Andert, S. *et al.* (1997) Toward a new reference method for the leukocyte five-part differential. *Cytometry* **30**, 72–84.

ICSH (1980) Recommended method for the determination of packed cell volume. WHO LAB/80.4.

ICSH (1994a) Guidelines for evaluation of automated blood cell analyzers including those used for differential leucocyte and reticulocyte counting and cell marker applications. *Clin. Lab. Haematol.* **16**, 157–74.

ICSH (1994b) Reference method for the enumeration of erythrocytes and leucocytes. *Clin. Lab. Haematol.* **16**,131–8.

Johnston, C.L. (1985) Leukocyte screening using the ELT-800WS. *Blood Cells* **1**, 241–55.

Kickler, T.S. (2000) Maximizing the utility of automated hematology systems for improved patient outcomes. XIIIth International Symposium on Technological Innovations in Laboratory Hematology. Banff, Canada. *Lab. Hematol.* **6**, 11.

Kienast, J. and Schmitz, G. (1990) Flow cytometric analysis of thiazole orange uptake by platelets: a diagnostic aid in the evolution of thrombocytopenic disorders. *Blood* **75**, 116–22.

Konno, T. and Kanda, T. (1996) The total hematology system based on laboratory information system and quick turn around time. *Sysmex J. Int.* **6**, 113–22.

Lebeck, L.K., Mast, B.J. and Houwen, B. (1993) Flow cytometric white blood cell differential: a proposed alternate reference method. *Sysmex J. Int.* **3**, 61–9.

Levy, W.C., Bull, B.S. and Koepke, J.A. (1986) The incorporation of red blood cell index mean data into quality control programs. *Am. J. Clin. Pathol.* **86**, 193–9.

Lewis, S.M. (1990) Standardization and harmonization of the blood count: the role of International Committee for Standardization in Haematology (ICSH). *Eur. J. Haematol.* **53**(Suppl), 9–13.

Mansberg, H.P., Saunders, AM. and Groner, W. (1974) The Hemalog-D white cell differential system. *Cytochemistry* **22**, 711–24.

Miale, J.B. (1982) *Laboratory Medicine Hematology*, 6th edn. St Louis: Mosby.

Mittman, N., Sreddhara, R. and Mushnick, R. *et al.* (1997) Reticulocyte hemoglobin content predicts functional iron deficiency in hemodialysis patients receiving rHuEPO. *Am. J. Kidney Dis.* **30**, 912–22.

Mohandas, N., Bunyataravey, A., Ballas, S. *et al.* (1992) Cell hemoglobin content and cell hemoglobin concentration: the forgotten red cell indices. *24th Congress of the International Society of Haematology* (Abstract 1007), London.

NCCLS (1991a) Procedures for the collection of diagnostic blood specimens by skin puncture, 3rd edn. Approved Standard. *NCCLS document H4-A3*. Wayne, PA: NCCLS.

NCCLS (1991b) Procedures for the collection of diagnostic blood specimens by venipuncture, 3rd edn. Approved Standard. *NCCLS document H3-A3*. Wayne, PA: NCCLS.

NCCLS (1992) Reference leukocyte differential count (proportional) and evaluation of instrument methods. Approved Standard. *NCCLS document H20-A*. Wayne, PA: NCCLS.

NCCLS (1993a) Procedure for determining packed cell volume: the microhematocrit method, 2nd edn. Approved Standard. *NCCLS document H7-A2*. Wayne, PA: NCCLS.

NCCLS (1993b) Reticulocyte counting by flow cytometry. *NCCLS document H44-P*. Wayne, PA: NCCLS.

NCCLS (1996) Performance goals for the internal quality control of multichannel hematology analyzers. Approved standard. *NCCLS document H26-A*. Wayne, PA: NCCLS.

NCCLS (1998) Calibration and quality control of automated hematology analyzers. Proposed standard. *NCCLS document H38-P*. Wayne, PA: NCCLS.

Orfao, A., Schmitz, C., Brando, R. *et al.* (1999) Clinically useful information provided by the flow cytometric immunophenotyping of hematological malignancies: current status and future directions. *Clin. Chem.* **45**, 1708–17.

Paterakis, G.S., Laoutaris, N.P., Alexia, S.V. *et al.* (1994) The effect of red cell shape on the measurement of red cell volume. A proposed method for the comparative assessment of this effect among various haematology analyzers. *Clin. Lab. Haematol.* **16**, 235–45.

Payne, B.A., Pierre, R.V. and Lee, W.K. (1987) Evaluation of the TOA E-5000 automated hematology analyzer. *Am. J. Clin. Pathol.* **88**, 51–7.

Pegels, J.G., Bruynes, E.C., Engelfriet, C.P. and von dem Borne, A.E. (1982) Pseudothrombocytopenia: an immunologic study on platelet antibodies dependent on ethylene diamine tetra-acetate. *Blood* **59**, 157–61.

Richardson-Jones, A., Hellman, R. and Twedt, D. (1985) The Coulter Counter leukocyte differential. *Blood Cells* **11**, 203–38.

Schumacher, H.R. (1997) The automated leukocyte count and differential: the future approach to diagnosis. In: Schumacher, H.R. (ed.), *Acute Leukemia*. Baltimore: Williams and Wilkins.

Smith, F.A. and Kroft, S.H. (1997) Optimal procedures for detecting analytic bias using patient samples. *Am. J. Clin. Pathol.* **108**, 254–68.

Thalhammer-Scherrer, R., Knobl, P., Korninger, L. and Schwarzinger, I. (1997) Automated five-part white blood cell differential counts. Efficiency of software-generated white blood cell suspect flags of the hematology analyzers Sysmex SE-9000, Sysmex NE-8000, and Coulter STKS. *Arch. Pathol. Lab. Med.* **121**, 573–7.

Thom, R. and Kachel, V. (1970) Fortschritte für die elektronischen Grössenbestimmung von Blutkörperchen. *Blut* **21**, 48–50.

Thom, R. (1969) Die elektronischen Volumenbestimmung von Blutkörperchen und ihre Fehlerquellen. *Z. Ges. Exp. Med.* **151**, 331–49.

Tsuji, T., Sakata, T., Hamaguchi, Y. *et al.* (1999) New rapid flow cytometric method for the enumeration of nucleated red blood cells. *Cytometry* **37**, 291–301.

US-Canadian consensus recommendations on the immunophenotypic analysis of hematologic neoplasia by flow cytometry. *Cytometry* **30**, 213–74.

van Assendelft, O.W. (1991) Interpretation of the quantitative blood cell count. In: Koepke, J.A. (ed.), *Practical Laboratory Hematology*. Edinburgh: Churchill Livingstone, 69–78.

Weber, N., Mast, B.J. and Houwen, B. (1995) Performance evaluation of hematology analyzers: an outline for clinical laboratory testing. *Sysmex J. Intl.* **5**(2), 103–13.

3

The differential cell count

BEREND HOUWEN

INTRODUCTION

Differential cell counts are typically considered as an enumeration of the different white blood cell (WBC) types circulating in the blood. However, as we will see later in this chapter, differential counts can also apply to other cell lineages, such as red blood cells (RBCs), or to cells within the same lineage but at different maturation levels. The WBC differential count has become widely accepted and used by clinicians and is generally considered to yield clinically useful information in health and disease.

As a procedure, the differential count is unlike almost all other tests in the clinical laboratory. It provides a pathology report on the morphological appearance of blood cells and on the frequency in which they appear, not in a descriptive manner but in a highly stylized, quantitative format. It is called a 'differential' count because all enumerated cells are brought into a common mathematical context, i.e. a frequency distribution for the different cell types present. The total number of cells counted may vary, but in most clinical situations this is 100, and specific cell types are commonly expressed as a percentage of the total count. Thus, there is within this context a particular distribution of cell types for healthy, normal individuals and there are distribution patterns associated with disease states.

Over time, the information derived from the WBC differential count has become a cornerstone in laboratory haematology and is widely used for screening, case finding, diagnosis and monitoring of haematological and non-haematological disorders. Examples include bacterial or viral infectious disease, evaluation of allergic conditions, diagnosis and monitoring of malignant disease such as leukaemia, and staging of HIV infection. The WBC differential count is often also used to monitor a patient's progress and/or response to treatment. For example, a decrease from elevated neutrophil counts in patients treated for (bacterial) infectious disease is generally regarded as a positive response.

However, the test is not without its problems. The traditional procedure for the differential WBC count by manual microscopy is time-consuming and labour-intensive and is therefore one of the most expensive routine tests in the clinical haematology laboratory. The 100-cell differential count is also often criticized for its statistical shortcomings because of its small sampling size. Despite all this, most clinicians still consider the manual WBC differential count to be effective, perhaps not in a direct decision-making manner, but more as a source of collateral information, like taking a patient's body temperature. The manual differential count thus shows a combination of poor statistical reliability, high expense, but definite clinical utility which has made it a prime target for automation and alternative approaches. Those efforts date back to the 1960s, and to date continue to push the boundaries of differential cell counting forward.

Newer technologies have enabled WBC differential counts to be obtained electronically from automated analysers, at much lower cost, with greater statistical reliability, often with greater overall accuracy, and with faster availability to the clinician. Moreover, these technologies have enabled laboratory workers to measure cellular differentiation and quantify cell types other than WBCs, with sometimes surprising clinical utility as outcomes.

3.1 THE EVOLUTION OF THE DIFFERENTIAL CELL COUNT

The introduction of aniline dyes in the second half of the 19th century made it possible to study individual blood cells by microscopy after a small amount of blood had been placed onto glass slides, dried and fixed and then stained. Eosin was the first of these dyes, in 1856, followed by haematoxylin in 1865, and later by the metachromatic Romanowsky dyes. Amazingly, up to the present day, the practice of manual leucocyte differential counting essentially has not changed in more than a century, although a few refinements have been made. These consist mainly of improvements in dye quality, staining procedures, automation of slide preparation and staining, and the microscopes used.

Attempts to automate WBC differential counting began in the 1960s with image analysis, using computer-based algorithms (Mahouy et al., 1973; Mui et al., 1977). At the time, building automated microscope systems capable of morphological analysis appeared to be an attractive solution for replacing manual differential counting: a consistent algorithm to replace subjective observer interpretation of morphology, coupled with automated sample handling to create a hands-off, 'walk away' system. In practice, most image analysis systems were capable of identifying the majority of, if not all, blood cells in normal specimens, but failed in preparations from patients with significant disease. This meant that the operator was required to interact with the system to resolve the identification of the remaining cells, which were typically difficult to classify. The reality with image analysis systems was that they were slow, even compared with manual microscopy, and they were not truly 'walk away' systems, because of often poorly executed automation and cell 'pattern' recognition algorithms requiring constant operator interaction. In addition, a number of countries have regulatory requirements that make it mandatory for all results to be reviewed before being released. These factors, plus stringent requirements for blood film preparation and staining as well as the small number of cells analysed with its inherent statistical problems, have led in most situations to replacement of image analysis systems by alternative technologies. The popularity of image analysis still persists, mainly in Japan and in certain European countries, but given the current sophistication of flow-based analysers, its role in the clinical laboratory environment is much reduced. The future development of such systems could become more directed towards high-quality image capture, storage and distribution to other workstations for review.

Another altogether different approach to differential counting was the development of flow-based systems that could analyse blood cells in suspension (Crosland-Taylor, 1953). This requires the use of a combination of a centre stream, containing the sample's cells, and an outside sheath fluid surrounding the sample stream. The sheath flow narrows the sample stream and forces the cells into single file, thus enabling passage of single cells through a sensing zone, optical or otherwise. The next step was the development of multi-parameter analysis on the same cell by combining the signals from several biosensors, e.g. forward and side scatter, fluorescence signals (Kamentsky et al., 1965) (see Fig. 2.4, p. 25). This led to the development of flow cytometers and, later, fluorescence-activated cell sorters (FACS) (Bonner et al., 1972). The earliest developments in automated flow-based haematology differential cell counters were based on continuous-flow systems, where individual samples were separated by air bubbles, similar to chemistry analysers then in existence (Skeggs, 1957). The combination of continuous flow with sample separation and enzyme cytochemical treatment of patient samples led to the first automated 5-cell differential introduced in the mid-1970s (Saunders, 1972; Mansberg et al., 1974). While results showed impressive improvement in statistical terms over manual microscopy WBC differential counting, it was not practical to operate the analyser on a 24-hr basis because of prohibitive reagent cost and because calibration of the continuous flow system proved delicate.

Many technological developments have occurred since, aimed at making differential WBC counting accessible by automated electronic analysis. The primary goal of these developments was to provide a differential count of the five 'normally appearing' WBCs (i.e. neutrophils, lymphocytes, monocytes, eosinophils and basophils) or, at a minimum, to provide a 'screening' differential that could eliminate the need for manual microscopy. Other than the already mentioned combination of continuous-flow and enzyme cytochemistry, systems were developed that analysed WBC based on light scattering properties (optical flow systems) or cell sizing (impedance). At first these systems yielded partial differential counts: enumeration of lymphocytes and granulocytes, with a third population of monocytes, usually mixed in with other cells (Cox et al.,1985; Johnston, 1985; Burgi and Marti, 1989) (Fig. 3.1). Eosinophils and basophils were not enumerated separately by these systems. These so-called three-part differentials were used for screening purposes, typically in combination with their own flagging systems and review criteria for selected parameters derived from the blood count. Such rule-based systems were surprisingly good at predicting abnormalities in patient specimens that required manual review or enumeration (Table 3.1). In unflagged specimens the differential count results would simply consist of the electronic three-part count, with the inherent assumption that the eosinophil and basophil count would be normal and therefore should not require separate reporting. The major benefit for the laboratory was that a significant reduction of 30–45% in manual reviews and differential counts could be obtained without compromising patient care. This resulted in lower costs and higher throughput (shorter 'turnaround times'). In the study quoted in Table 3.1, as well as in other studies, there

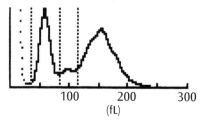

Fig. 3.1 *Histogram of a three-part white blood cell differential with three discriminators. The first discriminator separates debris from lymphocytes; the second separates lymphocytes from a central, mixed-cell population, consisting mostly of monocytes and eosinophils; and a third discriminator separates granulocytes from the central population.*

Table 3.1 *Numerical review criteria*

	Reference interval	Review criteria
WBCs ($\times 10^9$/L)	4.0–10.0	< 3.5 or > 12.0
Hgb (g/L)		
Female	120–160	< 100 or > 180
Male	140–180	
MCV (fL)	80–100	< 80 or > 102
MCHC (g/L)	310–360	< 310 or > 360
Platelets ($\times 10^9$/L)	140–440	< 100 or > 50
Lymphocytes (%)	16–48	< 16 or > 48
Monocytes (%)	1–10	< 1 or > 15
Granulocytes (%)	35–75	< 45 or > 78

WBCs, white blood cells; Hgb, haemoglobin; MCV, mean cell volume; MCHC, mean corpuscular haemoglobin concentration.

These 'review criteria' were used to screen for morphological abnormalities in addition to the analyser's own 'flagging' criteria (2194 specimens tested; 45.6% of specimens were without distributional or morphological abnormalities). In this study (Houwen *et al.*, 1985), evaluating three different instruments, the false normal rate ranged from 1.5 to 2.1%, and the false abnormal rate from 1.1 to 3.8%. The reduction in manual review of blood specimens using these rules was 30%.

was no significant difference in outcome between optical- or impedance-based systems (Houwen *et al.*, 1985; Pierre, 1991).

The next development came with further evolution of the enzyme cytochemical five-cell method, and with the availability of other systems capable of five-cell differentials, using different forms of analysis and cytochemical treatment (Brigden *et al.*, 1993; Cornbleet *et al.*, 1993; Houwen *et al.*, 1994; Fournier *et al.*, 1996; Kessler *et al.*, 1997; Jones *et al.*, 1998; Corberand *et al.*, 1999). This was made possible by the introduction of reagents that interact with WBCs and make these recognizable on the basis of cell volume and cellular contents. Purely optical methods and combinations of technologies such as impedance, radio frequency and optical sensors have been used for a variety of analysers from different manufacturers. For representation of the data, the histograms used for the mostly single parameter three-part differential were largely abandoned, and replaced by bivariate scatterplots, often in multiple representations (Fig. 3.2). Over the years, major improvements have been made in the methods that analyse the five-part differential multiparameter signals. Adaptable cluster analysis algorithms have largely displaced the earlier use of fixed discriminators as boundaries between cell populations. This was made possible by huge increases in computing power available at low cost. The development of 'diagnostic assist' systems is seen as a further improvement in the laboratory's ability to interpret electronic differential findings.

Both three- and five-part differential systems are equipped with flagging algorithms, alerting the user to possible morphological or other abnormalities, requiring review of the data or some other form of intervention such as morphology review. The advantage of five-part over three-part systems is a potential for further reduction in manual review rates. However, in reality, laboratory adherence to a combination of the five-part differential, the analyser's own flagging system plus blood count criteria such as those as set forth in Table 3.1 often led to an increased review rate. A more rational approach in analysers with a five-part differential count plus flagging system would be to discontinue the use of review criteria based on blood count parameters. Primarily those were developed as a safety net for three-part differential systems that generally have rather primitive differential count flags. Several current electronic differential counters have flags that are either user-adjustable or that flag at

DIFF

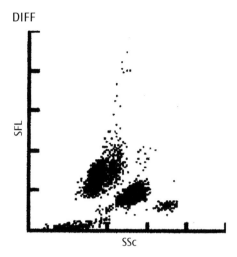

SFL

SSc

Fig. 3.2 *Bivariate scattergram of a five-cell white blood cell differential based on an adaptive cluster algorithm (SFL, side fluorescence; SSc, side scatter). These algorithms have largely replaced older methods of separating cell populations by fixed or moving discriminators. This scattergram contains the following populations: debris, lymphocytes, monocytes, basophils, neutrophilic granulocytes and eosinophils.*

several levels. This enables the user to adapt the system to the laboratory's specific caseloads and needs, and to decrease unnecessary morphology reviews further.

A logical next step in this evolution is the replacement of instrument flagging of abnormal cell populations by an actual count of such cells: the extended differential count (EDC). The EDC includes cell types other than the five normally present in blood, as listed in Table 2.5, p. 36. A task force, initiated by the International Society for Laboratory Hematology (ISLH), with representation from experts, industry and regulators, has formulated an approach that can enable clinical implementation of the EDC. The task force has also made recommendations that blood cell counts from bone marrow and body fluid specimens be included in the EDC.

The EDC will make immature granulocytes and nucleated red blood cells (NRBCs) an integral part of the electronic differential, and will replace flagging for these frequently observed cell types. While atypical or variant lymphocytes are also expected to be part of the EDC, at this moment 'left shift' is not included, due to lack of agreement on the morphology of left-shifted cells. Other cell types that can be included in the EDC are blast cells and haematopoietic progenitor cells. Once the EDC is fully implemented on haematology analysers, manual review rates are expected to drop to very low numbers and should be needed only in highly abnormal specimens, e.g. from patients with haematological malignancies or suspected of patients with conditions such as malaria.

An expected problem for EDC is validation of its performance: many of the cell types represented in the EDC are often present in blood in low numbers. Yet these low numbers can constitute the critical decision level which requires validation of analyser performance at 1/100 WBCs or less. In these situations it is not possible to use the manual 400-cell reference count for validation because of the enormous imprecision at such levels (Table 3.2). Alternative reference methods will have to be used, mostly monoclonal antibody-based flow cytometry. (Manufacturers must validate electronic differential counts by comparison against a 'reference' method, or at minimum against a predicate device that was validated earlier; this is part of the regulations for use as a clinical device. Analyser performance must be equal to or better than reference or predicate methods and must be tested in specimens from normal, healthy individuals as well as in patient specimens.)

Table 3.2 *Imprecision of the differential count at different levels*

Cell type	N	100	500	1000	10 000
Basophil	1	0–5.4*	0.3–2.3*	0.5–1.8*	0.8–1.3*
Eosinophil	4	1.1–9.9*	2.5–6.1*	2.9–5.4*	3.6–4.5
Monocyte	9	4.2–16.4*	6.6–11.9*	7.3–10.9	8.4–9.6
Lymphocyte	45	35–55.3*	40.6–49.5	41.9–48.1	44.0–46.0
Neutrophil	60	49.7–69.7*	55.6–64.3	56.9–63.1	59.0–61.0

The proportional cell counts for the individual white blood cell types have been chosen arbitrarily, and these do not represent a 100-cell differential. Results marked with an asterisk (*) show at least one confidence limit outside reference intervals. (For reference intervals, see Table 2.5, p. 37.)

Although there remains a role for morphological analysis of blood and other tissues such as bone marrow, for many routine purposes it is gradually being replaced by other technologies. In most developed countries, the traditional investigation of WBC and RBC morphology on a blood film has largely been substituted by some form of electronic analysis in combination with cytochemical or enzyme cytochemical treatment of blood cells. Recent developments in monoclonal antibody-based flow cytometry have made significant inroads in other areas of traditionally morphological blood, bone marrow and lymph node analysis, particularly for malignancies. The degree to which flow cytometry has replaced morphological analysis varies from institution to institution, even within a single country, but has been substantial over the past decade and a half. This has been supported by the development of a wide range of monoclonal antibodies and an increasingly better understanding of the cellular physiology of cluster designations (CDs) and epitopes against which the antibodies are directed. Not only has the diagnostic potential for monoclonal antibodies grown enormously, but the objectivity of flow-based results is often preferable to a morphological interpretation coloured by the observer's own subjectivity. Lastly, the relative ease of analysing large numbers of cells gives much better precision to data obtained by flow cytometry than by visual microscopy.

All this, plus much improved instrumentation and computer analysis, has made flow cytometry a superb tool for clinical use. Additionally, flow cytometry is capable of providing information that can offer insights into cellular physiology such as cell metabolism, apoptosis and drug response, not available by traditional morphological analysis (Garrido *et al.*, 2000; Selleri and Maciejewski, 2000). Another methodology that is replacing parts of traditional morphology practice is molecular analysis of tissues or even of individual cells. Examples include detection of minimal residual disease, multiple drug resistance detection by polymerase chain reaction (PCR) and diagnosis of chromosomal abnormalities in individual cells by fluorescent in-situ hybridization (FISH) techniques (Kobayashi *et al.*, 2000; Seong *et al.*, 2000). As the role for traditional visual microscopy is diminishing, electronic cell analysis by haematology analysers, flow cytometry using monoclonal antibodies and other probes and molecular diagnostics will play increasingly important roles in diagnostic approaches involving blood cells, whether in blood, bone marrow or body fluids.

3.2 STATISTICAL CONSIDERATIONS

As was pointed out for the blood cell count, low numbers of cells enumerated in a differential cell count lead to uncertainty about the results obtained. Typically, in a manual microscopy WBC differential count, a total of 100 cells are counted. This means that, almost always, far fewer than 100 cells are counted for each of the main five WBC categories present in blood films from normal, healthy adult individuals (in order of decreasing frequency: neutrophils, lymphocytes, monocytes, eosinophils and basophils). While more than 50 out of 100 WBCs may be neutrophils in a normal blood film, typically only one basophil per 100 WBCs will be found. Imprecision for routine manual differential counting is significant and its wide confidence limits seriously affect clinical decision-making (Rümke, 1985). Even if the total number of cells enumerated were doubled or quadrupled, reproducibility would be just mediocre, even for the most frequently appearing cell types, and still poor for cells that are less frequently observed. Assuming that the frequency of a certain cell type (N) remains constant regardless of how many cells are counted on a blood film, the standard deviation of its estimate will show stochastic convergence towards zero based on $1/\sqrt{N}$ with increasing sample size of N. However, this requires large numbers of cells to be counted, far exceeding the potential of even the most persistent morphologist. The statistical uncertainty of the 100-cell WBC differential count and its effect on assumptions of cell type distribution in a patient sample are shown in Table 3.2. The five WBC categories (with arbitrarily chosen cell counts for each individual cell type) and 95% confidence limits are shown at various total WBC differential counts. The cell counts represent typical levels within the reference interval for each cell type. When 100 WBCs are counted, all cell types show an upper confidence limit that is outside the reference interval. Even at 10 000 cells counted, the cell type with the lowest frequency (basophils) shows an upper confidence limit exceeding the reference interval. Such results would be deemed abnormal, and if no morphological abnormalities were found, distributionally abnormal. Those specimens or patients might be subjected to unnecessary further testing, driving up health care costs without any benefit to the patient. Similarly, when distributional abnormalities in reality are present, they can easily go undetected by visual microscopy. Since many automated analysers count around 8000 WBCs, the model in Table 3.2 clearly shows the statistical superiority of the electronic cell count over the visual count. It is unlikely that electronic WBC differential counts result in significant errors in determining distributional abnormalities.

A classic study illustrates this point, involving 73 examiners each performing a 100-cell WBC differential count on 496 patient specimens with distributional abnormalities present in 169 specimens (34%). Distributional abnormalities were 'detected' in 1.6% of samples without a distributional abnormality (false positives), while in 14.1% of samples with such abnormality present, none was found by the examiners (false negatives) (Koepke et al., 1985). This is probably one of the most poignant examples of the limitations of the visual 100-cell differential count.

3.3 THE REFERENCE WBC DIFFERENTIAL COUNT

This method was introduced to enable manufacturers and users to validate automated electronic WBC differentials (NCCLS, 1992). It is used widely for evaluation of electronic differential cell counts and leads to satisfactory results for most normal cell types (in this chapter the focus will be on reference WBC differential counting, while recognizing that instrument validation comprises more than just a manual, microscopic WBC differential count). When the manual reference method was developed it was well recognized that this could have all, or at least some, of the same problems as the routine differential count. To contain some of the imprecision of the routine count, it was decided that two independent observers each would count 200 WBCs on two separately prepared blood films. Instrument results should not be available to the observers, and their microscopy results should be adjudicated (if necessary) by a third independent observer with access to all information, including clinical data. For this purpose the availability of one or two additional slides is recommended. Problems are frequently encountered with the monocyte count, in part due to distributional problems and in part due to misidentification. The process of judgment allows for resolving discrepancies between observers as well as between instruments and observers, whether in morphology or in counts, and overcomes issues of sample switching, clerical errors, etc.

Despite these improvements, the method is still too imprecise to allow method comparison for cell categories that are present in low numbers, such as basophils. When applied to cell types with similar or lower frequency, the method essentially falls apart and alternative methods must be used. These are not always readily available, however, and there is a great need for the development and homologation of such methods, if available at all.

Several attempts have been made to develop monoclonal antibody-based flow cytometry methods for such purposes. The rationale behind this is simple: when cells appear in the blood in low or very low numbers, the method comparison becomes, in fact, 'rare event' analysis. Poisson error will be large when the sample size is small, and it will be impossible to judge from side-by-side comparison whether either method is correct. The solution is to increase the sample size, which can easily be done using flow cytometry.

Monoclonal antibody-based five-cell differential counts can readily and reproducibly be obtained by using CD45, CD14 and CD13 or other antibody combinations (Lebeck *et al.*, 1993; Hubl *et al.*, 1997). Similar approaches have been developed for NRBCs and reactive immature granulocytes (Lund-Johansen and Terstappen, 1993; Paterakis *et al.*, 1998; Tsuji *et al.*, 1999; Fujimoto *et al.*, 2000).

An example of the problems caused by imprecision of the visual count for low cell counts is shown in Figure 3.3. The purpose of this particular investigation was to test low range performance of NRBC identification (< 5/100 WBCs) by a new haematology analyser. The analyser was compared with the manual 400-cell reference count and a 20 000-cell flow cytometry count on 37 blood samples with known presence of NRBCs. It was impossible to decide on the basis of a microscopy reference 400-WBC differential count whether the analyser was correct or not. However, the results from comparison with the flow cytometry method clearly showed that the analyser gave the correct counts for NRBCs.

3.4 BLOOD FILM PREPARATION

Guidelines for blood film preparation and staining can be found in many laboratory and haematology textbooks and have recently been reviewed (Houwen, 2000). A well prepared and stained blood film is essential for good quality morphological analysis of blood cells. The most commonly used method for blood film preparation is the wedge-push type with Wright or Wright–Giemsa staining in North America. May–Grünwald–Giemsa type staining is more popular in European and some other countries. For good quality cell recognition, it is necessary to use the area of the blood film suitable for morphological analysis since part of the blood film will be too thick or too thin (Fig. 3.4). For a representative count of all cells it is necessary to cover the entire width of the examination area, because WBCs do not distribute evenly over the entire glass surface. Large cells such as monocytes and neutrophils are pushed towards the tail end of the blood film ('feather edge') and to the sides. This can lead to under-representation in the differential count if the side areas of the film are not included in the examination. A battlement track scan will avoid such problems and at the same time will avoid repeat analysis of the same cells (Fig. 3.4).

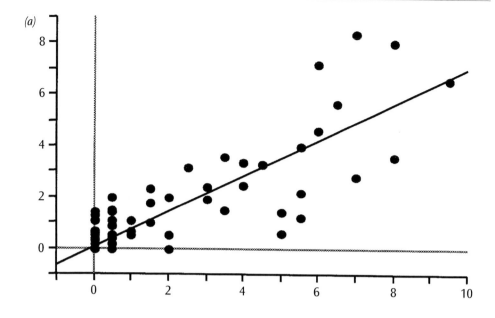

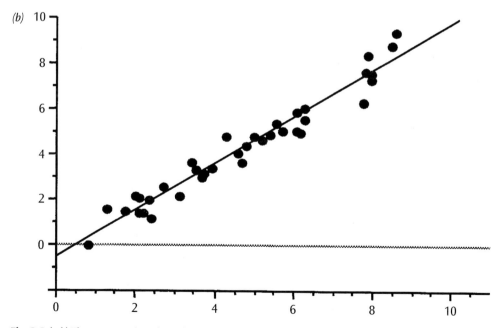

Fig. 3.3 *(a,b) These scatterplots show the correlation between instrument nucleated red blood cell (NRBC) enumeration (y-axis), visual NRBC counts from blood films (a: 400 white blood cells [WBCs] counted) and flow cytometric NRBC counts on the same specimens (b: 20 000 events counted). The interval chosen is from 0 to 10 NRBCs per 100 WBCs. Flow cytometric enumeration resulted in much better correlation than by the visual method due to higher numbers of NRBCs counted, but also because of better NRBC identification.*

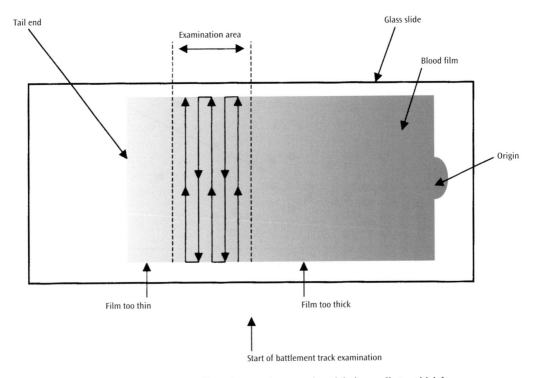

Fig. 3.4 *Schematic example of a blood film. The part closest to the origin is usually too thick for morphological use, and the tail end is too thin especially for evaluation of red blood cell morphology. When performing a differential leucocyte count, it is paramount that white blood cells be counted only once – hence the often used method of a 'battlement track', covering the entire width of the blood film.*

It is important to realize that for all types of blood film analysis the following issues apply. First, the process by which the cells are applied to the slide (spreading, smearing, spinning) may cause changes in their distribution and appearance. Secondly, the cells will flatten from their original spherical appearance due to air drying. Lastly, the cell contents will undergo changes because of fixation and subsequent staining. Thus, the morphological analyses of fixed and stained blood cells carry a large amount of artefacts, and direct comparison with untreated live cells in suspension may not always be possible, or is not very good. As an example, the fragile lymphocytes from patients with chronic lymphocytic leukaemia are often damaged beyond recognition by the methods used to apply blood cells onto the slides.

3.5 CELL IDENTIFICATION ISSUES

Manual microscopy differential counts are subject to a variety of cell identification errors, some of which are attributable to the observer's training level and experience, and others to motivation, fatigue, stress or level of distraction. Currently used practices of cross-training of technologists can also lead to problems, mainly because of insufficient regular practice of microscopic analysis. Colour blindness can play a role, although this should not *a priori* disqualify someone as a morphologist. A commonly used practice to 'skip' counting cells the observer is unsure about should be strongly discouraged, as this may lead to ignoring significant morbidity.

It should also be recognized that certain cell types lead to greater discordance between observers than others: observers rarely disagree on eosinophil counts, but quite often disagree about monocyte or band neutrophil counts. This is because morphological criteria can be easily defined for eosinophils, while it can be difficult to distinguish a small monocyte from a large, granular lymphocyte (NK cell). Generally the poorest reproducibility and accuracy results are obtained for counting cells with different maturation levels within the same lineage. Examples are band and segmented neutrophils, and to a lesser degree immature granulocytes: promyelocytes, myelocytes and metamyelocytes. It has proved very difficult to apply morphological criteria consistently by multiple observers and even more so across different institutions or countries. Thus the rather subjective differentiation of cell types by morphology leads to inconsistent results; there is much less chance for inconsistency when electronic cell analysis, monoclonal antibody-based flow cytometry or image analysis algorithms are applied to WBC populations.

3.6 APPLICATIONS OF THE DIFFERENTIAL CELL COUNT

The WBC differential count applies equally to blood, bone marrow or body fluids, although cell types may differ and also the presence of various cell types may be quantitatively different. In most institutions, clinicians use the proportional cell count of peripheral blood WBCs, despite efforts that have illustrated a laboratory preference for a count in absolute numbers. This reluctance to change is probably caused by the origins of the WBC differential count: results obtained on enumeration of 100 WBCs on a stained blood film, without a recalculation to absolute counts.

The foundation for the WBC differential count dates back to the days of Paul Ehrlich and others, more than a century ago, with the application of aniline dyes to blood cell preparations, rendering blood cells visible for microscopic identification (Ehrlich, 1891). And while some of the WBC differential count applications may seem antiquated now, and while reliance by clinicians upon its numbers may not always be fully warranted, there is no denying that the test can deliver powerful supportive data for clinical information and decision-making. This ambivalence is further underscored by the morphological uncertainties of the manual, microscopic differential count. One of the results of a WBC differential, often reviled by laboratory workers but considered by many clinicians as very valuable, is expressed as a 'left shift'. The morphological identification of 'left shifted' cells has been one of the most inconsistent and controversial aspects of the visual differential and is therefore no longer used by many institutions (Cornbleet and Novak, 1994). Ironically, the term 'left shift' finds its origins in the manual count itself. The devices used to punch in the numbers for the various cell types had the keys for immature WBC types on the left side of the keyboard – hence 'left shift' in a blood specimen when immature WBCs were found to be increased.

When observing the haematopoietic 'tree', from primitive stem cell to fully differentiated, functional 'end' cells, one can distinguish the differentiating pathways and can apply a differential count to the functional end-products of the tree's branches (Fig. 3.5a). In this chapter the terms 'differentiation' and 'maturation' will be considered loosely equivalent and are used to indicate an ongoing physiological process of cellular change, either by cell division plus cellular change or by cellular change alone, one that leads from immature to a mature, functional 'end' cell stage. A differential count of functional 'end' cells separates different lineages and can indicate changes in the distribution of these lineages in a blood or bone marrow sample. When compared with an established reference interval, this can provide clinically useful information. For example, increased numbers of eosinophils may be the result of allergies. Increased numbers of lymphocytes, especially with atypical or variant morphology, may be associated with certain viral infections such as infectious mononucleosis. Other viral infections, e.g. human immunodeficiency virus (HIV), can result in low numbers of circulating lymphocytes.

It is important to realize that the differential count is not just restricted to separation of blood cells into different types of functional end cells (the lineages); it can also give an indication of the distribution of cells at different levels of maturation within a single lineage (Fig. 3.5b). However, when this is done by purely morphological identification, there are significant pitfalls. While lineages can usually be easily differentiated from each other (the 'horizontal' differential count; Fig. 3.5c), it is not so simple to apply stepwise morphological criteria (i.e. segmented neutrophils vs. band or stab cells) onto a biological continuum of differentiation within a single lineage (the 'vertical' differential count; Fig. 3.5d). This is why 'left shift' is difficult to quantitate by morphological means. Proper identification of left shift can be useful in identifying bacterial infection, especially in newborns and in the elderly, but the lack of consensus about the morphological characteristics of what constitutes 'left shift' has severely damaged its reputation among laboratory workers (Cornbleet and Novak, 1994).

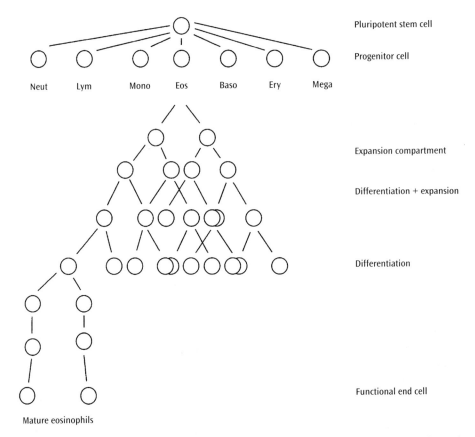

Fig. 3.5 *(a) Schematic representation of the stem cell model for haematopoiesis, in this case the formation of eosinophils. While the pluripotent stem cell has self-renewal capacity without entering a differentiation pathway ('lineage commitment'), progenitor cells have a limited proliferative potential. At first, expansion predominates, gradually replaced by differentiation without mitotic activity, resulting in mature end cells entering the circulation.*

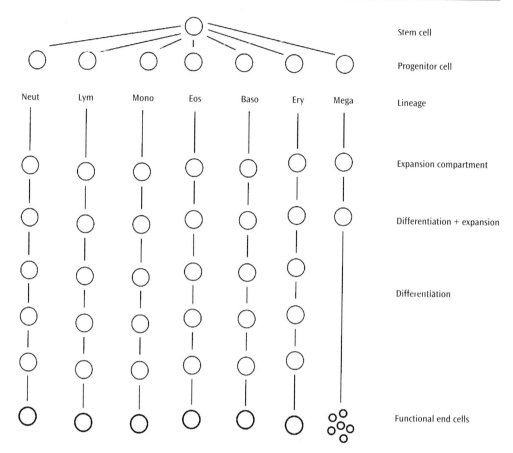

Fig. 3.5 *(b) Although the exact processes of expansion and differentiation differ per lineage, the basic process remains the same. Typically, under steady-state conditions, blood cells are not released from the haematopoietic marrow until mature. Release of earlier stages points towards accelerated or disordered production.*

Another form of 'vertical' differential counting is represented by the identification of even more immature neutrophils, such as promyelocytes, myelocytes and metamyelocytes. This can lead to difficulties among these specific cell types themselves, but as a group ('immature granulocytes') they are sufficiently different in morphology that they can be separated from mature neutrophils and band forms (Fig. 3.5d).

Recently, several efforts have been made to analyse bone marrow by haematology blood cell analysers. One application is to determine more effectively the myeloid to erythroid (M:E) ratio. Others include blast cell counts and myeloid differentiation patterns (d'Onofrio *et al.*, 1998; Schumacher *et al.*, 1998). New technological developments have made it possible to study maturation patterns in the erythroid series as well (Wang *et al.*, 1998; Zini *et al.*, 1999). With the introduction of the EDC in the clinical laboratory, it is expected that electronic analysis of bone marrow and body fluid specimens will rapidly increase and will replace, to a major extent, visual microscopy.

Vertical differential counting might become an important tool in assessing maturation and differentiation processes in the haematopoietic marrow. One of the roles of vertical differential counting can be viewed as similar to that of the immature reticulocyte fraction

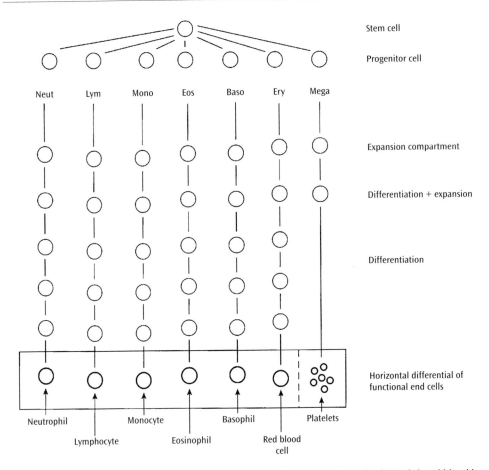

Fig. 3.5 *(c) Under normal, steady-state conditions, the differential count of cells in the peripheral blood is restricted to mature, functional end cells: the 'horizontal' differential of blood cells at the same level of maturation.*

(IRF). The IRF expresses the number of the most immature reticulocytes as a proportion of all reticulocytes, themselves immature RBCs. While it is well established that reticulocyte counts represent the production rate of RBCs (erythropoiesis), to many the exact role of IRF has not been as clearly defined. Based on the kinetic relationship between changes in IRF and reticulocyte counts, it is evident that the IRF is dissimilar from the reticulocyte count: changes often do not occur at the same time or on the same scale. This is illustrated in a patient receiving an autologous bone marrow reinfusion as part of cancer treatment (Fig. 3.6). Upon receiving the cytotoxic conditioning regimen, the IRF values drop to below normal before the reticulocyte counts fall below normal. Conversely, as engraftment takes place, the IRF increases to normal before the reticulocyte counts respond. When such changes and relationships between parameters are applied to generally accepted interpretations of what governs a production process, it is clear that the reticulocyte count represents the first derivative of erythropoiesis, i.e. the RBC production rate. Changes in maturity of the reticulocytes (IRF) thus reflect the rate of change in the RBC production rate, i.e. the second derivative of the production process. Greater immaturity indicates an increase in RBC production rates, and less immaturity a decrease. Similarly, left shifted neutrophils indicate an

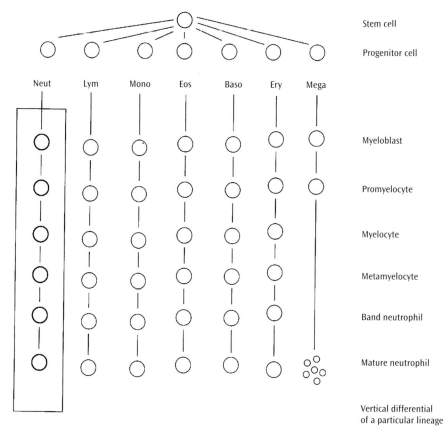

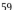

Fig. 3.5 *(d) During accelerated or disordered production of cell types of one or more lineages, immature cells belonging to those lineages may be found in the peripheral blood. The enumeration of immature cells in relation to its mature, functional end-product is deemed 'vertical' differential count. Although rarely used extensively, normal and pathological haematopoietic marrow will lend itself by nature to 'vertical' differential counts. The 'vertical' differential count of a particular lineage is a reflection of the dynamics of cell production within that lineage. Neut, neutrophil; Lym, lymphocyte; Mono, monocyte; Eos, eosinophil; Baso, basophil; Ery, erythrocyte; Mega, megakaryocyte.*

increase in neutrophil production rate, typically caused by infection or by the administration of haematopoietic growth factors such as G- or GM-CSF.

When expressed appropriately, i.e. as the proportion of immature cells within any specific lineage, the 'vertical' differential ratio can thus become an indication of the second derivative of the production process for that lineage: the rate of change in its production rate. The importance of second derivative measurements is that changes occur in advance of changes in the actual bone marrow output, i.e. the specific cell counts themselves, and in the case of IRF have a strong predictive value (Spanish Multicentric Study Group for Haematopoietic Recovery, 1994; Davis, 1996). It is exciting that such measurements may become available for myeloid and other lineages (Wang *et al.*, 2000), although they are certainly not yet mainstream.

Vertical differential counting for the erythroid and myeloid lineage will probably become routinely possible on haematology analysers, and the challenge is going to be how to incorporate such parameters into the laboratory and particularly how to make these accessible and useful to clinicians.

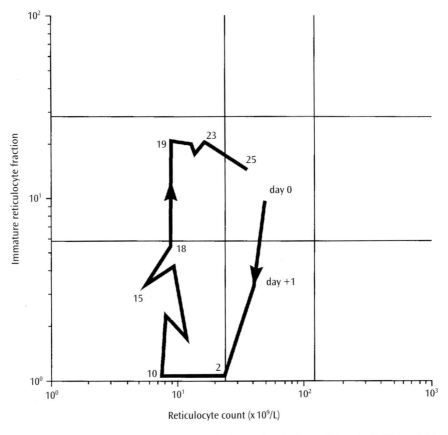

Fig. 3.6 *This bivariate plot brings the number of reticulocytes in relation to its 'vertical' differential, in this case the immature reticulocyte fraction (IRF). The data are represented on a log/log scale for easier interpretation and contain reference intervals for the reticulocyte count and IRF. The resulting division of the scatterplot into six quadrants means that the central quadrant represents normal values for both reticulocyte count and IRF. The data were obtained from a patient undergoing autologous marrow reinfusion and represent the patient's course during 25 days from initiation of treatment to full recovery. The first noticeable effect from high-dose myeloablative therapy was a drop in IRF, not reticulocytes, indicating a severe reduction in marrow erythroid proliferation. Reticulocytes continued to mature without mitosis from the remaining reservoir of red blood cell (RBC) precursors until depleted (day 2). After a period of bone marrow suppression where both parameters are suppressed, recovery is indicated by (first) a rise in IRF, followed almost 10 days later by a return of the reticulocyte count to normal. The 'vertical' differential of peripheral blood cells (reticulocytes), in this case IRF, can thus reflect events in the haematopoietic marrow relating to cell production in the erythroid lineage. It is important to note that in situations such as this case, changes in IRF precede those in actual reticulocyte counts.*

3.7 CONCLUSIONS

Electronic cell identification and enumeration has reached a point of sophistication that often matches or surpasses that of the routine bench morphology count. WBC differential counts obtained electronically have much better precision than their manual counterparts, and accuracy is mostly equal or better. Both cost and turnaround times are lower for electronic differentials. The extended differential will enable laboratories to perform counts on complex specimens, including bone marrow and body fluid samples. Manual review is likely to become greatly reduced, and new parameters may emerge. These could include methods to measure the kinetics of haematopoiesis without ever performing a bone marrow aspirate or biopsy.

Compared with electronic differential counts, relatively little information is obtained by routine morphological analysis of blood cell populations and their precursors. However, while manual, optical (morphological) WBC differential counting has been the mainstay for the analysis of WBC subpopulations for much of the twentieth century, it has become clear that the limitations posed by morphological analysis of Romanowsky stained blood films are impacting its potential for clinical use.

REFERENCES

Bonner, W.A., Hulett, H.R., Sweet, R.G. *et al.* (1972) Fluorescence activated cell sorter. *Rev. Sci. Instr.* **43,** 404–9.

Brigden, M.L., Page, N.E. and Graydon, C. (1993) Evaluation of the Sysmex NE-8000 automated hematology analyzer in a high-volume outpatient laboratory. *Am. J. Clin. Pathol.* **100,** 618–25.

Burgi, W. and Marti, H.R. (1989) Automated blood count analysis by trimodal size distribution with the Sysmex E-5000. *J. Clin. Chem. Clin. Biochem.* **27,** 365–8.

Corberand, J.X., Segonds, C., Fontanilles, A.M. *et al.* (1999) Evaluation of the Vega haematology analyzer in a university hospital setting. *Clin. Lab. Haematol.* **21,** 3–10.

Cornbleet, P.J., Myrick, D. and Levy, R. (1993) Evaluation of the Coulter STKS five-part differential. *Am. J. Clin. Pathol.* **99,** 72–81.

Cornbleet, P.J. and Novak, R.W. (1994) Classifying segmented and band neutrophils. *CAP Today* **8,** 37–41.

Cox, C.J., Habermann, T.M., Payne, B.A. *et al.* (1985) Evaluation of the Coulter counter model S-Plus IV. *Am. J. Clin. Pathol.* **84,** 297–306.

Crosland-Taylor, P.J. (1953) A device for counting small particles suspended in fluid through a tube. *Nature* **17,** 37–8.

D'Onofrio, G., Zini, G., Tommasi, M. *et al.* (1998) Automated analysis of bone marrow: routine implementation and differences from peripheral blood. *Lab. Hematol.* **4,** 71–9.

Davis, B.H. (1996) Immature reticulocyte fraction: by any name, a useful clinical parameter of erythropoietic activity. *Lab. Hematol.* **1,** 2–8.

Ehrlich, P. (1891) *Farbenanalytische Untersuchungen für Histologie und Klinik des Blutes.* Berlin, Germany: Hirschwald.

Fournier, M., Gireau, A., Chretien, M.C. *et al.* (1996) Laboratory evaluation of the Abbott Cell DYN 3500 5-part differential. *Am. J. Clin. Pathol.* **105,** 286–92.

Fujimoto, H., Sakata, T., Hamaguchi, Y. *et al.* (2000) Flow cytometric method for enumeration and classification of reactive immature granulocyte populations. *Cytometry,* **42,** 371–8.

Garrido, S.M., Willman, C., Appelbaum, F.R. and Banker, D.E. (2000) Three-color versus four-color multiparameter cell cycle analyses of primary acute myeloid leukemia samples. *Cytometry* **42,** 83–94.

Houwen, B. (2000) Blood film preparation. *Lab. Hematol.* **6,** 1–7.

Houwen, B., Mast, B.J., Lebeck, L.K. *et al.* (1994) Performance evaluation of the Sysmex SE-9000 hematology workstation. *Sysmex J. Int.* **4,** 5–18.

Houwen, B., Tisdall, P.A., Croucher, B. *et al.* (1985) Automated histogram differential analysis: a comparison of 3 instruments and strategies for clinical implementation. *Sysmex J.* **8,** 14–21.

Hubl, W., Wolfbauer, G., Andert, S. *et al.* (1997) Toward a new reference method for the leukocyte five-part differential. *Cytometry* **30,** 72–84.

Johnston, C.L. (1985) Leukocyte screening using the ELT-800WS. *Blood Cells* **11**, 241–55.

Jones, R.G., Faust, A., Glazier, J. *et al.* (1998) Cell-DYN 4000: Utility within the core laboratory structure and preliminary comparison of its expanded differential with the 400-cell manual differential count. *Lab. Hematol.* **4**, 34–44.

Kamentsky, L.A., Melamed, M.R. and Derman, H. (1965) Spectrophotometer: a new instrument for ultrarapid cell analysis. *Science* **150**, 630–1.

Kessler, C., Sheridan, B., Charles, C. *et al.* (1997) Performance of the Coulter Gen•S System's white cell differential on an abnormal specimen data set. *Lab. Hematol.* **3**, 32–40.

Kobayashi, H., Takemura, Y., Kawai, Y. *et al.* (2000) Competitive reverse transcription-polymerase chain reaction assay for quantification of human multidrug resistance 1 (MDR 1) gene expression in fresh leukemic cells. *J. Lab. Clin. Med.* **135,** 199–209.

Koepke, J.A., Dotson, M.A. and Shifman, M.A. (1985) A critical evaluation of the manual/visual differential leukocyte counting method. *Blood Cells* **11**, 173–86.

Konno, T. and Kanda, T. (1996) The total hematology system based on laboratory information system and quick turn around time. *Sysmex J. Int.* **6**, 113–22.

Lebeck, L.K., Mast, B.J. and Houwen, B. (1993) Flow cytometric white blood cell differential: a proposed alternate reference method. *Sysmex J. Int.* **3**, 61–9.

Lund-Johansen, F. and Terstappen, L.W. (1993) Differential expression of cell adhesion molecules during granulocyte maturation. *J. Leukoc. Biol.* **54**, 47–55.

Mahouy, G., Lund, P.R., Chinn, S. and Barnes, R.D. (1973) The use of automated image analysis in differential white cell counting. *Scand. J. Haemat.* **10**, 315–8.

Mansberg, H.P., Saunders, A.M. and Groner, W. (1974) The Hemalog-D white cell differential system. *J. Histochem. Cytochem.* **22**, 711–24.

Mui, J.K., Fu, K.S. and Bacus, J,W. (1977) Automated classification of blood cell neutrophils. *J. Histochem. Cytochem.* **25**, 633–40.

NCCLS (1992) Reference leukocyte differential count (proportional) and evaluation of instrument methods. Approved Standard. *NCCLS document H20-A.* Villanova, PA: NCCLS.

Paterakis, G., Kossivas, L., Kendall, R. *et al.* (1998) Comparative evaluation of the erythroblast cell count generated by three-color fluorescence flow cytometry, the Abbott Cell DYN 4000 hematology analyzer, and microscopy. *Lab. Hematol.* **4,** 64–70.

Pierre, R.V. (1991) Leukocyte differential counting. In: Koepke, J.A. (ed.), *Practical Laboratory Hematology.* Edinburgh: Churchill Livingstone, 131.

Rümke, C.L. (1985) The imprecision of the ratio of two percentages observed in differential white blood cell counts. *Blood Cells* **11**, 137–40.

Saunders, A.M. (1972) Development of automation of differential leukocyte counts by the use of cytochemistry. *Clin. Chem.* **18**, 783–8.

Schumacher, H., Glazier, J., Ismail, S. and Mazella, F. (1998) Bone marrow analysis provided by the Cell DYN 4000 hematology analyzer. *Lab. Hematol.* **4**, 94.

Selleri, C. and Maciejewski, J.P. (2000) The role of FAS-mediated apoptosis in chronic myelogenous leukemia. *Leuk. Lymphoma* **37**, 283–97.

Seong, C.M., Giralt, S., Kantarjan, H. *et al.* (2000) Early detection of relapse by hypermetaphase in situ hybridization after allogeneic bone marrow transplantation for chronic myeloid leukemia. *J. Clin. Oncol.* **18**, 1831–6.

Skeggs, L.T. (1957) An automatic method for colorimetric analysis. *Am. J. Clin. Pathol.* **28**, 311–22.

Spanish Multicentric Study Group for Hematopoietic Recovery (1994) Flow cytometric reticulocyte quantification in the evaluation of hematologic recovery. *Eur. J. Haematol.* **53**, 293–7.

Tsuji, T., Sakata, T., Hamaguchi, Y. *et al.* (1999) A new rapid flow cytometric method for the enumeration of nucleated red blood cells. *Cytometry* **37**, 291–301.

Wang, F.-S., Itose, Y., Sagoaga, O. *et al.* (2000) Development and clinical application of nucleated red blood cell staging with hematology analyzer XE-2100. *Lab. Hematol.* **6**, 33–4.

Wang, F.-S., Tsuji, T., Sakata, T. *et al.* (1998) Counting and staging of peripheral and cord blood nucleated red blood cells by flow cytometry. *Lab. Hematol.* **4**, 96.

Zini, G., Mistretta, G., Crollari, L. *et al.* (1999) Automated counting of nucleated red blood cells (NRBC): evaluation of the Sysmex XE-2100 system. *Lab. Hematol.* **5,** 94.

4

Instrumental flagging and blood film review

JOHN A. KOEPKE

INTRODUCTION

The blood count is one of the most frequently performed laboratory tests in both the in-patient and the outpatient setting. While in the past it was undertaken using a number of manual techniques which routinely included a blood film examination, instrument analysis is now the most common method used. In the United States up to 40 different instruments can perform leucocyte differential counts according to the College of American Pathologists (CAP) proficiency testing programme (CAP, 1991). In order to assess the accuracy of these methods, the CAP has developed eight different survey kits because of differences in the technology being used in these instruments.

While the quantitative measurements performed by this array of instruments, in general, are quite precise and accurate, the qualitative or morphological performance has varied from one manufacturer's instrument to another (Koepke, 1986, 1993). As noted above, most qualitative tests on the blood count were undertaken by microscopy of the blood film. However, with escalating workloads and decreasing technical staff numbers, methods for safely eliminating those unproductive components of blood counting have received increasing attention. A major effort has been devoted to determining if there are qualitative measurements which might be useful to triage blood specimens to identify those in which, most likely, no significant blood film abnormality is present (Brigden et al., 1990; Koepke, 1994). With such information the blood film would not require examination, thus saving significant amounts of time and effort in the laboratory.

4.1 THE THEORY OF BLOOD SPECIMEN FLAGGING

Flagging is defined in the *Illustrated Encyclopedic Dictionary* as 'signaling or communicating a message with, or as if with, a flag'. In the haematology laboratory a flag is a signal to the instrument operator that the specimen being analysed may have a significant abnormality (Houwen and Koepke, 1990). Automated instruments are programmed in a number of different ways in order to flag or issue a 'suspect' message for such specimens which may require additional study, most often the examination of a well-prepared blood film before a report is released from the laboratory (Koepke *et al.*, 1985; Brigden *et al.*, 1990; Birch *et al.*, 1991a,b; Lewis and Rowan, 1991). However, there may be significant differences among the various instruments as to which possible abnormalities are flagged as well as the efficiency of the flagging procedures.

The development of a reference method for leucocyte differential counting (NCCLS, 1992) included all nucleated cells normally present in the peripheral blood. For cells present in either increased or decreased numbers (quantitative or distributional abnormalities), the standard calls for identification of such specimens by the instrument. Table 4.1 lists such quantitative abnormalities which may require action by the laboratory and the clinician (NCCLS, 1996).

Several general statements can be made regarding quantitative flagging. The quantitative flags which are originally set by the manufacturer can be redefined by the user if desired. But it must be recognized that some reference ranges may vary according to age, gender, pregnancy and probably also race (van Assendelft, 1991). Therefore, quantitative flagging must take into account such differences. Unfortunately it is common for such demographic information not to be known to the laboratory and therefore such systems may not be able to be fully implemented. More importantly, the laboratory staff will most probably wish to use local action (i.e. quantitative) values rather than healthy reference ranges in its flagging programme. Table 4.2 catalogues action, sometimes called 'panic', values for quantitative haematology parameters. When these limits are exceeded, additional studies such as a blood film review may be indicated. If the quantitative values are confirmed, the patient's physician should be made aware of these findings if they are not already known.

Table 4.1 *Suggested quantitative flags. (Adapted from NCCLS, 1992.)*

Finding	Definition	Clinical relevance
Left shift/immature granulocytes	$> 0.9 \times 10^9$/L bands/metamyelocytes	Early inflammation or bacterial infection?
Variant lymphocytes	$> 0.7 \times 10^9$/L variant lymphocytes	Viral infection?
Fragile leucocytes	See text	HIV infection, other infections, prolonged specimen storage
Blasts	$> 0.1 \times 10^9$/L	Leukaemia, metastatic tumour?
Nucleated RBCs	$> 0.02 \times 10^9$/L	Severe anaemia/metastatic tumour?
Anisocytosis	$> 15\%$ RDW	Anisocytosis, dimorphic cell population
Red cell aggregation	MCV > 125	Cold agglutinins?
Platelet aggregation	MPV > 10 fL	Cold agglutinins?

RBC, red blood cell; RDW, red cell distribution width; MCV, mean cell volume; MPV, mean platelet volume.

The qualitative or morphological abnormalities present a more complex problem since, except for the imaging systems, there is a 'disconnect' between the morphology of the cells in question and the parameter(s) being measured by the haematology analyser. Table 4.2 lists those qualitative or morphological abnormalities which have clinical significance and which are ordinarily discovered when the patient's physician orders a complete blood count.

To be useful, qualitative flagging should ideally have a low false-positive rate coupled with a low false-negative rate with a resulting high efficiency for identifying potentially abnormal blood specimens. However, it is recognized that there will be compromises between false-negative and false-positive flagging rates which are unavoidable. Nevertheless, minimally acceptable rates of false results are goals towards which one should strive if they are not presently attainable. The method of Lacombe *et al.* (1995) provides a very useful way to maximize the efficiency of flagging and should be applied when evaluating haematology instruments. This group, in addition to presenting the usual comparisons of automated to visual differential counts, developed a likelihood ratio (LR) which helped to determine the optimum set points for flagging which minimizes false-negative and false-positive results. This method would be applicable to most haematology analysers.

The ultimate goal is to reduce the number of clinically non-contributory blood film examinations. As a result, the laboratory will become more productive, and average turn-around times for patient results will be shortened. (It is likely, however, that most patients in haematology services will still have more frequent blood film reviews than is absolutely necessary.) On the down side, the reduction in blood film review may result in a decrease in

Table 4.2   *Suggested action limits. (Reproduced with permission from NCCLS, 1996.)*

Analyte (units)	Action limits	Clinical relevance: abnormal results may reflect the following conditions
WBC (10^9/L)	< 3	Sepsis, chemotherapy, radiotherapy, agranulocytosis, marrow hypoplasia, cobalamin, folate, iron deficiency
	> 12	Acute stress (including surgery), infection, malignancy, lymphoma, leukaemia
RBC (10^{12}/L) Hb (g/L) Hct (L/L)	> 6.2 (M), > 5.2 (F) > 180 (M), > 160 (F) > 5.4 (M), > 0.48 (F)	Dehydration, polycythaemia, shock, chronic hypoxia
RBC (10^{12}/L) Hb (g/L) Hct (L/L)	< 4.4 (M), > 3.9 (F) < 120 (M), < 110 (F) < 0.39 (M), < 0.30 (F)	Anaemia from blood loss, cobalamin, folate, iron deficiency, malignancy, chronic inflammation, chronic liver disease, renal disease, marrow hypoplasia, chemotherapy, radiotherapy, haemolysis, haemoglobinopathy, thalassaemia
MCV (fL)	< 80	Microcytosis from iron deficiency, chronic blood loss, chronic inflammation, haemoglobinopathy, thalassaemia, sideroblastic anaemia
	> 100	Macrocytosis from chronic liver disease, cobalamin or folate deficiency, sprue, smoking, haemolysis
PLT (10^9/L)	< 50	Risk of bleeding, idiopathic, chemotherapy, radiotherapy
	> 800	Risk of thrombosis, polycythaemia, post-splenectomy, thrombocythaemia

WBC, white blood cells; RBC, red blood cells; Hb, haemoglobin; Hct, haematocrit; MCV, mean cell volume; PLT, platelets; M, male; F, female.

laboratory revenues which could pose a significant short-term cash flow problem. A further potential problem may be the gradual loss of morphological expertise by the laboratory staff since they will be examining fewer cases and may become less proficient in this important skill.

4.2 STATE OF THE ART FOR FLAGGING

In our laboratories we began the development of a flagging system by interfacing a small Apple computer with an Ortho ELT-8 haematology analyser (US Copyright, 1982). With the prototype system in place, it was found that about one-third of blood counts had insignificant blood film review abnormalities and these could be reported promptly. The instrument was later replaced by new analysers which included acceptable flagging systems (Koepke, 1994). With the increasing acceptance by the clinical staff, our laboratory service was able, over several years, to reduce the rate of blood film review from 82% to less than 40%. This low rate of review has continued up to the present day.

The more popular haematology instruments reveal reasonably good performance for quantitative abnormalities (Hallowell *et al.*, 1991; Anonymous, 1992; Cornbleet *et al.*, 1992, 1993; Lacombe *et al.*, 1995). With time and experience, the laboratory staff may safely broaden the flagging limits beyond the initial narrow quantitative reference ranges. So, for example, as confidence builds that the instrument correctly counts neutrophils in the mild to moderately abnormal range, a film review can be safely eliminated if this is the only quantitative flag. Also, if a patient's blood film has been examined recently and the quantitative count and the flag(s) are unchanged, there is no need to repeat the blood film review (Lewis and Rowan, 1991). As an example, patients undergoing cardiopulmonary bypass procedures have frequent blood counts in the immediate postoperative hours. These counts typically show thrombocytopenia and anaemia. There is no need to re-examine a blood film on consecutive specimens if the quantitative results are only mildly abnormal or if no marked changes have occurred.

Haematology analysers perform quite acceptably insofar as quantitative measurements are concerned and frequently there is little to be gained from a supplementary blood film examination. Therefore a great deal of skilled technical effort can be diverted to other more useful endeavours. The following discussion will focus on clinically meaningful qualitative abnormalities. In this case, gender, age or even racial differences are of less importance (except perhaps in the case of variant lymphocytes which are more frequent in children). The user has much less control over the qualitative flagging processes, which are proprietary for the most part.

It is difficult to compare the flagging efficiencies of the various instruments since the majority of evaluation studies have been undertaken using single instruments. However, a few studies have been published which compare multiple earlier instrument models on the same set of patient specimens (Buttarello *et al.*, 1992; Bentley *et al.*, 1993). More recent studies of the performance of several popular automated haematology analysers for the identification and/or flagging of qualitative abnormalities show false-positive rates up to 30% (Lacombe *et al.*, 1995; Fournier *et al.*, 1996; Kessler *et al.*, 1997) and false-negative rates up to 15% (Sana *et al.*, 1996; Thallhammer-Scherrer *et al.*, 1997). These data must be interpreted with caution since often the case mix of the study population was not well defined or varied from one study to another. It is almost impossible to reach firmer conclusions since the case mix in these studies in which false-positive and false-negative rates are determined profoundly affects the results. Because of this, the rate of flagging errors may reflect variation in the composition of the study group rather than the instrument performance. The NCCLS standard for differential leucocyte counting (NCCLS, 1992) recommends the number and types of cases to be included in the clinical sensitivity studies.

Examination of the overall trends in these data usually shows an inverse relationship between the false-negative and false-positive results, i.e. when the latter rate increases, the former decreases and vice versa. The studies by Lacombe *et al.* (1995) sought to develop a method to minimize the false rates, if at all possible. While intriguing, the method may not completely solve this problem without technological advancements such as the use of specific monoclonal antibodies for certain cell populations. Finally, if the clinician suspects conditions which have associated qualitative abnormalities, a blood film review should probably be ordered since the instrument performance may not be entirely satisfactory, i.e. the false-negative rate may be relatively high.

4.2.1 Flagging for qualitative red cell abnormalities

Traditionally, red cell abnormalities have been categorized by their number, size and variability, i.e. the red cell indices. Thus, microcytic, normocytic and macrocytic anaemias and polycythaemias have been quite adequately identified and categorized by haematology laboratories for many years.

More recently, red cell anisocytosis has been measured by the so-called red cell distribution width (RDW) with some success and additional categories of anaemia have been developed (Bessman *et al.*, 1983). However, this parameter has not been as helpful as originally proposed (Brittenham and Koepke, 1987). In the recent past, there have been efforts to screen for haemoglobinopathies (in addition to thalassaemias) which have shown promise (Lamb *et al.*, 1991; Honda *et al.*, 1994). However, this capability has not yet been incorporated into many haematology analysers.

4.2.2 Flagging for qualitative platelet abnormalities

While the quantitation of platelets has improved considerably in the recent past, the detection of qualitative platelet abnormalities by instruments is not always well done. Two additional platelet parameters have been proposed (Rowan, 1986). The first, the mean platelet volume (MPV), is conceptually similar to the mean cell volume (MCV), i.e. immature platelets are thought to be larger. Thus, in reactive thrombocytosis there is an increase in the MPV which reflects an increase in younger platelets (Bessman *et al.*, 1981). The presence of so-called giant platelets may increase the MPV somewhat but more often they are detected by examining the platelet histogram. The platelet histogram and/or the MPV may also be useful in the recognition of platelet cold agglutinins in which case the platelet count may be artefactually decreased. The MPV is reduced in myelosuppression for any cause. Unfortunately the MPV is unstable in EDTA; significant platelet swelling (up to 20%) occurs during the first 3 hours after venous sampling (Rowan and Fraser, 1982). This largely precludes use of the MPV as a clinical parameter. The second platelet parameter is the platelet distribution width (PDW) which is the platelet equivalent of the RDW. This measurement is stable in EDTA over time. The presence of giant platelets/megakaryocytic fragments in chronic myeloproliferative disease is well recognized (Levin and Conley, 1964; Zeigler *et al.*, 1978). This can result in an increase in the PDW which may thus serve to differentiate the thrombocytosis in chronic myeloproliferative disease from that in reactive processes.

4.2.3 Flagging for qualitative leucocyte abnormalities

Studies have confirmed the accuracy and reliability of the leucocyte count including the neutrophil, lymphocyte and eosinophil count (Hallowell *et al.*, 1991; Anonymous, 1992; Cornbleet *et al.*, 1992, 1993; Lacombe *et al.*, 1995). However, sometimes monocyte differentiation has been problematic but this is probably of minor clinical significance (Goosens *et al.*, 1991). With at least one manufacturer the problem was solved by a redesign of the monocyte counting system (Hallowell *et al.*, 1991).

For the common qualitative leucocyte reactions, e.g. left shift and variant (atypical) lymphocytosis, the instrument correlations with reference visual counts have been less than satisfactory. In some laboratory quarters, this is considered to be a shortcoming of the instruments, while others have taken the stance that there is little to be gained from discovery of these reactive patterns (Brigden and Page, 1990; Andron *et al.*, 1994). But many clinicians, especially surgeons and paediatricians, continue to rely on documenting these leucocyte reactions for the diagnosis of acute inflammation (e.g. appendicitis) or infections (viral or bacterial) (Mathy and Koepke, 1974; Dick, 1978).

More recently, a number of investigators have published data from the evaluation of newer models of several instruments. One study, using the Coulter GEN-S, indicated an efficiency of between 72 and 78% for morphological abnormalities, which improved substantially when qualitative or distributional criteria were added (Kessler *et al.*, 1997). An Austrian group (Thalhammer-Scherrer *et al.*, 1997) compared Sysmex and Coulter instruments using 467 randomly selected in-patient and outpatient specimens and determined that the efficiency of these instruments varied between 72 and 78%, similar to the above study. A Japanese evaluation of the Sysmex SF-3000 system showed excellent correlation with visual reference counts for the five common leucocytes. Sensitivity studies were analysed by histogram plots but no numerical results were given. However, the qualitative data were judged as good (Sana *et al.*, 1996).

Early studies (Koepke and Landay, 1989; Koepke and Smith-Jones, 1992) indicated that in patients with HIV infection there can be inaccurate leucocyte counts due to fragility of lymphocytes, particularly if the specimens are not counted promptly after the blood sample is collected. A survey of flow cytometry laboratories taken several years ago indicated that significant delays in testing occurred. In fact, they were more common and of longer duration in cytometry laboratories which perform the most CD34+ studies, i.e. referral laboratories (Koepke, 1996).

Inaccurate lymphocyte counts can significantly affect the diagnosis and treatment of HIV-infected individuals. Therefore a large study was developed to determine the effect of various haematology analysers, testing time delays, shipping and storage conditions on the CD4+ T cells when measured in the interlaboratory testing/accreditation programmes of the Centers for Disease Control and Prevention (Analytical Sciences, 1995). This cell fragility is apparently a manifestation of a process called apoptosis which is defined as programmed cell death. Leucocyte apoptosis has been associated with HIV (Gougeon and Montagnier, 1994), as well as other infections, diabetes mellitus, neoplasia, trauma and postoperative status (Shidham *et al.*, 1997).

The problem has been approached in several ways. First of all, prompt measurement of the absolute lymphocyte count is mandatory. In the case of referral laboratories where specimen delays are the rule, other solutions must be developed. Although earlier generations of flow cytometer only determined the proportional count, later models such as the Ortho CytoronAbsolute or the Beckton-Dickinson FACSCount have been developed which count lymphocytes in absolute terms. In such cases, the haematology laboratory would no longer be involved with CD4+ testing. Another solution has been the development of the so-called

WIC/WOC technology. In this case, the leucocyte count is determined in two ways, i.e. by the white cell impedance count (WIC) and by the white cell optical count (WOC). Leucocyte lysis rates are obtained on the specimen and the rate of change of the count is back-calculated to zero time. If the kinetic counting rate is outside the expected limits the sample is re-analysed. If the impedance (WIC) count is significantly greater than the optical (WOC) count, a message for suspected fragile leucocytes is reported and the impedance (WIC) count is reported, presuming that this is the correct leucocyte count.

4.3 UNEXPECTED CHANGES IN HAEMATOLOGICAL PARAMETERS

A significant change (delta check) in any of the patient's quantitative or qualitative results, even if they have occurred within the flagging limits, has been used as a method to detect laboratory blunders (Houwen, 1990). For example, if the platelet count drops significantly within a relatively short period of time (hours or days) there is reason to investigate. A blood film review is commonly done in such cases. Platelet clumping may account for the fall, but early disseminated intravascular coagulation might present in a similar way. Delta-checking systems are also useful in discovering specimen mix-ups due to blood collection errors. Although not yet well developed or widely available in laboratory information systems, undoubtedly there will be advances in this area and delta checking will most likely be incorporated into future systems.

4.4 QUALITY ASSURANCE PROCEDURES FOR FLAGGING

Quality assurance practices in haematology include careful attention to specimen collection, transport and storage. Problems such as red cell and platelet agglutination can be related to the delay in specimen analysis as well as specimen temperature. Cell fragility problems may be avoided if blood films are made at the bedside when the specimens are collected. However, biohazard protocols frequently preclude such procedures to the detriment of ideal blood films.

Since the flagging procedure, by definition, results in additional studies which usually include a blood film examination to confirm or rule out the presence of an abnormality, there is, in fact, an ongoing quality assurance programme in place. A comprehensive discussion of quality assurance strategies for automated haematology analysers suggests that blood film differential leucocyte reports be analysed on a continuing basis (Bull, 1991). However, in order to ensure that no significant abnormalities are missed, a representative sampling of non-flagged specimens should also be examined. Records should be kept of these checks. Such programmes will also help to maintain the morphological expertise of the laboratory staff.

4.5 THE BLOOD FILM REVIEW OF FLAGGED SPECIMENS

A recent book devoted to haematology laboratory management includes a chapter which outlines a system for the hierarchical review of flagged specimens (Koepke and Bull, 1995). The basis of this system includes the concept that more common flags such as left shift or red cell abnormalities can be confirmed by junior technologists while 'diagnostic cells' should be confirmed by the laboratory physician before being reported (Fig. 4.1).

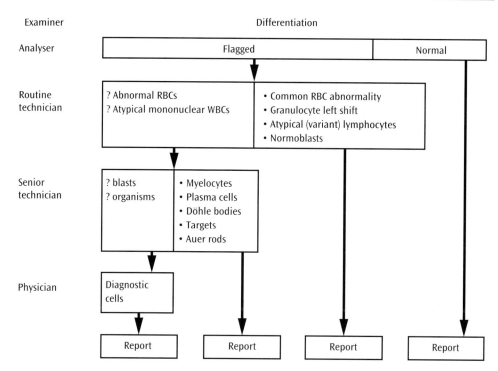

Examiner

Differentiation

Analyser

Routine technician

Senior technician

Physician

Fig. 4.1 *Hierarchical blood film evaluation.*

The blood film review process is similar in concept to the *modus operandi* in cytopathology laboratories where the screening technologist reviews all cases. If there is a suspicious cell or population of cells, the Papanicolaou smear is reviewed by a more experienced cytologist. If the smear is diagnostic of malignancy, the film is reviewed by the cytopathologist and a report to the patient's physician is generated.

For the blood film review process to be satisfactory, the blood film should be prepared from a fresh blood sample, and a technically satisfactory film should be prepared and properly stained with a Romanowsky stain (NCCLS, 1992). A number of devices which prepare blood films are marketed. Acceptable wedge or spun films can be made quickly. If spinners are used it is important to avoid potentially hazardous blood aerosols.

Appropriately trained and experienced laboratory workers should perform the blood film review. An observant worker with less experience may make the initial examination. If one of the more common abnormalities is found, but no suspicious cells, the report can be generated. But if there is any doubt, an examiner with wide experience of haematological disorders and/or more complex cases should review the blood film. Reference to an authoritative haematology atlas such as the one by Bessis (1977) can be very helpful.

If there are findings diagnostic of a specific haematological disorder, particularly if the disorder is malignant, these should be confirmed by the medical director of the laboratory. A recent discussion on blood film review outlines a practical yet comprehensive method for this procedure, which has been called the 'primary diagnostic tool of haematology' (Shively, 1995). The question of reimbursement for physician-performed microscopy (a moderately complex procedure) is debated.

Medical students in general do not receive training to justify their opinions as experts on blood film review. Residents and/or fellows in clinical pathology or haematology usually develop expertise in reviewing blood films during their training so that when entering practice they can satisfactorily perform this important service.

4.6 CONTEMPORARY CONSIDERATIONS

4.6.1 Reference methods

Early in the deliberations of the NCCLS committee which developed the leucocyte differential counting standard (NCCLS, 1992), it was hoped that a suitable reference method could be determined. But the then current cytochemical and imaging systems were, for one reason or another, not thought to be satisfactory. Therefore the 400-cell visual microscopy differential leucocyte count was finally adopted. But since this is a subjective method dependent on the training and experience of the morphologist, other more objective methods are still being investigated. It is conceivable that imaging systems could be adapted to serve as a reference method but presently this is not the case.

Two proposed reference methods for the five-part differential count have been published. The first method (Lebeck et al., 1995) uses flow cytometry with three monoclonal antibodies (anti-CD45 FITC, anti-CD14 PE and anti-CD13 PE). Analysis of the approximately 2000 patient specimen comparisons in this study correlated well with blood film differentials. A second reference method was published which used a somewhat different set of antibodies (anti-CD45 FITC, anti-CD14 PE and a cocktail of anti-CD2 PE, anti-CD16 and anti-HLA-DR antibodies). These investigators (Hübl et al., 1997a) compared their results with 1000-cell visual differential leucocyte counts. They concluded that this is a highly suitable reference method for the five-part differential. Reference methods for other cell types in the qualitative sphere are still under study. Certain of these may well be done using various cell-specific monoclonal antibodies (Hübl et al., 1997b). Others, such as the nucleated red cell count, may be done accurately with visual microscopy methods provided statistically appropriate numbers of cells are counted (see below).

4.6.2 Quantitation of flagged cell populations

The qualitative flags noted in Table 4.2 are presently under review by a NCCLS working group whose charge is to add qualitative flagging performance goals to the previously published differential leucocyte counting standard (NCCLS, 1992). The following section, however, discusses how this mission may be evolving into one that converts the qualitative flags into quantitative action limits, thus bypassing this difficult stage in the standardization of leucocyte counting.

For several years there has been a movement to extend the differential leucocyte count generated by automated haematology analysers beyond the basic five-part (mature neutrophils, lymphocytes, monocytes, eosinophils and basophils) differential count. In the past, nucleated blood cells other than these five types were to be flagged. A flagged blood sample then required additional evaluation, usually a microscopy examination. This was the process outlined in the NCCLS H20-A document (1992) and subsequently approved by the American Food and Drug Administration (FDA) which regulates medical devices as an acceptable standard for differential leucocyte counting. Such acceptance resulted in the movement of these blood cell counters from class III devices (for which there is insufficient information to establish a performance standard assuring safety and effectiveness) to class II devices (for which performance standards assure safety and effectiveness).

However, with advances in the flow cytometry capabilities of newer haematology analysers, analytical methods have been developed which can satisfactorily identify and even quantitate additional cell populations. For example, a method that quantitates nucleated red blood cells (NRBCs) in clinical specimens has been developed (Sher *et al.*, 1997). The sensitivity for NRBCs at a 1–4% level was 71% and the specificity was 100%, with a false-negative rate of 29%. Based on this work, Abbott Laboratories petitioned the FDA to reclassify their instruments from class III to class II insofar as NRBCs were concerned. This reclassification essentially legitimizes the reporting of this measurement without requiring individual laboratories to prove that the instrument indeed can quantitate NRBCs. This being the case, a blood film examination is not required on specimens that have NRBCs unless there might be other reasons for such a review. This breakthrough has caused the NCCLS subcommittee which is currently considering any revisions of *H-20* (particularly in regard to flagging methods) to rethink the direction of this review (NCCLS standards are normally reviewed approximately every 5 years).

The analytical goals for quantitative flags, including total leucocyte, red cell and platelet counts, are found in the NCCLS quality control standard *H26-A*, since that document includes the required precision and accuracy for quantitative results (NCCLS, 1996).

It should be pointed out that almost all the cells listed in Table 4.1 are normally present in the bone marrow or lymph nodes but can be found in the peripheral blood as a reaction to disease. They are not abnormal cells, but rather normal cells in an abnormal location. The lineage of these immature cells is sometimes difficult to determine. They are 'diagnostic' only by virtue of their location, not their morphology. Exceptions would be leukaemic cells or circulating malignant tumour cells such as occur, for example, in carcinoma of the breast or lung, or Sézary cells in lymphoproliferative malignancy (Mayer, 1985). At least one automated haematology analyser has been shown to be able to detect virtually all cases of acute leukaemia with either suspect flags or qualitative alerts which require blood film review (Hoyer *et al.*, 1996). A recent study indicates that these devices are capable of accurately identifying rare blast forms in the peripheral blood (Glazier *et al.*, 1997).

The now proven ability accurately to quantitate one of the qualitatively flagged cell types (NRBCs) has led to the notion that perhaps many or even all of the qualitative flags can, with appropriate technical advances, be converted into quantitative measurements, essentially skipping over the difficulties in standardizing qualitative flagging (Sher *et al.*, 1997).

Currently, work is being done on so-called 'immature granulocyte' quantitation. This would be useful clinically, e.g. in infection, acute surgical problems, etc., but it is not without controversy (Banez, 1990; Andron *et al.*, 1994; Koepke, 1995). If granulocyte reactions, expressed as either left shifts (i.e. increased band forms) or the presence of immature granulocytes (i.e. bands, metamyelocytes, myelocytes), can be accurately and precisely measured by an objective instrument rather than a subjective human observer, significant improvements in medical care would most likely result. But criteria for the identification of these cells used by the several instrument manufacturers vary and therefore any standardization initiatives will be difficult.

4.7 CURRENT INITIATIVES

These technology advances have resulted in proposals to extend the differential count in a stepwise fashion. Discussions between interested manufacturers and haematologists were held in 1996 and 1997, after which Abbott Laboratories initiated a proposal to the FDA to reclassify haematology analysers from class III to class II for specific cell populations of the extended differential based on the development of data which would validate the accuracy of such quantitation. Abbott, therefore, at the request of the FDA, recruited the other major manufacturers to join in this petition. Preliminary work on the so-called extended differential count was undertaken by an expert panel of the International Society of Laboratory Hematology (ISHL). Concurrently, the Hematology and Pathology Device Panel of the American FDA recommended that devices that could satisfactorily perform part or all of the components of the extended differential count be reclassified from class III to class II devices. In May 2001, the FDA published in the Federal Register a proposed rule to reclassify automated differential cell counters from class III to class II, provided that special controls, including voluntary standards and guidance documents, as well as published references, provide reasonable assurance for the safety and efficacy of these instruments. The NCCLS, which earlier had published a method for the evaluation of instrumental differential counters (NCCLS, 1992), has appointed a working group, which will revise and update that standard to include those cell types in the extended differential.

4.8 SUMMARY

When selecting a haematology instrument for the laboratory, in addition to the requirement for acceptable precision and accuracy for normal leucocytes (Koepke, 1993), there is a growing need for instruments that can efficiently flag or even count qualitatively abnormal cells. The more efficiently the instruments perform this task, the more cost- and time-effective the laboratory can become. Several haematology analysers are able to perform these tasks acceptably but further refinements are anticipated (Anonymous, 1992; Lacombe et al., 1995; Buttarello et al., 1997; Kessler et al., 1997). However, there are no studies which compare several of the latest models of instruments performing cell counts on the same set of patient specimens.

In the meantime, the laboratory staff should be well acquainted with the strengths and weaknesses of their particular haematology analyser. An important variable is the case mix being analysed. By and large, an instrument's sensitivity and specificity depend upon the case mix being studied. Outpatient specimens characteristically have fewer false-positive and false-negative results than in-patient specimens.

Finally, there usually is a direct relationship between the cost of the instrument and its efficiency. Initially, more advanced electronics are found in the 'top of the line' instruments. Thus, complicated scattergram analyses and secondary analyses (e.g. RDW, MPV, etc.) are only found in the more expensive analysers. Some studies, e.g. Veillon et al. (2000), provide guidance to the laboratory staff to help choose a haematology analyser and the College of American Pathologists periodically publishes a very detailed listing of high-volume haematology instruments which is helpful in comparing these instruments (Aller and Pierre, 2000).

REFERENCES

Aller, R.D. and Pierre, R.V. (2000) Getting better all the time – a comparison of high volume haematology analysers. *CAP Today* **14**, 27-34.

Analytical Sciences, Inc. (1995) *Recommendations for Conducting a Nation-wide CD4+ Testing Proficiency Testing/Accreditation Program*. Atlanta, GA: Centers for Disease Control and Prevention.

Andron, M.J., Westengard, J.C. and Dutcher, T.F. (1994) Band neutrophil counts are unnecessary for the diagnosis of infection in patients with normal total leucocyte counts. *Am. J. Clin. Pathol.* **102**, 646–9.

Anonymous (1992) Miles Technicon H-2 automated hematology analyzer evaluation. *Health Devices* **21**, 387–412.

Banez, E.I. (1990) Hematologic response to acute inflammation: the band neutrophil revisited. *Tex. Med.* **86**, 26–8.

Bentley, S.A., Johnson, A. and Bishop, C.A. (1993) A parallel evaluation of four automated hematology analysers. *Am. J. Clin. Pathol.* **100**, 626–32.

Bessis, M. (1977) *Blood Smears Revisited*. New York: Springer International.

Bessman, J.D., Williams, L.J. and Gardner, F.H. (1983) Improved classification of anemias by MCV and RDW. *Am. J. Clin. Pathol.* **80**, 322–6.

Bessman, J.D., Williams, L.J. and Gilmer, P.R. (1981) Mean platelet volume. The inverse relationship of platelet size and count in normal subjects and an artifact of other particles. *Am. J. Clin. Pathol.* **76**, 289–93.

Birch, A.J., Brozovic, M., Lewis, S.M. *et al.* (1991a). Role of the blood film with automated blood counting systems. In: Roberts, B. (ed.), *Standard Haematology Practice*. Oxford: Blackwell Scientific Publications, 19–22.

Birch, A.J., Brozovic, M., Lewis, S.M. *et al.* (1991b). Assessment of the need for blood film examination with blood counts by second generation light scatter counters. In: Roberts, B. (ed.), *Standard Haematology Practice*. Oxford: Blackwell Scientific Publications, 23–33.

Brigden, M.L. and Page, N.E. (1990) The lack of clinical utility of white blood cell differential counts and blood morphology in elderly individuals with normal hematology profiles. *Arch. Pathol. Lab. Med.* **114**, 394–8.

Brigden, M.L., Preece, E.V. and Page, N.E. (1990) 'Diff/if': a differential policy that works. *Medical Laboratory Observer*, **22**, 45–8.

Brittenham, G.M. and Koepke, J.A. (1987) Red blood cell volume distributions and the diagnosis of anemia: help or hindrance? *Arch. Pathol. Lab. Med.* **111**, 1146–8.

Bull, B.S. (1991) Quality assurance strategies. In: Koepke, J.A. (ed.), *Practical Laboratory Hematology*. Edinburgh: Churchill Livingstone, 3–29.

Buttarello, M., Bulian, P., Temporin, V. *et al.* (1997) Sysmex SE-9000 hematology analyzer. *Am. J. Clin. Pathol.* **108**, 674–86.

Buttarello, M., Gadotti, M., Lorenz, C. *et al.* (1992). Evaluation of automated hematology analysers. *Am. J. Clin. Pathol.* **97**, 345–52.

College of American Pathologists (1999) *CAP Surveys Manual – Hematology*. Northfield, IL: College of American Pathologists.

Cornbleet, P.J., Myrick, D. and Judkins, S. (1992) Evaluation of the Abbott Cell-Dyn 3000. *Am. J. Clin. Pathol.* **98**, 603–14.

Cornbleet, P.J., Myrick, D. and Levy, R. (1993) Evaluation of the Coulter STKS five-part differential. *Am. J. Clin. Pathol.* **99**, 72–81.

Dick, F.R. (1978) The lymphocyte differential count: Does it have potential? In: Koepke, J.A. (ed.), *Differential Leukocyte Counting*. Northfield, IL: College of American Pathologists, 61–8.

Federal Register (2001) Hematology and pathology devices: reclassification of automated differential cell counters. **66**(90). Washington DC: Food and Drug Administration.

Fournier, M., Gireau, A., Chretian, M.C. *et al.* (1996) Laboratory evaluation of the Abbott Cell DYN 3500 5-part differential. *Am. J. Clin. Pathol.* **105**, 286–92.

Glazier, J., Mazzaella, F., Roberts, L. *et al.* (1997) Recovery of cultured leukaemic blast cells by the Abbott Cell-Dyn 4000 automated hematology analyzer. *Lab. Hematol.* **3**, 138–45.

Goosens, W., van Hove, L. and Verwilghen, R.L. (1991) Monocyte counting: discrepancies obtained with different automated instruments. *J. Clin. Pathol.* **44**, 224–7.

Gougeon, M-L. and Montagnier, L. (1994) Apoptosis in peripheral T lymphocytes during HIV infection. In: Tomei, L.D. and Frederick, O. (eds) *Apoptosis II: The Molecular Basis of Apoptosis in Disease*. Plain View, NY: Cold Spring Harbor Laboratory Press, 5–19.

Hallowell, R., O'Malley, C., Hussein, S. *et al.* (1991) An evaluation of the Sysmex NE-8000 hematology analyzer. *Am. J.Clin. Pathol.* **96**, 594–601.

Honda, S.A.A., Bhagavan, V.N.V., Sugiyama, C.E. *et al.* (1994) Hemoglobinopathies detected by CBC analysis and HPLC Hemoglobin A$_{1c}$. *Lab. Med.* **25**, 176–81.

Houwen, B. (1990) Random errors in haematology tests: a process control approach. *Clin. Lab. Haematol.* **12**(Suppl.), 157–68.

Houwen, B. and Koepke, J. A. (1990) The classic manual differential count and current multiparameter electronic blood cell analysis: the end of an era? *Sysmex J.* **13**, 47–57.

Hoyer, J.D., Fisher, C.P., Soppa, V.M. *et al.* (1996) Detection and classification of acute leukemia by the Coulter SM hematology analyzer. *Am. J. Clin. Pathol.* **106**, 352–8.

Hübl, W., Andert, S., Thum, G. *et al.* (1997a) Value of neutrophil CD16 expression for detection of left · shift and acute-phase response. *Am. J. Clin. Pathol.* **107**, 187–96.

Hübl, W., Wolfbauer, G., Andert, S. *et al.* (1997b) Toward a new reference method for the leucocyte five-part differential. *Cytometry* **30**, 72–84.

Kessler, C., Sheridan, B., Charles, C. *et al.* (1997) Performance of the Coulter GEN-S® System's white cell differential on an abnormal specimen data set. *Lab. Hematol.* **3**, 32–40.

Koepke, J.A. (1986) Automation in the hematology laboratory. In: Fairbanks, V.F. (ed.), *Current Hematology and Oncology IV*. St Louis: Year Book Medical Publishers, 63–90.

Koepke, J.A. (1993) Fitting the cell counter to the bed count. In: Ward, P.C.J. (ed.), *Routine Hematologic Testing*. Clinics in Laboratory Medicine 13: 4. Philadelphia: W.B. Saunders, 817–29.

Koepke, J.A. (1994) Let's improve the flagging of abnormal hematology specimens. *Medical Laboratory Observer* **26**, 22–26.

Koepke, J.A. (1995) How should neutrophil reactions be measured? (editorial) *Lab. Hematol.* **1**, 87–8.

Koepke, J.A. (1996) Survey of quality assurance/quality control practices for CD4+ lymphocyte counting. *Cytometry* **26**,178–81.

Koepke, J.A. and Bull, B.S. (1995) The intralaboratory control of quality. In: Lewis, S.M., Koepke, J.A. (eds), *Hematology Laboratory Management and Practice*. Oxford: Butterworth Heinemann, 183–98.

Koepke, J.A., Dotson, M.A., Shifman, M.A. *et al.* (1985) A flagging system for multichannel hematology analysers. *Blood Cells* **11**, 113–21.

Koepke, J.A. and Landay, A.L. (1989) Precision and accuracy of absolute lymphocyte counts. *Clin. Immunol. Immunopathol.* **52**, 19–25.

Koepke, J.A. and Smith-Jones, M. (1992) Lymphocyte counting in HIV-positive individuals. *Sysmex J. Int.* **2**, 71–4.

Lacombe, F., Cazaux N., Briais, A. *et al.* (1995) Evaluation of the differential flags on a hematology analyzer (Cobas Argos 5 Diff). *Am. J. Clin. Pathol.* **104**, 495–502.

Lamb, A., Mallelian, S. and Freedman, J.J. (1991) Detection of abnormal hemoglobinopathies by the Sysmex NE~8000 automated cell counters (Letter to the editor). *Br. J. Haematol.* **77**, 567–8.

Lebeck, L.K., Chang, L., Chen, W. *et al.* (1995). White blood cell five-part subpopulation estimations. A flow cytometric based reference method. *Sysmex J. Int.* **5**, 77–84.

Levin, J. and Conley, C.L. (1964) Thrombocytosis associated with malignant disease. *Arch. Int. Med.* **114**, 497–501.

Lewis, S.M. and Rowan, R.M. (1991) Assessment of the need for blood film examination with blood counts by aperture-impedance systems. In: Roberts, B. (ed.), *Standard Haematology Practice*. Oxford: Blackwell Scientific Publications, 34–42.

Mathy, K. A. and Koepke, J. A. (1974) The clinical usefulness of segmented vs stab neutrophil criteria for differential leucocyte counts. *Am. J. Clin. Pathol.* **91**, 947–58.

Mayer, K. (1985) Presence of abnormal cells. *Blood Cells* **11**, 25–30.

NCCLS (1992) Reference leukocyte differential count (proportional) and evaluation of instrumental methods; Approved standard. *NCCLS Document H20-A*. Villanova, PA: NCCLS.

NCCLS (1996) Performance goals for the internal quality control of multichannel hematology analysers; Approved standard. *NCCLS Document H26-A*. Wayne, PA: NCCLS.

Rowan, R.M. (1986) Platelet size distribution analysis: principles, techniques and potential clinical utility. *Haematol. Rev.* **1**, 109–44.

Rowan, R.M. and Fraser, C. (1982) Platelet size distribution analysis. In: van Assendelft, O.W., England, J.M. (eds), *Advances in Hematology Methods: The Blood Count*. Boca Raton, Florida: CRC Press, 125–41.

Sana, S., Koyanagi, I., Tsuchi, M. *et al.* (1996) Fundamental study on the automated hematology analyzer SF-3000. *Sysmex J. Int.* **6**, 16–27.

Sher, G., Viltisano, B., Schisano, T. *et al.* (1997) Automated NRBC count, a new parameter to monitor, in real time, individualized transfusion needs in transfusion-dependent thalassemia major. *Lab. Hematol.* **3**,129–37.

Shidham, V.B., Gupta, D.C., Liu, C. *et al.* (1997) Apoptotic leukocytes in peripheral blood smears (abstract). *Am. J. Clin. Pathol.* **108**, 343.

Shively, J.A. (1995) Interpretive aspects of hematology tests with a focus on the blood film. In: Lewis, S.M., Koepke, J.A. (eds), *Hematology Laboratory Management and Practice*. Oxford: Butterworth Heinemann, 12–9.

Thalhammer-Scherrer, R., Knobl, P., Korninger, L. *et al.* (1997) Automated five-part white blood cell differential counts. *Arch. Pathol. Lab. Med.* **121**, 573–7.

United States Copyright TXu 112-345 (1982) A system for flagging blood film hematology specimens for review out of limit cell counts and abnormal cytograms (8 Dec).

van Assendelft, O. W. (1991) Interpretation of the quantitative blood cell count. In: Koepke, J.A. (ed.), *Practical Laboratory Hematology*. Edinburgh: Churchill Livingstone, 61–98.

Veillon, D.M., Curry, S., Tubbs, K. *et al.* (2000) Decision dilemma: how do we choose a new hematology analyser. *Lab. Hemat.* **6**, 151–6.

Zeigler, Z., Murphy, S. and Gardner, F.H. (1978) Microscopic platelet size and morphology in various hematologic disorders. *Blood* **51**, 479–84.

5

Reticulocyte counting: methods and clinical applications

GIUSEPPE D'ONOFRIO, GINA ZINI AND R. MARTIN ROWAN

INTRODUCTION

Within the apparently uniform circulating red cells, there exists a subpopulation in which supravital staining reveals a variable network of basophilic grains and strands: the reticulocytes. The role of the reticulocyte and the most convenient method for its demonstration has intrigued haematologists for more than a century. Gradually the real nature of these cells emerged and their biological and clinical significance became clear. Enumeration of reticulocytes entered the diagnostic armamentarium during the first half of the twentieth century (Seip, 1953; Koepke and Koepke, 1986; Rapaport, 1986; Houwen, 1992). The advent of automation in haematology greatly increased general productivity, however the reticulocyte count remained a visual microscopy procedure and until recently was relegated, with few exceptions, to the diagnosis of certain types of anaemia. Flow cytometric methods for reticulocyte counting have changed this, resulting in renewed interest in the clinical applications of the reticulocyte count.

5.1 NATURE AND PATHOPHYSIOLOGY OF RETICULOCYTES

5.1.1 Properties of reticulocytes

PHYSICAL PROPERTIES

Reticulocytes are larger and less dense than mature red cells. On electron microscopy they are irregular and lobular in appearance (Bessis, 1972), reflecting their motility, necessary for migration across the sinusoid wall by diapedesis or emperipolesis. Reticulocytes are less deformable and more adhesive to fibronectin than mature red cells: alteration in these characteristics may be involved in their release into the circulation (Patel *et al.*, 1985).

CONTENT

The distinctive feature of reticulocytes is the presence of ribosomal RNA in the cytoplasm. This is visible on electron microscopy as both polyribosomes and monoribosomes scattered uniformly throughout the cytoplasm of unstained reticulocytes or as aggregates after supravital staining. Reticulocytes contain other cytoplasmic organelles, such as mitochondria, remnants of the Golgi apparatus, centrioles, ferritin molecules, etc.

BIOCHEMICAL CHARACTERISTICS

Reticulocytes are biochemically more active than mature red cells – e.g. hexokinase, pyruvate kinase, glucose-6-phosphate dehydrogenase, catalase and carbonic anhydrase activities are all increased (Lakomek *et al.*, 1989) – and certain metabolic pathways exist which are not present in mature red cells, e.g. the tricarboxylic acid cycle. Resting oxygen consumption is 30 times higher and water content is increased by 5%. Reticulocytes absorb radiolabelled iron and amino acids *in vitro*, incorporating both into newly synthesized haemoglobin (London *et al.*, 1950). Haem synthesis, on the other hand, occurs exclusively during the bone marrow phase (Gavosto and Rechenman, 1954): the haemoglobin content of circulating reticulocytes and erythrocytes, when measured by laser cytometry (d'Onofrio *et al.*, 1995), are very similar.

THE THREE TYPES OF BASOPHILIC SUBSTANCE IN ERYTHROCYTES

When pre-fixed, as in Romanowsky staining, reticulocytes cannot generally be distinguished from mature erythrocytes. However, some can be recognized by a diffuse grey-bluish cytoplasm. Such polychromatophilic red cells are, on average, 27% larger (Perrotta and Finch, 1972), strongly absorb light at a wavelength of 260 nm typical for nucleic acids, but do not contain DNA, as indicated by a negative Feulgen reaction (Marshall, 1978). More rarely, in fixed films, reticulocytes are identified as red cells with basophilic stippling. Polychromasia, basophilic stippling and substantia granulofilamentosa are all manifestations of ribosomal RNA. All disappear after treatment by ribonuclease (Dustin, 1944). On electron microscopy all three correspond at the ultrastructural level to the presence of ribosomes and polyribosomes: homogeneously distributed in polychromatophilic erythrocytes, but precipitated and aggregated in punctate basophilia and in supravitally stained preparations.

Polychromatophilia is an expression of high RNA content, a feature of the youngest reticulocytes and named Heilmeyer class I, or stress macroreticulocytes. The proportion of these cells can be used as an indicator of erythropoietic response to anaemia (Crouch and Kaplow, 1985). Basophilic stippling, on the other hand, is possibly an artefact produced by drying and fixation. It also occurs in lead intoxication and in thalassaemia. Basophilic stippling must be distinguished from siderotic granules or Pappenheimer bodies: these are usually single, darker in colour and give a positive Perls' reaction.

SURFACE MOLECULES

Reticulocytes possess the same surface molecules as the mature red cell membrane, e.g. glycophorin A and blood group antigens (Serke and Huhn, 1993). However, reticulocytes are capable of absorbing iron molecules (Finch *et al.*, 1949) and transferrin receptors have been identified on their membrane (Frazier *et al.*, 1982; Seligman *et al.*, 1983). Their concentration decreases with, and disappears upon, maturation (Noble *et al.*, 1989). In flow cytometry using the monoclonal antibody anti-CD71 with double fluorescence, transferrin receptors can be shown only in the less mature fraction of circulating reticulocytes (Serke and Huhn, 1992). Similarly, the surface antigen of human erythroid cells identified by the monoclonal antibody HAE9 is present on an even smaller, still less mature subpopulation, corresponding to 5–10% of reticulocytes (Mechetner et al., 1991).

5.1.2 Definition of reticulocytes

Reticulocytes may be defined on the basis of their morphological, biochemical or functional characteristics. Physiologically, they are cells in the penultimate stage of the erythroid maturation, following extrusion of the nucleus but still containing residual cytoplasmic ribosomal RNA. The classical definition derives from their morphological appearance on supravital staining of unfixed blood as those erythrocytes characterized by the appearance of granulofilamentous substance (ranging from isolated granules to a dense network of granules and filaments). The term 'proerythrocyte' would be physiologically more correct (Bessis, 1972).

In 1976, Gilmer and Koepke defined minimum morphological criteria for identifying a reticulocyte. This definition, although basically adopted by standardizing organizations, has been subjected to various revisions (NCCLS, 1985; ICSH, 1992, 1998). In the joint NCCLS-ICSH standard (1997), the definition of a reticulocyte remains essentially morphological:

> A reticulocyte is an erythrocyte that, when stained with a supravital dye, (e.g. NMB), contains stainable nucleic acids i.e. cellular RNA. To be identified as a reticulocyte, the cell must contain two or more distinct blue-staining granules (NMB-reticulocyte) that are visible without requiring fine microscope adjustment on the individual cell to confirm their presence. The granules should be away from the cell margin to avoid confusion with Heinz bodies.

This definition should probably be revised, yet again, to include the affinity of reticulocyte RNA for fluorochromes.

5.2 MICROSCOPY METHODS FOR RETICULOCYTE COUNTING

5.2.1 Principles of methodology

Classical methods for counting reticulocytes are based on transformation of ribosomal RNA in the reticulocyte cytoplasm into a visible form. The technique used is 'supravital', i.e. the dye is added before fixation to fresh, vital cells so that it may cross the red cell membrane, interact with ribosomal structures and promote their aggregation and precipitation. The formation of the granulofilamentous substance is immediately followed by cell death.

5.2.2 Dyes for reticulocytes

Many chemical compounds have been used to stain reticulocytes, but the most widely used now are brilliant cresyl blue, new methylene blue and azure B. Fluorescent dyes have also been used with visual microscopy and are now employed in flow cytometry methods. The morphological appearance of stained reticulocytes depends not only on the dye employed, but also on its concentration, pH, mode of application, duration of staining and type of film. Moreover, there can be unpredictable variability in the staining characteristics of different batches of dye, and occasionally heavy dye deposits occur which severely interfere with accurate counting (Marshall, 1978).

Brilliant cresyl blue (Colour Index or CI 51010) is an oxazine dye which renders the reticulocyte cytoplasm weakly blue-green and the reticulum deep blue. Optimal results can be obtained with a dilute solution (0.1%) and a staining time of 30 seconds. Commercial solutions consist of variable mixtures of dye components and metal salts, whose chromatic yield can vary widely from one manufacturer to another.

New methylene blue (NMB: CI 52030) is a thiazine dye whose performance is very similar to brilliant cresyl blue (Brecher, 1949). There is, however, greater contrast between clear cytoplasm and blue reticulum. Reticulocyte counts performed with NMB preparations are approximately 5% higher than with brilliant cresyl blue (Terada *et al.*, 1965). Batch to batch composition is more stable and staining is more consistent; for these reasons it was selected by ICSH and NCCLS as the standard dye for microscopy reference measurement procedures. Although normally used in saline solution, it has been reported that admixture of 10% isopropyl alcohol may improve staining of the granulofilamentous material and the precipitation of unstable haemoglobin and haemoglobin H inclusion bodies (Ezzat and Al-Turki, 1990).

Azure B (CI 52010) is a purified component of polychrome methylene blue, the basis of panoptic stains, e.g. Giemsa or May–Grünwald solutions. Azure B provides reproducible, deposit-free preparations (Marshall *et al.*, 1976). In blood smears stained with azure B the reticulum appears dark violet and the cytoplasm very light greyish-pink, resulting in optimal contrast (Wittekind and Schulte, 1987). Haemoglobin H inclusions, Heinz bodies and Howell–Jolly bodies are as well stained by azure B as with brilliant cresyl blue or NMB.

5.2.3 Techniques of preparation

Many different techniques have been used for reticulocyte counting (Marshall, 1978). In the most commonly used method, a saline dye solution is mixed with fresh blood and incubated directly on the slide, on a watch glass, in the bulb of a cell counting pipette or, more commonly, in a test tube (Chanarin, 1989; Dacie and Lewis, 1995). The NCCLS and ICSH methods specify incubation of fresh blood with new methylene blue in a test tube.

One disadvantage of these methods is the limited stability of reticulocyte preparations over time. Permanent preparations can only be obtained by counterstaining supravitally stained smears by a Romanowsky method. The granulofilamentous substance is preserved but with some loss of contrast and definition. Stain precipitate may cause confusion. Heinz bodies are not visible in counterstained preparations. This method should never be used routinely.

5.2.4 Counting

All methods in use today for visual microscopy counting are indirect. The proportion of reticulocytes is expressed as a percentage of the total number of red cells (including those classified as reticulocytes):

$$\text{Reticulocytes (\%)} = \frac{\text{reticulocytes counted}}{\text{(red cells + reticulocytes) counted}} \times 100$$

The absolute number of reticulocytes per unit volume can then be calculated from the reticulocyte percentage and the red cell count obtained by an automated blood cell counter:

$$\text{Reticulocytes } (\times 10^{12}/\text{L}) = \frac{\text{reticulocytes (\%)} \times \text{red blood cells } (\times 10^{12}/\text{L})}{100}$$

or, since the absolute count is generally expressed $\times 10^9$L:

$$\text{Reticulocytes } (\times 10^9/\text{L}) = \frac{\text{Reticulocytes (\%)} \times \text{red blood cells } (\times 10^{12}/\text{L})}{100} \times 1000$$

Blood films must be well spread to ensure even distribution of cells over successive fields. An area of the film should be chosen at low magnification where the cells are well stained, not distorted and touch but do not overlap. In an average film, a suitable area is located between the centre and the feathered edge. The count should be carried out using an oil-immersion 100× objective on consecutive fields according to a 'battlement' pathway (Fig. 5.1). Spun films are particularly suitable for reticulocyte counting, owing to their very homogeneous and reproducible red cell distribution (May and Sage, 1976). Safety requirements concerning droplet and aerosol formation must be satisfied.

Most texts recommend counting 1000 red cells, regardless of the reticulocyte proportion. Since measurement precision depends on the number of reticulocytes counted, this number of 1000 is adequate only when the reticulocyte proportion is high. A more acceptable approach is to count to 100 reticulocytes, regardless of the number of red cells. The ICSH reference measurement procedure (ICSH, 1998) specifies the cell count requirements for stated coefficients of variation (CVs) at different reticulocyte counts (Table 5.1).

Several methods can increase the number of reticulocytes counted without proportionally increasing the red cell count requirements. This is achieved by means of area-reducing devices

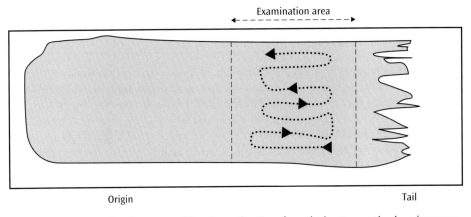

Fig. 5.1 *The correct examination area and 'battlement' pattern for reticulocyte counting by microscopy (modified from ICSH, 1998)*

Table 5.1 *ICSH proposed reference method for reticulocyte counting (1998): the number of cells to be counted for coefficients of variation (CVs) of 2, 5 and 10%. Reticulocyte proportion is expressed as unit fraction. For initial calibration of automated reticulocyte counter, a very precise count is required (CV = 2%), whereas for routine quality control purposes, CV = 5% is adequate (NCCLS/ICSH, 1997).*

	Target CV		
Reticulocyte proportion	**2%**	**5%**	**10%**
0.01	247 500	39 600	9 900
0.02	122 500	19 600	4 900
0.05	47 500	7 600	1 900
0.10	22 500	3 600	900
0.20	10 000	1 600	400
0.50	2 500	400	100

such as the Miller disk (Brecher *et al.*, 1950; ICSH, 1992) which divides the field for proportional counting into an entire square and a small square one-ninth the area, producing a ratio 9:1. Proportional counting is then carried out, i.e. the number of reticulocytes in the entire square and the number of red cells in the one-ninth area. Strict compliance with edge rules is of utmost importance to reduce imprecision. However, use of the Miller disk is not free from risk. In the College of American Pathologists surveys of external quality assessment (1988–1990), 25% of respondents used the Miller disk. Although correlation between the two methods was high, laboratories using the disk invariably obtained reticulocyte counts one-third lower. Similar results were obtained in later surveys, leading to the conclusion that use of the Miller disk might, in fact, be detrimental to precision (Davis *et al.*, 1997).

In order to improve precision for reference measurement procedures, it is possible to carry out the count using a video monitor attached to a microscope, or a double-headed microscope for multiple observations (ICSH, 1998). A potentially more accurate method, although impractical at the present time for routine use, could be based on computerized analysis of the image (Perel *et al.*, 1980; Rowan, 1986; Schimenti *et al.*, 1992).

5.2.5 Methods for correction of reticulocyte count

Reticulocyte counts are commonly expressed in proportional numbers, i.e. the number of reticulocytes per 100 red cells, and in certain situations this may be misleading, e.g. in patients with anaemia or during periods of intense erythropoietic stimulation. Several investigators have suggested that the clinical value of the reticulocyte count as an index of erythropoietic activity could be increased by introducing corrections: (i) for severity of anaemia (haematocrit correction), and (ii) for increased time of stress reticulocytes in the circulation (shift correction) (Hillman and Finch, 1969; Crosby, 1981; Koepke and Koepke, 1986).

For haematocrit correction, the observed proportional reticulocyte count is corrected to an arbitrary normal haematocrit (based on age and gender) to produce a reticulocyte index:

$$\text{Reticulocyte index} = \text{observed reticulocytes (\%)} \times \text{patient haematocrit}/0.45$$

Similar results are obtained using the haemoglobin concentration or red cell count values (Houwen, 1992). Unfortunately this correction is not widely used in routine practice, resulting in interpretation errors. The advent of automated counters which generate an absolute reticulocyte count obviates the need for this correction.

Shift correction should be considered during periods of intense erythropoietic stress when very young reticulocytes (stress macroreticulocytes) are released into the circulation prematurely (Hillman and Finch, 1969; Perrotta and Finch, 1972). The maturation time of these reticulocytes in the bone marrow is shortened, while the maturation time in the peripheral blood is lengthened. Therefore the number of reticulocytes in the peripheral blood may be increased without any corresponding increase in erythropoietic activity. There is no practical way to determine the age of the reticulocyte population during visual counting; however, Hillman and Finch (1969) proposed a 'shift correction' to compensate for increased duration in the circulating blood. This empirical correction for reticulocyte maturation is based on the haematocrit. This maturation time, calculated from measurements in healthy subjects undergoing repeated phlebotomies (Hillman, 1969), is as follows:

Haematocrit	Peripheral blood maturation time (days)
0.45	1.0
0.35	1.5
0.25	2.0
0.15	2.5

A reticulocyte count corrected for both 'haematocrit' and 'shift' is referred to as the 'reticulo-cyte production index', which was proposed as an effective means of evaluating erythropoietic activity and of classifying anaemias.

The principles laid down by Hillman and Finch (1969) have now been rendered unneces-sary by the introduction of flow cytometric measurement of the immature reticulocyte fraction (IRF), which utilizes the immature reticulocytes to evaluate erythropoiesis, rather than compensate for their presence (Davis, 1996).

5.2.6 Performance of microscope reticulocyte count

The clinical usefulness of reticulocyte counting by visual microscopy is limited by high imprecision and unpredictable inaccuracy. Intralaboratory reproducibility is poor, with CVs of between 20 and 50% on samples of normal to low reticulocyte counts (Tichelli et al., 1990). Interlaboratory reproducibility is even worse, as demonstrated in studies of the College of American Pathologists (Gilmer and Koepke, 1976; Rabinovitch, 1993; Davis et al., 1997). Generally the CVs obtained were so high that the diagnostic usefulness of the measurement was questioned (Savage et al., 1985).

One of the main reasons for such poor performance probably lies in subjective differences between observers (Peebles et al., 1981), mainly related to the morphological identification of the more mature reticulocytes containing minimal blue staining substance. Inconsistency in applying the approved definition of a reticulocyte is aggravated by incompetence, lack of motivation, fatigue and carelessness.

The number of cells counted also influences imprecision. Reticulocyte counting follows the statistical laws of the binomial distribution, and therefore the number of cells counted during the procedure has a major effect on the precision of the result. For example, in a sample with a reticulocyte count of 1%, the 95% confidence limits are 0.03–5.45% if 100 red cells are counted, but 0.48–1.84% when 1000 red cells are counted (Greenberg and Beck, 1984).

Other sources of variability include technical factors, such as the type of smear (wedge or spun), the method of supravital staining and the inconsistent use of area reducing devices. Attempts to standardize the microscope reticulocyte count have not been successful in spite of standards published by the ICSH (1992, 1998) and NCCLS/ICSH (1997). In a recent study, conducted by the Canadian Laboratory Proficiency Testing Program, interlaboratory CVs ranged from 25 to 30% (Lohmann et al., 1994), showing lack of improvement from 1983 to 1992 in contrast to the other cell count parameters. These results were confirmed in the CAP 1994–1995 Reticulocyte Proficiency Testing Program, which for the first time used surrogate blood for visual microscopy (Davis et al., 1997).

5.2.7 Reference method for reticulocyte counting by visual microscopy

Reference measurement procedures for reticulocyte counting based on the determination of reticulocyte to red cell ratio by visual microscopy of supravitally stained preparations have recently been published (NCCLS/ICSH, 1997; ICSH, 1998). The essential difference between the two methods is use of the Miller graticule. The NCCLS/ICSH (1997) document permits use of the graticule as an option whereas the ICSH (1998) document states 'this approach does not allow accurate classification on a cell by cell basis within the large area of the graticule and so cannot qualify as a reference method'. Otherwise the methods are identical. The intended use of the reference measurement procedure is the initial calibration and subsequent validation of reticulocyte flow cytometers. An outline of the method is presented in Box 5.1.

Box 5.1 An outline of the ICSH proposed reference method for reticulocyte counting based on determination of the reticulocyte to red cell ratio (1998)

Principle
Cell by cell classification by careful microscope examination of a supravitally stained blood film. Reticulocytes are identified as non-nucleated cells that contain at least two blue staining particles or one particle linked to a filamentous strand. The ratio of reticulocytes to red cells is converted to an absolute reticulocyte count ($\times 10^9$/L) using the red cell count as determined by the ICSH reference method (ICSH, 1994).

Specimen
Whole blood into K_2EDTA 3.7–5.4 μmol (1.5–2.2 mg/mL).

Stain
New methylene blue 1.0 g dissolved into 100 mL iso-osmotic phosphate buffer pH 7.4, filtered and stored in the dark at 2–6°C (stable 1 month).

Staining procedure
Mix 100 μL of blood in a tube with 100 μL of filtered stain solution.
Stain at room temperature for 3–5 minutes.
Resuspend the cells and make films on glass slides.
Dry films rapidly in warm air. Do not fix.

Counting
Check at microscope low power (100×) to ensure an even distribution of cells and the absence of interferents.
Using oil immersion microscopy, classify every cell within each field of view as a red cell or as a reticulocyte, moving field to field in a battlement pattern (see Fig. 5.1). The number of red cells to be counted depends on precision requirements (see Table 5.1).
The best results are achieved if two experienced morphologists simultaneously view the cells on a video monitor or on a two-headed microscope.

Results
Reticulocyte proportion (unit fraction) is calculated using the equation:

$$\text{Reticulocyte proportion} = \frac{\text{no. of reticulocytes counted}}{\text{no. of red cells} + \text{no. of reticulocytes counted}}$$

The reticulocyte count is expressed as the number of reticulocytes per litre of blood $\times 10^9$/L. This number is obtained by multiplying the fraction of reticulocytes expressed to three decimal places by the reference red cell count.

5.3 FLOW CYTOMETRIC RETICULOCYTE COUNTING

The introduction of automated methods for reticulocyte counting has radically modified the formerly limited range of clinical applications (Houwen, 1992; Cavill, 1993a) due to a striking improvement in precision and sensitivity to small differences, even within the normal to low range.

5.3.1 History of reticulocyte counting by flow cytometry

Staining of reticulocyte granulofilamentous substance can be performed using fluorescent molecules which specifically link to nucleic acids. RNA remnants can then be observed using ultraviolet light microscopy (Schlosshardt and Heilmeyer, 1942; Joossens and Hendrickx, 1946). The first fluorochrome used was auramine O, a basic phenylmethane dye. Subsequently, acridine orange became popular for fluorescence microscopy (Kosenow, 1952; Marmont, 1960; Vander et al., 1963). Acridine orange stains both RNA and DNA. It binds to RNA and causes denaturation of the RNA molecule, forming acridine orange–RNA complexes which typically exhibit metachromatic red fluorescence under ultraviolet light. Precipitated reticulocyte RNA appears bright reddish-orange against a greenish cytoplasmic background. Complexes of acridine orange with DNA fluoresce green-yellow, thus permitting easy differentiation of reticulocytes from nucleated red blood cells (NRBCs). This method proved to be simple and accurate for reticulocyte counting and was characterized by improved sensitivity: average counts obtained with acridine orange were slightly higher than those obtained with brilliant cresyl blue.

Using acridine orange with fluorescence microscopy, Thaer and Becker (1975) demonstrated a link between the RNA content of reticulocytes and their maturation status. The less mature forms fluoresced more strongly and quantitation of this effect was possible. This observation was supported by clinical studies in patients with pernicious anaemia during treatment with vitamin B_{12} and autoimmune haemolytic anaemia treated with prednisone. Thus, for the first time, the clinical usefulness of the short-term kinetics of reticulocyte release from the bone marrow was demonstrated. Recently, fluorometric microscopy with acridine orange has been automated using computer-based technology (Eder and Fritsche, 1989).

These pioneering studies led to the development of flow cytometric reticulocyte counting (Tanke et al., 1980; Wallen et al., 1980; Tanke et al., 1983). During the last 20 years, technical advances in this field have been continuous, leading to a wide range of clinical applications in new areas of medicine and to the development of increasingly complex instruments and methods. At present there are many instruments capable of counting reticulocytes, including multipurpose flow cytometers, semi-automated and fully automated discrete reticulocyte counters, and fully automated multiparameter haematology analysers. Each has an individual stain, its own thresholds and its own method of calibration and quality control. As a result, standardization and harmonization have become major issues in modern flow cytometric reticulocyte counting.

5.3.2 Fluorescent dyes

Fluorescent dyes, also called fluorochromes or fluorophores, are molecules with specific properties: they absorb light at a certain wavelength, possess a stated excitation wavelength, and emit light at a longer wavelength (emission wavelength). They are used as probes to visualize very small cell structures (even a few molecules) with great sensitivity and specificity. Fluorochromes for reticulocyte analysis must be capable of crossing the cell membrane, possibly without preliminary fixation, and binding to nucleic acids. Their excitation wavelength must be compatible with the laser source used in the flow cytometer: typically 488 nm wavelength argon lasers. Their quantum yield, defined as the increase in fluorescence produced when they bind to nucleic acids in suspension, should be sufficient to provide acceptable separation of reticulocytes from mature red cells, the latter possessing slight autofluorescence due to haemoglobin molecules. Additional important properties determining the efficiency of fluorochromes are the length of incubation and the photostability after staining. With acridine orange and thioflavine T, the fluorescence intensity in reticulocytes significantly increases with the length of incubation (Metzger and Charache, 1987). With such instability, any absolute measurement, such as for maturation assessment, must be performed under strictly controlled incubation times. Some fluorochromes, e.g. acridine orange, have a tendency to adhere to tubing and flow system components (Wearne *et al.*, 1985). Unless this residual dye is removed by washing with detergents, subsequent samples will take up the dye, exhibit fluorescence and lead to misinterpretation.

At the moment, the most widely used fluorochrome for reticulocyte counting with 488 nm multipurpose laser flow cytometers is thiazole orange. Thiazole orange has many advantages in terms of speed and simplicity both of sample preparation and of flow cytometric analysis (Lee *et al.*, 1986; Chin-Yee *et al.*, 1991). It is a vital stain which does not require fixation of cells. Optimal incubation time is only 30 minutes. The thiazole orange–RNA complex has a quantum yield suitable for good separation of reticulocytes from mature red cells; its fluorescence is sufficiently stable to permit quantitative measurement of reticulocyte sub-populations with high RNA content. Incubation with thiazole orange increases the background fluorescence of the entire red cell population 1.7 times that of unstained samples, while fluorescence of stained reticulocytes is 22 times brighter than in mature red cells. A recent multicentre study has shown that thiazole orange provides similar and comparable results on different flow cytometers, regardless of the methodology used (Davis *et al.*, 1997). Other fluorochromes used in flow cytometry of reticulocytes are auramine O and CD4K530, a proprietary cyanine dye which is excited at 488 nm and emits enhanced green fluorescence at 530 nm on binding to RNA or DNA (Van Bockstaele and Peetermans, 1989; d'Onofrio *et al.*, 1997; Kim *et al.*, 1997).

Non-fluorescent supravital dyes are used to stain ribosomal RNA in other haematology analysers, e.g. Oxazine 750, chemically related to brilliant cresyl blue, and different solutions of new methylene blue.

5.3.3 Principles of flow cytometric reticulocyte analysis

Although many different types of flow cytometer can be used to count reticulocytes, some general principles are common to all methods. Particularly with multipurpose flow cytometers, some preliminary manual steps are necessary to produce fluorochrome binding and staining of RNA. Concentration of the reagent, incubation time and temperature and other variables must be strictly controlled to obtain optimal separation of stained reticulocytes and unstained autofluorescing red cells from nucleated red cells, leucocytes and platelets which also produce various levels of cytoplasmic and nuclear fluorescence.

The first phase of flow cytometric analysis involves isolation of the cells of interest, e.g. red cells and reticulocytes, from cells which have to be excluded. This separation is usually obtained on a two-dimensional cytogram, in which the *x*-axis represents forward scattered light (FSc) and the *y*-axis side scattered light (SSc). FSc is a function of cell volume, while SSc mainly reflects cell structure. On the scattergram, red cells and reticulocytes form a tight homogeneous cluster, clearly distinct from other cell populations. This cluster can be gated electronically (Fig. 5.2b). Fluorescent signals obtained from the gated population are then converted to a one-dimensional histogram of fluorescence intensity (Fig. 5.2a). At this stage reticulocytes are separated from red cells by means of a threshold on the *x*-axis, located at fluorescence intensity previously determined on an autologous blank unstained sample. Owing to both autofluorescence of red cells and progressive decline in fluorescence in maturing reticulocytes, separation between red cells and reticulocytes is not clear-cut: location of the threshold is thus crucial (Schmitz and Werner, 1986). An additional upper fluorescence threshold is usually also set, to exclude interference from other fluorescent elements similar in size to erythrocytes, e.g. large platelets or small lymphocytes.

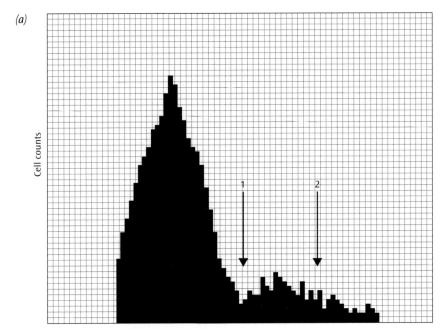

Channels of fluorescence or light scatter/absorbance

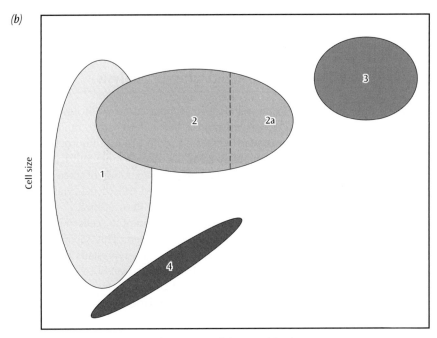

Fluorescence or light scatter/absorbance

Fig. 5.2 *Schematic representation of flow cytometric separation of reticulocytes from the red cell population. (a) Histogram of fluorescence (or light scatter/ absorbance) versus cell counts. Threshold 1 separates reticulocytes from unstained red cells, while threshold 2 separates immature reticulocytes on the right. (b) Two-dimensional cytogram of light scatter (proportional to cell size) versus cell fluorescence or light scatter/absorbance (proportional to RNA content). 1, mature red cells; 2, reticulocytes; 2a, immature reticulocytes (IRF); 3, leucocytes and erythroblasts; 4, platelets.*

Table 5.2 *Method for reticulocyte counting and new reticulocyte parameters.*

Method of detection	Level of automation	RNA staining	Name of the method	Immature reticulocytes	Reticulocye indices	References
Fluorescence	Manual preparation, automatic gating and reading	Thiazole orange	Retic-count kit for Becton Dickinson flow cytometers (FACScan)			Kojima *et al.* (1989) Tichelli *et al.* (1990) Shoustal (1992)
Fluorescence	Fully automated (dedicated)	Auramine O	Sysmex R-1000 Sysmex R-3000	Three fractions (LFR, MFR, HFR)		
Fluorescence	Fully automated with CBC	Auramine O	Sysmex SE-9000 with RAM-1 module	Three fractions (LFR, MFR, HFR)		
Fluorescence	Fully automated with CBC	Proprietary fluorochrome	Sysmex XE-2100	Three fractions and IRF		Inoue (1999)
Light scatter and absorption	Manual preparation automatic analysis with CBC	Oxazine 750	Bayer H*3	Three fractions (LR, MR, HR)	MCVr, CHCMr, CHr	d'Onofrio *et al.* (1995)
Light scatter and absorption	Fully automated with CBC	Oxazine 750	Bayer ADVIA 120	Three fractions (LR, MR, HR)	MCVr, CHCMr, CHr	
Light scatter	Manual preparation automatic analysis with CBC	New methylene blue on sphered cell	Coulter models STKS, MAXM, HMX			Davies *et al.* (1997) Buttarello *et al.* (1996)
Light scatter	Fully automated with CBC	New methylene blue on sphered cell	Coulter model GEN-S	Three fractions (LR, MR, HR) IRF, HLR	MRV	Kessler *et al.* (1997) Fourcade *et al.* (1999)
Light scatter	Manual preparation automatic analysis with CBC	New methylene blue	Abbott Cell-Dyn 3500 and 3700	IRF (3700 only)		
Fluorescence	Fully automated with CBC	CD530K (cyanine dye)	Abbott Cell-Dyn 4000	IRF (unit fraction)		Kim *et al.* (1997)
Fluorescence	Fully automated with CBC	Thiazole orange	ABX Pentra 120	Three fractions (RET, L, M, H), IRF (unit fraction)	MRV, MFI, IMM%, CRC	

IRF, immature reticulocyte fraction; MCVr or MRV, mean reticulocyte volume; MFI, mean fluorescence index obtained as the mean channel of fluorescence; CRC, reticulocyte count corrected by haematocrit; CBC, complete blood count; CHr, reticulocyte haemoglobin concentration; CHCMr, reticulocyte haemoglobin concentration mean; IMM, immature reticulocytes.

5.3.4 Blood cell counters incorporating the reticulocyte count

The most recent advance in reticulocyte count is the development of fully automated analytical methods incorporated in the latest generation of multiparameter haematological analysers. Some of these systems measure reticulocyte and related parameters using fluorescent dyes for RNA and laser light (Takubo *et al.*, 1989; Tichelli *et al.*, 1990; Davis *et al.*, 1996; d'Onofrio *et al.*, 1996c, 1997; Kim *et al.*, 1997), while others utilize supravital basic dyes causing precipitation and staining of reticular substance, which is then recognized by light absorbance or scattering (Buttarello *et al.*, 1995, 1996; d'Onofrio *et al.*, 1995; Davies *et al.*, 1997; Ghevaert *et al.*, 1997; Kessler *et al.*, 1997; Rudensky, 1997) (Table 5.2).

5.3.5 Interferences

Some interferences in reticulocyte counting affect both visual microscopy and automated methods, while others specifically influence flow cytometry measurements (Box 5.2). High leucocyte counts can falsely increase flow cytometry counts owing to invasion of the reticulo-cyte counting area by highly fluorescent white blood cells (Ferguson *et al.*, 1990; Bartels *et al.*, 1993; Serke and Huhn, 1993; Van Houte *et al.*, 1994; Bigelow and Davis, 1995). This occurs especially with small lymphocytes in chronic lymphocytic leukaemia. Removal of buffy coat in samples with elevated white cell count may result in a statistically significant decrease (20%) in the total and immature highly fluorescent reticulocyte counts measured (d'Onofrio *et al.*, 1996a). Another source of interference is thrombocytosis, particularly when accompanied by large platelets or platelet clumps. On the other hand, in sickle cell anaemia and cold agglutinin disease, irreversibly sickled cells or aggregated erythrocytes may not be included in the red cell gated area (Davis and Bigelow, 1994a). Scrutiny of cytograms and histograms is often useful in detecting the presence of interferences (Fig. 5.3).

Among red cell inclusions (ICSH, 1992), Pappenheimer bodies which contain iron do not show affinity for fluorochromes, but are stained by supravital dyes, usually as single dots with a darker shade of blue than the granulofilamentous material of the reticulocytes. If there is any doubt, Pappenheimer bodies can be identified by post-staining films for iron. DNA remnants, e.g. Howell–Jolly bodies are, on the other hand, intensely stained by both fluorochromes and supravital stains, producing a false increase in reticulocyte count (Lofsness *et al.*, 1994). With some methods, however, Howell–Jolly bodies may be more fluorescent than reticulocytes and are excluded by the upper reticulocyte threshold (Sher *et al.*, 1997). If necessary, counter-staining of films by a Romanowsky method permits identification. Falsely increased flow cytometric reticulocyte counts can also be observed in patients with Heinz bodies (Espanol *et al.*, 1999), haemoglobin H disease (Lai *et al.*, 1999) and unstable haemoglobins (Zini *et al.*, 1991; Hinchliffe, 1993), since some of these unstable variants may precipitate when exposed to supravital dyes. Some flow cytometric methods appear more susceptible to these interferences than others, as a function of the stain, incubation time or thresholding (Lai *et al.*, 1999).

Red cells containing malaria parasites can also be counted as reticulocytes (Makler *et al.*, 1987). Both intra-erythrocytic trophozoites and extracellular gametocytes, regardless of species, can cause pseudoreticulocytosis and marked increase in IRF associated with typically abnormal cytograms and histograms (Hoffman and Pennings, 1999). Wernli *et al.* (1991) suggested that this phenomenon may be used as a quantitative index of parasitaemia. False increases in reticulocyte count also occur with erythrocytes infested by Babesiosis parasites (Lofsness *et al.*, 1994).

Certain substances are characterized by spontaneous fluorescence, e.g. ascorbic acid, cyanocobalamin, phenolphthalein, flavine adenine dinucleotide and bilirubin, but this does

Box 5.2   Potential interferents in reticulocyte counting

Leucocytosis (especially lymphocytosis)
Leucocyte fragments (leukaemias)
Nucleated red blood cells
Thrombocytosis
Giant platelets
Platelet clumping
Red cell agglutination
Haemolysis and cryoagglutination
Platelet/red cell coincidence
Basophilic stippling
Howell–Jolly bodies
Heinz bodies
HbS, HbH and unstable haemoglobins
Pappenheimer bodies
Malaria parasites
Babesiosis
Porphyria (increased red cell fluorescence)
Paraproteins
Cryoglobulins
Fluorescent drugs (?) (ascorbid acid, cyanocobalamin)
Hyperbilirubinaemia (?)
Fluorescein (retinoic angiography)

not appear to interfere with flow cytometric reticulocyte counts (Kojima *et al.*, 1989). Interference has, however, been reported following intravenous infusion of fluorescein during retinoic fluorangiography (Hirata *et al.*, 1992).

5.3.6 Performance of flow cytometric reticulocyte count

The many advantages of flow cytometric reticulocyte counting have been responsible for its rapid dissemination into an expanding range of clinical fields. The procedure is objective and requires less time and labour. Many evaluation studies, moreover, have demonstrated improvements in linearity, precision, carryover, time stability, accuracy and comparability compared with visual microscopy.

PRECISION

This is greatly improved with average overall CVs generally below 5–10% for all flow cytometry methods, compared with 20–40% CVs with microscopy (Carter *et al.*, 1989; Kojima *et al.*, 1989; Tatsumi *et al.* 1989; Ferguson *et al.*, 1990; Bowen *et al.*, 1991; Hansson *et al.*, 1992; Schimenti *et al.*, 1992; Cavill, 1993b). The level of imprecision of cytometric methods depends, like all others, on the count level: it varies from CVs of 20–30% for very low reticulocyte counts (0.1–0.2%) to 3–7% within the normal range and below 3% for increased counts (Tichelli *et al.*, 1990; Nobes and Carter, 1990; Van Petegem *et al.*, 1993; Sandberg *et al.*, 1998). The improvement in precision is easily explained. Flow cytometers count and classify from 10 000 to more than 30 000 cells per sample, minimizing statistical error. They analyse cells in liquid suspension, avoiding sampling error due to irregular distribution of cells on a blood

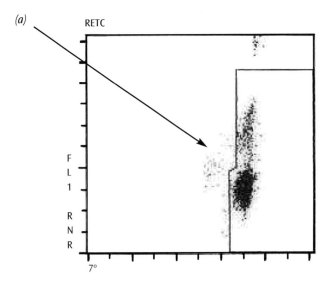

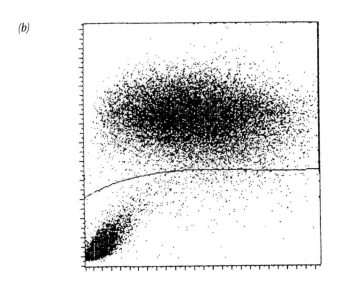

Fig. 5.3 *Two rare examples of false reticulocytosis: (a) due to the presence of trophozoites of* Plasmodium falciparum *measured on the Cell Dyn 4000: reticulocyte count of 5% or 185 × 10⁹/L, immature reticulocyte fraction (IRF) = 0.70; and (b) due to unstable haemoglobin Hammersmith measured on the Sysmex R 1000 where the reticulocyte count is 100%.*

film or incorrect application of edge rules for area-reducing devices. Moreover, they replace human subjectivity and variability with the uniform and objective criteria of automated analysis. Interlaboratory variability of the flow cytometric reticulocyte count, however, is still far from being ideal. In a recent study involving eight US laboratories with 11 instruments, global CVs among all laboratories ranged from 69% for samples with reticulocytes below 0.5%, to 24% for samples with reticulocytes above 2.5% (Davis *et al.*, 1994). Lower CVs were observed in subgroups formed by homogeneous instruments. Interlaboratory and inter-method variability of flow cytometric methods has recently been quantified in the reticulocyte proficiency testing programme of the College of American Pathologists (Davis *et al.*, 1997). This wide survey involved more than 2000 laboratories, using all technologies available at that time and receiving commercial stabilized surrogate material originally developed from human blood. Results confirmed that automated flow cytometry counts reticulocytes much more precisely than by microscope, generally achieving CVs below 20%, but it also demonstrated a clear bias between different flow cytometric methods (Davis *et al.*, 1997).

CARRYOVER

Flow cytometric reticulocyte counters do not usually have problems with carryover between samples.

ACCURACY

Accuracy of reticulocyte counting is assessed by comparison with the microscopy reference method. The level of agreement, usually measured by linear regression, is reported as excellent by most authors, with very high coefficients of correlation, close to 1.0 for all methods (Carter *et al.*, 1989; Nobes and Carter, 1990; Schimenti *et al.*, 1992).

However, some studies have shown that thiazole orange methods tend to overestimate reticulocytes, with percentages 1.5–2 times higher than the microscope reference method (Ferguson *et al.*, 1990; Van Hove *et al.*, 1990; Hansson *et al.*, 1992), especially in samples with leucocytosis (Bartels *et al.*, 1993). This can depend in part on a greater sensitivity of the fluorescence method, which can include among reticulocytes red cells with very low amounts of RNA, below the minimum microscopy criteria for reticulocyte identification. Some instruments, on the other hand, tend to underestimate reticulocyte counts, especially at values higher than 10% (Kojima *et al.*, 1989), probably because the most intensely stained cells with very high RNA content fall beyond the upper threshold and are excluded from the count.

At very low reticulocyte counts many flow cytometric methods tend to overestimate reticulocyte percentages. Most cytometers, in fact, never obtain reticulocyte counts of 0%, even in samples in which no reticulocyte at all can be seen on the peripheral blood film (Nobes and Carter, 1990; Tichelli *et al.*, 1990). This is probably due to difficulties in threshold location in the absence of a defined reticulocyte population and may be caused by the dim auto-fluorescence of mature red cells.

Inter-method agreement between flow cytometric systems is even better than with the reference microscopy method, with coefficients of correlation higher than 0.9 regardless of the instruments and the different dyes or fluorochromes (Bowen *et al.*, 1991; Cavill, 1993b; Van Petegem *et al.*, 1993).

LINEARITY

The linearity of flow cytometric reticulocyte counters is excellent in terms of correlation between expected and obtained results on diluted and/or concentrated samples over a wide range of values. As mentioned above, however, some methods have limited linearity at very low values.

STABILITY

All methods have been subjected to time lapse studies to define the period during which the reticulocyte count remains sufficiently stable for clinical use. With microscopy, the reticulocyte percentage does not significantly change in the first 24 hours (Lampasso, 1968), even in the paediatric age group (Shaffer *et al.*, 1993). Similar results have been obtained with flow cytometry methods. In general, when blood samples are stored at 2–6°C, the reticulocyte count remains unchanged for at least 72 hours; according to some studies, refrigerated samples may be analysed safely for up to 120 hours after collection (Cavill *et al.*, 1996). More variable results are obtained with storage at room temperature, sometimes resulting in significant change after 24 hours regardless of whether K_2 or K_3 EDTA anticoagulant is used (Cavill *et al.*, 1996). This may depend on the counting method: generally the reticulocyte count tends to decrease with auramine O, possibly as a result of *in vitro* maturation (Tichelli *et al.*, 1990), but tends to increase with thiazole orange methods, probably as the result of red cell membrane changes which enhance non-specific fluorochrome binding (Ferguson *et al.*, 1990; Bowen *et al.*, 1991).

5.3.7 Quality control

Intralaboratory quality control (QC) of the reticulocyte count is based on repeated analysis, on a daily basis or more frequently, of suitable control materials (Rowan, 1991). These are presently available from commercial sources in the form of stabilized human or animal blood, usually at three levels of reticulocyte count: low, normal and high. Human red blood cells encapsulated with RNA by a hypo/hypertonic dialytic process can also be used as a stable control material (Ebrahim and Ryan, 1996). Commercial preparations are usually supplied with assay target and limit values, but these should be verified by each laboratory (NCCLS/ICSH, 1997). A control preparation similar to those available commercially can be prepared by any laboratory, using human blood collected with ACD or CPD anticoagulants and stored at 4°C for 3 weeks. In such a material, the reticulocyte count has been shown to decrease slowly, but in a predictable and reproducible way thus permitting its use in quality control (Tsuda and Tatsumi, 1990).

Alternatively, for short-term QC it is possible to store (at 4°C) patient samples collected in CPD at three different count levels, to check instrument performance on the day of collection and the following day. Since the reticulocyte percentage under these conditions is stable up to 48 hours, this procedure allows recognition of instrument shifts (Davis and Bigelow, 1989; NCCLS/ICSH, 1997). It is also possible to obtain microscope reticulocyte counts on a small number of selected samples from the daily routine work using the reference method and to compare them with flow cytometry results (NCCLS/ICSH, 1997).

Interlaboratory quality assessment for reticulocyte counting is possible using commercial stabilized control preparations (Davis *et al.*, 1997) and also, on a local basis, using fresh blood stored at 4°C and analysed within 48 hours of phlebotomy (Davis *et al.*, 1995).

5.3.8 Reference values and biological variability

Reference values in health published before the introduction of flow cytometry methods show considerable heterogeneity (Seip, 1953; Lowenstein, 1959). This results from differences in methods, dyes and errors inherent in visual microscopy. The most widely accepted reference intervals for proportional reticulocyte counts ranged from 0.5% to 1.5 or 2.0% (NCCLS, 1985), independent of gender and race. After the advent of flow cytometry, published reference values have, in general, become more homogeneous and show a narrower range

(Tarallo *et al.*, 1994; Kraaijenhagen, 1996). Certain variability, however, still persists, mainly as a result of differences in methods, dyes and fluorochromes. In general, reference reticulocyte values obtained using fluorochromes tend to be higher than visual methods or automated methods using supravital dyes. Table 5.3 provides a summary of ranges from different authors using a wide selection of flow cytometric methods.

For this reason it is important that every laboratory establishes its own reference values, specific for its dye, method and cytometer. According to NCCLS/ICSH (1997), reference values should be determined on a reference population of at least 100 normal adults, equally divided between men and women, who should have a normal blood count, including red and white cell parameters. Since the data are invariably distributed lognormally, reference values for the reticulocyte count should be calculated as the central 95% of results, excluding the lower and upper 2.5% extremes of the distribution.

Reticulocyte counts show significant biological variability (Sandberg *et al.,* 1998). This can be a reflection of the low frequency of these cells and their short intravascular life span. Diurnal variation was as high as 20% (Jones *et al.*, 1996), in contrast to the much smaller variance of red blood cell count and indices. Previous studies described seasonal variation in reticulocyte percentage, with higher values in June than in January, March and October. This was ascribed to increased ultraviolet irradiation during summer (Seip, 1953). Significant within-day differences, on the other hand, have not been confirmed by others in relation to either the time of venepuncture or the hour of the day (Tarallo *et al.*, 1994). The reticulocyte count is not influenced by oral contraceptive drugs, meals or smoking (Tarallo *et al.*, 1994), but increases slightly following intense physical exercise or at high altitude.

Some authors have not found significant differences between males and females, either in percentage or in the absolute count (Bowen *et al.*, 1991; Hansson *et al.*, 1992; Lofsness *et al.*, 1994). These results are at odds with what would be expected taking into account the known differences in red cell counts between the sexes. In fact, if reticulocyte percentages were similar in males and females, absolute counts would be more elevated in males than in females. Such male prevalence in absolute count has been reported recently (Tatsumi *et al.*, 1989; Paterakis *et al.*, 1991; Tarallo *et al.*, 1994). Other studies, however, using microscopy (Deiss and Kurth, 1975) and cytofluorimetry (Carter *et al.*, 1989) have reported significantly higher proportional counts in females. This is related to erythropoietic stimulation caused by cyclic menstrual loss (Ninni, 1949). During pregnancy, reticulocyte counts either do not change or decrease very slightly until weeks 24–28 and then tend to increase moderately. This persists during the first weeks postpartum (Lurie, 1993). The decrease in mature reticulocytes is more significant in smoking pregnant women and is associated with an increase in the immature fraction (Mercelina Roumans *et al.*, 1995). Menarche and menopause do not have any effect on the reticulocyte count (Tarallo *et al.*, 1994).

Many authors have reported changes with age. The reticulocyte percentage is very high in prenatal life: in the 3 month fetus reticulocytes comprise 90%, but this falls to 15-20% by the sixth month. Using flow cytometry a progressive decrease has been demonstrated from about week 20 (mean values: 8.3% or 252×10^9/L) to week 34 (4% or 140.5×10^9/L) (Lahary *et al.*, 1995). Values at birth remain elevated; in both full-term and premature neonates counts between 2 and 6% are found. Reference values in cord blood by flow cytometry are significantly higher than in adults, with mean counts of 2.5–3% (mean absolute counts 150×10^9/L) (Paterakis *et al.*, 1993; Bock and Herkner, 1994a,b; Walka *et al.*, 1998). Neonatal reticulocytosis is independent of gender and type of delivery and has been ascribed to hypoxia at the time of delivery. Reticulocyte counts remain elevated during the first week of extrauterine life, then quickly fall to adult levels (Castriota-Scandenberg *et al.*, 1992; Bock and Herkner, 1994a,b; Tarallo *et al.*, 1994). The adult reference range is maintained in the elderly (Scola *et al.*, 1992; Tarallo *et al.*, 1994).

Table 5.3 *Reference ranges for absolute reticulocyte count ($\times 10^9$/L) as reported by different authors*

Central 95% range	Fluorochrome/ stain	Number of subjects	Age	Reference
50–100	New methylene blue (microscope)	NR	Adults	Dacie and Lewis (1995)
23–93	New methylene blue (microscope)	NR	Adults	Bick (1993)
10–110	New methylene blue (microscope)	NR	Adults	NCCLS/ICSH (1997)
20.0–110.0	New methylene blue (microscope)			
15–135	Thiazole orange	NR	Adults	NCCLS (1997)
12–60	Thiazole orange	154	Adults	Carter *et al.* (1989)
19.4–59.2	Thiazole orange	30	Adults	Nobes and Carter (1990)
19.0–98.0	Thiazole orange	29	Adults	Bowen *et al.* (1991)
30.2–133.6	Thiazole orange	60	Adults	Hansson *et al.* (1992)
24.3–77.4	Auramine O	166 (M)	Adults	Tatsumi *et al.* (1989)
19.2–57.2		99 (F)		
19.0–88.0	Auramine O	89	Adults	Bowen *et al.* (1991)
20–95	Auramine O	NR	Adults	NCCLS/ICSH (1997)
16.3–77.4	Auramine O	285	Adults	Tsuda and Tatsumi (1989)
30.0–70.0	Auramine O	43	18–49	Scola *et al.* (1992)
32.3–95.6	Auramine O	184 (M)	20–29	Tarallo *et al.* (1994)
23.5–88.0		207 (F)		
32.4–104.2	Auramine O	103 (M)	> 50	Tarallo *et al.* (1994)
26.6–90.2		73 (F)		
26.3–96.3	Auramine O	180	Adults	Paterakis *et al.* (1991)
22.7–66.9	Oxazine 750	64	Adults	d'Onofrio *et al.* (1995)
24.4–65.8		32 (M)		
25.4–66.6		32 (F)		
33.2–124.7	Oxazine 750	200	17–60	Chararuks *et al.* (1998)
37.1–144.7		100 (M)		
30.9–110.2		100 (F)		
35.1–112.0	Oxazine 750	133	Adults	Buttarello *et al.* (1995)
19.0–90.0	New methylene blue (automated)	159	Adults	Buttarello *et al.* (1996)
27.0–95.0	Auramine O	159	Adults	Buttarello *et al.* (1996)
22.5–112.5	CD4K530	100	Adults	Kim *et al.* (1997)
22.0–98.0	New methylene blue (automated)	66	Adults	Fourcade *et al.* (1999)
70.7–303.9	Auramine O	35	Cord blood	Paterakis *et al.* (1993)
24.2–124.2	Auramine O	150	Full term Newborns	Bock and Herkner (1994)
14.2–129.4	Auramine O	30	Premature Newborns	Bock and Herkner (1994a)
34.1–83.3	Auramine O	750	1 week– 16 years	Bock and Herkner (1994b)
25.8–89.3	Auramine O	369	4–19	Tarallo *et al.* (1994)

NR, not reported; M, male; F, female.

5.4 MATURATION STUDIES ON RETICULOCYTES: IMMATURE RETICULOCYTE FRACTION

The life span of reticulocytes lasts from the time the orthochromatic erythroblast loses its nucleus to the moment RNA is no longer detectable in the red cell. Kinetic studies with radioactive iron have shown that reticulocyte maturation under conditions of stable haematopoiesis, lasts, on average, 4 days (Papayannopoulou and Finch, 1975). Three of these are normally in the bone marrow. The average intravascular life span of a reticulocyte is thus about 24 hours. Maturation of reticulocytes is associated with a number of morphological, biochemical and functional changes (Lowenstein, 1959; Bessis, 1972; Coulombel *et al.*, 1979):

- disappearance of the granulofilamentous substance;
- reduction and disappearance of mitochondria and ribosomes (Gasko and Danon, 1972);
- reduction in the surface area of the cytoplasmic membrane through remodelling by endocytosis and of exocytosis of vesicles containing water, enzymes and organelles (Gasko and Danon, 1974; Chasis *et al.*, 1989; Johnstone and Ahn, 1990; Brugnara *et al.*, 1993b);
- formation of autophagocytic vacuoles (Simpson and Kling, 1968);
- decrease in cell size and increase in cell density;
- decreased adhesiveness and deformability (Mel *et al.*, 1977);
- decrease and disappearance of transferrin (Frazier *et al.*, 1982) and fibronectin (Patel *et al.*, 1985) receptors;
- decreased activity of many enzymes (Noble *et al.*, 1989; Lakomek *et al.*, 1989);
- change from an irregular polylobed shape to the biconcave shape of mature erythrocytes (Gronowicz *et al.*, 1984).

5.4.1 Reticulocyte differential count

Morphologically, circulating reticulocytes can be divided into various subpopulations by the amount and distribution of granulofilamentous material in their cytoplasm. Among the many methods of morphological differentiation, the best known is that proposed by Heilmeyer (Heilmeyer and Westharer, 1932). This divides reticulocytes into four groups, designated by Roman numerals, together with a group 0 designating erythroblasts which have not yet expelled their nuclei. The other Heilmeyer groups are characterized by a progressive reduction in the amount and compactness of reticulum. A simpler three-stage maturity classification was proposed by Astaldi and Bernardelli (1946) and is possibly closer to modern maturation indices derived from flow cytometry. All classifications relate the quantity of granulofilamentous substance present to the age of the cell. A left shift in reticulocyte maturation, with a relative increase of categories I, II and III, is an early sign of erythroid regeneration. The physiopathological and clinical value of this classification has been confirmed by flow cytometry using RNA dyes and fluorochromes (see below). These new methods have led to a reappraisal of the importance of such measurements, neglected for decades because of technical difficulty and poor reproducibility.

5.4.2 Premature or stress macroreticulocytes

Young reticulocytes (Heilmeyer I and II or Astaldi class B), are rare in the peripheral blood of healthy subjects or patients with hyporegenerative anaemia. A marked increase in this type of reticulocyte is observed experimentally following phenylhydrazine-induced haemolysis or haemorrhage. The intense erythroid stimulation thus produced is reflected by a sustained increase in reticulocytes (30–40% of red cells) and premature release into the circulation of large cells, clearly with a greater volume than both mature red cells and normal reticulocytes. These giant reticulocytes are very rich in RNA and have abundant, dense granulofilamentous substance. They have been defined as 'shift' or 'stress macroreticulocytes'. After fixation and staining of peripheral blood films with panoptic methods (May–Grünwald–Giemsa or Wright), they appear as polychromatic red cells (Brecher and Stohlman, 1961; Perrotta and Finch, 1972). Stress macroreticulocytes have specific properties differing from normal reticulocytes:

- cell volume is 25–100% greater (Brecher and Stohlman, 1962);
- water and haemoglobin content are increased (Ganzoni et al., 1969), although density and haemoglobin concentration are decreased;
- they contain increased amounts of haemoglobin F (Blau et al., 1993), ribosomes and mitochondria (Noble et al., 1990) and membrane antigens like CD36 and CD71 (Himmelfarb et al., 1995; Browne and Hebbel, 1996);
- they are less deformable, more rigid and adhesive (Patel et al., 1985);
- their survival in the circulating blood has been variably reported as longer than the normal 24 hours (Hillman, 1969) but may be shorter owing to more rapid splenic sequestration (Noble et al., 1990).

Shift or stress macroreticulocytes are seen during regenerative anaemia like acute auto-immune haemolysis (Baldini and Panacciulli, 1960), as a response to the administration of haematinic agents in nutritional anaemia, following the administration of recombinant erythropoietin (Brugnara et al., 1993a) and in bone marrow regeneration after chemotherapy-induced haematopoietic aplasia (Kuse, 1993) or stem cell transplantation (Davies et al., 1992). Their production results from accelerated erythroid maturation caused by a sudden intense erythropoietic stimulus. This may lead either to the omission of one or more mitotic divisions or, more simply, to the premature release of reticulocytes into the circulation.

Shift reticulocytes are, at least in part, identical to so-called F reticulocytes. These are characterized by an increased concentration of fetal haemoglobin produced in addition to adult haemoglobin, when there is intense erythroid stimulation associated with expansion of the erythroid compartment (Blau et al., 1993). F reticulocytes can be enumerated accurately by immunofluorescence microscopy or image cytometry (Osterhout et al., 1996; Maier-Redelsperger et al., 1998). This is increasingly used to monitor treatment of sickle cell disease and other types of anaemia. The induction of modifications in haemoglobin synthesis seems to suggest that these cells are the result of an unusual rapid pathway of erythroid maturation. The more immature reticulocytes are more common in the bone marrow than in the peripheral blood (Inoue and Tatsumi, 1991).

5.4.3 Reticulocyte maturation with flow cytometric methods

One of the great advantages of flow cytometry for reticulocyte counting is the reliable measurement of RNA content as fluorescence intensity, light absorption or scattering after supravital staining. Fluorescence or staining intensity is directly proportional to the quantity of RNA in reticulocytes; it thus provides a quantitative and objective direct estimate of the reticulocyte maturity. Quantitation of reticulocyte fluorescence or staining is now established as a supplementary measurement extending and completing the diagnostic value of the reticulocyte count (Houwen, 1992; Davis and Bigelow, 1993; Davis and Bigelow, 1994b,c; Davis, 1996). Flow cytometric studies of reticulocyte maturation have followed two different technical approaches: (i) the determination of an average index, designated reticulocyte maturation index (RMI), i.e. measurement of the average fluorescence or staining of the entire reticulocyte population; or (ii) the division of reticulocytes into two or three subpopulations with different amounts of RNA, corresponding to reticulocytes in different stages of maturation.

RETICULOCYTE MATURATION INDEX (RMI)

This method of measuring the intensity of reticulocyte fluorescence initially used pyronin Y (Tanke *et al.*, 1983) but was subsequently improved by the use of thiazole orange. With the latter dye, more stable fluorescence is obtained and therefore more reliability and consistency of results (Davis and Bigelow, 1989, 1994a). The maturity of the entire reticulocyte population is expressed in arbitrary units indicating the channel which corresponds to the average intensity of fluorescence. When reticulocytes are immature, the maturation curve is shifted towards the right with an increase in the RMI. Although this approach has led to interesting observations following bone marrow transplantation (Davis *et al.*, 1989) and in iron deficiency anaemia (Wells *et al.*, 1992), the limited inter-method comparability and transferability of results is a disadvantage.

RETICULOCYTE SUBPOPULATIONS

This method identifies different subpopulations of reticulocytes, characterized by increasing intensity of fluorescence or staining. They are separated from each other by electronic thresholds which are positioned either automatically or manually (Davis *et al.*, 1993). Different types of reticulocytes are identified: (i) a population with low intensity of fluorescence or staining, referred to as LFR (low fluorescence ratio) or LR which, in subjects with normal haemopoiesis, includes 70–80% of reticulocytes (corresponding to Heilmeyer's class IV); and (ii) a second population with a greater degree of fluorescence or staining that can be further subdivided into cells with intermediate (MFR or MR) or high (HFR or HR) fluorescence or staining. These correspond to Heilmeyer's other classes and include, at least in the case of HFR, stress reticulocytes. This second approach has yielded results of great interest for diagnostic haematology.

IMMATURE RETICULOCYTE FRACTION (IRF)

The quantitation of RNA content as a means to assess reticulocyte maturation, however, does not solve the problems of interlaboratory comparability and standardization. To achieve a greater degree of harmonization of results between methods and between laboratories, Davis *et al.* (1993) proposed a method by which a single fraction of more highly fluorescent or immature reticulocytes can be referenced to a normal healthy adult reticulocyte population, yielding a normal reference range (approximately 0.2–0.45) that allows detection of changes in both the low and high ranges. General agreement has recently been obtained among experts that the IRF concept (i.e. quantitation of the youngest reticulocyte population and expression as a fraction) is the best flow cytometry indicator of erythropoietic activity (Davis, 1997). The IRF is available on many latest generation automated multiparameter analysers.

Standardization of IRF, however, is still far from being accomplished because of the great heterogeneity in terminology, software algorithms and reference values. Since reticulocyte maturation represents a continuum of RNA levels and different reagents have differing sensitivity, it is difficult to adopt a uniform definition and threshold level at which reticulocytes should be considered immature. Moreover, there is, as yet, no stable universally recognized reference material, nor an accepted reference method. However, a level of inter-method agreement, acceptable from a clinical standpoint, can be achieved, with a correlation coefficient ranging from 0.70 to 0.87 (Davis *et al.*, 1994, 1996). Finally, it must be remembered that most potential interferences with the flow cytometry reticulocyte count (see Section 5.3.5) may have an even greater effect on the IRF (Villamor *et al.*, 1996).

5.4.4 Reference values for immature reticulocyte fraction

Definition of reference ranges for immature reticulocytes is necessary for clinical use (Kraaijenhagen, 1996), but is hampered by lack of standardization due to the heterogeneity of methods. Available data (Table 5.4) suggest that there may be statistically significant differences related to gender and age, with a slightly higher percentage of stronger fluorescing reticulocytes in males (Takubo *et al.*, 1989; Tarallo *et al.*, 1994). Immature reticulocyte levels are high in antenatal blood (Lahary *et al.*, 1995), in cord blood (Paterakis *et al.*, 1993) and during the first days of life (Bock and Herkner, 1994a,b); they also tend to increase slightly during pregnancy (Belfiore *et al.*, 1993; Mercelina Roumans *et al.*, 1995). Within-subject biological variability for immature reticulocytes (HFR and MFR) was found to be about 10% (Sandberg *et al.*, 1998).

IRF reference ranges differ significantly between methods (Davis, 1997). It is therefore necessary that each laboratory establishes its own reference range for its particular method.

Table 5.4 *Reference ranges for immature reticulocyte fraction (IRF, transformed into unit fraction) reported by different authors. For methods that measure three classes of reticulocytes according to their RNA content, IRF is calculated as the sum of high and medium fluorescence/stain ratios. M, male; F, female*

Central 95% range	Fluorochrome/ stain	Number of subjects	Age (years, unless noted otherwise)	Reference
0.11–0.41 (M)	Auramine O	40	Adults	Takubo *et al.* (1989)
0.01–0.28 (F)		42		
0.06–0.25	Auramine O	285	Adults	Tsuda and Tatsumi (1989)
0.03–0.16	Auramine O	180	Adults	Paterakis *et al.* (1991)
0.01–0.15 (M)	Auramine O	184	20–29	Tarallo *et al.* (1994)
0.01–0.12 (F)		207		
0.01–0.17 (M)	Auramine O	103	> 50	Tarallo *et al.* (1994)
0.01–0.13 (F)		73		
0.05–0.21	Auramine O	250	Adults	Buttarello *et al.* (1999)
0.03–0.33 (M+F)	Oxazine 750	200	17–60	Charuruks *et al.* (1998)
0.04–0.36 (M)		100		
0.02–0.29 (F)		100		
0.04–0.25	Oxazine 750	250	Adults	Buttarello *et al.* (1999)
0.06–0.23	Thiazole orange	250	Adults	Buttarello *et al.* (1999)
0.15–0.35	CD4K530	250	Adults	Buttarello *et al.* (1999)
0.09–0.31	CD4K530	100	Adults	Kim *et al.* (1997)
0.20–0.37	New methylene blue (automated)	250	Adults	Buttarello *et al.* (1999)
0.20–0.49	New methylene blue (automated)	66	Adults	Fourcade *et al.* (1999)
0.26–0.46	Auramine O	35	Cord blood	Paterakis *et al.* (1993)
0.24–0.30	Auramine O	147	1–3 days	Bock and Herkner (1994a)
0.05–0.06	Auramine O	670	1 month– 16 years	Bock and Herkner (1994b)
0.01–0.16	Auramine O	369	4–19	Tarallo *et al.* (1994)

This is confirmed by a recent study of Buttarello *et al.* (1999) on five latest generation blood cell counters with reticulocyte count and IRF count capability (Table 5.4).

5.5 RETICULOCYTE INDICES

Although knowledge of the physical properties of reticulocytes (shape, size, density and osmotic resistance) has existed since the mid-twentieth century, this has not, until recently, translated into clinical practice. A number of publications have recently described flow cytometric measurements of reticulocyte volume and haemoglobin concentration and suggested clinical uses (Brugnara *et al.*, 1994a; Buttarello *et al.*, 1995; d'Onofrio *et al.*, 1998).

5.5.1 Experimental studies

RETICULOCYTE SIZE (DIAMETER, SURFACE AREA, VOLUME)

Reticulocytes are larger than mature red blood cells and their size gradually diminishes during maturation (Lowenstein, 1959). By visual microscopy of dry smears, the average diameter of reticulocytes is 1.0–1.5 μm greater than the mature red cell. This difference is maintained in pathological conditions, such as megaloblastic and microcytic anaemias. The mean diameter of bone marrow reticulocytes is normally greater than its peripheral blood counterpart. Diameter reduction correlates with progression through the Heilmeyer classes towards full maturation (Paolino, 1946). These early studies, however, were subject to a number of artefacts induced by absorption of supravital dyes and subsequent drying on glass slides.

On wet preparations stained by brilliant cresyl blue, planimetry of highly magnified (×4000) photographs was used to measure the mean area of reticulocytes (Killman, 1964). The CV of the method ranged from 0.41 to 0.98%. These studies showed that the area of normal reticulocytes is on average 13.0% larger than that of mature erythrocytes (range 7.7–22.0%); the calculated reticulocyte volume was 20% larger. The mean reticulocyte/erythrocyte area ratio was 1.13 and the calculated mean volume ratio was 1.2. These measurements were expressed in arbitrary rather than metric units. Clarkson and Moore (1976), again using planimetry, confirmed these results; in their studies mean reticulocyte volume, calculated from an average mean cell volume (MCV) of 88 fL measured with a Coulter Model S, was 106 fL in normal subjects, 79 fL in iron deficiency (mean MCV 73 fL) and 139 fL in megaloblastic anaemia (mean MCV 103). The presence of microreticulocytes or macroreticulocytes in the peripheral blood appeared to be an early finding during the development of iron deficiency or vitamin B_{12}/folate deficiency, respectively.

Several authors have estimated the mean volume of reticulocytes from the ratio of packed cell volume to cell number in samples with very high reticulocyte concentrations. Reticulocyte enrichment up to 100% was obtained in experimental animals treated with phlebotomies and/or haemolytic agents. This comparatively crude and inaccurate method estimated reticulocyte volumes from 1.2 to 3 times larger than those of mature red cells (Betke and Rodig, 1955; Weicker and Fichsel, 1955). These workers did not measure the volume of normal reticulocytes, but that of the much larger stress reticulocytes produced under very intense erythropoietic stimulation. The mean corpuscular haemoglobin concentration (MCHC) of these oversized reticulocytes, moreover, was much lower than that of normal mature red cells.

Such changes in reticulocyte volume can be detected indirectly by changes in the red cell size distribution curves obtained by automated haematology analysers (Weiser and Kociba,

1982). Reticulocyte macrocytosis can also be induced by more physiological models of erythropoietic stimulation, such as bleeding, exposure to simulated altitude and the injection of erythropoietin (Brecher and Stohlman, 1962), and after successful treatment of iron deficiency anaemia (Bessman, 1977).

Recently a different experimental model exploited erythropoietic stimulation following temporary suppression of erythropoiesis with thiamphenicol and phlebotomy (Noble et al., 1989). The stress reticulocytes produced were larger (mean diameter 9.66 ± 1.10 µm, compared with 7.04 ± 1.10 µm for normal reticulocytes and 6.66 ± 0.34 µm for mature red cells); their immaturity was also indicated by a very rich content in ribosomes, mitochondria and other cellular organelles (Noble et al., 1990).

On Romanowsky-stained blood films, stress macroreticulocytes appear as polychromato-philic erythrocytes: on average their diameter was found to be 27% larger than mature erythrocytes (Perrotta and Finch, 1972). Polychromatophilia is abolished following treatment with ribonuclease. As stated by Ferrata (1912), all polychromatophilic red cells are reticulo-cytes in which preliminary alcohol fixation has not permitted the precipitation of ribosomes with formation of the reticulum. On the other hand, not all reticulocytes are polychromato-philic with panoptic stains: this reaction only occurs with the most immature Heilmeyer class I and II reticulocytes. The polychromatophilic red cell count corresponds to a 'shift reticulo-cyte count'; this was proposed as a useful indicator of bone marrow response to anaemia (Crouch and Kaplow, 1985), analogous to the immature reticulocyte fraction recently obtained by flow cytometry. Macroreticulocytes produced during abrupt erythroid expansion are also characterized by the co-expression of adult and fetal haemoglobin (so-called F reticulocytes) (Blau et al., 1993; Nagel et al., 1993).

RETICULOCYTE DENSITY AND HAEMOGLOBIN CONCENTRATION

Reticulocytes are less dense than mature red cells. Reticulocytes from anaemic rabbits were estimated to have a density of 1.105 g/mL cells, compared with 1.122 g/mL cells for mature anaemic red cells (Lowenstein, 1959; Bosch et al., 1993). It was demonstrated that this difference largely depended on the lower haemoglobin concentration and higher water content of reticulocytes compared with mature red cells. It has been shown using an automated haematology analyser that the percentage of reticulocytes in a blood sample correlates with the percentage of hypochromic macrocytes (Bain and Cavill, 1993). The lower density of reticulocytes permits the recovery of enriched fractions of these cells from mature erythrocytes using centrifugation and density separation on Percoll columns (Leif and Vinograd, 1964; Murphy, 1973; Salvo et al., 1982; Bosch et al., 1993). A method for quantify-ing reticulocytes based on density medium fractionation and size assessment has been reported as more objective and precise than microscope reticulocyte counting (Burns et al., 1987).

5.5.2 Automated measurement of reticulocyte indices

Certain reticulocyte indices have recently emerged as automated measurements. With laser based technology, simultaneous measurement of volume and haemoglobin concentration is possible on red blood cells and reticulocytes (Brugnara et al., 1994a). Reticulocyte analysis is based on the measurement of scatter and absorption of helium-laser light by isovolumetrically sphered red cells. In the erythrocyte flow cell three detectors measure laser light scatter at low angle (2°–3°) and high angle (5°–15°) together with light absorption. Stained reticulocytes are separated from unstained red cells through an absorption threshold and their mean corpuscular volume (MCVr, in fL) and corpuscular haemoglobin concentration mean (CHCMr, in g/dL) are measured separately from MCV and CHCM of mature erythrocytes. Mean haemoglobin content of reticulocytes (CHr) and red blood cells (CH) are calculated from the product of the volume and haemoglobin concentration of single cells.

The measurement of reticulocyte indices has shown excellent precision both in normal subjects and in patients with reticulocytosis. In one reported study, coefficients of variation for MCVr, CHCMr and CHr were 0.8–1.6% after 21 repeated determinations (Brugnara *et al.*, 1994a). The MCVr remains stable up to 72 hours storage at 4°C, while CHr and CHCMr show a small but statistically significant decrease. Biological variability of automated reticulocyte indices is below 2% within subject, and below 4% between subjects (Sandberg *et al.*, 1998).

5.5.3 Reference values for reticulocyte indices

There are now several published studies concerning the unexplored area of reference intervals of reticulocyte indices in healthy subjects (Table 5.5). In all subjects the reticulocyte parameters showed a Gaussian distribution and no statistically significant difference between sexes. Average MCVr was 24% higher than the corresponding MCV of mature erythrocytes, while CHCMr was 16.7% lower. The MCVr/MCV ratio was on average 1.24. Similar reference values were obtained in other studies on adult normal subjects (Buttarello *et al.*, 1995; Chararuks *et al.*, 1998).

Reticulocyte indices were also measured in 110 paediatric outpatients (51 males and 59 females, aged 1–10 years) with normal haematological parameters according to the age-adjusted reference range (Brugnara *et al.*, 1994a). Paediatric reference values show good general agreement with those in adults; although the average volumes are lower, the MCVr/MCV ratio is again greater than 1 (1.24), the average CHCMr/CHCM ratio is lower than 1 (0.81) and the CHr/CH ratio is 0.96. Thus, in children, as in adults, reticulocytes have a larger volume, a reduced cell haemoglobin concentration and a similar haemoglobin content compared with mature red blood cells.

Measures of dispersion for the reticulocyte indices have also been reported (d'Onofrio *et al.*, 1995); the RDW of reticulocytes, expressed as the coefficient of variation of volumes, is on average very close to that of mature erythrocytes (14.3 vs. 14.0%), while the variability of haemoglobin concentration (HDW), expressed as the standard deviation, is greater in reticulocytes than in red cells (3.3 vs. 2.6 g/dL).

Reticulocyte and red blood cell indices have also been measured in anaemic patients with abnormalities of red cell size. The microcytic anaemia group included 58 patients with overt iron deficiency anaemia before iron treatment and 40 with heterozygous β-thalassaemia and no iron deficiency. The macrocytic anaemia group included 28 patients with anaemia of different aetiologies and MCV above 100 fL. In these subjects, the average values of reticulocyte indices showed the same relationship with erythrocyte indices as in healthy subjects (d'Onofrio *et al.*, 1995). Thus regardless of the final red blood cell size, reticulocytes appear consistently larger than their mature counterparts, whereas their haemoglobin concentration is consistently lower; as a consequence of these changes, haemoglobin content is almost the same. These results have been confirmed using different flow cytometric methods (Fourcade *et al.*, 1999). They are in surprisingly good agreement with the data obtained by planimetry (Killman 1964; Clarkson and Moore, 1976).

Finally, it must be noted that, although reticulocytes are capable of haemoglobin synthesis while in the bone marrow (Gavosto and Rechenman, 1954), their haemoglobin content does not change significantly after entry into the peripheral circulation.

Table 5.5 *Reference ranges (central 95% ranges) for reticulocyte indices reported by different authors*

MCVr (fL)	CHCMr (g/dL)	CHr (pg)	Fluorochrome/ stain	Number of subjects	Age	Reference
103.2–126.3	23.5–28.7	25.9–30.6	Oxazine 750	64	Adults	d'Onofrio *et al.* (1995)
92.4–120.2	26.7–33.0	27.1–33.9	Oxazine 750	133	Adults	Buttarello *et al.* (1995)
99.9–120.7 (M+F)	23.4–28.5 (M+F)	24.3–31.2 (M+F)	Oxazine 750	200	17–60	Charruruks *et al.* (1998)
98.3–120.6 (M)	23.7–28.7 (M)	24.5–31.1 (M)		100		
101.6–119.6 (F)	23.2–28.2 (F)	24.2–30.9 (F)		100		
100.0–125.0			New methylene blue (automated)	66	Adults	Fourcade *et al.* (1999)
88.2–107.0	25.4–31.0	23.5–29.9	Oxazine 750	110	1–10 years	Brugnara *et al.* (1994a)

MCVr, mean reticulocyte volume; CHCMr, corpuscular haemoglobin concentration mean; CHr, mean haemoglobin content of reticulocytes.

5.6 CLINICAL APPLICATIONS OF RETICULOCYTE MEASUREMENTS

The introduction in 1926 of liver extracts for the treatment of pernicious anaemia represented one of the most significant advances in clinical haematology, and reticulocyte counting occupied an important support role (Wintrobe, 1985). The reticulocyte count had already been defined as an indicator of erythropoiesis in patients with anaemia, in terms of amount, rate and efficacy of red cell production. Recently the reticulocyte count has, once more, assumed clinical prominence with the development of bone marrow/stem cell transplantation and erythropoietin (rhu-EPO) therapy.

The classic radioisotope study by Cline and Berlin (1963) determined that a reticulocyte count of 40×10^9/L represents an effective threshold level to distinguish anaemias associated with an effective erythropoietic response from those which are hypoproliferative in nature. At reticulocyte counts below 10×10^9/L, marked reduction of bone marrow erythropoiesis is certain. Increased reticulocyte counts are a consistent finding in anaemia associated with decreased red cell survival and increased red cell destruction or loss by haemorrhage, provided that effective erythropoietic function is preserved in the bone marrow.

The introduction of flow cytometry methods has resulted in realistic reticulocyte counting. In addition to improved precision, sensitive indicators of maturation have significantly extended the range of clinical applications. Increased sensitivity to minimal differences and the ability to measure RNA content as an indicator of reticulocyte maturation permit real-time assessment of small deviations of bone marrow erythropoietic activity. More recently, the flow cytometric determination of IRF and reticulocyte indices, such as volume and haemo-globin content, has extended such diagnostic potential.

In the last decade an increasing number of reports in the medical literature testify to the increasingly widespread usefulness of measurement of reticulocyte parameters in clinical haematology and internal medicine.

HAEMOLYTIC ANAEMIA

Reticulocytes are markedly increased in most haemolytic anaemias, the highest reticulocyte counts being seen in haemolytic crises in chronic hereditary haemolytic anaemias, e.g. red cell enzyme deficiency, immunohaemolytic anaemias or malaria infestation. In aplastic crisis, frequently caused by parvovirus B19 infection in chronic haemolytic anaemias, particularly hereditary spherocytosis and sickle cell disease, the sudden disappearance of reticulocytes is a very early sign (Rao *et al.*, 1996). B19 parvovirus infection is also implicated in aplastic episodes associated with reticulocytopenia, which occur in childhood acute leukaemia, other malignant diseases (Carstenen *et al.*, 1989; Yoto *et al.*, 1993) and HIV infection (Griffin *et al.*, 1991).

In haemolytic anaemia, the total reticulocyte count and the immature reticulocyte fraction are both increased (Fourcade *et al.*, 1999) as expression of the normal compensatory response of a hyperplastic and functional erythropoietic marrow to massive erythropoietin production due to acute peripheral red cell destruction. In haemolytic anaemia, there is an inverse correlation between reticulocyte count and haemoglobin concentration, similar to normal non-anaemic subjects (d'Onofrio *et al.*, 1996a), confirming the compensatory significance of reticulocytosis. An elevated reticulocyte count may also provide a clue to an unsuspected haemolytic state, e.g. haemolytic-uraemic syndrome associated with some anticancer drugs (Serke *et al.*, 1999) or toxic haemolysis caused by cis-platinum (Tanke *et al.*, 1986).

During haemolytic crises in G6PD-deficiency or chronic PK-deficiency, reticulocytes have a higher enzymatic activity than mature erythrocytes, and the reticulocyte count must be taken into account when assessing enzyme activity (Lakomek *et al.*, 1989).

POST-HAEMORRHAGIC ANAEMIA

Some degree of reticulocytosis is observed after significant blood loss due to acute or subacute haemorrhage. In anaemia due to chronic prolonged blood loss, reticulocyte counts tend to be normal or even low, reflecting the decreased erythropoietic function due to iron depletion.

MEGALOBLASTIC ANAEMIA

In typical megaloblastic anaemia due to vitamin B_{12} or folate deficiency, the reticulocyte count tends to be normal or decreased, with the immature reticulocyte fraction variably reported as decreased, normal or increased (Lin *et al.*, 1993). The so-called 'reticulocyte crisis' is the early, specific and consistent sign of erythropoietic response to vitamin B_{12} or folic acid administration. The massive and rapid increase in circulating reticulocytes reflects normoblastic transformation of erythroblasts in bone marrow. Using microscopy methods, the reticulocytosis was seen to occur after 4–6 days of treatment, reaching a peak of 20% after 8–10 days. The first reticulocytes to be released are almost all very immature stress macroreticulocytes (Heilmeyer classes I and II). Flow cytometry methods show a very early increase in immature reticulocytes with high RNA content, as early as 2–4 days from the start of therapy.

Reticulocyte indices also change in megaloblastic erythropoiesis. For example, administration of methotrexate, a potent inhibitor of dihydrofolate reductase, causes an abrupt and sustained increase in reticulocyte volume, often exceeding 140 fL, and specific replacement therapy induces a rapid normalization of reticulocyte size, without any early change in red cell MCV (Clarkson and Moore, 1976). Release into the peripheral blood of reticulocytes, which are smaller than the mature, pre-existing macrocytes, has been confirmed using automated flow cytometric methods (d'Onofrio *et al.*, 1995).

IRON DEFICIENCY

The total reticulocyte count is usually low to normal in untreated iron deficiency anaemia and provides very limited information for differential diagnostic purposes. Even here, however, interesting observations result from the indicators of reticulocyte maturation. In patients with iron deficiency anaemia, reticulocytes show increased fluorescence as compared with non-anaemic subjects, indicating increased amounts of cytoplasmic RNA (Wells *et al.*, 1992; Davis *et al.*, 1995). It should be possible to exploit this observation to differentiate between iron deficiency and anaemia of chronic disorders, e.g. rheumatoid arthritis, malignancies. It has also been found that the reticulocyte count and IRF are significantly lower in elderly subjects with iron deficiency anaemia than in middle-aged iron-deficient patients (Matsuo *et al.*, 1995).

Reticulocyte indices appear useful in iron deficiency anaemia, because the characteristics of reticulocytes released into the peripheral blood during the previous 24 hours represent an indicator of marrow erythropoietic activity. Using microscope planimetry, Clarkson and Moore (1976) demonstrated in experimentally induced iron deficiency that 2 days after the fall of the transferrin saturation, the mean reticulocyte volume diminished abruptly, preceding decrease of the red cell MCV by several weeks. With iron supplementation, the mean reticulocyte volume increases rapidly. Using flow cytometric methods, recent studies have shown that reticulocytes in patients with iron deficiency also have an abnormally low haemoglobin content, especially in children. A reduced CHr has been reported as the strongest predictor of iron deficiency in a group of 210 children with mean age of 2.9 years (Brugnara *et al.*, 1999); serum ferritin proved of little or no diagnostic value in this study.

In chronic haemodialysis patients, diagnosis of iron deficiency is difficult because of the frequent non-specific increase in serum ferritin. However, the diagnosis is critical and can predict the therapeutic efficiency of the most effective and expensive anti-anaemic treatment, i.e. rhu-EPO. In adult haemodialysis patients, reports have suggested that a decreased CHr, i.e. < 26 pg, predicts depletion of iron stores with higher sensitivity and specificity than serum ferritin, transferrin saturation or the percentage of hypochromic red cells (Fishbane *et al.*, 1997; Bhandari *et al.*, 1998; Cullen *et al.*, 1999; Giacomini *et al.*, 1999; Schaefer and Schaefer, 1999).

Response to iron administration in iron deficiency anaemia is characterized by a prompt and sustained increase in reticulocyte count with a peak reticulocytosis of 10–15% by 8–10 days. The mean reticulocyte volume increases rapidly in the phlebotomized iron-deficient subjects (Clarkson and Moore, 1976). Flow cytometric studies have demonstrated that the response to iron administration is associated, within 1–2 weeks, with an increase of the absolute reticulocyte count (pretreatment mean value of 65×10^9/L increasing to 130×10^9/L) and of the CHr (pretreatment mean value of 18.1 pg increasing to 23.4 pg), the RBC indices remaining unchanged (Brugnara *et al.*, 1994c, 1998; Ashenden *et al.*, 1998). Persistence of low CHr values identifies patients not responding to oral iron administration and who may require intravenous iron. In a study on uraemic patients, the mean CHr increased rapidly within 2 days of administration of intravenous iron (Fishbane *et al.*, 1997).

INFLAMMATORY PROCESSES

In patients with chronic inflammatory disease, reticulocyte count and serum erythropoietin levels are lower than expected for the degree of anaemia (Souweine *et al.*, 1995).

THALASSAEMIA SYNDROMES

In subjects with heterozygous β-thalassaemia, the reticulocyte count is moderately increased and is inversely correlated with haemoglobin concentration (Paterakis *et al.*, 1991). This might aid in discriminating microcytic anaemias; reticulocyte counts are usually lower in iron deficiency than in heterozygous β-thalassaemia, although threshold levels and sensitivity/specificity patterns have not yet been defined. Patients with thalassaemia inter-media and major usually show higher reticulocyte counts and IRF, reflecting extreme marrow erythroid hyperplasia and ineffective erythropoiesis. Reticulocyte counts are even higher after splenectomy (Khuhapinant *et al.*, 1994). The presence of inclusion bodies in HbH disease has been shown to cause interference with some automated methods for reticulocyte counting (Lai *et al.*, 1999).

SICKLE CELL ANAEMIA

Reticulocytes are increased in homozygous sickle cell disease. A reticulocyte count higher than 2% has been suggested as a sensitive discriminator between heterozygous sickle cell trait and homozygous sickle cell anaemia (Losek *et al.*, 1992). Automated methods can be used to identify the proportion of dehydrated hyperdense reticulocytes with CHCMr > 38 g/dL (Mohandas, 1993). The administration of hydroxyurea to induce fetal haemoglobin synthesis results in a decrease or disappearance of these hyperdense reticulocytes. Oral magnesium supplements in patients with sickle cell disease has a similar effect (De Franceschi *et al.*, 1997) and reduces reticulocyte volume distribution width (RDWr) and haemoglobin distribution width (HDWr).

RENAL FAILURE ANAEMIA

In anaemic patients with chronic renal failure and uraemia, the reticulocyte count and IRF are both moderately decreased and show a direct relationship with plasma levels of erythropoietin (Kendall *et al.* 1993; Chang and Kass, 1997). Mean reticulocyte volumes tend to be higher in patients with end-stage renal disease treated with haemodialysis, while their reticulocyte haemoglobin concentration tends to be lower (Giacomini *et al.*, 1999). The reticulocyte/red cell volume ratio is > 1 in uraemic patients. In these patients the determination of reticulocyte indices is useful to monitor iron status and response to rhu-EPO.

PREDICTION OF ERYTHROPOIESIS IN RENAL TRANSPLANT

The increase in plasma erythropoietin levels which follows successful kidney transplantation is associated with a significant increase in IRF, and precedes, by several days, the subsequent increase in the reticulocyte count. These changes represent an early, sensitive predictor of erythropoietic improvement following renal transplantation (Serre *et al.*, 1994; Moulin *et al.*, 1995). The simultaneous measurement of serum EPO and immature reticulocytes also allows separation of poor graft function (with low EPO and low IRF) from other causes of decreased erythropoiesis with elevated EPO and low IRF, e.g. iron deficiency, inflammation, aluminium intoxication, hyperparathyroidism (Moulin *et al.*, 1995).

MYELODYSPLASTIC SYNDROMES (MDS)

Reticulocytopenia with a low reticulocyte production index has been reported in MDS (Cazzola *et al.*, 1987). Using flow cytometry, the reticulocyte count is normal or low, regardless of the haemoglobin concentration, while the percentage of highly fluorescent reticulocytes (variously reported as HFR or IRF) is increased (Daliphard *et al.*, 1993; Tsuda and Tatsumi, 1989; Watanabe *et al.*, 1994; d'Onofrio *et al.*, 1996a). This pattern appears to be typical of MDS. Among the different types of MDS, the absolute reticulocyte count is lower in refractory anaemia with ringed sideroblasts (Bowen *et al.*, 1996). The IRF correlates inversely with haemoglobin (d'Onofrio *et al.*, 1996a) and is directly proportional to plasma erythropoietin concentration (Bowen *et al.*, 1994). Therefore when there is an ineffective erythropoietic response to anaemia, reticulocyte counts are lower than normal and the inverse correlation with the severity of anaemia is lost, but there is an increased output of early, RNA-rich reticulocytes reflecting the intensity of erythropoietin stimulation on an ineffective bone marrow. Reticulocyte size (MCVr) is larger in patients with MDS than in normal subjects, corresponding to the average larger MCV of mature red cells (Bowen *et al.*, 1996).

Serial reticulocyte and IRF measurements monitor the effect of treatment in MDS, e.g. rh-EPO administration (Musto *et al.*, 1994). Reticulocyte responses have also been reported in some MDS patients during treatment with G-CSF (Nagler *et al.*, 1995).

In occasional MDS patients, a marked, persistent increase in reticulocyte count has been described in the absence of a corresponding increased erythrocyte turnover: this results from persistence of RNA in circulating red blood cells due to defective degradation (Tulliez *et al.*, 1982; Lofters *et al.*, 1987; Hertenstein *et al.*, 1993; Sher *et al.*, 1994; de Pree *et al.*, 1995; Garulli *et al.*, 1998). This pseudoreticulocytosis can mimic other causes of increased reticulocyte production.

ACUTE LEUKAEMIA

In untreated acute leukaemia, the reticulocyte count tends to be slightly lower than normal and the IRF is increased (d'Onofrio *et al.*, 1996a); a normal reticulocyte count with high IRF has, however, also been described (Lin *et al.*, 1993).

APLASTIC ANAEMIA

In primary aplastic anaemia, reticulocyte counts are usually very low (Lin *et al.*, 1993). The IRF is usually low as well, but can occasionally be normal or slightly increased (Tsuda and Tatsumi, 1989; Watanabe *et al.*, 1994; Lin *et al.*, 1993).

CHRONIC MYELOPROLIFERATIVE DISEASES

The reticulocyte count and IRF are moderately increased in myelofibrosis. A similar pattern is found in primary polycythaemia and there is a direct correlation with haemoglobin concentration (d'Onofrio *et al.*, 1996b). This accords with the presence of autonomous rather than compensatory increase in erythropoietic activity.

PAROXYSMAL NOCTURNAL HAEMOGLOBINURIA (PNH)

Reticulocyte counts and IRF are moderately increased in PNH (Watanabe *et al.*, 1994), due to intravascular haemolysis resulting from an acquired membrane protein defect. However, PNH reticulocytes are more susceptible to acid haemolysis *in vitro* and are destroyed more rapidly *in vivo* than older red cells (Kan and Gardner, 1965).

ANAEMIA OF PREMATURITY

Reference values for total reticulocyte count and different maturity fractions in neonates have been published (Bock and Herkner, 1994a). Flow cytometric reticulocyte maturity analysis is useful to follow erythropoietic change in anaemic newborns (Bock and Herkner, 1994b; Newman and Easterling, 1994; Herkner, 1996), to monitor response to rhu-EPO therapy (Ohls *et al.*, 1995) and to gauge transfusion needs. The percentage of the most immature reticulocytes shows a direct correlation with the haemoglobin concentration in anaemic neonates (Kakuya *et al.*, 1991).

EXERCISE AND SPORT

Recent reports have demonstrated a significant increase in reticulocyte counts in the anaemia which develops during intense training in long-distance runners (Dressendorfer *et al.*, 1991). This anaemia can be prevented by wearing cushioned shoes (Dressendorfer *et al.*, 1992), indicating that a probable microhaemolytic process coexists with the known dilutional pseudo-anaemia of athletes caused by increased plasma volume. Fitness-type exercising also increases the reticulocyte count in young females (Kondo *et al.*, 1995), demonstrating an independent facilitating effect on erythropoiesis. There is growing interest in using reticulocyte parameters to detect illegal use of rhu-EPO in athletes (Audran *et al.*, 1999; Parisotto *et al.*, 2000).

CHEMOTHERAPY

The behaviour of reticulocytes and their immature fractions during cytotoxic therapy is a further example of clinical utility, particularly in the low range of counts. It is well known that the first indicator of bone marrow regeneration following aplasia caused by anti-neoplastic cytotoxic chemotherapy is the reappearance of reticulocytes with increased RNA content (Kuse, 1993; Lesesve *et al.*, 1995). Early recovery can be detected when the reticulocyte count remains very low (Kuse *et al.*, 1996). With some cytotoxic drugs, e.g. cis-platinum, a small increase in reticulocyte count may unmask a toxic, haemolytic effect producing anaemia (Tanke *et al.*, 1986).

HAEMOPOIETIC PROGENITOR CELL TRANSPLANTATION

Monitoring the success of haemopoietic progenitor cell (HPC) transplantation is based on sequential peripheral blood cell counts. Initially the earliest practical measure to detect engraftment was the absolute neutrophil count; the visual reticulocyte count was too imprecise (Thomas *et al.*, 1972).

More recently several reports have demonstrated that serial flow cytometric reticulocyte counts provide an early and accurate index of engraftment (Lazarus *et al.*, 1992), especially if the youngest and most RNA-rich reticulocytes are quantified (Davis *et al.*, 1989, 1992; Vannucchi *et al.*, 1992; Kanold *et al.*, 1993; Greinix *et al.*, 1994; Spanish Multicentric Study Group for Hematopoietic Recovery, 1994; Dalal *et al.*, 1996; d'Onofrio *et al.*, 1996b; Grotto *et al.*, 1999). The majority of these reports show that IRF, regardless of the method of measurement used, is the earliest indicator of engraftment. The characteristics of haematopoietic recovery vary according to the type of HPC transplantation. Peripheral blood HPC transplantation is universally characterized by the fastest recovery of reticulocytes and IRF, as well as neutrophil and platelet counts (Santamaria *et al.*, 1997; Testa *et al.*, 1997; Sica *et al.*, 1998). The IRF starts to rise less than 2 weeks after HPC infusion. A rapid decline of reticulocyte number thereafter has been reported as a useful predictor of early graft failure in non-HLA-identical bone marrow transplantation in children (Gerritsen *et al.*, 1996), allowing early immunosuppressive intervention with higher probability of success.

Reticulocyte counts after HPC transplant correlate inversely with serum erythropoietin and the observed to expected serum erythropoietin level (Davies *et al.*, 1995).

During the follow-up of transplant patients, significant changes in measurable reticulocyte indices, namely MCVr and the MCVr/MCV ratio, occur (d'Onofrio *et al.*, 1995). After conditioning chemotherapy, a marked decrease in reticulocyte number occurs. This is associated with progressive decrease in MCVr and transitory inversion of the MCVr/MCV ratio. Erythroid regeneration, on the other hand, is heralded by an abrupt increase of MCVr, to values above normal.

Reticulocytes persist during refrigerated storage and are detectable in the circulation of most recipients after transfusion (Perry *et al.*, 1996). Therefore, when flow-cytometric measurements are carried out at subnormal reticulocyte counts, such as during the aplastic phase which precedes HPC transplant engraftment, transfused reticulocytes may contribute to the overall picture (Ortola *et al.*, 1993).

STEM CELL COLLECTION

According to recent reports, the IRF is significantly increased in peripheral blood during HPC mobilization, and precedes the presence of circulating CD34+ cells by about 2 days in patients treated with chemotherapy and G-CSF (Remacha *et al.*, 1996) or G-CSF alone (Gonzalez *et al.*, 1996). Moreover, the IRF shows a linear correlation with CD34+ cells and with the colony-forming units mixed (CFU-Mix) counts in peripheral blood (Mougi *et al.*, 1997). Thus the IRF can be used as an indirect marker for timing stem cell harvesting.

MONITORING EFFECTIVENESS OF THERAPEUTIC USE OF HUMAN RECOMBINANT ERYTHROPOIETIN (RHU-EPO)

The use of rhu-EPO has grown rapidly in recent years, particularly in the treatment of anaemias associated with low endogenous erythropoietin production. Because of high cost and possible refractoriness to rhu-EPO, sensitive laboratory methods are needed for early assessment of response to therapy. In most patients, measurement of reticulocyte parameters may provide this (Goodnough *et al.*, 2000).

The earliest response to erythropoietin administration in mice is a shift of young reticulocytes from the marrow to the peripheral blood (Himmelfarb *et al.*, 1995). This response is dose-related and can be detected within 12–24 hours of a single dose of erythropoietin and before the total number of reticulocytes has increased significantly. The immaturity of these 'shift' reticulocytes is confirmed by their increased fluorescence with thiazole orange (due to high RNA content) and by the presence on their membrane of the CD71 antigen, i.e. cell surface transferrin receptor (Himmelfarb *et al.*, 1995). In normal human volunteers, rhu-EPO produces a characteristic sequence of events (Major *et al.*, 1994; Breymann *et al.*, 1996). The initial response, within 12 hours of intravenous administration, is a significant increase in the proportion of young RNA-rich reticulocytes in the circulation, probably reflecting the premature release of pre-existing immature reticulocytes from the bone marrow. At this stage there is no noticeable increase in the total reticulocyte count; this follows 2 or 3 days later. Reticulocyte indices of haematologically healthy subjects consistently show significant change after even a single dose of subcutaneous rhu-EPO (Brugnara *et al.*, 1994b). Reticulocytes produced after rhu-EPO have a larger volume, decreased haemoglobin concentration and also a significant decrease in haemoglobin content (CHr). These changes become evident after 5–13 days, depending on the dose and schedule of administration (Breymann *et al.*, 1996). Similar changes were observed preoperatively in non-anaemic patients undergoing elective cardiac surgery treated with high-dose rhu-EPO intravenously to reduce blood transfusion needs (Sowade *et al.*, 1997). During the first week of treatment, parallel increases in the fraction of the most immature reticulocytes, in the reticulocyte mean volume and in the reticulocyte distribution width (rRDW) occurred associated with a decrease in reticulocyte haemoglobin concentration. During the second week the reticulocyte mean haemoglobin content (CHr) decreased, independently of all iron parameters (Sowade *et al.*, 1997; Sowade *et al.*, 1998). The increase in the percentage of hypochromic reticulocytes, i.e. cells with CHr < 23 pg, was associated with a decrease in transferrin saturation even in the presence of normal iron stores. This was considered an early sign of functionally iron-deficient erythropoiesis (Brugnara *et al.*, 1994c). This hypothesis, however, does not fully explain the initial simultaneous increase in reticulocyte volume reported by the same authors.

The ability to predict rhu-EPO responsiveness is an important economic and clinical issue, especially in patients with chronic renal failure on dialysis. In patients with chronic renal disease, the treatment of anaemia with rhu-EPO initially induces an increase in the reticulocyte count and mean fluorescence with thiazole orange (Zachée *et al.*, 1992). The increase in immature reticulocytes after a single dose of rhu-EPO in uraemic subjects was proposed as an early biological test of sensitivity (Tatsumi *et al.*, 1990). The reticulocyte count, by flow cytometry, increases within 1 week of treatment with rhu-EPO (Beguin *et al.*, 1995), reflecting a sudden output of shift reticulocytes into the bloodstream. After this early response the reticulocyte count levels off.

The capability of the IRF to indicate within a few days those patients adequately responding to rhu-EPO has been confirmed (Kendall *et al.*, 1993; Pradella *et al.*, 1996). Moreover, total absolute reticulocyte counts and serum transferrin (TfR) levels have been reported to increase significantly over baseline in patients who are going to respond with an improvement of their haemoglobin concentration to an increased rhu-EPO dosage (Ahluwalia *et al.*, 1997). The sensitivity of the association of > 20% increase in serum TfR and absolute reticulocyte count was 92% in this study. In a few patients with end-stage renal failure treated with rhu-EPO, however, the haemoglobin level may not increase despite a brisk reticulocyte response. Gastrointestinal blood loss has been consistently found in this group (Jeffrey *et al.*, 1995).

The administration of rhu-EPO can be useful in some hyporegenerative anaemias not associated with renal failure. In these cases the proportion of responders is smaller, so that serial monitoring of reticulocyte count and related parameters can be a valuable tool to distinguish responders from non-responders at an early stage.

Monitoring by reticulocyte count and IRF has also been described during treatment with rhu-EPO in premature babies (Ohls *et al.*, 1995; Bader *et al.*, 1996; Meister *et al.*, 1998). In myelodysplastic syndromes an early increase in the most fluorescent young reticulocytes was shown as an early specific and consistent event only in the minority of patients who subsequently showed a significant clinical response to rhu-EPO (Musto *et al.*, 1994). In anaemic cancer patients, an early increase in reticulocyte count ($> 40 \times 10^9$/L) from baseline predicts responsiveness to rhu-EPO after 2–4 weeks, especially when associated with an increase in haemoglobin level by > 10.0 g/L (Henry *et al.*, 1995). Simple predictive algorithms based on the reticulocyte count have been proposed (Cazzola *et al.*, 1996, 1997).

Accelerated erythropoiesis during treatment with rhu-EPO may cause functional iron deficiency in subjects with normal iron stores, since rhu-EPO stimulates erythroid proliferation and differentiation to such an extent that demand for iron exceeds the body's ability to release it from stores. Functional iron deficiency is one of the most common causes of poor response to rhu-EPO administration. It can be detected in uraemic patients by monitoring transferrin saturation or the percentage of hypochromic red blood cells (Macdougall *et al.*, 1992; Macdougall, 1995a,b). More recently, reticulocyte measurements have shown excellent sensitivity and specificity as indicators of functional iron deficiency under rhu-EPO administration (Brugnara, 1998; d'Onofrio *et al.*, 1998). Functional iron deficiency can be observed even when rhu-EPO is administered to non-anaemic subjects, such as normal subjects undergoing multiple blood donations for autotransfusion schedules (Brugnara *et al.*, 1993a).

Besides increased reticulocyte volume and decreased haemoglobin concentration, which are typical features of acute erythropoietic response to rhu-EPO (Breymann *et al.*, 1996), the measurement of CHr seems to represent the most sensitive and specific indicator of functional iron deficiency; in particular, the percentage of reticulocytes with CHr < 23 pg is an effective indicator of iron-deficient erythropoiesis and is inversely correlated with the log value of baseline serum ferritin (Brugnara *et al.*, 1994b; Mittman *et al.*, 1997).

Reticulocytosis and reticulocyte haemoglobin content can be increased by the administration of intravenous iron saccharate to healthy volunteers, autologous blood donors or patients with renal failure receiving rhu-EPO (Mercuriali *et al.*, 1993). The flow cytometric study of reticulocyte indices (especially CHr) in such cases provides a method of evaluating erythropoietic response to iron and rhu-EPO administration (Major *et al.*, 1997; Bhandari *et al.*, 1998; Cullen *et al.*, 1999; Schaefer and Schaefer, 1999). In patients with functional iron deficiency under rhu-EPO, the mean CHr has been shown to increase rapidly after the administration of intravenous iron (Fishbane *et al.*, 1997).

Functional iron deficiency may also develop as a consequence of increased endogenous erythropoietin production, e.g. in immunohaemolytic anaemia. In these cases, a sudden and unexpected fall of reticulocyte count associated with the production of small reticulocytes with reduced mean corpuscular volume can be the first manifestation (d'Onofrio *et al.*, 1995).

The measurement of IRF and reticulocyte indices thus seems very useful to assess response to rhu-EPO. Their value in comparison or in association with new effective methods for measuring erythropoietic activity, such as the determination of plasma soluble transferrin receptor (Cazzola *et al.*, 1996), needs to be studied further.

MISCELLANEOUS

A number of recent reports point out potential new applications of sensitive and accurate reticulocyte parameters. Splenectomy, shock and other conditions characterized by acute hypoxaemia induce a mild and transitory reticulocytosis. Higher levels of circulating reticulocytes have been found in workers exposed to solvents (Cardoso *et al.*, 1999). A moderate reticulocyte increase, with increased IRF indicating erythropoietic stimulation, takes place at the beginning of the postpartum period (Richter *et al.*, 1995). Lower reticulocyte counts without changes in reticulocyte subgroups have been reported in the cord blood of neonates of mothers who smoke (Marcelina-Roumans *et al.*, 1996). Acclimatization to high altitude is associated with a significant increase in reticulocytes and plasma erythropoietin when compared with sea-level values (Savourey *et al.*, 1996). A significantly increased number of reticulocytes has been reported in subjects with major depression (Maes *et al.*, 1996). In patients with chronic inflammatory disease, reticulocyte count and serum EPO are lower than expected for the degree of anaemia.

BIVARIATE PLOTTING OF RETICULOCYTE COUNT VERSUS IRF

The characteristics of erythropoiesis in different types of anaemia can effectively be appreciated by simultaneously assessing reticulocyte count and IRF. The absolute reticulocyte count, in fact, is an indicator of the efficiency of erythrocyte production (Cline and Berlin, 1963; Cazzola and Beguin, 1992), while the IRF more closely reflects the presence of immature reticulocytes prematurely released from bone marrow following intense erythropoietinic stimulation (d'Onofrio et al., 1996c). A graphical representation in the form of a bivariate plot (Fig. 5.4) reveals specific erythropoietic patterns in different haemopoietic disorders and provides a useful means for anaemia classification (Davis *et al.*, 1993; Davis, 1996, 1997; d'Onofrio *et al.*, 1996c; Kim *et al.*, 1997).

Thus a simultaneous increase in reticulocyte count and IRF, as occurs in acute haemolytic anaemias, reflects the compensatory response of a normally functional marrow to massive erythropoietin stimulation, while in hyporegenerative anaemia, as in uraemia, both reticulocyte count and IRF are simultaneously decreased owing to depressed erythropoietin

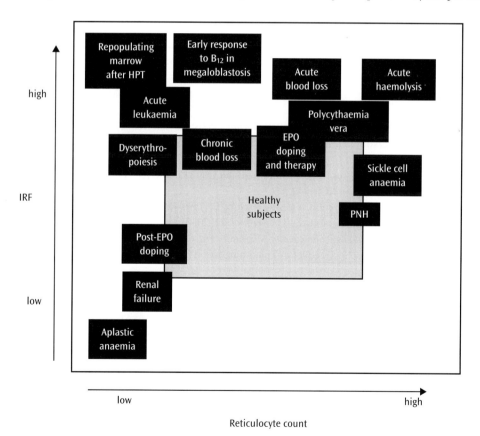

Fig. 5.4 *Bivariate plotting of reticulocyte count versus immature reticulocyte fraction (IRF): specific erythropoietic patterns in different haematopoietic disorders. HPT, haemopoietic progenitor cell transplant; PNH, paroxysmal nocturnal haemoglobinuria.*

production. In myelodysplastic syndromes and dyserythropoietic anaemia, on the other hand, the reticulocyte count is not increased and IRF tends to be high, the typical pattern of ineffective erythropoiesis.

REFERENCES

Ahluwalia, N., Skikne, B.S., Savin, V. and Chonko, A. (1997) Markers of masked iron deficiency and effectiveness of EPO therapy in chronic renal failure. *Am. J. Kidney Dis.* **30**, 532–41.

Ashenden, M.J., Dobson, P.J. and Hahn, A.G. (1998) Sensitivity of reticulocyte indices to iron therapy in an intensely training athlete. *Br. J. Sports Med.* **32**, 259–60.

Astaldi, G. and Bernardelli, L. (1946) La maturazione dei reticolociti. *Boll. Soc. It. Biol. Sper.* **22**, 1165–79.

Audran, M., Gareau, R., Matecki, S. *et al.* (1999) Effects of erythropoietin administration in training athletes and possible indirect detection in doping control. *Med. Sci. Sports Exerc.* **31**, 639–45.

Bader, D., Blondheim, O., Jonas, R. *et al.* (1996) Decreased ferritin levels, despite iron supplementation, during erythropoietin therapy in anaemia of prematurity. *Acta Paediatr.* **85**, 496–501.

Bain, B. and Cavill, I.A.J. (1993) Hypochromic macrocytes: are they reticulocytes? *J. Clin. Pathol.* **46,** 963–64.

Baldini, M. and Panacciulli, I. (1960) The maturation rate of reticulocytes. *Blood* **15**, 614–29.

Bartels, P.C.M., van Houte, A.J. and Schoorl, M. (1993) Discrepancies in current automated methods for reticulocyte enumeration. *Sysmex J. Int.* **3**, 75–9.

Beguin, Y., Loo, M., R'Zik, S., Sautois, B. *et al.* (1995) Quantitative assessment of erythropoiesis in haemodialysis patients demonstrates gradual expansion of erythroblasts during constant treatment with recombinant human erythropoietin. *Br. J. Haematol.* **89**, 17–23.

Belfiore, P., Moscarelli, G., Virzi, G. *et al.* (1993) Magnesio ed eritropoiesi in gravidanza. *Giorn. It. Ost. Gin.* **4,** 549–50.

Bessis, M. (1972) *Cellules du Sang Normal et Pathologique.* Paris: Masson, 166–278.

Bessman, J.D. (1977) Erythropoiesis during recovery from iron deficiency: normocytes and macrocytes. *Blood* **50**, 987–93.

Betke, K. and Rodig, I. (1955) Zur Frage des Volumens der vital-granulierten Erythrocyten (Reticulocyten). *Klin. Wschr.* **33**, 911–2.

Bhandari, S., Turney, J.H., Brownjohn, A.M. and Norfolk, D. (1998) Reticulocyte indices in patients with end stage renal disease on hemodialysis. *J. Nephrol.* **11**, 78–82.

Bick, R.L. (ed.) (1993) *Hematology: Clinical and Laboratory Practice.* St Louis: Mosby.

Bigelow, N. and Davis, B.H. (1995) Leukocyte contamination in flow cytometric reticulocyte analysis. *Lab. Hematol.* **1**, 71–5.

Blau, A.C., Constantoulakis, P., Al-Khatti, A. *et al.* (1993) Fetal hemoglobin in acute and chronic states of erythroid expansion. *Blood* **81**, 227–33.

Bock, A. and Herkner, K.R. (1994a) Reticulocyte maturity pattern analysis as a predictive marker of erythropoiesis in paediatrics. Part I: evaluation of age-dependent reference values. *Clin. Lab. Haematol.* **16**, 247–51.

Bock, A. and Herkner, K.R. (1994b) Reticulocyte maturity pattern analysis as a predictive marker of erythropoiesis in paediatrics. Part II: pilot study for clinical applications. *Clin. Lab. Haematol.* **16**, 343–8.

Bosch, F.H., Were, J.M., Roerdinkholder-Stoelwinder, B. *et al.* (1993) Young red blood cells; observations about the cytometry and morphologic alterations in the beginning of their life. *Clin. Lab. Haematol.* **15**, 265–74.

Bowen, D., Bentley, N., Hoy, T. and Cavill, I. (1991) Comparison of a modified thiazole orange technique with a fully automated analyser for reticulocyte counting. *J. Clin. Pathol.* **44**, 130–3.

Bowen, D.T., Culligan, D., Beguin, Y. *et al.* (1994) Estimation of effective and total erythropoiesis in myelodysplasia using serum transferrin receptor and erythropoietin concentrations, with automated reticulocyte parameters. *Leukemia* **8**, 151–5.

Bowen, D., Williams, K., Phillips, I. and Cavill, I. (1996) Cytometric analysis and maturation characteristics of reticulocytes from myelodysplastic patients. *Clin. Lab. Haematol.* **18**, 155–60.

Brecher, G. (1949) New methylene blue as a reticulocyte stain. *Am. J. Clin. Pathol.* **19**, 895–903.

Brecher, G. and Stohlman, F. (1961) Reticulocyte size and erythropoietic stimulation. *Proc. Soc. Exp. Biol. Med.* **107**, 887–91.

Brecher, G. and Stohlman, F. (1962) The macrocytic response to erythropoietin stimulation. In: Jacobson, L. and Doyle, M. (eds), *Erythropoiesis*. New York: Grune and Stratton, 216.

Brecher, G., Schneidermann, M. and William, G.Z. (1950) A time saving device for counting reticulocytes. *Am. J. Clin. Pathol.* **20**, 1079–84.

Breymann, C., Bauer, C., Major, A. *et al.* (1996) Optimal timing of repeated rh-erythropoietin administration improves its effectiveness in stimulating erythropoiesis in healthy volunteers. *Br. J. Haematol.* **93**, 295–301.

Browne, P.V. and Hebbel, R.P. (1996) CD36-positive stress reticulocytosis in sickle cell anemia. *J. Lab. Clin. Med.* **127**, 340–7.

Brugnara, C. (1998) Use of reticulocyte cellular indices in the diagnosis and treatment of hematological disorders. *Int. J. Clin. Lab. Res.* **28**, 1–11.

Brugnara, C., Chambers, L.A., Malynn, E. *et al.* (1993a) Red cell regeneration induced by subcutaneous recombinant erythropoietin: iron-deficient erythropoiesis in iron-replete subjects. *Blood* **81**, 956–64.

Brugnara, C., Kruskall, M.S. and Johnston, R.M. (1993b) Membrane properties of erythrocytes in subjects undergoing multiple blood donations with or without recombinant erythropoietin. *Br. J. Haematol.* **84**, 118–30.

Brugnara, C., Hipp, M.J., Irving, P.J. *et al.* (1994a) Automated reticulocyte counting and measurement of reticulocyte cellular indices. Evaluation of the Miles H*3 blood analyzer. *Am. J. Clin. Pathol.* **102**, 623–32.

Brugnara, C., Colella, G.M., Cremins, J.C. *et al.* (1994b) Effects of subcutaneous recombinant human erythropoietin in normal subjects: development of decreased reticulocyte hemoglobin content and iron-deficient erythropoiesis. *J. Lab. Clin. Med.* **123**, 660–667.

Brugnara, C., Laufer, M.R., Friedman, A.J. *et al.* (1994c) Reticulocyte hemoglobin content (CHr): early indicator of iron deficiency and response to therapy. *Blood* **83**, 3100.

Brugnara, C., Zurakowski, D., DiCanzio, J., Boyd, T. and Platt, O. (1999) Reticulocyte hemoglobin content to diagnose iron deficiency in children. *J. Am. Med. Assoc.* **281**, 2225–30.

Burns, E.R., Goldberg, S.N. and Wenz, B. (1987) A new assay for quantifying human reticulocytes. *Am. J. Clin. Pathol.* **88**, 338–42.

Buttarello, M., Bulian, P., Farina, G. *et al.* (1999) Immature reticulocyte fraction (IRF): reference intervals obtained with different automated analysers (Abstract). *Proceedings of the XLIX National Congress of the Italian Association of Clinical Pathologists*, p. 19.

Buttarello, M., Bulian, P., Pra, M.D. *et al.* (1996) Reticulocyte quantification by Coulter MAXM VCS (volume, conductivity, light scatter) technology. *Clin. Chem.* **42**, 1930–7.

Buttarello, M., Bulian, P., Venudo, A. and Rizzotti, P. (1995) Laboratory evaluation of the Miles H.3 automated reticulocyte counter. A comparative study with manual reference method and Sysmex R-1000. *Arch. Pathol. Lab. Med.* **119**, 1141–8.

Cardoso, E., Cazenave, J.P., Schoch, H. *et al.* (1999) Reticulocytes and solvents: an epidemiological study. *Hematol. Cell. Ther.* **41**, 39–45.

Carstensen, H., Ornvold, K. and Cohen, B.J. (1989) Human parvovirus B19 infection associated with prolonged erythroblastopenia in a leukemic child. *Ped. Infect. Dis. J.* **8**, 56.

Carter, J.M., McSweeney, P.A., Wakem, P.J. and Nemet, A.M. (1989) Counting reticulocytes by flow cytometry: use of thiazole orange. *Clin. Lab. Haematol.* **89**, 267–71.

Castriota-Scandenberg, A., Pedrazzi, G., Mercadanti, M. *et al.* (1992) Normal values of total reticulocytes and reticulocyte subsets in children and young adults. *Haematologica* **77**, 363–4.

Cavill, I. (1993a) The rejected reticulocyte. *Br. J. Haematol.* **84**, 563–5.

Cavill, I. (1993b) Performance characteristics of the H*3 and comparison with the R-1000 reticulocyte counter. In: *Conference Proceedings 'H*3: New Perspectives for Hematology*. Tarrytown, USA: Bayer Diagnostics.

Cavill, I., Kraaijenhagen, R., Pradella, M. *et al.* (1996) In vitro stability of the reticulocyte count. *Clin. Lab. Haematol.* **18**(Suppl. 1), 9–11.

Cazzola, M. and Beguin, Y. (1992) New tools for clinical evaluation of erythron function in man. *Br. J. Haematol.* **80**, 278–84.

Cazzola, M., Mercuriali, F. and Brugnara, C. (1997) Use of recombinant human erythropoietin outside the setting of uremia. *Blood* **89**, 4248–67.

Cazzola, M., Ponchio, L., Pedrotti, C. *et al.* (1996) Prediction of response to recombinant human erythropoietin (rHuEpo) in anemia of malignancy. *Haematologica* **81**, 434–41.

Cazzola, M., Pootrakul, P., Heubers, H.A. *et al.* (1987) Erythroid marrow function in anaemic patients. *Blood* **69**, 96–101.

Chanarin, I. (ed.) (1989) *Laboratory Hematology*. Edinburgh: Churchill Livingstone, 15–16.

Chang, C. and Kass L. (1997) Clinical significance of immature reticulocyte fraction determined by automated reticulocyte counting. *Am. J. Clin. Pathol.* **108**, 69–73.

Charuruks, N., Limpanasithikul, W., Voravud, N. *et al.* (1998) Reference ranges of reticulocytes in adults. *J. Med. Assoc. Thai.* **81**, 356–64.

Chasis J.A., Prenant, M., Leung A. and Mohandas, N. (1989) Membrane assembly and remodeling during reticulocyte maturation. *Blood* **74**, 1112–20.

Chin-Yee, I., Keeney, M. and Lohmann, R.C. (1991) Flow cytometric reticulocyte analysis using thiazole orange; clinical experience and technical limitations. *Clin. Lab. Haematol.* **13**, 177–88.

Clarkson, D.R. and Moore, E.M. (1976) Reticulocyte size in nutritional anemias. *Blood* **48**, 669–77.

Cline, J.M. and Berlin, N.I. (1963) The reticulocyte count as an indicator of the rate of erythropoiesis. *Am. J. Clin. Pathol.* **39**, 121–7.

Coulombel, L., Tchernia, G. and Mohandas, N. (1979) Human reticulocyte maturation and its relevance to erythropoietic stress. *J. Lab. Clin. Med.* **94**, 467–74.

Crosby, W.H. (1981) Reticulocyte counts. *Arch. Intern. Med.* **141**, 1747–8.

Crouch, J.Y. and Kaplow, L.S. (1985) Relationship of reticulocyte age to polychromasia, shift cells, and shift reticulocytes. *Arch. Pathol. Lab. Med.* **109**, 325–9.

Cullen, P., Soffker, J., Hopfl, M. *et al.* (1999) Hypochromic red cells and reticulocyte haemoglobin content as markers of iron-deficient erythropoiesis in patients undergoing chronic haemodialysis. *Nephrol. Dial. Transplant* **14**, 659–65.

Dacie, J.V. and Lewis, S.M. (1995) *Practical Haematology*, 8th edn. Edinburgh: Churchill Livingstone, 65–8.

Dalal, B.I., Stockford, G.R., Naiman, S.C. *et al.* (1996) Criteria for marrow engraftment: comparison of reticulocyte maturity index with conventional parameters. *Bone Marrow Transplant* **17**, 91–2.

Daliphard, S., Bizet, M., Callat, M.P. *et al.* (1993) Evaluation of reticulocyte subtype distribution in myelodysplastic syndromes. *Am. J. Hematol.* **44**, 210–1.

Davies, S.V., Cavill, I., Bentley, N. *et al.* (1992) Evaluation of erythropoiesis after bone marrow transplantation: quantitative reticulocyte counting. *Br. J. Haematol.* **81**, 12–7.

Davies, S.V., Fegan, C.D., Kendall, R. *et al.* (1995) Serum erythropoietin during autologous bone marrow transplantation: relationship to measures of erythroid activity. *Clin. Lab. Haematol.* **17**, 139–44.

Davies, J.I., Smyth, M.S. and Martin, J.H.J. (1997) Automated reticulocyte counting: evaluation of the Coulter STKS haematology analyser reticulocyte counting function. *Clin. Lab. Haematol.* **19**, 89–92.

Davis, B.H. (1996) Immature reticulocyte fraction (IRF): by any name, a useful clinical parameter of erythropoietic activity. *Lab. Hematol.* **2**, 2–8.

Davis, B.H. (1997) Report of the ISLH-sponsored immature reticulocyte fraction (IRF). *Lab. Hematol.* **3**, 261–3.

Davis, B.H. and Bigelow, N.C. (1989) Flow cytometric reticulocyte quantification using thiazole orange provides clinically useful reticulocyte maturity index. *Arch. Pathol. Lab. Med.* **113**, 684–9.

Davis, B.H. and Bigelow, N.C. (1993) Flow cytometric reticulocyte analysis and the reticulocyte maturity index. *Ann. NY Acad. Sci.* **677**, 281–92.

Davis, B.H. and Bigelow, N.C. (1994a) Automated reticulocyte analysis. Clinical practice and associated new parameters. *Hematol. Oncol. Clin. North. Am.* **8**, 617–30.

Davis, B.H. and Bigelow, N.C. (1994b) Reticulocyte analysis and reticulocyte maturity index. In: Darzynkiewicz, Z., Crissman, H.A. and Robinson, J.P. (eds), *Methods in Cell Biology: Flow Cytometry, Vol. 42.* New York: Academic Press, 263–74.

Davis, B.H. and Bigelow, N.C. (1994c) Reticulocyte analysis and reticulocyte maturity index. *Methods Cell Biol.* **42** (Pt B), 263–74.

Davis, B.H., Bigelow, N., Ball, E.D. *et al.* (1989) Utility of flow cytometric reticulocyte quantification as a predictor of engraftment in autologous bone marrow transplantation. *Am. J. Hematol.* **32**, 81–7.

Davis, B.H., Bigelow, N.C., Koepke, J.A. *et al.* (1994) Flow cytometric reticulocyte analysis: multi-institutional interlaboratory correlation study. *Am. J. Clin. Pathol.* **102**, 468–77.

Davis, B.H., DiCorato, M., Bigelow, N.C. and Langweiler, M.H. (1993) Proposal for standardization of flow cytometric reticulocyte maturity index (RMI) measurement. *Cytometry* **14**, 318–36.

Davis, B.H., Ornvold, K. and Bigelow, N.C. (1995) Flow cytometric reticulocyte maturity index: a useful laboratory parameter of erythropoietic activity in anemia. *Cytometry* **22**, 35–9.

Davis, B.H., Bigelow, N.C. and van Hove, L. (1996) Immature reticulocyte fraction (IRF) and reticulocyte counts: comparison of Cell-Dyn 4000, Sysmex R-3000, thiazole orange flow cytometry and manual counts. *Lab. Hematol.* **2**, 144–9.

Davis, B.H., Spier, C., Kachin, J. and Cornbleet, P. (1997) College of American Pathologists' Reticulocyte proficiency testing program using surrogate blood: insights into contemporary clinical practice. *Lab. Hematol.* **3**, 84–91.

De Franceschi, L., Bachir, D., Galacteros, F. *et al.* (1997) Oral magnesium supplements reduce erythrocyte dehydration in patients with sickle cell disease. *J. Clin. Invest.* **100**, 1847–52.

de Pree, C., Cabrol, C., Frossard, J.L. and Beris, P. (1995) Pseudoreticulocytosis in a case of myelodysplastic syndrome with translocation t(11;14) (q42;q32). *Semin. Hematol.* **32**, 232–6.

Deiss, A. and Kurth, D. (1975) Circulating reticulocytes in normal adults as determined by the new methylene blue method. *Am. J. Clin. Pathol.* **53**, 481–4.

d'Onofrio, G., Chirillo, R., Zini, G. *et al.* (1995) Simultaneous measurement of reticulocyte and red cell indices in healthy subjects and patients with microcytic and macrocytic anemia. *Blood* **85**, 818–23.

d'Onofrio, G., Kuse, R., Foures, C. *et al.* (1996a) Reticulocytes in haematological disorders. *Clin. Lab. Haematol.* **18**(Suppl 1), 29–34.

d'Onofrio, G., Tichelli, A., Foures, C. *et al.* (1996b) Indicators of haematopoietic recovery after bone marrow transplantation: the role of reticulocyte parameters. *Clin. Lab. Haematol.* **18**(Suppl 1), 45–54.

d'Onofrio, G., Zini, G., Tommasi, M. and Van Hove, L. (1996c) Integration of fluorescence and hemocytometry in the Cell-Dyn 4000: reticulocyte, nucleated red blood cell, and white blood cell viability study. *Lab. Hematol.* **2**, 131–8.

d'Onofrio, G., Kim, Y.R., Schulze, S. *et al.* (1997) Evaluation of the Abbott Cell Dyn 4000 automated fluorescent reticulocyte measurements: comparison with manual, FACScan and Sysmex R1000 methods. *Clin. Lab. Haematol.* **19**, 253–60.

d'Onofrio, G., Zini, G. and Brugnara, C. (1998) Clinical applications of automated reticulocyte indices. *Hematology* **3**, 165–76.

Dressendorfer, R.H., Keen, C.L., Wade, C.E. *et al.* (1991) Development of runner's anemia during a 20-day road race: effect of iron supplements. *Int. J. Sports Med.* **12**, 332–6.

Dressendorfer, R.H., Wade, C.E. and Frederick, E.C. (1992) Effect of shoe cushioning on the development of reticulocytosis in distance runners. *Am. J. Sports Med.* **20**, 212–6.

Dustin, P. (1944) Contribution à l'étude histophysiologique et histochimique des globules rouges des vértebrés. *Arch. Biol.* **55**, 285–99.

Ebrahim, A. and Ryan, W.L. (1996) Encapsulation of ribonucleic acid in human red blood cells for use as a reticulocyte quality control material for flow cytometric analysis. *Cytometry* **25**, 156–63.

Eder, H. and Fritsche, H. (1989) Automated microfluorometric absolute count and maturation analysis of reticulocytes. *Klin. Wochenschr.* **67**, 1048–57.

Espanol, I., Pedro, C. and Remacha, A.F. (1999) Heinz bodies interfere with automated reticulocyte counts. *Haematologica* **84**, 373–4.

Ezzat, H.G. and Al-Truki, N. (1990) Staining of inclusion bodies and reticulocytes: a modified procedure. *Med. Lab. Sci.* **47**, 49–51.

Ferguson, D.J., Lee, S.F. and Gordon, P.A. (1990) Evaluation of reticulocyte counts by flow cytometry in a routine laboratory. *Am. J. Hematol.* **33**, 13–7.

Ferrata, A. (1912) *Le Malattie del Sangue.* Milano: Società Editrice Libraria.

Finch, C.A., Wolff, J.A., Rath, C.E. and Fluharty, R.G. (1949) Iron metabolism. Erythrocyte iron turnover. *J. Lab. Clin. Med.* **34**, 1480–90.

Fishbane, S., Galgano, C., Langley, R. *et al.* (1997) Reticulocyte hemoglobin content in the evaluation of iron status of hemodyalisis patients. *Kidney Int.* **52**, 217–22.

Fourcade, C., Jary, L. and Belaouni, H. (1999) Reticulocyte analysis provided by the Coulter GEN.S: significance and interpretation in regenerative and nonregenerative hematologic conditions. *Lab. Hematol.* **5**, 153–8.

Frazier, J.L., Caskey, H.J., Yoffe, M. and Seligman, P.A. (1982) Studies on the transferrin receptor on both human reticulocytes and nucleated cells in culture. *J. Clin. Invest.* **69**, 853–65.

Ganzoni, A., Hillman, R.S. and Finch, C.A. (1969) Maturation of the macroreticulocyte. *Br. J. Haematol.* **16**, 119–35.

Garulli, G., Marini, A., Azzarà, A. *et al.* (1998) Pseudoreticulocytosis in a case of myelodysplastic syndrome. *Acta Haematol.* **100**, 156–8.

Gasko, O. and Danon, D. (1972) Deterioration and disappearance of mitochondria during reticulocyte maturation. *Exp. Cell Res.* **75**, 159–69.

Gasko, O. and Danon, D. (1974) Endocytosis and exocytosis in membrane remodelling during reticulocyte maturation. *Br. J. Haematol.* **28**, 463–70.

Gavosto, F. and Rechenman, R. (1954) In vitro incorporation of glycine-1-^{14}C in reticulocytes. *Biochim. Biophys. Acta* **13**, 583–6.

Gerritsen, E.J., Stam, E.D., Van den Berg, H. *et al.* (1996) Follow-up of leucocyte and reticulocyte counts for the prediction of early graft failure after non-HLA identical BMT in children. *Bone Marrow Transpl.* **17**, 781–7.

Ghevaert, C., Fournier, M., Reade, V. *et al.* (1997) Laboratory evaluation of the Coulter STKS reticulocyte method in a children's hospital. *Lab. Hematol.* **3**, 92–7.

Giacomini, A., Legovini, P., Urso, M. *et al.* (1999) Measurement of reticulocyte mean cell volume and hemoglobin indices in healthy subjects and hemodialysis patients. *Eur. J. Lab. Med.* **7**, 111–6.

Gilmer, P.R. and Koepke, J.A. (1976) The reticulocyte. An approach to definition. *Am. J. Clin. Pathol.* **66**, 262–7.

Gonzalez, F.A., Sanchez, J., Llorente, L. and Villegas, A. (1996) Changes in reticulocyte fractions during peripheral stem cell harvesting exclusively mobilized with rhG-CSF. *Bone Marrow Transplant* **18**, 673.

Goodnough, L.T., Skikne, B. and Brugnara, C. (2000) Erythropoietin, iron, and erythropoiesis. *Blood* **96**, 823–33.

Greenberg, R.E. and Beck, J.R. (1984) The effect of sample size on reticulocyte counting and stool examination. *Arch. Pathol. Lab. Med.* **108**, 396–8.

Greinix, H.T., Linkesch, W., Keil, F. *et al.* (1994) Early detection of hematopoietic engraftment after bone marrow and peripheral blood stem cell transplantation by highly fluorescent reticulocyte counts. *Bone Marrow Transplant* **14**, 307–13.

Griffin, T.C., Squires, J.C., Timmons, J.F. and Buchanan, G.R. (1991) Chronic human parvovirus B19-induced erythroid hypoplasia as the initial manifestation of human immunodeficiency virus infection. *J. Pediatrics* **118**, 899–903.

Gronowicz, G., Swift, H. and Steck, T.L. (1984) Maturation of the reticulocyte in vitro. *J. Cell Sci.* **71**, 177–97.

Grotto, H.Z.W., Vigoritto, A.C., Noronha, J.F.A. and Lima, G.A.L.M. (1999) Immature reticulocyte fraction as a criterion for marrow engraftment. Evaluation of a semi-automated reticulocyte counting method. *Clin. Lab. Haematol.* **21**, 285–7.

Hansson, G.K., Andersson, M., Jarl, H. and Stemme, S. (1992) Flow cytometric analysis of reticulocytes using an RNA-binding fluorochrome. *Scand. J. Clin. Lab. Invest.* **52**, 35–41.

Heilmeyer, L. and Westharer, R. (1932) Reifungsstadien an überlebenden Reticulocyten in vitro und ihre Bedeutung für die Schätzung der täglichen Hämoglobinproduktion in vivo. *Zeitschr. Klin. Med.* **121**, 361–9.

Henry, D., Abels, R. and Larholt, K. (1995) Prediction of response to recombinant human erythropoietin (r-huEPO/Epoetin) therapy in cancer patients. *Blood* **85**,1676–8.

Herkner, K.R. (1996) Clinical applications of reticulocyte maturity grading in paediatrics: an overview. *Clin. Lab. Haematol.* **18**(Suppl 1), 55–9.

Hertenstein, B., Kurrle, E., Redenbacher, M. *et al.* (1993) Pseudoreticulocytosis in a patient with myelodysplasia. *Ann. Hematol.* **67**, 127–8.

Hillman, R.S. (1969) Characteristics of marrow production and reticulocyte maturation in normal man in response to anemia. *J. Clin. Invest.* **48**, 443–52.

Hillman, R.S. and Finch, C.A. (1969) The misused reticulocyte. *Br. J. Haematol.* **17**, 313–4.

Himmelfarb, J., Connerney, M., Mitchell, J. *et al.* (1995) Increased transferrin receptor expression on reticulocytes is an early indicator of response to erythropoietin. *Lab. Hematol.* **1,** 105–11.

Hinchliffe, R.F. (1993) Errors in automated reticulocyte counts due to Heinz bodies. *J. Clin. Pathol.* **46**, 878–9.

Hirata, R., Morita, Y., Hirai, N. and Seki, M.(1992) The effects of fluorescent substances on the measurement of reticulocytes using automated reticulocyte analyzers R-1000 and R-3000. *Sysmex. J. Int.* **2**, 10–5.

Hoffman, J.J.M.L. and Pennings, J.M.A. (1999) Pseudo-reticulocytosis as a result of malaria parasites. *Clin. Lab. Haematol.* **21**, 257–60.

Houwen, B. (1992) Reticulocyte maturation. *Blood. Cells* **18**, 167–86.

ICSH (1992) Guidelines for reticulocyte counting by microscopy on supravitally stained preparations. *WHO/LBS/92.3.* Geneva: World Health Organization.

ICSH (1998) Proposed reference method for reticulocyte counting based on the determination of the reticulocyte to red cell ratio. *Clin. Lab. Haematol.* **20**, 77–9.

Inoue, H. (1999) Overview of an automated hematology analyzer XE-2100™. *Sysmex J. Int.* **9**, 58–64.

Inoue, T. and Tatsumi, N. (1991) Evaluation of erythropoiesis by New Methylene Blue staining to establish reticulocyte maturity in bone marrow aspirates and peripheral blood. *Acta Cytol.* **35**, 479–80.

Jeffrey, R.F., Khan, A.A., Kendall, R.G. *et al.* (1995) Quantitative reticulocyte analysis may be of benefit in monitoring erythropoietin treatment in dialysis patients. *Artificial Organs* **19**, 821–6.

Johnstone, R.M. and Ahn, J. (1990) A common mechanism may be involved in the selective loss of plasma membrane functions during reticulocyte maturation. *Biomed. Biochim. Acta* **49**, S70–5.

Jones, A.R., Twedt, D., Swaim, W.R. and Gottfried, E. (1996) Diurnal change of blood count analysis in normal subjects. *Am. J. Clin. Pathol.* **106**, 723–7.

Joossens, J.V. and Heindrickx, M. (1946) Une nouvelle méthode de numération des réticulocytes en fluorescence. *Presse Méd.* **54**, 536–8.

Kakuya, F., Ishioka, T., Shirai, M. *et al.* (1991) Studies on differential reticulocyte count by laser flow cytometry in relation to hemoglobin and erythropoietin in normal neonates. *Sysmex J. Int.* **1**, 29–33.

Kan, S.Y. and Gardner, F.H. (1965) Life span of reticulocytes in paroxysmal nocturnal hemoglobinuria. *Blood* **25**, 759–66.

Kanold, J., Bezou, M.J., Coulet, M. *et al.* (1993) Evaluation of erythropoietic reconstitution after BMT by highly fluorescent reticulocyte counts compares favorably with traditional peripheral blood cell counting. *Bone Marrow Transplant* **11**, 313–18.

Kendall, G.R., Jeffries, R., Lyden, C.A. *et al.* (1993) Relationships between endogenous erythropoietin levels, reticulocyte count and reticulocyte RNA distribution: a study of anaemic patients with and without renal failure. *Sysmex J. Int.* **3,** 116–20.

Kessler, C., Machin, S., Pollard, Y. *et al.* (1997) Reticulocyte performance on the Coulter GEN-S system. *Lab. Hematol.* **3**, 41–7.

Khuhapinant, A., Bunyaratvej, A., Tatsumi, A. *et al.* (1994) Number and maturation of reticulocytes in various genotypes of thalassaemia assessed by flow cytometry. *Acta Haematol.* **91**, 119–25.

Killman, S.A. (1964) On the size of normal human reticulocytes. *Acta Med. Scand.* **176**, 529–33.

Kim, Y.R., Kantor, J., Landayn, M. *et al.* (1997) A rapid and sensitive reticulocyte method on a high throughput hematology instrument. *Lab. Hematol.* **3**, 19–26.

Koepke, J.F. and Koepke, J.A. (1986) Reticulocytes. *Clin. Lab. Haematol.* **8**, 169–79.

Kojima, K., Niri, M., Setoguchi, K. *et al.* (1989) An automated optoelectronic reticulocyte counter. *Am. J. Clin. Pathol.* **92**, 57–61.

Kondo, S., Fuke, T., Tokiwa, M. *et al.* (1995) The effects of fitness-type exercise on iron status and hematological status for female college students. *Rinsho. Byori* **43**, 953–9.

Kosenow, W. (1952) Über den Strukturwandel der basophilen Substanz junger Erythrozyten im Fluoreszensmikroskop. *Acta. Haematol.* **7**, 360–8.

Kraaijenhagen, R.J. (1996) Reticulocyte reference values by the Bhattacharya method: results of a pilot study. *Clin. Lab. Haematol.* **18**(Suppl 1), 15–16.

Kuse, R. (1993) The appearance of reticulocytes with medium or high RNA content is a sensitive indicator of beginning granulocyte recovery after aplasiogenic cytostatic drug therapy in patients with AML. *Ann. Hematol.* **66**, 213–14.

Kuse, R., Foures, C., Jou, J.M. *et al.* (1996) Automated reticulocyte counting for monitoring patients on chemotherapy for acute leukaemias and malignant lymphomas. *Clin. Lab. Haematol.* **18**(S1), 39–43.

Lahary, A., Labadie, G., Duval, C. *et al.* (1995) Normal reticulocyte count and subtype HFR in antenatal blood. *Am. J. Hematol.* **48**, 69–70.

Lai, S.K., Yow, C.M.N. and Benzie, I.F.F. (1999) Interference of Hb-H disease in automated reticulocyte counting. *Clin. Lab. Haematol.* **21**, 261–4.

Lakomek, M., Schroter, W., De Maeyer, G. and Winkler, H. (1989) On the diagnosis of erythrocyte enzyme defects in the presence of high reticulocyte counts. *Br. J. Haematol.* **72**, 445–51.

Lampasso, J.A. (1968) Changes in hematologic values induced by storage of ethylenediamine tetraacetate human blood for varying periods of time. *Am. J. Clin. Pathol.* **38**, 443–7.

Laurenti, L., Sica, S., Salutari, P. *et al.* (1998) Assessment of hematological and immunological function during long-term follow-up after peripheral blood stem cell tranplantation. *Haematologica* **83**, 138–42.

Lazarus, H.M., Chahine, A., Lacerna, K. *et al.* (1992) Kinetics of erythrogenesis after bone marrow transplantation. *Am. J. Clin. Pathol.* **97**, 574–83.

Lee, L.G., Chen, C.H. and Chiu, L.A.(1986) Thiazole orange: a new dye for reticulocyte analysis. *Cytometry* **7**, 508–17.

Leif, R.C. and Vinograd, J. (1964) The distribution of buoyant density of human erythrocytes in bovine albumin solutions. *Proc. Natl Acad. Sci.* **51**, 520–8.

Lesesve, J.F., Lacombe, F., Marit, G. *et al.* (1995) High fluorescence reticulocytes are an indicator of bone marrow recovery after chemotherapy. *Eur. J. Haematol.* **54**, 61–3.

Lin, C.K., Hsu, H.C., Chay, W.K. *et al.* (1993) Reticulocyte counts with maturation fractions in pancytopenic evaluation by a fully automated cell counter. *J. Clin. Lab. Anal.* **7**, 371–5.

Lofsness, K.G., Kohnke, M.L. and Geier, N.A. (1994) Evaluation of automated reticulocyte counts and their reliability in the presence of Howell–Jolly bodies. *Am. J. Clin. Pathol.* **101**, 85–90.

Lofters, W.S., Ali, M.A.M. and Pineo, G.F. (1978) Preleukemia and leukocytosis: a case report with in vitro evidence of abnormal maturation. *Scand. J. Haematol.* **20**, 417–20.

Lohmann, R.C., Crawford, L.N. and Wood, D.E. (1994) Proficiency testing in reticulocyte counting. *Clin. Lab. Haematol.* **16**, 57–64.

London, I.M., Shemin, D. and Rittenberg, D. (1950) Synthesis of heme in vitro by the immature non-nucleated mammalian erythrocytes. *J. Biol. Chem.* **183**, 749–56.

Losek, J., Hellmich, T. and Hoffman, G. (1992) Diagnostic value of anemia, red blood cell morphology, and reticulocyte count for sickle cell disease. *Ann. Emerg. Med.* **21**, 915–18.

Lowenstein, L.M. (1959) The mammalian reticulocyte. *Int. Rev. Cytol.* **8**, 135–74.

Lurie, S. (1993) Changes in age distribution of erythrocytes during pregnancy: a longitudinal study. *Gynecol. Obstet. Invest.* **36**, 141–4.

Macdougall, I.C. (1995a) Poor response to erythropoietin: practical guidelines on investigation and management. *Nephrol. Dial. Transplant* **10**, 607–14.

MacDougall, I.C. (1995b) How to get the best out of r-HuEpo. *Nephrol. Dial. Transplant* **10**(S2), 85–91.

Macdougall, I.C., Cavill, I., Hulme, B. *et al.* (1992) Detection of functional iron deficiency during erythropoietin treatment: a new approach. *Br. Med. J.* **304**, 225–6.

Maes, M., Van de Vyvere, J., Vandoolaeghe, E. *et al.* (1996) Alterations in iron metabolism and the erythron in major depression: further evidence for a chronic inflammatory process. *J. Affect. Disord.* **40**, 23–33.

Maier-Redelsperger, M., Elion, J. and Girot, R. (1998) F reticulocyte assay: a method to evaluate fetal hemoglobin production. *Hemoglobin* **22**, 419–25.

Major, A., Bauer, C., Breyman, C. *et al.* (1994) Rh-erythropoietin stimulates immature reticulocyte release in man. *Br. J. Haematol.* **87**, 605.

Major, A., Mathez-Loic, F., Rohling, R. *et al.* (1997) The effect of intravenous iron on reticulocyte response to recombinant human erythropoietin. *Br. J. Haematol.* **98**, 292–4.

Makler, M.T., Lee, L.G. and Rechtenwald, D. (1987) Thiazole orange: a new dye for Plasmodium species analysis. *Cytometry* **8**, 568–70.

Marmont, A. (1960) Acridine orange fluorescence microscopy in haematology. In: Bernard, J., Discombe, G. (eds), *Proceedings of the 7th Congress of the European Society of Haematology*, London 1959, part 2. Basel: Karger, 361–4.

Marshall, P.N., Bentley, S.A. and Lewis, S.M. (1976) Purified Azure B as a reticulocyte stain. *J. Clin. Pathol.* **29**, 1060–3.

Marshall, P.N. (1978) Reticulation, polychromasia and stippling of erythrocytes. *Microscopica Acta* **8**, 89–106.

Matsuo, T., Kario, K., Kodoma, K. and Asada, R. (1995) An inappropriate erythropoietic response to iron deficiency anaemia in the elderly. *Clin. Lab. Haematol.* **17**, 317–21.

May, J.A. and Sage, B.H. (1976) Spinner films for reticulocyte counts. *Am. J. Med. Technol.* **42**, 357–60.

Mechetner, E.B., Sedmak, D.D. and Barth, R.F. (1991) Heterogeneity of peripheral blood reticulocytes: a flow cytometric analysis with monoclonal antibody HAE9 and thiazole orange. *Am. J. Hematol.* **38**, 61–3.

Meister, B., Khoss, A., Burda, G. *et al.* (1998) Decreasing reticulocyte counts associated with declining post-dose erythropoietin plasma levels in anaemia of prematurity. *Biol. Neonate* **74**, 409–15.

Mel, H.C., Prenant, M. and Mohandas, N. (1977) Reticulocyte motility and form: studies on maturation and classification. *Blood* **49**, 1001–9.

Mercelina Roumans, P.E., Ubachs, J.M. and van Wersh, J.W. (1995) The reticulocyte count and its subfractions in smoking and non-smoking pregnant women. *Eur. J. Clin. Chem. Biochem.* **33**, 263–5.

Mercuriali, F., Zanella, A., Barosi, G. *et al.* (1993) Use of erythropoietin to increase the volume of autologous blood donated by orthopedic patients. *Transfusion* **33**, 55–60.

Metzger, D.K. and Charache, S. (1987) Flow cytometric reticulocyte counting with thioflavine T in a clinical hematology laboratory. *Arch. Pathol. Lab. Med.* **111,** 540–4.

Mittman, N., Sreedhara, R. and Mushnick, R. (1997) Reticulocyte hemoglobin content predicts functional iron deficiency in hemodialysis patients receiving rHuEpo. *Am. J. Kidney Dis.* **30**, 912–22.

Mohandas, N. (1993) Reticulocyte biology in red blood cell disorders. In: *New Perspective for Hematology – Conference Proceedings*. Tarrytown, NY: Bayer Diagnostics, 46–7.

Mougi, H., Shinmyozu, K. and Osame, M. (1997) Determining the optimal time for peripheral blood stem cell harvest by detecting immature cells (immature leukocytes and immature reticulocytes) using two newly developed automatic cell analyzers. *Int. J. Hematol.* **66**, 303–13.

Moulin, B., Ollier, J., George, F. *et al.* (1995) Serum erythropoietin and reticulocyte maturity index after renal transplantation: a prospective longitudinal study. *Nephron* **69**, 259–66.

Murphy, J.R. (1973) Influence of temperature and method of centrifugation on the separation of erythrocytes. *J. Lab. Clin. Med.* **82**, 334–41.

Musto, P., Modoni, S., Alicino, G. *et al.* (1994) Modifications of erythropoiesis in myelodysplastic syndromes treated with recombinant erythropoietin as evaluated by soluble transferrin receptor, high fluorescence reticulocytes and hypochromic erythrocytes. *Haematologica* **79**, 493–9.

Nagel, R.L., Vichinsky, E., Shah, M. *et al.* (1993) F reticulocyte response in sickle cell anemia treated with recombinant human erythropoietin: a double-blind study. *Blood* **81**, 9–14.

Nagler, A., MacKichan, M.L., Negrin, R.S. *et al.* (1995) Effects of granulocyte colony-stimulating factor therapy on in vitro hemopoiesis in myelodysplastic syndromes. *Leukemia* **9**, 30–9.

NCCLS (1985) Method for reticulocyte counting; proposed standard. *NCCLS Document H16-P*. Villanova, PA: NCCLS.

NCCLS/ICSH (1997) Methods for reticulocyte counting (flow cytometry and supravital dyes); approved guideline. *NCCLS Document H44-P*. Wayne, PA: NCCLS.

Newman, T.B. and Easterling, M.J. (1994) Yield of reticulocyte counts and blood smears in term infants. *Clin. Pediatr.* **33**, 71–6.

Ninni, M. (1949) I reticolociti. Morfologia, fisiologia, clinica. *Biblioteca "Haematologica" IX*. Pavia, Italy: Tipografio del libro.

Nobes, P.R. and Carter, A.B. (1990) Reticulocyte counting using flow cytometry. *J. Clin. Pathol.* **43**, 675–8.

Noble, N.A., Xu, Q.P. and Ward, J.H.(1989) Reticulocytes. I. Isolation and in vitro maturation of synchronized populations. *Blood* **74**, 475–81.

Noble, N.A., Xu, Q.P. and Hoge, L.L. (1990) Reticulocytes II: reexamination of the in vivo stress reticulocytes. *Blood* **75**, 1887–92.

Ohls, R.K., Osborne, K.A. and Christensen, R.D. (1995) Efficacy and cost analysis of treating very low birth weight infants with erythropoietin during their first two weeks of life: a randomized, placebo-controlled trial. *J. Pediatr.* **126**, 421–6.

Ortola, J., Aulesa, C., Olive, T. and Ortega, J.J. (1993) Transient reticulocyte increase in patients undergoing bone marrow transplantation after erythrocyte concentrate transfusions. *Sangre* **38**, 339–40.

Osterhout, M.L., Ohene-Frempong, K. and Horiuchi, K. (1996) Identification of F-reticulocytes by two-stage fluorescence image cytometry. *J. Histochem. Cytochem.* **44**, 393–7.

Paolino, W. (1946) Il comportamento dei diametri delle classi reticolocitarie ed il suo significato nella fisiopatologia della eritropoiesi. *Minerva. Med.* **18**, 327–33.

Papayannopoulou, T. and Finch, C. (1975) Radioiron measurements of red cell maturation. *Blood Cells* **1**, 535–47.

Parisotto, R., Gore, C.J., Emslie, K.R. *et al.* (2000). A novel method utilizing markers of altered erythropoiesis for the detection of recombinant human erythropoietin abuse in athletes. *Haematologica* **85**, 564–72.

Patel, V.P., Ciechanover, A., Platt, O. and Lodish, H.F. (1985) Mammalian reticulocyte lose adhesion to fibronectin during maturation to erythrocytes. *Proc. Natl Acad. Sci. USA* **82**, 440–59.

Paterakis, G.S., Voskaridou, E., Loutradi, A. *et al.* (1991) Reticulocyte counting in thalassemic and other conditions with the R-1000 Sysmex analyzer. *Ann. Hematol.* **63**, 218–22.

Paterakis, G.S., Lykopoulou, L., Papassotiriou, J. *et al.* (1993) Flow cytometric analysis of reticulocytes in normal cord blood. *Acta Haematol.* **90**, 182–5.

Peebles, D.A., Hochberg, A. and Clarke, T.D. (1981) Analysis of manual reticulocyte counting. *Am. J. Clin. Pathol.* **76**, 713–17.

Perel, I.D., Herrmann, N.R. and Watson, L.J. (1980) Automated differential leucocyte counting by the Geometric Data Hematrak system: eighteen months' experience in a private pathology laboratory. *Pathology* **12**, 449–69.

Perrotta, A.L. and Finch, C.A. (1972) The polychromatophilic erythrocyte. *Am. J. Clin. Pathol.* **57**, 471–7.

Perry, E.S., Moore, R.H., Berger, T.A. *et al.* (1996) In vitro and in vivo persistence of reticulocytes from donor red cells. *Transfusion* **36**, 318–21.

Pradella, M., Cavill, I. and d'Onofrio, G. (1996) Assessing erythropoiesis and the effect of erythropoietin therapy in renal disease by reticulocyte counting. *Clin. Lab. Haematol.* **18**(S1), 35–7.

Rabinovitch, A. (1993) Reticulocyte count. *CAP Today* **April**, 42–3.

Rao, S.P., Desai, N. and Miller, S.T. (1996) B19 parvovirus infection and transient aplastic crisis in a child with sickle cell anemia. *J. Pediatr. Hematol. Oncol.* **18**, 175–7.

Rapaport, S.M. (1986) *The Reticulocyte*. Boca Raton, FL: CRC Press.

Remacha, A.F., Martino, R., Sureda, A. *et al.* (1996) Changes in reticulocyte fractions during peripheral stem cell harvesting: role in monitoring stem cell collection. *Bone Marrow Transplant* **17**, 163–8.

Richter, C., Huch, A. and Huch, R. (1995) Erythropoiesis in the postpartum period. *J. Perinat. Med.* **23**, 51–9.

Rowan, R.M. (1986) Automated examination of the peripheral blood smear. In: Rowan, R.M., England, J.M. (eds), *Automation and Quality Assurance in Haematology*. London: Blackwell Scientific Publications, 129–77.

Rowan, R.M. (1991) Reference method, quality control and automation of reticulocyte count. *Pure Appl. Chem.* **63**, 1141–5.

Rudensky, B. (1997) Comparison of a semi-automated new Coulter methylene blue method with fluorescence flow cytometry in reticulocyte counting. *Scand. J. Clin. Lab. Invest.* **57**, 291–6.

Salvo, G., Caprari, P., Samoggia, P. *et al.* (1982) Human erythrocyte separation according to age on a discontinuous 'Percoll' density gradient. *Clin. Chim. Acta* **122**, 293–300.

Sandberg, S., Rustad, P., Johannesen, B. and Stoelsnes, B. (1998) Within subject biological variation of reticulocytes and reticulocyte-derived parameters. *Eur. J. Haematol.* **61**, 42–8.

Santamaria, A., Martino, R., Bellido, M. and Remacha, A.F. (1997) Reticulocyte recovery is faster in allogeneic and autologous peripheral blood stem cell transplantation than in bone marrow transplantation. *Eur. J. Haematol.* **58**, 362–4.

Savage, R.A., Skoog, D.P. and Rabinovitch, A. (1985) Analytic inaccuracy and imprecision in reticulocyte counting: a preliminary report from the College of American Pathologists Reticulocyte Project. *Blood Cells* **11**, 97–112.

Savourey, G., Garcia, N., Besnard, Y. *et al.* (1996) Pre-adaptation, adaptation and de-adaptation to high altitude in humans: cardio-ventilatory and haematological changes. *Eur. J. Appl. Physiol.* **73**, 529–53.

Schaefer, R.M. and Schaefer, L. (1999) Hypochromic red blood cells and reticulocytes. *Kidney Int.* **69**(Suppl), S44–8.

Schimenti, K.J., Lacerna, K., Wamble, A. *et al.* (1992) Reticulocyte quantification by flow cytometry, image analysis, and manual counting. *Cytometry* **13**, 853–62.

Schlosshardt, H. and Heilmeyer, L. (1942) Blutzellen im Fluoreszenslicht. *Jenaische Zeitschr. Med. Naturw.* **75**, 90–103.

Schmitz, F.J. and Werner, E.(1986) Optimization of flow-cytometric discrimination between reticulocytes and erythrocytes. *Cytometry* **7**, 439–44.

Scola, S., Di Lorenzo, G., Cutrò, S. *et al.* (1992) Valutazione delle popolazioni reticolocitarie per lo studio della riserva funzionale della serie eritroide nell'anziano anemico con analizzatore automatico (R-1000 Sysmex). *Il Patologo Clinico* **I**, 423–4.

Seip, M. (1953) Reticulocyte studies. *Acta Med. Scand.* **282**(Suppl), 9–164.

Seligman, P.A., Allen, R.H., Kirchanski, S.J. and Natale, P.J. (1983) Automated analysis of reticulocytes using fluorescent staining with both acridine orange and an immunofluorescent technique. *Am. J. Hematol.* **14**, 57–66.

Serke, S. and Huhn, D. (1992) Identification of CD71 (transferrin receptor) expressing erythrocytes by multiparameter flow-cytometry (MP-FCM): correlation to the quantitation of reticulocytes as determined by conventional microscopy and by MP-FCM using a RNA-staining dye. *Br. J. Haematol.* **81**, 432–9.

Serke, S. and Huhn, D. (1993) Improved specificity of determinations of immature erythrocytes (reticulocytes) by multiparameter flow-cytometry and thiazole orange using combined staining with monoclonal antibody (anti-glycophorin-A). *Clin. Lab. Haematol.* **15**, 33–4.

Serke, S., Riess, H., Oettle, H. and Huhn, D. (1999) Elevated reticulocyte count – a clue to the diagnosis of haemolytic-uraemic syndrome (HUS) associated with gemcitabine therapy for metastatic duodenal papillary carcinoma: a case report. *Br. J. Cancer* **79**, 1519–21.

Serre, A.F., Souweine, B., Evreux, O. *et al.* (1994) Reticulocyte response to endogenous erythropoietin after renal transplantation. *Clin. Transpl.* **8**, 353–8.

Shaffer, M., Kiser, G., Luban, N.L. and De Palma, L. (1993) Performance of reticulocyte counts in stored blood specimens in a pediatric population utilizing new methylene blue. *Pediatr. Pathol.* **13**, 591–5.

Sher, G.D., Pinkerton, P.H., Ali, M.A. and Senn, J.S. (1994) Myelodysplastic syndrome with prolonged reticulocyte survival mimicking hemolytic disease. *Am. J. Clin. Pathol.* **101**, 149–53.

Sher, G., Vitisallo, B., Schisano, T. *et al.* (1997) Automated NRBC count, a new parameter to monitor, in real time, individualized transfusion needs in transfusion-dependent thalassemia major. *Lab. Hematol.* **3**, 129–37.

Shoustal, A.M. (1992) Evaluation of the Sysmex R-3000 automated reticulocyte analyzer with comparison to the Sysmex R-1000. *Sysmex J. Int.* **2**, 16–25.

Sica, S., Salutari, P., Laurenti, L. *et al.* (1998) Highly fluorescent reticulocytes after CD34+ peripheral blood progenitor cell transplant. *Bone Marrow Transplant* **21**, 361–4.

Simpson, C.F. and Kling, J.M. (1968) The mechanism of mitochondrial extrusion from phenylhydrazine-induced reticulocytes in the circulating blood. *J. Cell Biol.* **36**, 103–9.

Souweine, B., Serre, A.F., Philippe, P. *et al.* (1995), Serum erythropoietin and reticulocyte counts in inflammatory process. *Ann. Med. Intern. Paris* **146**, 8–12.

Sowade, O., Sowade, B., Brilla, K. *et al.* (1997) Kinetics of reticulocyte maturity fractions and indices and iron status during therapy with epoetin beta (recombinant human erythropoietin) in cardiac surgery patients. *Am. J. Hematol.* **55**, 89–96.

Sowade, O., Sowade, B., Gross, J. *et al.* (1998) Evaluation of eryhropoietic activity on the basis of the red cell and reticulocyte distribution widths during eopetin beta therapy in patients undergoing cardiac surgery. *Acta Haematol.* **99**, 1–7.

Spanish Multicentric Study Group for Hematopoietic Recovery (1994) Flow cytometric reticulocyte quantification in the evaluation of hematologic recovery. *Eur. J. Haematol.* **53**, 293–7.

Takubo, T., Kitano, K., Ohto, Y. *et al.* (1989) The usefulness of the use of the R-1000 automated reticulocyte counter in a clinical hospital laboratory. *Eur. J. Haematol.* **43**, 88–9.

Tanke, H.J., Nieuwenhuis, I.A.B., Koper, G.J.M. *et al.* (1980) Flow cytometry of human reticulocytes based on RNA fluorescence. *Cytometry* **5**, 313–20.

Tanke, H.J., Rothbarth, P.H., Vossen, J.M.J.J. *et al.* (1983) Flow cytometry of reticulocytes applied to clinical hematology. *Blood* **61**,1091–7.

Tanke, H.J., van Vianen, P.H., Emiliani, F.M.F. *et al.* (1986) Changes in erythropoiesis due to radiation or chemotherapy as studied by flow cytometric determination of peripheral blood reticulocytes. *Histochemistry* **84**, 544–8.

Tarallo, P., Humbert, J.C., Mahassen, P. *et al.* (1994) Reticulocytes: biological variations and reference limits. *Eur. J. Haematol.* **53**, 11–5.

Tatsumi, N., Tsuda, I., Kojima, K. *et al.* (1989) An automated reticulocyte counting method: preliminary observations. *Med. Lab. Sci.* **46**, 157–60.

Tatsumi, N., Kojima, K., Tsuda, I. et al. (1990) Reticulocyte count used to assess recombinant human erythropoietin sensitivity in hemodialysis patients. *Contrib. Nephrol.* **82**, 41–8.

Terada, H., Hirano, K., Inoue, Y. *et al.* (1965) An examination of the reticulocyte staining method: a comparison of the Brecher method and a variation of the Kammerer method and also the use of the Miller ocular disk. *Jap. J. Clin. Pathol.* **13**, 403–6.

Testa, U., Rutella, S., Martucci, R. *et al.* (1997) Autologous stem cell transplantation: evaluation of erythropoietic reconstitution by highly fluorescent reticulocyte counts, erythropoietin, soluble transferrin receptors, ferritin, TIBC and iron dosages. *Br. J. Haematol.* **96**, 762–75.

Thaer, A. and Becker, H.(1975) Microscope fluorometric investigations on the reticulocyte maturation distribution as diagnostic criterion of disordered erythropoiesis. *Blut* **30**, 339–48.

Thomas, E.D., Storb, R., Fefer, A. *et al.* (1972) Aplastic anaemia treated by marrow transplantation. *Lancet* **i**, 284–9.

Tichelli, A., Gratwohl, A., Driessen, A. *et al.* (1990) Evaluation of the Sysmex R-1000. An automated reticulocyte analyzer. *Am. J. Clin. Pathol.* **93**, 70–8.

Tsuda, I. and Tatsumi, N. (1989) Maturity of reticulocytes in various hematological disorders. *Eur. J. Haematol.* **43**, 252–4.

Tsuda, I. and Tatsumi, N. (1990) Reticulocytes in human preserved blood as control material for automated reticulocyte counters. *Am. J. Clin. Pathol.* **93**, 109–10.

Tulliez, M., Testa, U., Rochart, H. *et al.* (1982) Reticulocytosis, hypochromia, and microcytosis: an unusual presentation of the preleukemic syndromes. *Blood* **59**, 293–5.

Van Bockstaele, D.R. and Peetermans, M.E. (1989) 1,3′-diethyl-4-2′-quinolylthiacyanine iodide as a "thiazole orange" analogue for nucleic acid staining. *Cytometry* **10**, 214–18.

Van Houte, A.J., Bartels, P.C., Schoorl, M. and Mulder, C. (1994) Methodology dependent variations in reticulocyte counts using a manual and two different flow cytometric procedures. *Eur. J. Clin. Chem. Clin. Biochem.* **32**, 859–63.

Van Hove, L., Goossens, W., Van Duppen, V. and Verwilghen, R. (1990) Reticulocyte count using thiazole orange. A flow cytometric method. *Clin. Lab. Haematol.* **12**, 287–99.

Van Petegem, M., Cartuyvels, R., De Schouwer, P. *et al.* (1993) Comparative evaluation of three flow cytometers for reticulocyte enumeration. *Clin. Lab. Haematol.* **15**, 103–11.

Vander, J.B., Harris, C.A. and Ellis, S.R. (1963) Reticulocyte counts by means of fluorescence microscopy. *J. Lab. Clin. Med.* **62**, 132–9.

Vannucchi, A., Bosi, A., Grossi, A. *et al.* (1992) Stimulation of erythroid engraftment by recombinant human erythropoietin in ABO-compatible, HLA-identical, allogeneic bone marrow transplant patients. *Leukemia* **6**, 215–19.

Villamor, N., Kirsch, A., Huhn, D. *et al.* (1996) Interference of blood leucocytes in the measurements of immature red cells (reticulocytes) by two different (semi-) automated flow-cytometry technologies. *Clin. Lab. Haematol.* **18**, 89–94.

Walka, M.M., Sonntag, J., Kage, A. *et al.* (1998) Complete blood counts from umbilical cords of healthy term newborns by two automated cytometers. *Acta Haematol.* **100**, 167–73.

Wallen, C.A., Higashikubo, R. and Dethlefsen, L.A. (1980) Comparison of two flow cytometric assays for cellular RNA: acridine orange and propidium iodide. *Cytometry* **3**, 155–61.

Watanabe, K., Kawai, W., Takeuchi, K. *et al.* (1994) Reticulocyte maturity as an indicator for estimating qualitative abnormality of erythropoiesis. *J. Clin. Pathol.* **47**, 736–9.

Wearne, A., Robin, H., Joshua, D.E. and Kronenberg, H.(1985) Automated enumeration of reticulocytes using acridine orange. *Pathology* **17**, 75–7.

Weicker, H. and Fichsel, H. (1955) Das Reticulocytenvolumen. *Klin. Wochenschr.* **33**, 1074–82.

Weiser, M.G. and Kociba, G.J. (1982) Persistent macrocytosis assessed by erythrocyte subpopulation analysis following erythrocyte regeneration in cats. *Blood* **60**, 295–303.

Wells, D.A., Daigneault-Creech, C.A. and Simrell, C.R.(1992) Effect of iron status on reticulocyte mean channel fluorescence. *Am. J. Clin. Pathol.* **97**, 130–4.

Wernli, M., Tichelli, A., von Planta, M. *et al.* (1991) Flow cytometric monitoring of parasitaemia during treatment of severe malaria by exchange transfusion. *Eur. J. Haematol.* **46**, 121–3.

Wintrobe, M. (1985) *Hematology, the Blossoming of a Science: a Story of Inspiration and Effort.* Philadelphia: Lea & Febiger.

Wittekind, D. and Schulte, E. (1987) Standardized Azure B as a reticulocyte stain. *Clin. Lab. Haematol.* **9**, 395–8.

Yoto, Y., Kudoh, T., Suzuki, N.M. *et al.* (1993) Retrospective study on the influence of human parvovirus B19 infection among children with malignant diseases. *Acta Haematol.* **90**, 8–12.

Zachée, P., van Hove, L., Hauglustaine, D. *et al.* (1992) Effect of recombinant human erythropoietin on reticulocyte age in hemodialysis patients. *Nephron* **62**, 366–7.

Zini, G., d'Onofrio, G., Tommasi, M. *et al.* (1991) Un caso di emoglobina Hammersmith: descrizione delle interferenze strumentali. In: Atti del V Incontro degli Utilizzatori dei sistemi ematologici Bayer Technicon, Montecatini Terme, 59–62.

6

Leucocyte immunophenotyping: the principles and key practical issues

JOHN T. REILLY AND DAVID BARNETT

INTRODUCTION

Monoclonal antibodies

Hybridoma technology, developed in the mid-1970s by Köhler and Milstein (1975), has made it possible to produce virtually limitless quantities of highly specific monoclonal antibodies that can detect distinct epitopes of cellular antigens, on both normal and neoplastic cells. In 1982 at the 'First International Workshop on Leucocyte Differentiation Antigens', the term 'cluster of differentiation' (CD) was introduced to help ensure that such reagents were accurately characterized, in terms of both specificity and tissue distribution. Six workshops have identified and characterized over 160 CDs (as shown in Table 6.1; Kishimoto *et al.*, 1997) (Bernard *et al.*, 1984; Reinherz *et al.*, 1986; McMichaels *et al.*, 1987; Knapp *et al.*, 1990; Schlossman *et al.*, 1995; Kishimoto *et al.*, 1997), with a further 90 CDs being added at a recent workshop in Harrogate, UK (July 2000). The monoclonal antibodies within each CD have similar tissue reactivity and recognize the same antigen as determined by serological, molecular, biochemical and histochemical studies. Concise summaries (CD guides) for each of the 190 antigens defined within the 160 CDs (Table 6.1) are available on the World Wide Web (http://www.ncbi.nlm.nih.gov/prow/). This large array of available antibodies, together with the development of the flow cytometer (see below), has enabled sophisticated immuno-logical cell marker analysis, or 'immunophenotyping', to become a routine diagnostic tool in many haematology laboratories.

Table 6.1 *Principal features of known cluster differentiation (CD) molecules*

Cluster	Main cellular distribution	Comments/function/diagnostic value
CD1a,b,c	Cortical thymocytes, dendritic cells, B-cells	Structurally similar to MHC class I
CD2	T-cells	Receptor for sheep erythrocytes and LFA
CD3	T-cells	Five chains (γ–η), associated with T-cell receptor
CD4	T-cell subset, monocytes, macrophages	Receptor for MHC class II and AIDS virus (HIV-1)
CD5	T-cells, B-cell subset (weak)	Member of 'scavenger' molecular family
CD6	T-cells, B-cells (weak)	Member of 'scavenger' family
CD7	Most T-cells	Earliest marker for T-cell lineage
CD8	T-cell subset	Receptor for MHC class I. Associated with $p56^{lck}$
CD9	Platelets, monocytes, pre-B-cells	Member of TM4 ('tetra-span') molecular family
CD10	Haematopoietic stem cells	Neutral endopeptidase, also termed cALLA
CD11a	Many leucocytes	α-chain of LFA-1, binds to ICAM-1 (CD54)
CD11b	Granulocytes, monocytes, NK cells	α-chain of Mac-1, receptor for C3bi, fibrinogen
CD11c	Macrophages, granulocytes, NK cells and hairy leukaemia cells	α-chain of p150,95. Receptor for fibrinogen
CD12	Myeloid cells	Little known
CD13	Granulocytes, monocytes	Aminopeptidase N
CD14	Monocytes, Kupffer cells, granulocytes	Useful monocytes/macrophage marker
CD15	Granulocytes, Reed–Sternberg cells	X hapten
CD16	Granulocytes, some macrophages, NK cells	Low affinity IgG receptor
CDw17	Granulocytes, monocytes, platelets	Lactosylceramide
CD18	Many leucocytes	β-chain of LFA/Mac-1 integrin family
CD19	Precursor B-cells, B-cells	B1
CD20	Subpopulations of precursor B-cells, B-cells	Member of TM4 'tetra-span' molecular family
CD21	B-cells	Receptor for C3d, EBV
CD22	Precursor B-cells, B-cells	Intracytoplasmic in early B-cells
CD23	Activated B-cells	Low affinity IgE receptor
CD24	Some B-cells, granulocytes	
CD25	Activated cells, macrophages	Low affinity IL-2 receptor (α-chain)
CD26	Activated T- and B-cells, macrophages	Dipeptidylpeptidase IV
CD27	T-cells, plasma cells	Belongs to NGFR family, binds to CD70
CD28	T-cell subset	Binds to B7 (expressed on activated B-cells)
CD29	T-cell subset	β1 integrin subunit
CD30	Activated lymphocytes, R-S cells	Belongs to NGFR family
CD31	Granulocytes, monocytes, platelets, B-cells	CEA-like molecule
CD32	Granulocytes, B-cells, monocytes, platelets	IgG receptor
CD33	Myeloid progenitors, monocytes	gp67
CD34	Haematopoietic progenitors	Binds to L-selectin
CD35	B-cells, red cells, granulocytes	Receptor for C3b and C4b
CD36	Monocytes/macrophages, platelets	Receptor for *Plasmodium falciparum* on RBCs
CD37	B-cells, monocytes, T-cells	Member of the TM4 ('tetra-span') family
CD38	Germinal centre cells, activated T-cells	T10
CD39	Activated B- and NK cells, macrophages	Little known
CD40	B-cells	Homologous to NGFR

Cluster	Main cellular distribution	Comments/function/diagnostic value
CD41	Megakaryocytes and platelets	GpIIb, αIIb integrin, binds fibronectin, fibrinogen
CD42a	Megakaryocytes and platelets	GpX, complexes with gpIb to form receptor for vWF
CD42b	Megakaryocytes and platelets	GpIb-α
CD42c	Megakaryocytes and platelets	GpIb-β
CD42d	Megakaryocytes and platelets	GpV
CD43	Leucocytes, erythrocytes	Leucosialin, defective in Wiskott–Aldrich syndrome
CD44	Leucocytes, erythrocytes	HERMES, Pgp-1
CD45	Most leucocytes	Leucocyte common antigen (LCA)
CD45RA	B-cells, T-cell subset, monocytes	Epitope coded by exon A
CD45RB	As CD45RA, but including granulocytes	Epitope coded by exon B
CD45RO	B-cells, T-cell subset, monocytes	Epitope not encoded by exons A, B or C
CD46	Many cell types	MCP, co-factor for cleavage of C3b/C4b
CD47	Many cell types	Integrin-associated protein (IAP)
CD48	Many leucocytes	Homologous to CD2 and CD58. GPI linked
CD49a	Lymphocytes	VLA1 alpha chain, receptor for collagen, laminin
CD49b	Platelets, lymphocytes, monocytes	VLA2 alpha chain, receptor for collagen, laminin
CD49c	Basal epidermis	VLA3 alpha chain, receptor for laminin, fibronectin
CD49d	Lymphocytes	VLA4 alpha chain, receptor for fibronectin
CD49e	Granulocytes, platelets, T-cells	VLA5 alpha chain
CD49f	Platelets	VLA6 alpha chain
CD50	Leucocytes	ICAM-3, binds LFA-1
CD51	Platelets	VNR α-chain, complexes with CD61
CDw52	Leucocytes	Campath-1, used in treatment of GVHD
CD53	Leucocytes	Member of TM4 ('tetra-span') molecule family
CD54	Endothelial cells, activated lymphocytes	ICAM-1, ligand for CD11a and CD11b
CD55	Many cell types	DAF, limits complement activation
CD56	NK cells	Isoform of neural cell adhesion molecule (N-CAM)
CD57	NK cells, T-cell subset	HNK1
CD58	Many cell types	LFA-3, ligand for CD2
CD59	Many cell types	MAC inhibitor, protectin
CDw60	T-cell subset, platelets	Sequence on gangliosides
CD61	Platelets, megakaryocytes	Glycoprotein IIIa, VNR β-chain
CD62E	Endothelium	E-selectin
CD62L	Lymphocytes	L-selectin, LAM-1
CD62P	Activated platelets, endothelium	P-selectin, PADGEM, GMP-140
CD63	Activated platelets, monocytes, basophils	Lysosome internal membrane protein (LIMP)
CD64	Monocytes	High affinity receptor for IgG, FcγR1
CDw65	Granulocytes, monocytes	Type II chain fucoganglioside
CD66a	Activated granulocytes	Biliary glycoprotein
CD66b	Activated granulocytes	CEA gene family members 6
CD66c	Activated granulocytes	Non specific cross reacting antigen (NCA)
CD66d	Activated granulocytes	CEA gene family members 1 (CGM1)
CD66e	Activated granulocytes	Carcino embryonic antigen (CEA)

Table 6.1 – *continued*

Cluster	Main cellular distribution	Comments/function/diagnostic value
CD67	(Now classified as part of CD66)	
CD68	Monocytes, macrophages, myeloid cells	Pan-macrophage marker
CD69	Activated cells, NK cells, platelets	Involved in early lymphocyte activation events
CD70	Activated lymphocytes, R-S cells	Ligand for CD27
CD71	Activated cells, macrophages	Transferrin receptor
CD72	B-cells, some macrophages	Ligand for CD5
CD73	B-cells and T-cell subset	Ecto-5' nucleotidase
CD74	B-cells, monocytes, macrophages	Invariant chain of MHC class II
CDw75	Mature B-cells	Carbohydrate antigen
CDw76	Mature B-cells, T-cell subset	Carbohydrate antigen
CD78	B-cells	Neutral glycosphingolipid
CD79a	B-cells, including plasma cells	Forms dimer with CD79b
CD79b	B-cells, excluding plasma cells	Forms dimers with CD79a
CD80	Activated B-cells, T-cells, monocytes	Binds to CTLA-4 and CD28
CD81	B-cells, T-cells, macrophages	Belongs to TM4 ('tetra-span') family
CD82	Broad cellular distribution	Belongs to TM4 ('tetra-span') family
CD83	Dendritic cells, activated lymphocytes	HB15
CD84	Monocytes, platelets	Upregulated following activation
CD85	Plasma cells, hairy cell leukaemia	Little known
CD86	Germinal centre cells, activated B-cells	FUN-1
CD87	Monocytes, macrophages	Receptor for urokinase/plasminogen activator
CD88	Lymphocytes, eosinophils, monocytes	Complement C5a receptor
CD89	Lymphocytes, granulocytes, monocytes	Medium affinity receptor for IgA
CDw90	Subset of CD34-positive cells	GPI-linked
CD91	Hepatocytes, monocytes	Receptor for α-2-macroglobulin
CDw92	Lymphocytes, monocytes, platelets	Little known
CD93	Lymphocytes, monocytes, endothelium	Little known
CD94	NK cells and some T-cells	Kp43, dimeric molecule found on NK cells
CD95	Activated lymphoid cells	Fas, induces apoptosis
CD96	Activated lymphoid cells	Tactile
CD97	Monocytes, granulocytes	F12, VIM3, an activation marker
CD98	Monocytes and activated cells	Di-sulphide-linked dimer
CD99	Most human cells	E2, MIC2
CD100	Restricted to leucocytes	Little known
CD102	Endothelial cells	ICAM-2, ligand for LFA-1
CD103	Intraepithelial lymphocytes (IEL)	α^E integrin subunit
CD104	Endothelium	β_4 integrin subunit
CD105	Endothelium	Endoglin, a component of the TGF-β receptor
CD106	Endothelial cells	VCAM-1, ligand for VLA-4 and $\alpha_4\beta_7$
CD107a	Activated platelets	Lysosome associated membrane protein (LAMP-1)
CD107b	Activated platelets	Lysosome associated membrane protein (LAMP-2)
CDw108	Malignant B-cells	GPI-linked
CDw109	Activated T-lymphocytes and platelets	GPI-linked
CD110–114	(Not yet assigned, reserved for molecules to be defined later)	
CD115	Monocytes, macrophages	c-fms, CSF-1 receptor
CD116	Myeloid progenitor cells	GM-CSF receptor

Cluster	Main cellular distribution	Comments/function/diagnostic value
CD117	Haematopoietic precursor cells	c-kit, stem cell factor receptor
CD118	Wide cell distribution	IFN-α receptor
CD119	T-cells, B-cells, monocytes	IFN-γ receptor
CD120a	Many cell types	Type I TNF receptor
CD120b	Many cell types, especially monocytes	Type II TNF receptor
CD121a	T-cells, fibroblasts, endothelial cells	IL-1 receptor type I
CD121b	B-cells, monocytes, macrophages	IL-1 receptor type II
CD122	T-cells, some B-cells, NK cells	IL-2 receptor β subunit
CD123	Haematopoietic precursors, monocytes	α chain of the IL-3 receptor
CD124	Lymphoid precursors	α chain of the IL-4 receptor
CD125	Eosinophils, basophils, T-cells	α chain of the IL-5 receptor
CD126	Activated B-cells, plasma cells	α chain of the IL-6 receptor
CD127	Monocytes, some early B-cells, T-cells	α chain of the IL-7 receptor
CD128	Granulocytes, subset of T-cells	High affinity receptor for IL-8
CD129	(Provisionally unassigned)	
CD130	Activated B-cells and plasma cells	gp130, signal transduction
CD131	Monocytes, granulocytes, eosinophils	Common β chain
CD132	T- and B-cell, haematopoietic precursors	Common γ chain
CD134	Activated T-cells	OX40, adhesion of activated T-cells to endothelium
CD135	CD34 cells, carcinoma cells	Flt3, Flk2, a tyrosine kinase receptor
CDw136	Not determined	Macrophage stimulating protein-receptor
CD138	B-cells	Syndecan-1, heparin sulphate proteoglycan
CD139	B-cells	(Limited details known)
CD140a	Endothelial cells	PDGF-receptor alpha, tyrosine kinase activity
CD140b	Endothelial cells	PDGF-receptor beta, tyrosine kinase activity
CD141	Myeloid, endothelial, smooth muscle cells	Thrombomodulin
CD142	Monocytes, endothelial cells	Tissue factor
CD143	Endothelial cells, macrophages	ACE (angiotensin-converting enzyme)
CD144	Endothelial cells	VE-Cadherin, adhesion molecule
CDw145	Endothelial cells	(Few details known)
CD146	Endothelial cells, activated T-cells	MUC18, S-Endo, homing of activated T-cells
CD147	Endothelial, myeloid and lymphoid cells	Neurothelin, Basigin, TCSF
CD148	Haematopoietic cells	HPTP-eta, DEP-1, contact inhibition of cell growth
CD149	Lymphocytes	MEM133, function unknown
CDw150	T-cells	SLAM, signalling molecule
CD151	Platelets, granulocytes, endothelial cells	PETA3, signalling complex with FcR IIa?
CD152	T-cells	CTLA-4, negative regulation for T-cell co-stimulation
CD153	T-cells	CD30L, co-stimulatory for T-cells
CD154	T-cells	CD40L, gp39, co-stimulatory molecule
CD155	Monocytes, macrophages, CNS neurones	Polio Virus R
CD156	Monocytes, macrophages, granulocytes	ADAM8 (MS2 mouse homologue)
CD157	Monocytes, neutrophils, endothelial cells	Bst-1, ADP-ribose cyclase
CD158a	NK, T-cells	p58.1, MHC class-1 specific NK receptors
CD158b	NK, T-cells	p58.2, MHC class-1 specific NK receptors
CD159	(Not assigned)	
CD160	(Not assigned)	
CD161	NK cells	NKRP1A, regulation of NK cell-mediated activity

Table 6.1 – *continued*

Cluster	Main cellular distribution	Comments/function/diagnostic value
CD162	Monocytes, granulocytes, T-cells	PSGL-1, leucocyte rolling on activated endothelium
CD163	Monocytes, some macrophages	M130, function unknown
CD164	Myeloid cells, progenitor cells, T-cells	MGC-24, adhesion of progenitor cells to stroma
CD165	T-cells, NK cells, platelets	AD2, gp37, adhesion of thymocytes to endothelium
CD166	Activated B- and T-cells	ALCAM, activated leucocyte adhesion molecule

Flow cytometers

The modern bench-top flow cytometers have their roots firmly linked to the development of the first cell counters, e.g. the early Coulter instruments. Indeed, such instruments have been in use since the late 1940s and are still the mainstay of many clinical laboratories for the determination of red cell, white cell and platelet counts. The modern day flow cytometer used for immunophenotyping consists of a number of key components (Fig. 6.1), namely the light source (laser), fluidics unit, photodetector and signal processing units, display and analysis units (computer work station) and sorter module (only on cell sorters). Essentially, cells are suspended in a liquid and then stained with fluorochrome conjugated antibodies, or dyes, that bind to the antigen(s) or protein to be analysed. The stained cells are then passed through a flow cell one at a time. This is achieved by the fluidics unit which introduces a 'sheath' of liquid that has a higher flow rate than the sample, a process termed 'hydrodynamic focusing'. The cells, which are now in single file, are then interrogated using a beam of light (usually generated by a laser) which is focused upon a specific point of the flow cell by lenses. As the cell passes through this laser beam, it will scatter light, whilst at the same time the attached fluorochrome(s) will be excited to emit a fluorescence signal. Discrimination of two, three or four colours of fluorescence emission is accomplished by optical filters placed in front of separate photodetectors, the signals of which are processed into data to be analysed by the computer workstation. Flow cytometers are able to collect data relating to both cell size and cell granularity, as well as information derived from the fluorochrome(s). Larger flow cytometers, termed cell sorters, also have the capability to sort cells individually based upon preselected characteristics of cell size, granularity and antigen expression. (For more detailed information on flow cytometry see Macey, 1994; Shapiro, 1995; Robinson *et al.*, 1997.)

The 1990s saw a further revolution in flow cytometric technology. The development of specific therapeutic protocols for HIV-positive patients highlighted the need for accurate determination of absolute CD4+ T lymphocyte counts. Traditionally, absolute CD4+ T lymphocyte counts were calculated using a dual-platform system, the percentage of CD4+ T lymphocytes being derived from the flow cytometer and the absolute lymphocyte, or total white cell, count derived from an haematology analyser. It became apparent, however, that such an approach can result in considerable variation (Robinson *et al.*, 1992) and, as a result, single-platform analysers have now been developed that are capable of producing data in both

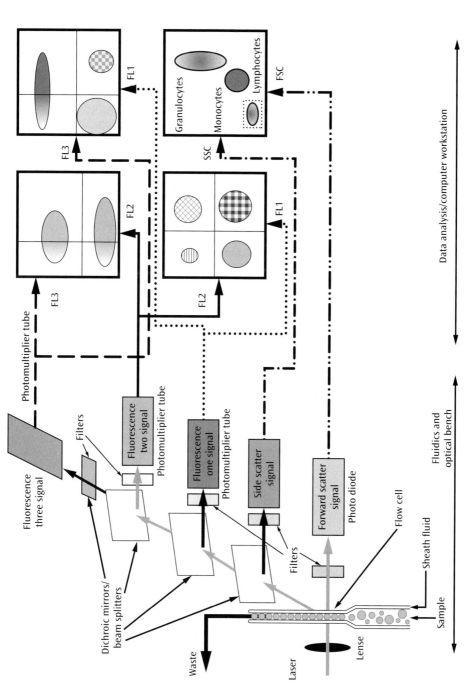

Fig. 6.1 *Simplified schematic representation of a bench-top flow cytometer, illustrating the transition from cell interrogation by the laser to the multi-parametric analysis.*

absolute and percentage formats (Mercolino *et al.*, 1995; Strauss *et al.*, 1996). UK NEQAS for Leucocyte Immunophenotyping has shown that, using single-platform analysers, the inter-laboratory coefficients of variation for absolute CD4+ T-lymphocytes are reduced from over 30% to approximately 15% (unpublished observations), a finding confirmed by Connelly *et al.* (1995). As a result, different approaches have been developed to enable flow cytometers to determine absolute values. True single-platform instruments include the FACSCount, Imagn 2000 system and the Ortho *Cytoron*Absolute, while the Coulter XL, Becton Dickinson FACSCalibur and FACScan can be adapted to offer such a facility. The Ortho *Cytoron*Absolute, for example, operates by delivering precise volumetric aliquots for analysis, while the Coulter XL, Becton Dickinson FACSCalibur and FACSCount use a known quantity of added beads to enable the accurate and precise measurement of percentage and absolute cell counts. There is, however, a very important practical issue to consider when operating such instruments and that is the requirement for accurate pipetting. It is recommended that 'reverse pipetting' techniques are used throughout.

Immunophenotyping is now the preferred method for lineage assignment, maturational characterization of malignant cells, clonality determination, detection of aberrant phenotypes, and the quantitation of haematopoietic cells (i.e. CD4+ T-lymphocytes, CD34+ stem cells). The aim of this chapter is to review the use of immunophenotyping techniques, selection of antibody combinations and fluorochromes, data analysis and quality assurance.

6.1 IMMUNOPHENOTYPING METHODOLOGY

6.1.1 Immunocytochemistry

Immunocytochemistry is routinely employed in haematological laboratories for the evaluation of leukaemic samples. This approach allows peripheral blood, bone marrow smears and cytospin preparations to be stained with specific antibodies. Samples are then counter-stained with a secondary reagent and, following the development of a colour reaction, visualized using a light microscope. A well established immunocytochemical technique is the APAAP (alkaline phosphatase anti-alkaline phosphatase) method, which enables the simultaneous examination of morphology and antigen expression (Erber *et al.*, 1986). The latter is of particular value when the cells of interest form a minor population, or when the morphology of the malignant cells differs only slightly from normal cells (see Tables 6.2 and 6.3 for the advantages and disadvantages of immunocytochemistry). Immunocytochemistry can be performed without the requirement for expensive equipment and can also provide a

Table 6.2   *Advantages of immunofluorescence and immunocytochemical staining*

Immunofluorescence	Immunocytochemistry
Antigen preservation	Retrospective studies
Quantitate antigenic sites	Simultaneous detection of both membrane and cytoplasmic antigens
Rapid analysis of high cell numbers by flow cytometry	Morphology of cells retained
Multi-parametric analysis (three or more antigens)	Slides can be stored until required
	Uses light microscope

Table 6.3 *Disadvantages of immunofluorescence and immunocytochemical analysis*

Immunofluorescence	Immunocytochemistry
Expensive apparatus	Fixation
Retrospective cell analysis not possible	Multi-parametric analysis very difficult
Interpretation difficulties	Membrane/cytoplasmic discrimination difficulties
	Antigenic quantitation not possible
	Lengthy procedure

permanent record of the staining pattern (Fig. 6.2). Furthermore, since the cells are fixed prior to staining, the resultant permeabilization also enables cytoplasmic antigen detection. Diagnostically important intracellular antigens can easily be detected using such an approach and include the myeloid lineage marker myeloperoxidase and lymphoid antigens, e.g. the T-cell marker CD3 and the B-cell marker CD22.

The practicalities of immunocytochemistry have been discussed in detail elsewhere (Moir *et al.*, 1983). Briefly, the smears are air-dried, preferably for a minimum of 1 hour, although storage at room temperature for up to 1 week is not deleterious (Forrest and Barnett, 1989; Mason and Erber, 1991). Slides can be stored for longer periods if they are wrapped in either clear polythene film or aluminium foil, and then stored below −20°C. It is important that slides stored in such a manner are allowed to reach room temperature before unwrapping (approximately 60 minutes), in order to prevent condensation formation and resultant cell lysis.

Prior to staining, it is recommended that an area of approximately 1.5 cm in diameter is inscribed, using either a diamond or a proprietary grease pen to: (i) enable the antibodies to be applied to the same area; (ii) facilitate the location of stained cells; and (iii) prevent antibodies from dissipating across the slide. The smears are then fixed in either acetone:methanol (ratio 1:1) for 90 seconds, or acetone for 10 minutes, at less than 4°C. Paraformaldehyde is best avoided, as weak antigens may be masked resulting in false-negative results (Forrest and Barnett, 1989). After fixation, the smears are washed in Tris-buffered saline (TBS), pH 7.6 for 5 minutes. The slides should not be allowed to become dry before adding the primary antibody and until the procedure has finished. The primary antibodies should have been titrated against samples known to be positive for the particular antigen (Reilly, 1996).

Following incubation, the slides are washed in TBS and incubated, using the same conditions as for the primary antibody, with the second stage antibody, an unconjugated rabbit-anti-mouse (RAM). The secondary antibody is best titred prior to use (usually in the range of 1/25–1/50). After washing, the APAAP complex is added for 30 minutes. This monoclonal antibody, raised against calf intestinal alkaline phosphatase, and then coupled to calf intestinal alkaline phosphatase (Cordell *et al.*, 1984), is added for 30 minutes. The second stage antibody (RAM) will bind the APAAP complex via its monoclonal antibody portion and thus complete the APAAP tower (Fig. 6.3). The RAM and APAAP steps are then repeated, with incubation times of 10 minutes, so that a latticework of alkaline phosphatase is built up. The presence of the enzyme is detected using an azo dye cytochemical substrate (naphthol-AS-MX phosphate and Fast Red TR) resulting in a vivid red colour detectable by light microscopy. Cellular morphology can be improved by counterstaining with haematoxylin (Fig. 6.2).

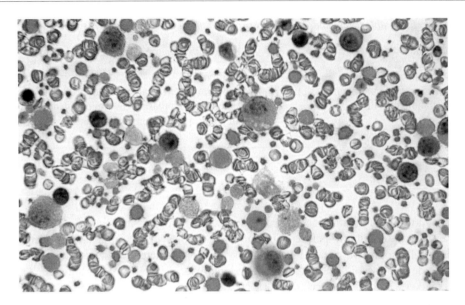

Fig. 6.2 *A case of acute myeloid leukaemia stained for myeloperoxidase using the alkaline phosphatase anti-alkaline phosphatase (APAAP) immunocytochemical technique.*

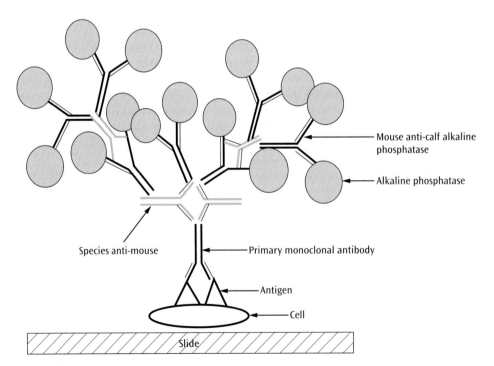

Fig. 6.3 *Schematic representation of the alkaline phosphatase anti-alkaline phosphatase (APAAP) immunocytochemical technique.*

6.1.2 Immunofluorescence staining

The second approach to detect cellular antigens, namely immunofluorescence, incorporates fluorochrome conjugated antibodies. Fluorescence microscopy was used to visualize the sites of antibody binding in the early 1980s (Janossy, 1982), a technique that was limited to single or dual colour staining on account of the restricted number of available fluorochromes (i.e. fluorescein isothiocyanate [FITC] or rhodamine [RITC]). An additional disadvantage with UV microscopy is that, following cellular staining, the cell suspension has to be 'wet mounted' on a glass slide and the positive and negative cells counted manually, a process which is time-consuming and which may limit the number of cells analysed.

Flow cytometry overcomes these limitations and enables rapid analysis of large numbers of cells using up to four antibody combinations (Camplejohn, 1994; Horvatinovich *et al.*, 1994; Lillevang *et al.*, 1995). The most widely used approach involves the direct labelling of peripheral blood or bone marrow leucocytes. The erythrocytes are subsequently eliminated by differential lysis, and the remaining cells are washed and analysed by flow cytometry. Briefly, fluorochrome conjugated antibodies are incubated with the test sample for 15 minutes in the dark at room temperature. The erythrocytes are then lysed, using a differential lysing solution that retains the leucocyte characteristics, washed and analysed by the flow cytometer. The advantages and disadvantages of the immunofluorescence technique are listed in Tables 6.2 and 6.3. Recently, whole blood 'no-lyse, no-wash' techniques have been developed which enable leucocyte analysis, even in the presence of unlysed erythrocytes, to be undertaken with minimal manipulation (McCarthy and Macey, 1993; Strauss *et al.*, 1996).

6.2 CLINICAL APPLICATIONS

6.2.1 Acute leukaemia

Immunophenotypic analysis should be undertaken in all cases of acute leukaemia, blast cell transformation of chronic myeloid leukaemia and other chronic myeloproliferative disorders (e.g. polycythaemia vera, idiopathic myelofibrosis). Gating is critical in the identification of the abnormal, or leukaemic, cells and data should be derived from as pure a population as possible. Borowitz *et al.* (1993) have proposed that the combination of CD45 expression with side scatter produces the best separation of blasts from promyelocytes, myelocytes, metamyelocytes and monocytes, especially when analysing bone marrow samples.

SAMPLE COLLECTION AND STORAGE

Blood and bone marrow samples must be obtained in anticoagulant. Preservative-free heparin is an acceptable reagent and such specimens are also suitable for cytogenetic analysis. Alternative reagents for cell marker analysis include K_2EDTA and K_3EDTA which, although unsuitable for cytogenetic analysis, will preserve the morphology, an important factor when interpreting leukaemia samples. Specimens should be processed as soon as possible after collection. However, samples may be stored for 24 hours, either at room temperature (whole blood) or at 4°C (isolated mononuclear cells), before immunophenotyping. When samples are not fresh (over 24 hours), it is advisable to perform a viability test to exclude dead cells (BCSH, 1994a).

MINIMUM PANELS

A 'minimum' primary panel may be used for lineage assignment of the blast population followed, if necessary, by a secondary panel of reagents to further define the maturational stage depending on the initial results. The 10 most useful reagents for a primary acute leukaemia panel, designed to characterize and distinguish acute myeloid leukaemia (AML) from B- and T-cell-derived acute lymphoblastic leukaemia (ALL), are as follows (BCSH, 1994a):

- three myeloid associated markers: CD33, cytoplasmic CD13 (cytCD13), anti-myeloperoxidase (anti-MPO);
- three B-cell associated markers: CD19, cytCD22 (and/or CD79a), CD10;
- three T-cell associated markers: CD2, cytCD3, CD7;
- the nuclear enzyme terminal deoxynucleotidyltransferase (TdT).

These 10 reagents will enable the detection and identification of all types of B-cell ALL (TdT+, CD19+, cytCD22+, CD10+/−), T-cell ALL (TdT+, CD7+, cytCD3+, CD2+/−) and AML (CD33+/−, cyCD13+/−, anti-MPO+/−). This 'primary' panel will identify more than 98% of acute leukaemias as myeloid, B-cell or T-cell, but will allocate approximately 2% of cases to the undifferentiated category.

A second panel of reagents can then be used to characterize the subtypes of AML (especially M0 and M7) and ALL further, or to help to establish the origin in cases classified as undifferentiated by the primary panel. These monoclonal antibodies, however, are not essential and are only useful in certain cases:

- the detection of the cytoplasmic μ chain (cyt μ) and surface immunoglobulins (SmIg) enables the subclassification of ALL into early B-ALL (CD19+, cyCD22+), common-ALL (CD10+), pre-B-ALL (cyt μ+) and B-ALL (SmIg+);
- anti-CD41 (glycoprotein IIb/IIIa) or/anti-CD61 (glycoprotein IIIa, vitronectin receptor β-chain) to detect acute megakaryoblastic leukaemia (M7);
- anti-glycophorin A to diagnose erythroleukaemias;
- additional T-associated markers (CD1, CD5, CD4 and CD8) to further characterize T-ALL.

An example of a practical three colour surface immunophenotyping panel, which will facilitate the phenotypic characterization of most acute leukaemias, whilst at the same time ensuring that the most frequent 'aberrant phenotypes' are detected, is shown in Tables 6.4 and 6.5.

Table 6.4 *Acute leukaemia panel for membrane staining*

Tube	FITC	PE	PerCP or PE/Cy5
1	IgG_1	IgG_{2a}	IgG_1
2	GpA	CD34	CD45
3	CD2	CD4	CD8
4	CD7	CD33	CD3
5	CD61	CD13	CD14
6	CD19	CD10	HLA-DR
7	CD5	CD1a	HLA-DR
Extra (if required)			

Table 6.5 *Panel for cytoplasmic/nuclear antigen staining*

Tube	FITC	PE
1	TdT Con	IgG_{2a}
2	TdT	CD13
3	MPOx	CD3
4	MPOx	CD22

IMMUNOPHENOTYPING OF THE FAB CLASSIFICATION OF AML (BENNETT *et al.*, 1976)

Acute undifferentiated leukaemia (M0) Immunophenotyping studies have been crucial in the recognition and characterization of AML with minimal myeloid differentiation (Bennett *et al.*, 1991). Features include: (i) negative myeloperoxidase and Sudan black reactions; (ii) negative B, T, megakaryocytic and erythroid lineage marker expression; and (iii) the expression of myeloid antigens recognized by at least one monoclonal antibody, such as anti-CD13, CD33 or MPO. Such cases frequently express CD34, have poor remission rates and have been reported to have a high incidence of cytogenetic abnormalities (Keenan *et al.*, 1992).

Acute myeloid leukaemia with maturation (M1) Morphological and cytochemical features are usually sufficient to identify this subtype of AML. However, M1 blasts are usually positive for CD13, CD33 and HLA-DR, but may exhibit weaker CD34 expression than that observed in cases of M0.

Acute myeloblastic leukaemia with maturation (M2) This type of AML is typically diagnosed by morphology and cytochemistry. However, 65% of all cases of M2 have the cytogenetic abnormality t(8;21)(q22;q22) with the corresponding AML1/ETO fusion transcript. Co-expression of CD19 and CD56 is unique to such patients (Hurwitz *et al.*, 1992). CD56, an isoform of the neural cell adhesion molecule, has been proposed to link the propensity of t(8;21) AML to develop granulocytic sarcomas, particularly cranial nerve chloromas (Tallman *et al.*, 1993).

Acute promyelocytic leukaemia (APML-M3) The immunophenotype of M3 is unique and represents a rare example of agreement between immunophenotype and morphological diagnosis. The findings (CD13+, CD9+, and HLA-DR–) are consistently associated with the RAR-α rearrangements found in both classical M3 and the 'microgranular' variant (M3v) (Lo Coco *et al.*, 1991). Given the different therapeutic approaches used in acute promyelocytic leukaemia, the identification of both M3/M3v is of particular clinical importance. Interestingly, the antigenic profile of APML is similar to that of basophils (CD34–, CD13+, CD33+, HLA-DR–, CD68+, CD9+), which has prompted the hypothesis that APML cells may be derived from a basophil precursor, rather than from the normal promyelocytic counterpart (Erber *et al.*, 1994). The retinoic acid syndrome, a serious complication of therapy for this disorder, has been correlated with the expression of CD13 by the leukaemic cells (Vahdat *et al.*, 1994).

Acute myelomonocytic and monoblastic leukaemias (M4/M5) Immunophenotyping, although of value in classifying leukaemias with monocytic differentiation, does not replace morphological and cytochemical analysis. Anti-CD14 and CD11b are the most helpful reagents, but while CD14-positive leukaemias are nearly always CD11b+, the reverse situation is not always true. Expression of the T-cell marker CD2 is characteristic of acute myelo-monocytic leukaemia with eosinophilia (M4Eo) and inv(16)(p13q22) (Adriaansen *et al.*, 1993).

Acute erythroleukaemia (M6) CD34 and HLA-DR are characteristically negative in most acute erythroleukaemias. Anti-glycophorin A is the most helpful marker (Gahmberg *et al.*, 1984) but, because it recognizes a sialoglycoprotein that appears shortly before the synthesis of haemoglobin, it can be negative if cells originate prior to the proerythroblast stage.

Acute megakaryoblastic leukaemia (M7) The lineage-specific immunological markers that aid the identification of M7 include monoclonal antibodies that react with the platelet glyco-protein IIIa (GpIIIa, CD61), GpIIb and the GpIIb/IIIa complex (CD41), GpIX and Ib (CD42a and b), and polyclonal reagents to von Willebrand antigen. However, CD61 and CD41 are generally considered to be the more sensitive and discriminatory (Erber *et al.*, 1987; San Miguel *et al.*, 1988). Nevertheless, caution must be exercised, as false-positive reactions may occur due to platelet adherence to leukaemic blasts (Betz *et* al., 1992).

PROGNOSTIC FACTORS IN AML

The contribution of immunophenotyping to prognosis in AML has been a controversial issue, with a large number of studies demonstrating significantly different results. This may be due, in part, to the use of different technical methods, monoclonal reagents and threshold values, as well as to the diversity of the patient population studied and the treatment protocols employed. In general, correlation of single antigen expression, rather than the total pheno-type, to clinical outcome is of dubious value. For example, lymphoid antigen expression in AML is associated with both favourable (t(8;21), t(15;17), inv(16)), and poor (t(9;22) and 11q23 rearrangements) prognostic chromosomal abnormalities.

CLASSIFICATION OF ALL SUBTYPES

Classification of ALL by immunophenotyping is shown in Table 6.6. As predicted from normal B-cell antigenic expression, the most consistent marker for B-lineage ALL is CD19 which is often brightly co-expressed with CD10. Interestingly, Hurwitz *et al.* (1988) studied the phenotype of 113 B-lineage ALL cases and compared them with cells from normal stages of B-cell ontogeny. They observed 16 different leukaemia phenotypes that were not found in normal marrow. These findings suggest that B-cell ALL may not accurately represent cells arrested at the stage where the leukaemogenic event occurred.

T-lineage ALLs are generally classified according to the three stages of thymocyte maturation. Early thymocytes express CD7, CD2, CD5 and CD38 (stage 1). In stage II, the

Table 6.6   *Immunophenotypic classification of acute lymphoblastic leukaemia (ALL)*

Cell type	Subclassification	Immunophenotype
B cell	Early B-cell precursor	CD19+, cCD22+, TdT+
	Common ALL	CD10+, CD19+, cCD22+, TdT+
	Pre-B ALL	CD19+, cCD22+, Cytμ+, TdT+
	B-cell ALL	CD19+, cCD22+, SmIg (κ/λ)+, TdT+
T cell	Pre-T cell ALL	cCD3+, CD7+, TdT+
	Early T cell ALL	CD2+, cCD3+, CD5+, CD7+, TdT+
	Cortical T cell ALL	CD1+, CD2+, cCD3+, CD4/8+, CD5+, TdT+
	Late T cell	CD2+, CD3+, CD4/8+, CD7+, TdT+

common thymocytes acquire expression of CD1 and co-express CD4 and CD8. In stage III, the medullary thymocytes lose CD1, express CD3 and retain either CD4 or CD8. Cytoplasmic CD3 (cCD3) can be identified in the earliest thymocyte and is therefore a specific and reliable marker for early T cells (van Dongen *et al.*, 1988). Most cases of T-lineage ALL are TdT+, CD7+ and HLA-DR–. Cases expressing CD7 and HLA-DR can be difficult to resolve and require additional study with further T-cell and myeloid markers. The expression of additional T-cell markers without myeloid antigens is probably T-cell ALL, while if more than one myeloid marker is present, in the absence of other T-cell markers excluding CD7, then the case is likely to be an acute myeloid leukaemia. It should be stressed that CD7 is not specific for T-cells, since up to 26% of acute myeloid leukaemias express this antigen (Bradstock *et al.*, 1989).

MINIMAL RESIDUAL DISEASE

Providing leukaemic cells express an unusual immunophenotype, cell marker analysis can be used to identify the presence of minimal residual disease (MRD). This is of particular value in monitoring leukaemic patients in remission, as well as detecting leukaemic contamination of bone marrow and/or peripheral blood progenitor cells collected for autologous bone marrow transplantation (Campana, 1994; Serui *et al.*, 1995; San Miguel *et al.*, 1997). The assessment of remission is important in determining therapy, although the sensitivity of conventional morphology for detecting residual blasts is only about 5%. The sensitivity of routine cytogenetics, as well as fluorescein in situ hybridization (FISH) techniques, lies within the range of routine morphology and patients with normal results may still possess as many as 10^{10} leukaemic cells. The sensitivity of MRD detection can be significantly improved by immunological and molecular methods, with less than one leukaemic cell in 10^4 normal cells being detectable. At present, it is well established that, with few exceptions, there are no leukaemic-specific antigens. However, the use of large panels of monoclonal reagents in double and triple combinations has identified aberrant phenotypic characteristics not usually observed in normal cells. It is the identification of such aberrant phenotypes that enables MRD to be detected by immunological methods. Firstly, some normal combinations of antigen expression are restricted to specific tissues, e.g. normal thymocytes express TdT, together with markers such as CD3, CD5 or CD1. While such expression is not normally found outside the thymus, it is characteristic of T-ALL. Therefore, even one CD3/TdT-positive cell in the peripheral blood or bone marrow suggests the presence of residual disease. Secondly, acute leukaemias may express normal differentiation antigens in combinations not present on normal haematopoietic cells, i.e. asynchronous antigen expression, CD13/TdT, CD33/TdT for B-lineage leukaemias, and CD34/CD56 and CD117/CD15 for acute myeloid leukaemia (San Miguel *et al.*, 1997). Further cases can be characterized by antigen over expression (Macedo *et al.*, 1995).

6.2.2 Chronic lymphoproliferative disorders

The value of immunophenotyping as a diagnostic aid in chronic lymphoproliferative disorders can be summarized as follows (BCSH, 1994b):

- to distinguish acute lymphoblastic leukaemias (TdT+) from mature chronic lymphoproliferative disorders (TdT–) (Burkitt's or L3-ALL being the exception);
- to enable the differentiation of clonal B-cell malignancies from non-clonal or polyclonal reactive lymphocytosis, by means of the surface expression patterns of immunoglobulin light chains (κ or λ);

K₃EDTA), and analysed within 6 hours. Specimens referred to a central laboratory for analysis must be accompanied by a total white cell count (WCC) (absolute lymphocyte counts are best derived from the total WCC and the flow cytometric differential, rather than from a haematology analyser alone). All samples should be dated, with the time of collection being documented, and fully processed within 18 hours to minimize the effect of anticoagulant. Storage and transportation should be between 10 and 30°C and specimens should not be subjected to temperatures below 10°C (Ekong *et al.*, 1992). Packaging and transportation of HIV-infected material should be in accordance with the regulations of the appropriate postal and/or courier service. Specimen integrity must be confirmed on receipt, and further specimens requested if there is evidence of gross haemolysis, clots, or if the sample is received after 18 hours from the time of venepuncture.

6.3.3 Gating strategies

In the late 1980s, the improvement in software coupled with the discovery of additional fluorochromes enabled lymphocyte identification and characterization by either light scatter gating procedures or differential staining with CD45 and CD14 (Loken *et al.*, 1990). These approaches, however, have several disadvantages: first, a forward/side scatter gate approach does not identify gate contaminants and may result in falsely low percentage values, while the need for larger panels (i.e. up to six tubes) increases analysis time, specimen handling and ultimately cost. Secondly, it is not possible to detect tube-to-tube variation when a light scatter gate is derived from CD45/CD14 'back-gating' and, in addition, the isotype control fails to control for CD45/CD14 staining. Therefore, it is recommended that CD4+ T lymphocyte enumeration is performed using three colour immunophenotyping by one of the three gating strategies highlighted below. A summary of the evolution of current gating techniques can be found in Mandy *et al.* (1997), while the advantages and disadvantages of each technique are detailed in the recently published BCSH guidelines (BCSH, 1997).

T-GATE METHOD

This technique uses whole blood lysis and is best suited to those flow cytometers that are capable of generating absolute counts (Mandy *et al.*, 1992). The absolute T-lymphocyte subset counts can be obtained from a single tube containing a mixture of FITC-conjugated anti-CD3, PE-conjugated anti-CD4 and anti-CD8 conjugated to a third fluorochrome (e.g. PerCP). Isotype controls are not required and, following staining, lysis and washing, the specimen is analysed using both right angle light scatter and the CD3 fluorescence channel. This allows the T-lymphocyte cluster to be identified and the relevant gate to be set. Events are collected and analysed through this T-gate using the first (FL1) and second (FL2) channels. The T-cell subsets are expressed as a percentage of total CD3+ lymphocytes, since B-lymphocytes, CD8+ NK (natural killer) cells, monocytes and debris are excluded. The antibody combinations are detailed in BCSH (1997).

LINEAGE GATING

Lineage gating, a development of T-gating, was first proposed by Mercolino *et al.* (1995). It combines both T- and B-lineage gating strategies so that all lymphocyte subsets are captured, including NK cells. The use of three tubes, including isotype controls, enables the analysis of T-, B- and NK lymphocytes, as well as obtaining duplicate T-lymphocyte analyses and a lymphosum (lymphosum is defined as the sum of T, B and NK values). The latter two features enable the verification of results, an important internal quality control parameter. The combination of antibodies and fluorochromes is detailed in BCSH (1997). Essentially, an isotype control tube is used to set a lymphocyte gate, using forward scatter (FSc) versus side scatter (SSc), and events within this region are used to identify negative and positive regions on the three fluorescence channels. The second tube, which contains fluorochrome-conjugated CD3, CD4 and CD8 antibodies, is then used to analyse T-lymphocytes, as in the T-gating method. The final tube, which contains an NK marker (e.g. anti-CD16), a B-lymphocyte marker (i.e. anti-CD19) and the T-lymphocyte marker anti-CD3, enables the lymphosum to be calculated, as well as obtaining a duplicate check on CD3+ T-lymphocytes.

CD45/SIDE SCATTER (SSC) GATING

Methods relying solely on light scatter gating may lead to problems with contamination. Consequently, approaches have been devised to optimize the placement of light scatter gates and, at the same time, provide details of gate contamination by non-lymphocytes and debris. The use of a combination of anti-CD45 and CD14 was initially proposed (Loken *et al.*, 1990), but has major disadvantages as detailed earlier. However, to overcome such limitations CD45/SSc techniques were devised and are the basis of the Centers for Disease Control (CDC) guidelines (Centers for Disease Control, 1992, 1993). As with T- and lineage gating, this approach uses fluorescence versus side scatter. CD45 expression is used to identify the lymphocyte population (CD45^{bright}, low linear SSc). The lymphocyte gate thus defined is relatively free from contaminating cells and debris. The remaining fluorescence channels are then analysed through this region. For an in-depth description of this procedure, see Nicholson *et al.* (1996).

6.3.4 Sample preparation and analysis

Sample preparation should be undertaken in a designated area, which requires thorough decontamination after use. Test tubes need to be individually capped in order to prevent spillage and to retain aerosols that may be created during mixing. Buffered paraformaldehyde (pH 7.0–7.4, 2% solution) or a proprietary cell fixing agent should be added to samples following staining, lysing and washing, in order to minimize the infection risk. All samples require an inactivation procedure before disposal, using, ideally, a combined viral inactivating and mycobactericidal reagent.

   Minimal manipulation of samples is desirable, and therefore to ensure no loss of cells, or their subsets, the whole blood lymphocyte staining method should be used. Briefly, peripheral blood is added to premixed three colour monoclonal antibodies at concentrations recommended by the manufacturer. If such premixed reagents are not commercially available, the user will need to determine the optimum working concentrations by titration of each antibody against each other and compare the results with that obtained when using single staining (Reilly, 1996). After incubation in the dark, the red cells are lysed using a proprietary lysing reagent, and washed in accordance with the manufacturer's recommendations. Several commercial systems now employ the 'lyse-no-wash' technique, thereby reducing specimen handling, cell disruption and loss due to centrifugation and washing. If a wash step is included, vortexing is advisable before analysis, to disrupt cell aggregates.

   The choice of gating strategy will influence the method of analysis. Manual gating techniques must be employed if computer-assisted analysis is not used. It is preferable that data are acquired ungated, with a minimum of 2500 lymphocyte events being collected. If data are acquired gated, e.g. by using CD45/SSc, then the gate placement should be checked for each tube, so that tube-to-tube variation can be reduced. Significant differences between tubes usually indicate sample preparation error and the tube (or panel) should be repeated. In addition, if monocyte contamination of more than 5% is obtained within the gate, then the tube should be repeated and, if still unacceptable, a new specimen requested.

6.3.5 Key points (see BCSH, 1997)

- Stream-in-air flow cytometers should not be used for CD4+ T-lymphocyte determination in HIV-positive individuals.
- Peripheral blood specimens should be collected into EDTA and fully processed within 18 hours. Total WCC enumeration on haematology analysers should be performed within 6 hours of collection.
- Specimens require storage at between 10 and 30°C.
- Samples should be fixed in 2% paraformaldehyde, or proprietary cell fixative, for a minimum of 30 minutes after staining and prior to analysis.
- Analysis should be by three or four colour lymphocyte immunophenotyping, incorporating either T-gating, lineage gating or CD45/SSc gating.
- Anti-CD4 and CD8 antibodies should be phycoerythrin-conjugated.
- Isotype controls are not required for T-gating and CD45/SSc gating methods.
- Process controls should be used at least once a week, and preferably daily.
- Analysis gates should have < 5% monocyte contamination.
- CD4+ T-lymphocytes should be reported as both percentage and absolute values. If T-gating is used, the clinician should be notified that the T-lymphocyte subset percentage values are expressed as a percentage of the total T-lymphocytes only.
- Wherever possible, calculation of absolute CD4+ T-lymphocytes numbers should be obtained using single platform technology.
- Participation in external proficiency testing schemes should be demonstrable.

6.4 CD34+ HAEMOPOIETIC STEM CELL ENUMERATION

It is well established that the 1–3% of cells in the bone marrow, expressing the CD34 antigen, a heavily glycosylated mucin-like structure, are capable of reconstituting long-term, multi-lineage haematopoiesis after ablative therapy (Berenson et al., 1988; Andrews et al., 1992). CD34+ cells are also found in the peripheral blood of normal individuals, but are extremely rare (approximately 0.01–0.05%). However, current treatment regimes, including chemo-therapy and/or haematopoietic growth factors, can significantly increase CD34+ stem cell counts in patients and donors. Peripheral blood stem cells (PBSCs) have now virtually replaced bone marrow as the primary source of stem cells for autologous transplantation after myeloablative therapy (Gratwohl et al., 1996). The procedure is also being increasingly used for allogeneic transplantation between HLA-identical siblings (Russell et al., 1996). Advantages of PBSCs include the generally shorter engraftment time, the reduced hospital-ization costs (Arger et al., 1995), the presence of large numbers of T-lymphocytes and NK cells which may reduce post-transplant relapse (Dreger et al., 1994), and the elimination of a general anaesthetic which extends the procedure's applicability. In addition, the PBSC product is also more suitable for ex vivo manipulation, including CD34+ cell selection (Brugger et al., 1994), tumour purging (Ross et al., 1995) and gene manipulation (Bregni et al., 1992).

Transplant centres routinely rely on CD34-positive cell quantitation by flow cytometry as a marker of pluripotential stem cells to facilitate the optimal timing and adequacy of haematopoietic progenitor cell harvests (Haas *et al.*, 1994). Assessment of haematopoietic progenitors in colony-forming assays, although reported by a number of groups to correlate with CD34 levels (Siena *et al.*, 1991), is handicapped by lack of reproducibility and prolonged assay time. A minimum threshold dose of between 2 and 5×10^6 CD34-positive cells/kg body weight has been observed in multiple clinical settings to result in adequate engraftment (Krause *et al.*, 1996), although the lack of standardization of the assay prevents a more exact definition of threshold level (Bender *et al.*, 1992). It is this lack of standardization with respect to reagents and gating strategies, as well as the use of haematology instruments to derive absolute counts, that has contributed to the widespread variation among reported results. There is, therefore, an urgent need for internationally agreed protocols to standardize the approach and to enable the comparison of clinical and laboratory data. Recently, a number of these issues have been addressed and the following recommendations can be made.

6.4.1 Monoclonal antibody selection

The CD34 antigen possesses epitopes that can be classified in three broad categories, depending on their sensitivity to neuraminidase and glycoprotease from *Pasteurella haemolytica* (Sutherland *et al.*, 1992). Epitopes recognized by class I antibodies (MY10, 12.8, Immu133, Immuno409, 43.A1) are sensitive to both enzymes. Those detected by class II antibodies (QBEND10, ICH3) are sensitive to glycoprotease only, while those detected by class III antibodies (Tük3, HPCA-2, BIRMA-K3) are insensitive to both enzymes. Class I antibodies fail to detect all glycoforms of the CD34 antigen, due to their dependence on negatively charged carbohydrate moieties, and consequently may miss CD34 expression in some leukaemias (Sutherland and Keating, 1992), while their lower avidity and reduced reactivity following conjugation further limit their use. Therefore, it is extremely important that class II or class III antibodies are used for CD34+ stem cell enumeration. The use of the brightest excitable fluorochromes with an argon laser, i.e. phycoerythrin (PE), is also recommended for detection of CD34+ cells (Johnsen, 1995; Sutherland *et al.*, 1996a,b). FITC conjugation, because of its induced negative charge, interferes with the binding properties of some class II antibodies such as QBEND10 and should not be used.

An FITC-conjugated monoclonal antibody to the CD45 antigen is used in combination with CD34-PE to provide an additional parameter in the identification of CD34+ cells (see the Mulhouse, ISHAGE and SIHON protocols below). Not only does it enable the identification of true CD34+ cells, but it is also a useful indicator of the effectiveness of the red cell lysis step and aids in the detection of white cells from contaminating events, such as platelets, platelet aggregates and other debris that can bind low levels of PE-conjugated CD34 antibodies (Sutherland *et al.*, 1996a,b).

6.4.2 Cell separation, lysis and counting techniques

Whole blood lysis techniques, using NH_4Cl-based reagents, are recommended for peripheral blood and apheresis products, as a number of groups have reported improved recovery when compared with cell separation techniques (Siena *et al.*, 1991; Owens and Loken, 1995). UK NEQAS data have revealed a marked variation in the number of CD45-positive cells routinely counted (10 000 to 1.2 million), with a number of laboratories counting significantly less than 50 000. Reduction of the number of events per test (tube) will reduce the reliability of the estimation to unacceptable levels. Given the fact that the standard error of the number of positive cells per analysis is given by the square root of the number of positive cells, the larger the acquisition, the smaller the coefficient of variation (Wunder *et al.*, 1992). It is therefore recommended that a minimum of 100 CD34+ events and at least 75 000 CD45+ events be collected (Sutherland *et al.*, 1996a).

6.4.3 Gating strategies

A number of gating strategies for flow cytometric enumeration of CD34+ cells have been published, the most important being the Milan, Mulhouse, ISHAGE and SIHON protocols:

The Milan Protocol (Siena *et al.*, 1991) is the simplest and involves the use of forward scatter (FSc) and side scatter (SSc) to gate out the red cells, debris and cell aggregates. The gated nucleated cell population is then plotted on CD34 versus SSc. Only CD34+ cells with low SSc are used to calculate the number of CD34+ cells expressed as a percentage of nucleated cells. However, this method suffers from a number of limitations (Sutherland *et al.*, 1996b):

- the reliance on an isotype-matched control to set the positive cell analysis region for CD34+ cells is unsatisfactory for rare event analysis;
- a reliance on simple FSc versus SSc to set the denominator;
- an absence of any means to exclude dead cells from the analysis.

Despite these limitations, the Milan protocol is probably adequate for analysing CD34+ cells in cytokine-mobilized peripheral blood and apheresis products providing the samples are in good viable condition and relatively free of debris.

The Mulhouse Protocol, proposed by Bender *et al.* (1994), is a logical development of the Milan protocol and uses CD45-positive events to identify the leucocytes. These are then plotted on CD34 versus SSc. Only CD34-positive events with low SSc are used to calculate the number of CD34+ cells expressed as a percentage of CD45+ cells. The use of anti-CD45 allows a more accurate resolution between leucocytes and other (irrelevant) cells and also enables the detection of stem cells with lower expression of CD45 than mature lymphocytes and monocytes (Borowitz *et al.*, 1993).

The ISHAGE protocol was first described by Sutherland *et al.* (1994) and takes advantage of the dim CD45 expression of CD34+ stem cells with low SSc and incorporates a sequential gating strategy; three tubes are set up containing the following antibodies: CD45-FITC/CD34-PE (two tubes), and CD45-FITC/isotype-PE (one tube). At least 75 000 CD45+ events per tube and a minimum of 100 CD34+ events should be counted. An initial gate is set on a CD45 versus SSc dot plot so as to contain all CD45+ events, ranging from dim to bright expression, and should include all events except those that are CD45-negative and dead cells that fluorescence well to the right of the brightest monocytes and lymphocytes. The events in gate R1 are then displayed on a CD34 versus SSc dot plot, which is used to place a second gate (R2) to include the cluster of CD34+ events. The third plot is CD45 versus SSc of CD34+ events that fulfil the criteria of gates R1 and R2 (i.e. sequential gating). Cells forming a cluster with characteristic low SSc and low to intermediate CD45 fluorescence are gated by a third region (R3). Finally, the events fulfilling the criteria of all three gates (R1, R2 and R3) are displayed on a FSc versus SSc dot plot. The region R4 identifies a cluster of events meeting all the fluorescence and light scatter criteria of CD34+ stem/progenitor cells. Any events falling outside region R4 are not included in the calculation of the percentage of CD34+ cells or the absolute number of CD34+ cells. The absolute CD34+ cell count is determined as follows: the number of non-specific events in R4 from the isotype control tube is subtracted from the average total number of events in the CD34-stained sample tubes to form the numerator. The denominator is provided by the average total number of CD45+ events from the CD45 FITC/CD34 PE replicate samples. The absolute CD34+ cell count in the sample, therefore, is calculated by multiplying this figure by the absolute total white cell count (WCC) as provided by the haematology analyser.

This strategy has been incorporated into the guidelines formulated by the Stem Cell Enumeration Committee of the International Society of Hematotherapy and Graft Engineering (ISHAGE) (Sutherland *et al.*, 1996a). A single platform version of this protocol is provided by the Stem-Kit assay (Coulter-Immunotech) in which a known amount of microbeads, at a known concentration (Stem-Count), is added to a known amount of stained, lysed whole blood. The absolute CD34+ cell count can be calculated from the observed ratio between the number of flow cytometrically counted beads and CD34+ cells.

The SIHON (Dutch Foundation for Immunophenotyping in Haemato-Oncology) Protocol (Gratama *et al.*, 1997a) incorporates the DNA/RNA laser excited dye (LDS-751) to identify nucleated cells during data collection (Terstappen *et al.*, 1988). In addition, monocytic (CD14+) and mature myeloid cells (CD66e+) are excluded during list-mode data analysis, in order to eliminate interference by their Fcγ receptor-mediated monoclonal antibody binding. The latter may be important as the expression and activity of these receptors to bind murine IgG has been shown to be upregulated by G-CSF and GM-CSF used to mobilize PBSCs (van de Winkel and Capel, 1993). A single-platform software-driven method, including thresholding on nucleated cells using a proprietary DNA/RNA stain, is offered by the ProCount kit (Becton Dickinson) (Chan *et al.*, 1994).

It is unlikely that standardization based on narrowly defined protocols will be achieved in the foreseeable future. As a result, Gratama *et al.* (1997a) have stated that:

> the most effective approach to reducing interlaboratory variation in CD34 enumeration consists of the adherence to consensus protocols formulated in general terms, combined with real-time evaluation of performance by the organizations for external quality assurance.

However, quality control issues may be further magnified in the future if quantification of CD34+ cell subsets becomes routine, since neutrophil and platelet recovery appears to correlate best with CD34+CD38+ and CD34+CD41+ subsets, respectively (Dercksen *et al.*, 1995).

6.4.4 Key points (see Barnett *et al.*, 1999)

- Whole blood staining, NH₄Cl-based erythrocyte lysis, no fixation, no washing techniques should be used (Bossuyt *et al.*, 1997; Macey *et al.*, 1997).
- Class II (which must be PE-conjugated) or class III conjugated anti-CD34 antibodies should be used.
- Single-platform enumerations are recommended, i.e. absolute CD34+ cell count derived directly without the need for an haematology analyser.
- Anti-CD45 should be used as an additional parameter for identifying the CD34+ cell population. Pan-CD45 reagents should be used that detect not only all isoforms but also all glycoforms, e.g. anti HLE-1 (BDIS), J33 (Immunotech) and KC56 (Coulter) (Sutherland *et al.*, 1996).
- Control tubes for non-specific antibody binding are not required.
- Acquisition of list mode data containing a fixed, statistically significant number of CD34+ cells.

6.5 QUALITY CONTROL ISSUES AND PITFALLS

Three common areas in which problems occur in immunophenotyping are: (i) specimen processing, (ii) data acquisition and (iii) data analysis/reporting.

6.5.1 Specimen processing

It is important that specimens are as fresh as possible (Ekong *et al.*, 1992, 1993), especially when undertaking antigen density quantification or cytoplasmic staining (see below). Several guidelines have been published which address the issues of specimen integrity (NCCLS, 1992; Nicholson, 1994; BCSH, 1997). Correct handling and transportation procedures need to be established, while the choice of anticoagulant is important. For example, K_3EDTA is preferred since it maintains the morphology and the flow cytometric profile of the cellular components (NCCLS, 1992; Nicholson, 1994; BCSH, 1997). Red cell lysis and cell separation procedures are frequent causes of analytical variation (Romeu *et al.*, 1992). Over-lysis may result in changes in forward and side scatter patterns, quenching of fluorochromes (particularly if aldehyde-based lysis reagents are used) and selective cell loss. In contrast, poorly lysed specimens retain red cells which may impair the identification of specific cell populations as well as producing tube-to-tube variation in forward and side scatter patterns, thus making consistent gate placement difficult. Inappropriate vortexing conditions may similarly cause tube-to-tube variation. For example, samples treated too vigorously exhibit excessive cell debris or develop separation of granulocyte populations, whilst under-vortexing may result in cell doublets that are excluded from routine gating strategies, termed 'escapees' (Jackson, 1990; Gratama *et al.*, 1997b). Centrifugation can be a major cause of cell loss and poor final sample preparation. Excessive centrifugation causes cell damage and alters the forward and side light scatter characteristics, as well as increasing the level of cell debris. It is also well recognized that washing undertaken after lysis incurs cell loss and is even more pronounced if the centrifugation speed is too slow.

6.5.2 Data acquisition

The number of events acquired and the configuration of the instrument are two important variables influencing the reproducibility of results. It is important that the flow cytometer is calibrated daily (Agrawal *et al.*, 1991) using commercial beads, in order to: (i) monitor the light scatter and fluorescence peak channel CVs; (ii) monitor light and fluorescence peak channel drift; (iii) monitor instrument sensitivity; and (iv) facilitate compensation setup to adjust for spectral overlap. All values should be logged daily, together with the instrument settings. All settings should be re-established following a change in bead batch, or after an instrument service. Commercial beads, however, only provide guidance for the final flow cytometer setup, and optimization of settings used in the analysis and acquisition of specimens is best achieved using a fresh normal sample (NCCLS, 1992; Schwartz and Fernandez-Repollet, 1993; Schwartz *et al.*, 1996; BCSH, 1997). The use of a process control is recommended to enable the monitoring of reagent performance, staining, lysis and analysis (Barnett *et al.*, 1996; Fay *et al.*, 1996; BCSH, 1997). Such controls must be run at least once a week (prior to any of the week's work being processed) and preferably on a daily basis. They should also be run: (i) if there has been a change in reagent and/or laboratory personnel; (ii) after instrument service and/or instrument calibration; or (iii) in any situation where the validity of the technique is suspect. Process controls, which should be stable for at least 30 days and have manufacturer-assigned target values, are used to test the labelling procedure and if possible the lysing step. Results obtained from these reagents should be plotted on a Levy–Jennings type plot, and provide a visual indication of drift or bias over time. Fresh normal specimens are not ideal as a daily process control, due to variability between individuals, although they may be used for instrument setup and correcting for spectral overlap (compensation).

6.5.3 Data analysis

A number of variables may affect data analysis, namely:

- the gating strategy and gate placement/analysis region used (Kromer and Grossmuller, 1994); (ii) the establishment of acceptability criteria;
- the use of automated gating;
- the need for quality control checks (within-assay replicates);
- the cursor placement for isotype controls; and
- the development of artefactual staining patterns.

The results issued from a laboratory depend on the gating strategy employed; for example, when using the T-gating approach (Mandy *et al.*, 1992) it is important that values for CD4+ and CD8 + T-lymphocytes are expressed as a percentage of the total T-lymphocyte population and not of the total lymphocyte population. The placement of the analysis region is a further factor for consideration, since if the gate is too tight there is a possibility of excluding relevant cells, while an over-generous gate will include contaminating cells (Kromer and Grossmuller, 1994) and give a falsely low result. Failure to establish acceptability criteria can lead to the release of erroneous results by the laboratory. Recent guidelines for CD4+ T-lymphocyte enumeration have suggested a monocyte contamination within a CD45/SSc gate of less than 5% (BCSH, 1997) and a lymphosum (CD3 + CD19 + NK cells [CD16 and/or CD56] = 100 ± 3%) (Nicholson, 1994; BCSH, 1997). Furthermore the tube-to-tube variation for replicate antigens should be less than 3%. Care should also be taken when using automated gating software, and individual operators need to be familiar with the strengths and weaknesses of such technology. Data analysis plots should be checked to ensure correct gate placement and that the software is not excluding specific cell populations.

It is important that if isotype control antibodies are used, they are matched to the test antibody, in both fluorochrome and antibody concentration, and that the cursor is correctly placed. In contrast to leukaemia immunophenotyping, enumeration of CD4+ T-lymphocytes and CD34+ cells may be undertaken without isotype controls (Sutherland *et al.*, 1996a,b; BCSH, 1997).

Finally, operators need to be aware of several causes of false-positive staining reactions. False positivity may result from non-specific antibody binding through Fc receptors, a situation characteristically seen in acute monoblastic leukaemia, or from a number of technical problems, such as using the wrong antibody or inclusion of dead cells in the analysis. Non-specific antibody binding can be reduced by blocking the Fc receptors by pre-incubating the cells with rabbit serum. In contrast, the identification of B-lymphocyte clonality by demonstrating light chain restriction may be masked by cytophilic antibody binding. This problem is overcome on removal of the immunoglobulin by suspending the cells in PBS at 37°C for 30 minutes and then washing several times in PBS at 37°C. More recently, this approach has been applied to whole blood techniques with good effect. Briefly, 0.5 mL of whole blood is suspended in 9.5 mL of PBS at 37°C for 30 minutes, with gentle inversion of the tube every 10 minutes, followed by washing three times in PBS. Care is needed when removing the supernatant so as not to disturb the cell pellet, which is then re-suspended in 0.5 mL of PBS before analysis as for whole blood. A further cause of false positivity has been described by Ekong *et al.* (1993), who demonstrated artefactual double staining CD4+CD8+ T-lymphocytes in 17% of HIV-positive and 6% of normal individuals. The group suggested that this results from a plasma/serum factor that can be precipitated with ammonium sulphate. Finally, inappropriate instrument setup can be a source of erroneous results and is usually attributed to inappropriate flow cytometer compensation (for further details, see Owens and Loken, 1995).

6.6 FUTURE DEVELOPMENTS

Flow cytometric analysis has, in recent years, been one of the most rapidly expanding areas in diagnostic haematology. The change from single colour immunofluorescence phenotyping by UV microscopy to multi-parametric four colour analysis by flow cytometry occurred in approximately 10 years. Thus the versatility of the flow cytometer has enabled new and innovative flow cytometric techniques to be added to this repertoire, the most important of which are surface membrane antigen quantification and intracellular antigen detection.

6.6.1 Antigen density quantification

Several studies have highlighted the clinical and research applications of antigen quantification or 'quantimetry'. Using such an approach, it has been possible not only to define antigen density on normal cells, but also to monitor changes in antigen expression that occur during viral infection (Lenkei and Andersson, 1995) and ageing (Storie *et al.*, 1995), and moreover to facilitate leukaemia diagnosis and minimal disease monitoring (Caldwell *et al.*, 1987; Lavabre-Bertrand *et al.*, 1994; Farahat *et al.*, 1995a,b). Recent studies (Lavabre-Bertrand *et al.*, 1994; Farahat *et al.*, 1995b), for example, have employed quantitative flow cytometry to distinguish normal B-cell precursors from their leukaemic counterparts by identifying the differentially high expression of CD10 and CD19 in ALL. In addition, Ginaldi *et al.* (1996) have reported that the combined quantification of CD3 and CD7 expression is of diagnostic value in distinguishing normal from malignant T-cells. Collectively, these studies suggest that quantimetry is of value in differentiating a variety of leukaemias from their normal cellular counterparts and providing additional information with regard to the developmental processes involved in lineage maturation. Finally, the Leucocyte Antigen Workshops have reported the use of antigen quantification as a means of assisting the assignment of antibodies to CD clusters (Poncelet *et al.*, 1986).

Four methods for antigen quantification or 'quantimetry' techniques have been developed; quantitative indirect immunofluorescence (QIFI) (Poncelet and Carayon, 1985), antibody binding capacity (ABC) (Schwartz *et al.*, 1996) and, more recently, calibration of the flow cytometer with molecules of equivalent soluble fluorescence (MESF) and the subsequent use of antibody conjugates with known MESF/antibody ratios (Davis *et al.*, 1996; Iyer *et al.*, 1996). The first two approaches are discussed below.

THE QIFI APPROACH

The QIFI method utilizes beads, coated with known amounts of murine monoclonal antibody (IgG anti-CD5), to serve as a control for indirect immunofluorescence analysis. These are then used to represent cells that express antigen at differing densities and thus form an external calibrant for construction of calibration curves. The manufacture and calibration of these beads were achieved by labelling a CD5-expressing cell line with increasing concentrations of radiolabelled anti-CD5 (clone T101). When the plateau of reactivity was reached (i.e. counts per minute versus increasing concentration of radiolabelled antibody), the number of monoclonal antibodies that bound to the cell could then be calculated. Once determined, an aliquot of the same CD5-bearing cells, labelled with anti-CD5 antibody, was then incubated with an FITC-conjugated secondary antibody and the mean fluorescence intensity measured. A linear relationship between the mean number of antibodies bound per cell and the mean fluorescence was observed. The experiment was then repeated using subclones of the CD5-bearing cell line (i.e. clones with different CD5 densities) in order to construct a calibration curve. This standard curve was then used to measure the amount of CD5 attached to various bead populations and thus achieve a quantification kit which could then be used to measure other antigen densities using an indirect staining approach.

The procedure employs a monovalent antibody in order to achieve a 1:1 antibody:antigen binding. It also retains the relationship between biological and non-biological (bead) standards. However, accuracy of the QIFI system is dependent on the same secondary antibody being used on both beads and test sample. Furthermore, the test cannot be used to measure antigen density with direct labelling procedures, i.e. monoclonal antibodies that are directly conjugated.

QUANTUM SIMPLY CELLULAR (ABC) APPROACH

A second approach, which is more widely used in clinical haematology, is the Quantum Simply Cellular (QSC) system. The ABC method employs a cocktail of five highly uniform microbead populations, one blank and four coated with defined (and varying) quantities of polyvalent goat anti-mouse antibody (Schwartz et al., 1996). The principle of the test is that the antibody-coated beads capture any mouse monoclonal antibody, independent of the fluorochrome or IgG subtype. Thus, under saturating conditions, the antigen density can be defined as the number of antibodies of a particular type that can bind to a cell and is termed antibody-binding capacity. The QSC approach is designed for use with monoclonal antibodies which are directly conjugated. Briefly, a calibration curve is constructed by incubating the monoclonal antibody with the beads under saturating conditions for at least 60 minutes. The beads are then analysed using a flow cytometer and the mean channel values for each individual peak are determined and plotted against the ABC value for the bead populations. The antigen density of the test sample is then determined by reading the mean channel obtained for the positive peak from the calibration curve. The QSC beads can also provide valuable information on flow cytometer performance.

However, despite the growing acceptance of antigen quantification techniques, there are a number of important technical and quality control issues which have yet to be addressed. For example, two studies have reported discrepant findings for CD10 expression in B-lineage acute lymphoblastic leukaemia (Lavabre-Bertrand et al., 1994; Farahat et al., 1995b). In view of the increasing interest in antigen quantification, UK NEQAS recently examined the technical issues involved. It was found that alterations in pH, incubation temperature, lysing reagent, fluorochrome and antibody titre can all have significant effects on the result of antibody-binding capacity (ABC) (Barnett et al., 1998). The antigen binding capacity for CD4 on normal lymphocytes, for example, was shown to be significantly lower at pH above and below 7.4 (differences greater than 40 000 molecules/cell being noted). In addition, the ABC for CD3 was dependent on the fluorochrome used and whether single, two or three colour analysis was undertaken. When antigens are normally distributed (e.g. CD3 and CD4), no significant differences are observed in their ABC values when using either mean or median channel. However, for antigens which do not have a normal distribution, such as CD8 (due to the presence of CD8[dim] cells), significant differences are found, with median channel values being consistently lower. Furthermore, Bikoue et al. (1996) found that different monoclonal antibodies to a given antigen (i.e. CD8) can give different ABC values when the same cells are analysed. To our knowledge, no such studies examining the inter- or intra-laboratory variation of antigen quantification on pathological samples have yet been undertaken. The studies by UK NEQAS highlight the urgent need for a standard approach to enable intra- and interlaboratory comparisons. It is our view that single colour staining using FITC-conjugated antibodies, with all reagents at pH 7.4 ± 0.1 and incubation and lysing at 20 ± 1°C, should be considered as the benchmark technique. Indeed, using this approach, an interlaboratory study conducted by UK NEQAS found a high degree of consensus for CD3, CD4, CD8 and CD19 ABC determinations (unpublished observations).

6.6.2 Intracellular antigen detection

It is widely recognized that during lineage maturation there is upregulation (or down-regulation) of certain antigens and enzymes. For example, in myeloid differentiation, the surface expression of HLA-DR is lost by the promyelocyte stage. However, there are antigens which are detectable in the cytoplasm of cells before being expressed on the cell surface, such as CD3, CD22 and CD79. In addition, intracellular enzymes (e.g. myeloperoxidase and terminal deoxynucleotidyl transferase [TdT]), which are of major importance in the immuno-phenotyping and classification of leukaemias, lymphomas and HIV, cannot be detected using conventional surface staining techniques. Consequently, because of the importance of such intracellular antigen detection, many laboratories routinely use the APAAP technique or UV microscopy. Early attempts at intracellular antigen detection by flow cytometry were labour-intensive and poorly quality controlled. Permeabilization/fixation solutions, for example, changed the light scatter patterns so that it was not possible to relate cells of interest to those in untreated samples or to samples stained for surface membrane antigens. Recently, however, the development of new permeabilization/fixation solutions (Pizzolo *et al.*, 1994; Tiirikainen, 1995) has enabled the technique to be reliably performed on a routine basis (Groeneveld *et al.*, 1996). Nevertheless, not all commercially available reagents are equally as effective for the detection of a given antigen and quality control, and standardization issues will need to be addressed in the near future.

In the clinical immunophenotyping laboratory, cytoplasmic antigen testing by flow cytometry is now being introduced for the detection of TdT, CD3, CD22, CD79 and myeloperoxidase. The nuclear enyzme TdT is an essential marker for the diagnosis of acute leukaemias, while the majority of precursor-B-ALL and T-ALL can be defined by the cyto-plasmic expression of the CD79 and CD3 antigens, respectively (van Dongen *et al.*, 1988; Verschuren *et al.*, 1993). In addition, the identification of cells which co-express TdT and CD79 or CD3, a feature of lymphoid immaturity, can aid the separation of leukaemic, or primitive, cells from mature lymphoid populations. Finally, T-helper cells can be further subclassified as T_{h1} and T_{h2} subtypes based on intracellular cytokine expression following stimulation. Recent studies suggest that an imbalance of these subsets may have prognostic significance in individuals infected with HIV.

REFERENCES

Adriaansen, H.J., te Boekhorst, P.A., Hagemeijer, A.M. *et al.* (1993) Acute myeloid leukaemia M4 with bone marrow eosinophilia (M4Eo) and inv(16)(p13q22) exhibits a specific immunophenotype with CD2 expression. *Blood* **81**, 3043–51.

Agrawal, Y.P., Mahlamaki, E.K. and Penttila, I.M. (1991) Use of quality control standards in clinical flow cytometry. *Ann. Med.* **23**, 127–33.

Andrews, R.G., Bryant, E.M., Bartelmez, S.H. *et al.* (1992) CD34+ marrow cells, devoid of T and B lymphocytes, reconstitute stable lymphopoiesis and myelopoiesis in lethally irradiated baboons. *Blood* **80**, 1693–701.

Ager, S., Scott, M.A., Mahendra, P. *et al.* (1995) Peripheral blood stem cell transplants after high-dose chemotherapy in patients with malignant lymphoma: a retrospective comparison with autologous bone marrow transplantation. *Bone Marrow Transplant* **16**, 79–83.

Barnett, D., Granger, V., Mayr, P. *et al*. (1996) Evaluation of a novel stable whole blood quality control material for lymphocyte subset analysis: results from the UK NEQAS immune monitoring scheme. *Cytometry* **26**, 216–22.

Barnett, D., Storie, I., Wilson, G. *et al*. (1998) Determination of leucocyte antibody binding capacity (ABC): the need for standardization. *Clin. Lab. Haematol*. **20**, 155–64.

Barnett, D., Janossy, G., Lubenko, A. *et al*. (1999) Guideline for the flow cytometric enumeration of CD34+ haematopoietic stem cells. Prepared by the CD34+ haematopoietic stem cell working party. General Haematology Task Force of the British Committee for Standards in Haematology. *Clin. Lab. Haematol*. **21**, 301–8.

BCSH (1994a) Immunophenotyping in the diagnosis of acute leukaemia. *J. Clin. Pathol*. **47**, 77–8.

BCSH (1994b) Immunophenotyping in the chronic (mature) lymphoproliferative disorders. *J. Clin. Pathol*. **47**, 871–5.

BCSH (1997) Guidelines for the enumeration of CD4+T lymphocytes in immunosuppressed individuals. *Clin. Lab. Haematol*. **19**, 231–41.

Bender, J., To, L.B., Williams, S. and Schwartzberg, L. (1992) Defining a therapeutic dose of peripheral blood stem cells. *J. Hematother*. **1**, 329–42.

Bender, J.G., Unverzagt, K. and Walker, D. (1994) Guidelines for determination of CD34+ cells by flow cytometry: application to the harvesting and transplantation of peripheral blood stem cells. In: Wunder, E., Sovalat, H., Henon, P.R., Serke, S. (eds), *Hematopoietic Stem Cells: The Mulhouse Manual*. Dayton, OH: AlphaMed Press, 23–43.

Bennett, J.M., Catovsky, D., Daniel, M.T. *et al*. (1976) Proposals for the classification of the acute leukaemias. *Br. J. Haematol*. **33**, 451–8.

Bennett, J.M., Catovsky, D., Daniel, M-T. *et al*. (1989) Proposals for the classification of chronic (mature) B and T lymphoid leukaemias. *J. Clin. Pathol*. **42**, 567–84.

Bennett, J.M., Catovsky, D., Daniel, M.T. *et al*. (1991) Proposal for the recognition of minimally differentiated acute myeloid leukaemia (AML-M0). *Br. J. Haematol*. **78**, 325–9.

Berenson, R.J., Andrews, R.G., Bensinger, W.J. *et al*. (1988). Antigen CD34-positive marrow cells engraft lethally irradiated baboons. *J. Clin. Invest*. **81**, 951–5.

Bernard, A., Boumsell, L., Dausset, J. *et al*. (eds) (1984) *Leucocyte Typing I*. Berlin: Springer-Verlag.

Betz, S.A., Foucar, K., Head, H.D. *et al*. (1992) False-positive flow cytometric platelet glycoprotein IIb/IIIa expression in myeloid leukaemias secondary to platelet adherence to blasts. *Blood* **79**, 2399–403.

Borowitz, M.J., Guenther, K.L., Schultz, K.E. *et al*. (1993) Immunophenotyping of acute leukaemia by flow cytometry: use of CD45 and right angle light scatter to gate on leukemic blasts in three colour analysis. *Am. J. Clin. Pathol*. **100**, 534–40.

Bossuyt, X., Marti, G.E. and Fleisher, T.A. (1997) Comparative analysis of whole blood lysis methods for flow cytometry. *Cytometry* **30**, 124–33.

Bikoue, A., George, F., Poncelet, P. *et al*. (1996) Quantitative analysis of leukocyte membrane antigen expression: normal adult values. *Cytometry* **26**, 137–47.

Bradstock, K.F., Kirk, J., Grimsley, P.G. *et al*. (1989) Unusual immunophenotypes in acute leukaemias: incidence and clinical correlations. *Br. J. Haematol*. **72**, 512–18.

Bregni, M., Magni, M., Siena, S. *et al*. (1992) Human peripheral blood haematopoietic progenitors are optimal targets of retroviral-mediated gene transfer. *Blood* **80**, 1418–22.

Brugger, W., Henschler, R., Heimfeld, S. *et al*. (1994) Positively selected autologous blood CD34+ cells and unseparated peripheral blood progenitor cells mediate identical hematopoietic engraftment after high-dose VP16, ifosfamide, carboplatin, and epirubicin. *Blood* **84**, 1421–6.

Caldwell, C.W., Patterson, W.P. and Hakami, N. (1987) Alterations of Hle-1 (T200) fluorescence intensity on acute lymphoblastic leukaemia cells may relate to therapeutic outcome. *Leukaemia Res*. **11**, 103–6.

Campana, D. (1994) Applications of cytometry to study acute leukemia: in vitro determination of drug sensitivity and detection of minimal residual disease. *Cytometry* **18**, 68–74.

Camplejohn, R.S. (1994) The measurement of intracellular antigens and DNA by multi-parametric flow cytometry. *J. Microsc.* **176**, 1–7.

Centers for Disease Control (1992) Guidelines for the performance of CD4+ T-cell determinations in persons with human immunodeficiency virus infection. *Morbidity and Mortality Weekly Report* **41**, 1–19.

Centers for Disease Control (1993) Revised classification system for HIV infection and expanded surveillance case definition for AIDS among adolescents and adults. *Morbidity and Mortality Weekly Report* **41**, 1–35.

Chan, C.H., Lin, W., Shye, S. *et al.* (1994) Automated enumeration of CD34+ cells in peripheral blood and bone marrow. *J. Hematother.* **3**, 3–13.

Connelly, M.C., Knight, M., Giorgi, J.V. *et al.* (1995). Standardization of absolute CD4+ lymphocyte counts across laboratories: an evaluation of the Ortho *Cytoron*Absolute flow cytometry system on normal donors. *Cytometry* **22**, 200–10.

Cordell, J.V., Fallen, B. and Erber, W.J. (1984) Immunoenzymatic labelling of monoclonal antibodies using immune complexes of alkaline phosphatase and monoclonal anti-alkaline phosphatase (APAAP complexes). *J. Histochem. Cytochem.* **32**, 219–29.

Davis, K.A., Abrams, B., Hoffman, R.A. *et al.* (1996) Quantitation and valence of antibodies bound to cells. *Cytometry* **8**(Suppl.),125.

Dercksen, M.W., Rodenhuis, S., Dirkson, M.K.A. *et al.* (1995) Subsets of CD34+ cells and rapid hematopoietic recovery after peripheral-blood stem-cell transplantation. *J. Clin. Oncol.* **13**, 1922–32.

Dreger, P., Haferlach, T., Eckstein, V. *et al.* (1994) G-CSF mobilised peripheral blood progenitor cells for allogeneic transplantation: safety, kinetics of mobilization, and composition of the graft. *Br. J. Haematol.* **87**, 609–13.

Ekong, T., Hill, A.M., Gompels, M. *et al.* (1992) The effect of the temperature and duration of sample storage on the measurement of lymphocyte sub-populations from HIV-1 positive and control subjects. *J. Immunol. Methods* **151**, 217–25.

Ekong, T., Kupek, E., Hill, A. *et al.* (1993) Technical influences on immunophenotyping by flow cytometry. The effect of time and temperature of storage on the viability of lymphocyte subsets. *J. Immunol. Methods* **164**, 263–73.

Erber, W.J., Mynheer, L.C. and Mason, D.Y. (1986) APAAP labelling of blood and bone marrow samples for phenotyping leukaemia. *Lancet* **I**, 761–5.

Erber, W.J., Breton-Gorius, J., Villeval, J.V. *et al.* (1987) Detection of cells of megakaryocyte lineage in haematological malignancies by immuno-alkaline phosphatase labelling cell smears with a panel of monoclonal antibodies. *Br. J. Haematol.* **65**, 87–94.

Erber, W. N., Asbahr, H., Rule, S.A. *et al.* (1994) Unique immunophenotype of acute promyelocytic leukaemia as defined by CD9 and CD68 antibodies. *Br. J. Haematol.* **88,** 101–4.

Farahat, N., Lens, D., Zomas, A. *et al.* (1995a) Differential TdT expression in acute leukaemia by flow cytometry: a quantitative study. *Leukemia* **9**, 583–7.

Farahat, N., Lens, D., Zomas, A. *et al.* (1995b) Quantitative flow cytometry can distinguish between normal and leukaemic B-cell precursors. *Br. J. Haematol.* **91**, 640–6.

Fay, S.P., Barnett, D., Brando, B. *et al.* (1996) Ortho *Absolute*Control, full process leukocyte immunophenotyping control, multi-site European trial. *Cytometry* **42**, 67–71.

Forrest, M.J. and Barnett, D. (1989) Laboratory control of immunocytochemistry. *Eur. J. Haematol.* **42**, 67–71.

Gahmberg, C.G., Ekblom, M. and Andersson, L.C. (1984) Differentiation of human erythroid cells is associated with increased O-glycosylation of the major sialoglycoprotein glycoprotein A. *Proc. Natl Acad. Sci. USA* **81**, 6752–6.

Ginaldi, L., Matutes, E., Farahat, N. *et al.* (1996) Differential expression of CD3 and CD7 in T-cell malignancies: a quantitative study by flow cytometry. *Br. J. Haematol.* **93**, 921–7.

Gratama, J.W., Kraan, J., Levering, W. *et al.* (1997a) Analysis of variation in results of CD34+ hematopoietic progenitor cell enumeration in multi-centre study. *Cytometry* **30**, 109–17.

Gratama, J.W., van der Linden, R., van der Holt, B. *et al.* (1997b) Analysis of factors contributing to the formation of mononuclear cell aggregates ('escapees') in flow cytometric immunophenotyping. *Cytometry* **29**, 250–60.

Gratama, J.W., Orfao, A., Barnett, D. *et al.* (1998) Flow cytometric enumeration of CD34+ stem cells. *Cytometry* **34**, 128–42.

Gratwohl, A. Baldomero, H. and Hermans, J. (1996) Haemopoietic precursor cell transplant activity in Europe 1994. *Bone Marrow Transplant.* **17,** 137–48.

Groeneveld, K., te Marvelde, J.C., van den Beemd, M.W. *et al.* (1996) Flow cytometric detection of intracellular antigens for immunophenotyping of normal and malignant leukocytes. *Leukemia* **10**, 1383–9.

Haas, R., Mohle, R., Fruehauf, S. *et al.* (1994) Patient characteristics associated with successful mobilizing and autografting of peripheral blood progenitor cells in malignant melanoma. *Blood* **83**, 3787–94.

Horvatinovich, J.M., Sparks, S.D. and Borowitz, M.J. (1994) Detection of terminal deoxy-nucleotidyl transferase by flow cytometry: a three colour method. *Cytometry* **18**, 228–30.

Hurwitz, C.A., Loken, M.R., Graham, M.L. *et al.* (1988) Asynchronous antigen expression in B lineage acute lymphoblastic leukaemia. *Blood* **72**, 299–307.

Hurwitz, C.A., Raimondi, S.C., Head, D. *et al.*, (1992) Distinctive immunophenotypic features of t(8;21)(q22;q22) acute myeloblastic leukemia in children. *Blood* **80**, 3182–8.

Iyer, S., Suni, M., Davis, K. *et al.* (1996) Quantitation of cellular expression of CD69 on activated T cells using R-phycoerythrin labelled beads. *Cytometry* (Suppl. 8), 113.

Jackson, A.L. (1990) Basic phenotyping of lymphocytes: selection and testing of reagents and interpretation of data. *Clin. Immunol. Newsletter* **10**, 43–55.

Janossy, G. (1982) Membrane markers in leukaemia. In: Catovsky, D. (ed.), *The Leukemic Cell.* Methods in Hematology. Edinburgh: Churchill Livingstone, 129–83.

Johnsen, H.E. (1995) Report from a Nordic workshop on CD34+ cell analysis: technical recommendations for progenitor cell enumeration in leukapheresis from multiple myeloma patients. *J. Hematother.* **4,** 21–8.

Keenan, F.M., Barnett, D. and Reilly, J.T. (1992) Clinico-pathological features of minimally differentiated acute myeloid leukaemia (M0). *Br. J. Haematol.* **81**, 458–9.

Kishimoto, T., Goyert, S., Kitutani, H. *et al.* (eds) (1997) *Leucocyte Typing VI: White Cell Differentiation Antigens.* Oxford: Garland.

Knapp, W., Dörken, B., Gilks, W.R. *et al.* (eds) (1989). *Leucocyte Typing IV.* Oxford: Oxford University Press.

Köhler, G. and Milstein, C. (1975) Continuous cultures of fused cells secreting antibody of predetermined specificity. *Nature* **256**, 495–7.

Krause, D., Fackler, M.J., Civin, C.I. *et al.* (1996) CD34: structure, biology, and clinical utility. *Blood* **87**, 1–13.

Kromer, E. and Grossmuller, F. (1994) Light scatter based lymphocyte gate – helpful tool or source of error? *Cytometry* **15**, 87–9.

Lavabre-Bertrand, T., Duperray, C., Brunet, C. *et al.* (1994) Quantification of CD24 and CD45 antigens in parallel allows a precise determination of B-cell maturation stages: relevance for the study of B-cell neoplasms. *Leukemia* **8**, 402–8.

Lenkei, R. and Andersson, B. (1995) High correlations of anti-CMV titers with lymphocyte activation status and CD57 antibody-binding capacity as estimated with three-color, quantitative flow cytometry in blood donors. *Clin. Immunol. Immunopathol.* **77**, 131–8.

Lillevang, S.T., Sprogoe-Jackson, U., Simonsen, B. *et al.* (1995) Three-colour flow cytometric immunophenotyping in HIV-patients: comparisons to dual-colour protocols. *Scand. J. Immunol.* **41**, 114–20.

Lo Coco, F., Avvisati, G., Diverio, D. *et al.* (1991) Rearrangement of the RAR-α gene in acute promyelocytic leukaemia: correlations with morphology and immunophenotype. *Br. J. Haematol.* **78**, 494–9.

Loken, M.R., Brosnan, J.M., Bach, B.A. *et al.* (1990) Quality control in flow cytometry: I. Establishing optimal lymphocyte gates for immunophenotyping by flow cytometer. *Cytometry* **11**, 453–9.

McMichaels, A.J., Beverley, P.L.C. and Cobbold, S. (eds) (1987). *White Cell Differentiation Antigens.* Oxford: Oxford University Press.

McCarthy, D.A. and Macey, M.G. (1993) A simple flow cytometric procedure for the determination of surface antigens on unfixed leucocytes in whole blood. *J. Immunol. Methods* **163**,155–160.

Macedo, A., Orfao, A., Gonzalez, M. *et al.* (1995) Immunological detection of blast cell sub-populations in acute myeloblastic leukemia diagnosis: implications for minimal residual disease studies. *Leukemia* **9**, 993–8.

Macey, M.G. (1994) *Flow Cytometry Clinical Applications.* Oxford: Blackwell Scientific Publications.

Macey, M.G., McCarthy, D.A., van Agthoven, A *et al.* (1997) How should CD34+ cells be analysed? A study of three classes of antibody and five leukocyte preparation procedures. *J. Immunol. Methods* **204**, 175–88.

Malone, J.L., Simms, T.E., Gray, G.C. *et al.* (1990) Sources of variability in repeated T-helper lymphocyte counts from human immunodeficiency virus type 1-infected patients: total lymphocyte count fluctuations and diurnal cycle are important. *J. Acquir. Immune Defic. Syndr.* **3**, 144–51.

Mandy, F.F., Bergeron, M., Recktenwald, D. *et al.* (1992) A simultaneous three-color T cell subset analysis with single laser flow cytometers using T cell gating protocol. Comparison with conventional two-color immunophenotyping method. *J. Immunol. Methods* **156**, 151–62.

Mandy, F.F., Bergeron, M. and Minkus, T. (1997) Evolution of leucocyte immunophenotyping as influenced by the HIV/AIDS pandemic: a short history of the development of gating strategies for CD4+ T-cell enumeration. *Cytometry* **30**, 157–65.

Mason, D.Y. and Erber, W.N. (1991) Immunocytochemical labelling of leukaemic samples with monoclonal antibodies by the APAAP procedure. In: Catovsky, D. (ed.), *The Leukemic Cell.* Methods in Haematology. Edinburgh: Churchill Livingstone, 196–214.

Mercolino, T.J., Connelly, M.C., Meyer, E.J. *et al.* (1995) Immunologic differentiation of absolute count with an integrated flow cytometric system: a new concept for absolute T cell subset determinations. *Cytometry* **22**, 48–59.

Moir, D.J., Ghosh, A.K., Abdulaziz, Z. *et al.* (1983) Immunoenzymatic staining of haematological samples with monoclonal antibodies. *Br. J. Haematol.* **55**, 395–410.

Nagakura, S., Nakakuma, H., Horikawa, S. *et al.* (1993) Expression of decay-accelerating factor and CD59 in lymphocyte subsets in healthy individuals and paroxysmal nocturnal haemoglobinuria patients. *Am. J. Hematol.* **43**, 14–18.

NCCLS (1992) Clinical applications of flow cytometry. Quality assurance and immunophenotyping of peripheral blood lymphocytes. *Publication H42-T.* Villanova, PA: NCCLS, 12.

Nicholson, J.K.A. (1994) Immunophenotyping specimens from HIV-infected persons: laboratory guidelines from the Centre for Disease Control and Prevention. *Cytometry* **18**, 55–9.

Nicholson, J.K.A., Hubbard, M. and Jones, B.M. (1996) Use of CD45 fluorescence and side-scatter characteristics for gating lymphocytes when using the whole blood lysis procedure and flow cytometry. *Cytometry* **26**, 16–21.

Owens, M.A. and Loken, M.P. (1995) Peripheral blood stem cell quantitation. In: *Flow Cytometry Principles for Clinical Laboratory Practice.* New York: Wiley-Liss, 111.

Pizzolo, G., Vincenzi, C., Nadali, G. *et al.* (1994) Detection of membrane and intracellular antigens by flow cytometry following ORTHO PermeaFix™ fixation. *Leukemia* **8,** 672–6.

Poncelet, P. and Carayon, P. (1985) Quantification of cell-surface antigens by indirect immunofluorescence using monoclonal antibodies. *J. Immunol. Methods* **85**, 65–75.

Poncelet, P., Lavabre-Bertrand, T. and Carayon, P. (1986) Phenotypes of B chronic lymphocytic leukaemia B cells established with monoclonal antibodies from the B cell protocol. In: Reinherz, E.L., Haynes, B.F., Nadler, L.M., Bernstein, D. (eds), *Leucocyte Typing II.* Berlin: Springer-Verlag, 329–43.

Reilly, J.T. (1996). Use and evaluation of leucocyte monoclonal antibodies in the diagnostic laboratory: a review. *Clin. Lab. Haematol.* **18**, 1–6.

Reinherz, E.L., Haynes, B.F., Nadler, L.M. and Bernstein, I.D. (eds) (1986) *Leucocyte Typing II*. Berlin: Springer-Verlag.

Robinson, G., Morgan, L., Evans, M. *et al.* (1992) Effect of type of haematology analyser on CD4 count. *Lancet* **340**(ii), 485.

Robinson, J.P., Darzynkiewicz, Z., Dean P.N. *et al.* (1997) *Current Protocols in Flow Cytometry*. Chichester: John Wiley.

Rollins, S.A. and Sims, P.J. (1990) The complement-inhibitory activity of CD59 resides in its capacity to block incorporation of C9 into membrane C5b-9. *J. Immunol.* **144**, 3478–83.

Romeu, M.A., Mestre, M., Gonzalez, L. *et al.* (1992) Lymphocyte immunophenotyping by flow cytometry in normal adults. Comparison of fresh whole blood lysis technique, Ficoll-Paque separation and cryopreservation. *J. Immunol.* **154**, 7–10.

Ross, A.A., Miller, G.W., Moss, T.J. *et al.* (1995) Immunocytochemical detection of tumour cells in bone marrow and peripheral blood stem cell collections from patients with ovarian cancer. *Bone Marrow Transplant.* **15**, 929–33.

Russell, N.H., Gratwohl, A. and Schmitz, N. (1996) The place of blood stem cells in allogeneic transplantation. *Br. J. Haematol.* **93**, 747–53.

San Miguel, J.F., Gonzalez, M., Canizo, M.C. *et al.* (1988) Leukemias with megakaryoblastic involvement: clinical, hematologic, and immunologic characteristics. *Blood* **72**, 402–7.

San Miguel, J.F., Martinez, A., Macedo, A. *et al.* (1997) Immunophenotyping investigation of minimal residual disease is a useful approach for predicting relapse in acute myeloid leukemia patients. *Blood* **90**, 2465–70.

Schlossman, S.F., Boumsell, L., Gilks, W. *et al.* (1995) *Leucocyte Typing V*. Oxford: Oxford University Press.

Schubert, J., Alvarado, M., Uciechowski, P. *et al.* (1991) Diagnosis of paroxysmal nocturnal haemoglobinuria using immunophenotyping of peripheral blood cells. *Br. J. Haematol.* **79**, 487–92.

Schwartz, A. and Fernandez-Repollet, E. (1993) Development of clinical standards for flow cytometry. *Ann. NY Acad. Sci.* **677**, 28–39.

Schwartz, A., Fernandez-Repollet, E., Vogt, R.F. *et al* (1996) Standardizing flow cytometry: construction of a standardised fluorescence plot using matching spectral calibrators. *Cytometry* **26**, 22–31.

Serui, T., Yokota, S., Nakao, M. *et al.* (1995) Prospective monitoring of minimal residual disease during the course of chemotherapy in patients with acute lymphoblastic leukemia, and detection of contaminating tumor cells in peripheral blood stem cells for autotransplantation. *Leukemia* **9**, 615–23.

Shapiro, H.M. (1995) *Practical Flow Cytometry*, 3rd ed. New York: Wiley-Liss.

Shichishima, T., Terasawa, T., Saitoh, Y. *et al.* (1993) Diagnosis of paroxysmal nocturnal haemoglobinuria by phenotypic analysis of erythrocytes using two-colour flow cytometry with monoclonal antibodies to DAF and CD59/MACIF. *Br. J. Haematol.* **85**, 378–86.

Siena, S., Bregni, M., Belli, N. *et al.* (1991) Flow cytometry for clinical estimation of circulating hematopoietic progenitors for autologous transplantation in cancer patients. *Blood* **77**, 400–9.

Storie, I., Wilson, G.A., Granger, V. *et al.* (1995) Circulating CD20[dim] T-lymphocytes increase with age: evidence for a memory cytotoxic phenotype. *Clin. Lab. Haematol.* **17**, 323–8.

Strauss, K., Hannet, I., Engel, S. *et al.* (1996) Performance evaluation of FACSCount: a dedicated system for clinical cellular analysis. *Cytometry* **26**, 52–9.

Sutherland, D.R. and Keating, A. (1992) The CD34 antigen: structure, biology and potential clinical applications. *J. Hematother.* **1**, 115–29.

Sutherland, D.R., Marsh, J.C.W., Davidson, J. *et al.* (1992) Differential sensitivity of CD34 epitopes to cleavage by pasteurella haemolytica glycoprotease: implications for purification of CD34-positive progenitor cells. *Exp. Hematol.* **20**, 590–9.

Sutherland, D.R., Keating, A., Nayar, R. *et al.* (1994) Sensitive detection and enumeration of CD34+ cells in peripheral blood and cord blood by flow cytometry. *Exp. Hematol.* **22**, 1003–10.

Sutherland, D.R., Anderson, L., Keeney, M. *et al.* (1996a) Toward a worldwide standard for CD34+ enumeration. *J. Hematother.* **6**, 85–9.

Sutherland, D.R., Anderson, L., Keeney, M. *et al.* (1996b) The ISHAGE guidelines for CD34+ cell determination by flow cytometry. *J. Hematol.* **5**, 213–26.

Tallman, M.S., Hakimian, D., Shaw, J.M. *et al.*, (1993) Granulocytic sarcoma is associated with the 8;21 translocation in acute myeloid leukaemia. *J. Clin. Oncol.* **11**, 690–7.

Terstappen, L.W.M.M., Shah, V.O., Conrad, M.P. *et al.* (1988) Discrimination between damaged and intact cells in fixed flow cytometric samples. *Cytometry* **9**, 477–84.

Tiirikainen, M.I. (1995) Evaluation of red blood cell lysing solutions for the detection of intracellular antigens by flow cytometry. *Cytometry* **20**, 341–8.

Vahdat, L., Maslak, P., Miller, W.H. *et al.* (1994) Early mortality and the retinoic acid syndrome in acute promyelocytic leukemia: impact of leukocytosis, low-dose chemotherapy, PML/RAR-α isoform, and CD13 expression in patients treated with all-trans retinoic acid. *Blood* **84**, 3843–9.

van de Winkel, J.G.J. and Capel, P.J.A. (1993) Human IgG Fc receptor heterogeneity: molecular aspects and clinical implications. *Immunol. Today* **14**, 131–42.

van Dongen, J.J.M., Krissansen, G.W., Wolvers-Tettero, I.L.M. *et al.* (1988) Cytoplasmic expression of the CD3 antigen as a diagnostic marker for immature T-cell malignancies. *Blood* **71**, 603–12.

Verschuren, M.C.M., Comans-Bitter, W.M., Kapteijn, C.A.C. *et al.* (1993) Transcription and protein expression of mb-1 and b29 genes in human hematopoietic malignancies and cell lines. *Leukemia* **7**, 1939–47.

Wunder, E., Sovalat, H., Fritsch, G. *et al.* (1992) Report on the European workshop on peripheral blood stem cell determination and standardization - Mulhouse, France. *J. Hematother.* **1,** 131–42.

2

Haemoglobinometry

7

Haemoglobinometry: the reference method[1]

ONNO W. VAN ASSENDELFT AND BEREND HOUWEN

INTRODUCTION

Blood is the body fluid of humans that has probably been studied the longest and most intensively. Even at an early stage, attention focused on haemoglobin, being one of many haem-containing proteins found in higher vertebrates. On the basis of the chemical structure of its four haem groups, the two alpha and two beta globin chains, human haemoglobin A is calculated to have a relative molecular mass of 64 458 (anhydrous; Braunitzer et al., 1961; Hill et al., 1962; Braunitzer, 1964), with a mass fraction of haemoglobin iron of 0.003 47.

Many methods have been developed to determine the total haemoglobin concentration (c_{tHb}) in human blood; comprehensive reviews have been published (Sunderman et al., 1953; van Assendelft, 1970). Around the 1950s, numerous methods, more or less inaccurate, were in use. These methods often yielded widely different results so that values obtained in different laboratories were not, or were hardly, comparable and a diagnosis of anaemia depended as much on the laboratory method as on the condition of the patient. The need for improvement was clear and several attempts at standardization were made.

Establishing a reference point for haemoglobinometry primarily involved two decisions. The first concerned the selection of a physical or chemical property of haemoglobin that can be measured accurately and easily. The second consideration was to adopt one or more methods to correlate exactly the results of the physicochemical measurement with a known amount of haemoglobin.

Among the physicochemical properties of haemoglobin that can be measured accurately and easily, absorption of visible light has been used most widely. With modern spectro-photometers, the absorbance of haemoglobins in solution (Fig. 7.1) can be easily measured

---

[1] The use of trade names is for identification only and does not constitute endorsement by the Public Health Service or the US Department of Health and Human Services.

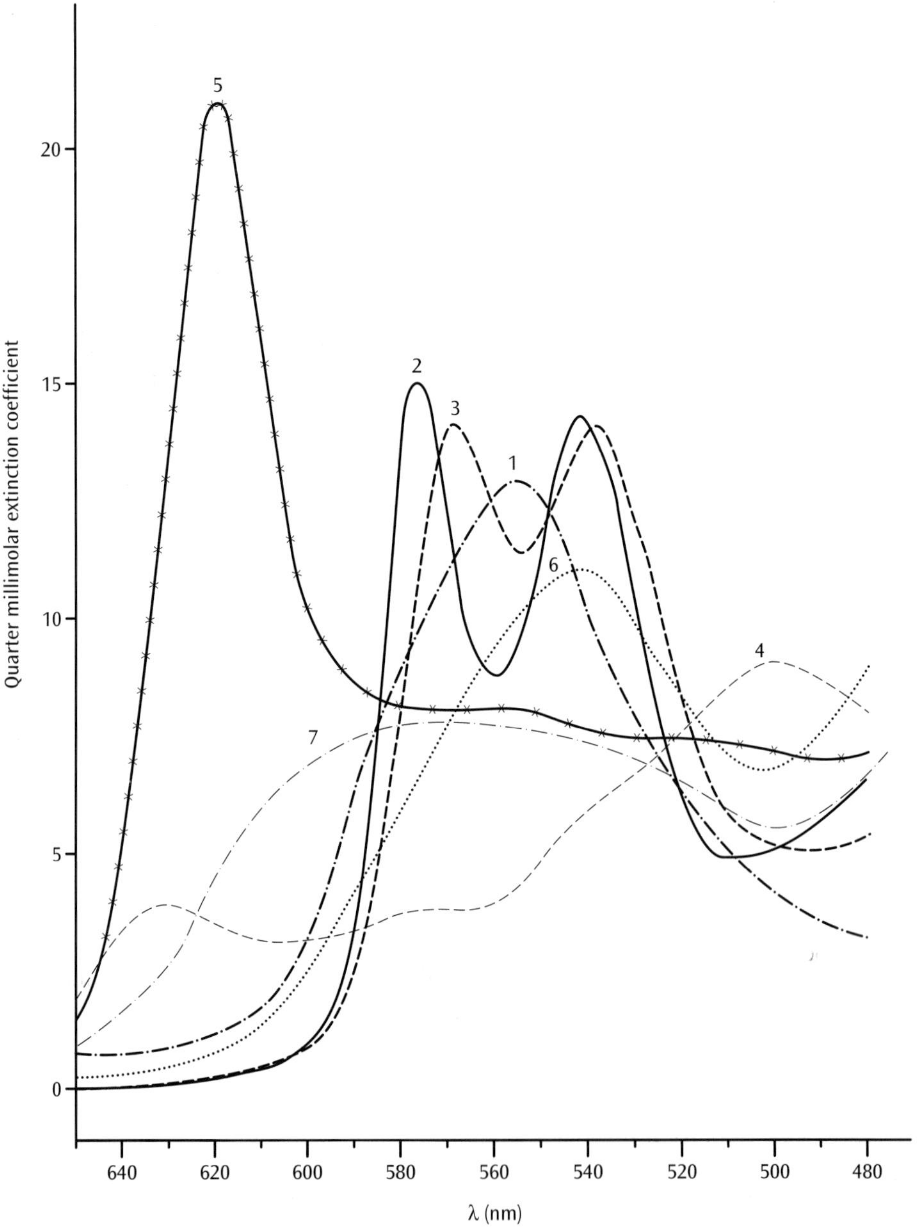

Fig. 7.1 *Light absorption spectra of common haemoglobin derivatives. 1, deoxyhaemoglobin, HHb; 2, oxyhaemoglobin, O₂Hb; 3, carboxyhaemoglobin, COHb; 4, haemiglobin (methaemoglobin), pH 7.0–7.4, Hi; 5, sulph-haemoglobin, SHb; 6, haemiglobincyanide (methaemoglobin-cyanide, cyanmethaemoglobin), HiCN; 7, sulph-haemiglobincyanide, SHiCN. Data from van Assendelft (1970) and van Kampen and Zijlstra (1983).*

within 0.5% reproducibility. It needs no argument, of course, that in such a solution all haemoglobins must be converted into one and the same haemoglobin derivative, or at least into derivatives that are photometrically indistinguishable at the wavelengths of measurement.

In the United States, in 1958, a National Academy of Sciences-National Research Council, Division of Medical Sciences Panel on the Establishment of a Hemoglobin Standard reviewed several photometric methods for the determination of c_{tHb} and concluded that it was best determined photometrically after conversion of all haemoglobins in the specimen to haemiglobincyanide (HiCN, methaemoglobincyanide; cyanmethaemoglobin) (Cannan, 1958a,b,c) for the following reasons (Cannan, 1958b):

> The method involves dilution with a single reagent. All forms of hemoglobin likely to occur in circulatory blood, with the exception of sulfhemoglobin, are determined. The color is suitable for measurement in filter as well as in narrow band spectrophotometers because its absorption band at a wavelength of 540 nm is broad and relatively flat. Standards prepared from either crystalline hemoglobin or washed erythrocytes and stored in a brown glass container and in sterile condition are stable for at least 9 months (change < 2%).

The Panel adopted a value of 11.5 for the quarter millimolar absorptivity of HiCN at a wavelength of 540 nm, ε_{HiCN}^{540}. This value of 11.5 dates back to the work of Drabkin and Austin (1932, 1935/36) and was based on photometric data and oxygen capacity measurements of 11 samples of human, nine of rabbit, and 14 of canine blood. Thus, in establishing a reference point, the measured quantity was to be the absorbance of HiCN solutions at a wavelength of 540 nm: A_{HiCN}^{540}.

The second decision in establishing a reference point was somewhat more difficult as one could choose either a method based on some functional property of haemoglobin, e.g. oxygen or carbon monoxide binding capacity, or an analytical method based on the chemical composition of the haemoglobin molecule. From a physiological point of view, standardization of haemoglobinometry on the basis of the oxygen binding capacity would seem to be desirable. However, the existence of (temporarily) inactive haemoglobins, such as haemiglobin, carboxyhaemoglobin and dyshaemoglobins, as well as technical difficulties and uncertainties in blood gas analysis, favoured the use of an analytical method aimed at the chemical composition of the haemoglobin molecule. The complete elucidation of the composition of haemoglobin A (Braunitzer et al., 1961; Hill et al., 1962) added a strong argument in favour of chemical analysis. Having made this choice, the next step was to determine the most suitable atomic species among the six (C, H, O, N, S and Fe) contained in the haemoglobin molecule: Fe has been the atom of choice.

The determination of 'absolute' chemical values must ultimately be based on a direct method of analysis, i.e. a gravimetric or a volumetric method. For the determination of haemoglobin Fe content, these criteria were met by the titrimetric method with titanous chloride ($TiCl_3$) (Zijlstra and van Kampen, 1960). Indirect methods of analysis are suitable only if properly prepared standard solutions based on weight analysis are used and if all interfering factors have been thoroughly studied, preferably by comparison with a direct method of analysis. These safeguards were taken in the spectrophotometric haemoglobin Fe determination using α,α'-dipyridyl and in haemoglobin Fe determination by X-ray emission spectrography (Zijlstra and van Kampen, 1960; Morningstar et al., 1966).

To establish a reference point there thus remained: relating A_{HiCN}^{540} (the absorbance of HiCN solutions at 540 nm) to the haemoglobin Fe content of these solutions, i.e. determining ε_{HiCN}^{540}. In Europe, the value of ε_{HiCN}^{540} was extensively investigated in the late 1950s (Meyer-Wilmes and Remmer, 1956; Remmer, 1956; Zijlstra and van Kampen, 1960). Based on the determination of haemoglobin Fe by a spectrophotometric method using a,a'-dipyridyl, and a titrimetric one using $TiCl_3$, a mean value of 11.0 L/mmol/cm was found for ε_{HiCN}^{540}. This value was further verified by other measurements of haemoglobin Fe (van Oudheusden et al., 1964; Morningstar et al., 1966), haemoglobin nitrogen (Tentori et al., 1966) and haemoglobin carbon (Itano, 1972), and by direct titration of haemiglobin (Hi, methaemoglobin) with cyanide (Hoek *et al.*, 1981). Taking all data together, $\varepsilon_{HiCN}^{540} = 10.99 \pm 0.01$ (standard error of the mean), $n = 521$ (van Kampen and Zijlstra, 1983).

At the ninth European Congress of Haematology, held in 1963, a Standardizing Committee of the European Society of Haematology was established. As one of its first recommendations, this committee proposed, at the European level, that the HiCN method (van Kampen and Zijlstra, 1961) be the method of choice to measure c_{tHb}, and that a value of 11.0 L/mmol/cm be adopted for ε_{HiCN}^{540}. Furthermore, it was proposed that the value of 64 458 for the relative molecular mass of human haemoglobin A be accepted (de Boroviczeny, 1964). At the 10th International Congress of Haematology in 1964 this Standardizing Committee was enlarged to form the International Committee (currently Council) for Standardization in Haematology (ICSH). The HiCN method was adopted as the method of choice for the determination of c_{tHb} at the European level and, provisionally, at the world level. The committee also issued recommendations for the preparation and use of HiCN reference solutions (de Boroviczeny, 1965; ICSH, 1966) and instituted an Expert Panel on Haemoglobinometry with the task of drawing up recommendations for haemoglobinometry and measuring and controlling HiCN reference solutions prepared by the Dutch Institute of Public Health.

Recommendations for haemoglobinometry, with the HiCN method as that of choice, were adopted at the world level during the 11th International Congress of Haematology in 1966 (ICSH, 1967), and in 1968 the World Health Organization (WHO) established HiCN solutions as WHO International HiCN Reference Preparations (now International HiCN Standards) (WHO, 1968).

7.1 THE REFERENCE MEASUREMENT PROCEDURE

Accurate determination of c_{tHb} is:

- required for the assignment of values to calibration and control materials in haemoglobin measurement procedures;
- required for whole blood calibration procedures of automated haematology analysers;
- necessary in the evaluation of instruments and alternative methods for the measurement of c_{tHb};
- applicable in the routine laboratory for diagnostic purposes and for monitoring patients or the progress of therapy;
- applicable when patient red cell measurement mean values are used in the quality control of haematology analysers (Bull and Korpman, 1982).

7.1.1 Principle

In the HiCN reference method, conversion of the common haemoglobin derivatives in blood takes place in two steps:

1 Oxidation of haemoglobin Fe by potassium hexacyanoferrate(III) [$K_3Fe(CN)_6$], so that all haemoglobins convert to Hi;
2 The addition of cyanide (CN^-) to form HiCN:

$$Hb(Fe^{2+}) + Fe^{(3+)}(CN)^{3-} \rightarrow Hi(Fe^{3+}) + Fe^{(2+)}(CN)^{4-}$$
$$Hi(Fe^{3+}) + CN^- \rightarrow Hi(Fe^{3+})CN$$

The oxidation reaction is rather slow, with the reaction velocity dependent on the pH of the solution. At pH = 8.5 and ambient (room) temperature (20–25°C) the reaction takes approximately 30 minutes to complete; at pH 7.2 this is less than 5 minutes. Oxidation of COHb takes much longer, about 90 minutes at pH 8.5, and about 30 minutes at pH 7.2 (van Kampen and Klouwen, 1954; Taylor and Miller, 1965; van Assendelft, 1970).

In Hi, the sixth coordination position of the iron, which in Hb binds the oxygen, is bound to water at low pH and to OH^- at high pH. Several other anions, e.g. fluoride, nitrite, azide and cyanide, are also readily bound to Hi and, because of differences in binding strength, a displacement series has been shown to exist: $OH^- < F^- < NO_2^- < N_3^- < CN^-$ (van Assendelft 1970). Of these, HiCN is the most stable compound. The binding of CN^- to Hi proceeds rapidly and is dependent mainly on the cyanide concentration in the reagent solution. However, a haemoglobin derivative that is not converted to HiCN is sulph-haemoglobin (SHb). SHb is a haemoglobin derivative with a sulphur atom irreversibly incorporated in the protoporphyrin ring (Nijveld, 1943; Liebecq, 1946). In the presence of $K_3Fe(CN)_6$, SHb iron is oxidized to form sulph-haemiglobin (SHi), which also readily binds cyanide to form SHiCN. The absorptivity of SHiCN is approximately 8 instead of 11 L/mmol/cm (Dijkhuizen et al., 1977), and can thus cause a slight underestimation of c_{tHb}. Clinically, SHb rarely occurs at significant concentrations, but formation can be induced by various drugs, e.g. phenacetin, phenylazoaminopyridin and sulphonamides.

After conversion of the haemoglobins, the resulting HiCN solutions are measured on a suitable (spectro)photometer and c_{tHb} is calculated from the absorbances, A, measured at 540 nm: A_{HiCN}^{540}.

7.1.2 Specimen

Although blood specimens could be obtained by skin puncture (capillary blood), vene-puncture is recommended. Venous blood should be anticoagulated by appropriate salts of ethylenediaminetetra-acetic acid (EDTA) or heparin. In principle, however, sodium-citrate or sodium, potassium, ammonium or lithium oxalate could be used to anticoagulate specimens. ICSH recommends K_2EDTA, 1.5–2.2 mg/mL (3.7–5.4 μmol/mL) blood as the anticoagulant of choice, especially for blood cell counting and sizing (ICSH, 1993). It should be borne in mind that, when liquid anticoagulants, e.g. a solution of K_3EDTA, are used, there is a dilution of the specimen by 1–2%.

Best results are obtained when fresh blood is analysed; c_{tHb} preferably should be determined on the day the specimen is drawn. It has, however, been shown that storage of blood for 1 week at ambient (room) temperature does not affect c_{tHb} obtained when using the reference method. Once the sample is mixed with reagent, the resulting HiCN solution is stable and its absorbance can be measured when convenient. Storage for periods longer than 6 hours should be at 4–10°C, in the dark, in tightly stoppered containers.

Lipaemia, the presence of significant amounts of (lipo)proteins, or white blood cell counts $> 20 \times 10^9$/L may falsely elevate c_{tHb} because of turbidity of the resulting HiCN solutions. Turbidity problems have also been described with platelet counts $> 700 \times 10^9$/L, with significant amounts of haemoglobin S, and in cases of severe microcytosis and hypochromia.

Before sampling, the specimen must be well-mixed by completely inverting the specimen container at least 12 times, making sure the container is no more than two-thirds filled with blood.

7.1.3 Reagent

The purpose of the reagent is threefold: dilution of the sample, lysis of all blood cells and conversion of haemoglobins to HiCN. Whole blood must be diluted in order to obtain an absorbance within the range of 0.090–0.700, a range that can be measured accurately with conventional (spectro)photometers with a sample lightpath of 1 cm. The usual dilution is 200- to 300-fold.

Ideally the reagent should cause instant cell lysis, including erythrolysis, convert all common haemoglobins rapidly into HiCN, and result in solutions free from any turbidity. No reagent has been described that fully meets all these requirements.

In the original determination of c_{tHb} as HiCN, separate solutions of $K_3Fe(CN)_6$ and KCN were used (Stadie, 1920). It soon became clear that these could be combined into a single reagent (Palmer, 1918). For many years the original 'Drabkin's' formulation [200 mg $K_3Fe(CN)_6$, 50 mg KCN, 1.0 g $NaHCO_3$, water to 1000 mL; pH = 8.6] and the modified 'Drabkin's' formulation (as previously, without $NaHCO_3$; pH = 9.6) were quite popular, although they required conversion times in excess of 15 min and frequently resulted in slightly turbid HiCN solutions. Green and Teal (1959) introduced modifications to avoid the occasional precipitation of globulins; van Kampen and Zijlstra (1961) introduced further modifications.

Reagent solutions used with the HiCN method all contain $K_3Fe(CN)_6$, usually 200 mg/L, and KCN, usually 50 mg/L. Because HCN is a weak acid (pK_a = 9.1), $K_3Fe(CN)_6$/KCN solutions have a high pH , around 9.6, and oxidation of oxyhaemoglobin (O_2Hb) and deoxy-haemoglobin (HHb) proceeds slowly. Thus, K_2HPO_4 was added to lower the pH and decrease the time required for oxidation of the haemoglobins to 3–5 minutes. However, lowering the pH favours precipitation of plasma proteins, primarily γ globulins with an isoelectric point near the pH of the reagent. This required the addition of a non-ionic detergent to effectively prevent the occurrence of turbidity in the majority of cases. The reagent solution recom-mended by ICSH (1967, 1978, 1987), and first described by van Kampen and Zijlstra (1961), thus contains the following: $K_3Fe(CN)_6$, 200 mg (0.607 mmol); KCN, 50 mg (0.769 mmol); KH_2PO_4, 140 mg (1.028 mmol); non-ionic detergent, 0.5–1.0 mL; and deionized or distilled water to 1000 mL.

The reagent is a clear, pale yellow solution with a pH of 7.0–7.4, an osmolality of 6–7 mOsm/kg (as measured by freezing point depression), and does not absorb light above 480 nm (Fig. 7.2). The conversion time of most haemoglobins to HiCN is 3–5 minutes. When stored at ambient (room) temperature in a tightly capped, amber borosilicate glass bottle, the shelf-life is 6–8 weeks. However, the reagent is unstable when exposed to light and $K_3Fe(CN)_6$ is destroyed by freezing (Weatherburn and Logan, 1964). On freezing and subsequent thawing, hexacyanoferrate(III), $Fe(CN)_6^{3-}$, is converted to hexacyanoferrate(II), $Fe(CN)_6^{4-}$, and oxidation to Hi cannot take place. Consequently the haemoglobins in the solution remain mainly as O_2Hb and, because ε_{O2Hb}^{540} = 14.32 (Zijlstra et al., 1991), c_{tHb} values up to 30% too high will be measured. During freezing of the reagent solution, the following reaction occurs:

$$2 \, (Fe(CN)_6^{3-}) + 2 \, CN^- \rightarrow 2 \, (Fe(CN)_6^{4-}) + (CN)_2$$

and $(CN)_2$ bubbles can be seen forming in the water–ice phase boundary (Zweens et al., 1979). This decomposition can be prevented by the addition of 20 mL/L ethanol, methanol or ethylene glycol, or 5 mL/L glycerol, because the transition from the liquid to the solid state then occurs abruptly after the reagent has become supercooled and no phase boundary develops. Turbidity of the resultant HiCN solutions is increased slightly by ethylene glycol, but not by ethanol or glycerol. Thus, under circumstances where freezing of the reagent is likely to occur, the addition of 20 mL ethanol should be considered.

Loss of CN^- from the reagent when stored in plastic containers has also been described (van Assendelft, 1971). In this case all haemoglobins will be oxidized to Hi, but the subsequent formation of HiCN will be incomplete or absent and, because ε_{Hi}^{540} = 7.14 (van Assendelft, 1970), c_{tHb} values up to 35% too low could be measured. The cyanide content of the reagent

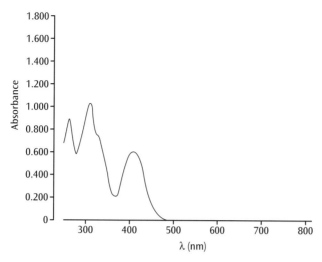

Fig. 7.2 *Light absorption spectrum of ICSH-recommended reagent for the haemiglobincyanide (HiCN) method. Recorded with Varian Cary 219 spectrophotometer, 1.000 cm lightpath, against water as blank.*

solutions can be measured directly using ion-selective electrodes (Zijlstra *et al.*, 1972) or, when in doubt, c_{tHb} can be remeasured after adding extra KCN to the reagent or to the 'HiCN' solution.

Although in the majority of cases HiCN solutions do not appear turbid, often some residual turbidity can be demonstrated, even in blood samples taken from normal, healthy individuals (Houwen *et al.*, 1996). In certain pathological conditions (e.g. severe lipaemia, paraprotein-aemia, increased γ globulins, high platelet or leucocyte counts), turbidity may cause a significant overestimation of c_{tHb}. To combat turbidity, several modified reagents have been proposed (Matsubara *et al.*, 1972, 1979; Vanzetti and Franzini, 1972) with increased ionic strength through the addition of NaCl or increasing the concentration of the phosphate buffer. Addition of one drop of 25% (v/v) ammonia solution (van Kampen and Zijlstra, 1983) has also been used. These modified reagents have not been widely used and it has proven more practical to clear HiCN solutions by other methods such as membrane filtration (Houwen *et al.*, 1996).

As stated above, the only haemoglobin derivative occurring in patients that is not converted to HiCN is SHb – SHiCN is formed instead. Generally, the effect on c_{tHb} of the presence of SHb is slight. Since $\varepsilon_{SHiCN}^{540} = 8.0$ (Dijkhuizen *et al.*, 1977), it can be calculated that the presence of 1% SHb in blood causes c_{tHb} to be underestimated by 0.27%. Since SHb fractions exceeding 5% are rarely, if ever, encountered in clinical practice, underestimation of c_{tHb} will be limited to $\leq 1.3\%$.

COHb is completely converted into HiCN, but the conversion time is considerably longer than for other haemoglobin derivatives (Taylor and Miller, 1965), and because $\varepsilon_{COHb}^{540} = 14.27$ (van Assendelft, 1970), non-conversion to HiCN would result in an overestimation of c_{tHb}. The upper limit of this error can be calculated if we suppose that no COHb is oxidized during the first 5 minutes after dilution with reagent. For example, for a sample with $c_{tHb} = 150$ g/L, a 10 or 20% COHb fraction will cause an overestimation of c_{tHb} by 3 and 6%, respectively. In practice the error will be less because COHb is present in only small amounts except in cases of CO intoxication. Any error can be prevented by increasing the time between mixing a suspect sample with reagent and its measurement from 5 to 30 minutes.

7.1.4 Diluting a blood sample with reagent

Although any convenient volume of blood and of reagent could be used, it is recommended that the resulting HiCN solutions give absorbance readings in the region where, for a given photometric error, the measurement error is the smallest. Thus, for single beam spectrophotometers and samples with c_{tHb} ranging from 120 to 160 g/L, the sample dilution should be between 200- and 250-fold, resulting in absorbance values of around 0.400. The concentration range that will give the best accuracy in photometric analyses can be determined for any (spectro)photometer by plotting a Ringbom curve (Eilers and Crocket, 1972).

For routine measurement of c_{tHb}, a 1:251 dilution is recommended, obtained by adding 20 µL blood to 5.0 mL of reagent, using calibrated glassware. The highest accuracy is obtained when calibrated 0.400 or 0.500 mL to deliver pipettes, or 0.500 mL Ostwald pipettes, and 100 mL class A volumetric flasks are used; this virtually eliminates all variance caused by dilution errors.

In practice, accurate dilutions with a reproducibility between absorbance readings on separate dilutions from the same blood sample with a coefficient of variation (CV) $\leq 0.5\%$ are obtained by: (i) diluting 100 µL well-mixed blood (calibrated to deliver pipette) with 25.0 mL of reagent (calibrated class A volumetric flask) (NCCLS, 1994); or (ii) diluting 40 µL well-mixed blood (calibrated positive displacement pipette) with 10 mL of reagent (calibrated class A volumetric flask) (Houwen et al., 1996). After aspirating the blood, wipe the pipette in the upright position. Ensure that the meniscus at the pipette tip is flat. Deliver the contents of the pipette into the reagent and rinse the pipette by aspirating and delivering the blood–reagent mixture at least five times. Allow 3–5 minutes for conversion of haemoglobins to HiCN. Because HiCN solutions are stable, absorbance measurement may be postponed for hours, even days, if the solutions are stored in a cool, dark environment and evaporation is prevented.

7.1.5 Filtration of HICN solutions

The recommended reagent (ICSH, 1967, 1978) contained 0.5 mL Sterox SE, an alkyl-phenol (thiol) polyethylene oxide, as non-ionic detergent; this detergent, however, is no longer available. Other detergents (ICSH, 1987), nonidet P-40 (a polyethylene glycol P-ethyl/phenyl ether, 1.0 mL/L – also no longer available) or Triton X-100 (registered trademark of Union Carbide Chemical and Plastics Co., Int.), an octyl phenyl polyethylene glycol ether, 1.0 mL/L, have been tested. However, neither of these is as effective in preventing residual turbidity as was Sterox SE (Houwen et al., 1996), and, in practice, many HiCN solutions show some marginal residual turbidity (A^{750} up to 0.005) because of the presence of protein aggregates and/or erythrocyte stroma remnants. Because an error of 0.001 in the absorbance measurement at 540 nm equates to a c_{tHb} error of 0.37 g/L, the reference method requires membrane filtration of the HiCN solutions before measuring. The use of Triton X-100 at 1.0 mL/L is now recommended, despite its limitations, because it is still widely available (ICSH, 1996). However, it is recommended (NCCLS, 1994; Houwen et al., 1996; ICSH, 1996) to filter the HiCN solutions using a syringe and a 25-mm diameter, low-binding, low-release membrane filter, 0.20–0.25 µm mean pore diameter. The filtered solution should stand for at least 1 minute to allow air bubbles to escape. Use of filters with a smaller diameter can lead to considerable pressure build-up with some samples, posing a potential hazard to the user because of dislodging of the filter with resulting accidental spray of the HiCN solution. Low-binding, low-release properties of candidate membrane filters can be determined in the laboratory by serial filtration of HiCN solutions and absorbance measurements at 750, 540, and 504 nm; non-turbid, pure HiCN solutions give A^{750} values ≤ 0.003 and $1.59 \leq A^{540}/A^{504}$

≤ 1.63. Unwanted release by candidate filters is checked by filtration of reagent only and verifying zero absorbance at 750 and 540 nm. Excellent results have been obtained with 0.22 µm polyvinylidene difluoride Millex-GV (Millipore Corp., Bedford, MA) and with 0.20 µm polypropylene Puradisc 25 PP (Whatman Inc., Fairfield, NJ) membrane filters (Houwen et al., 1996). Another filter that was found to be satisfactory is the Microprep 0.22 µm PVDF filter (Osmonics Laboratory and Speciality Products Group, Livermore, CA) (Van Assendelft et al., 1997, unpublished results).

7.1.6 Measurement

Using a calibrated (as to absorbance and wavelength) spectrophotometer and matched 1.000 cm cuvettes, read the absorbance of the diluted blood–reagent mixture at 540 nm against the reagent or water as blank. Single-beam spectrophotometers may require only one cuvette. Accurate spectrophotometric measurement of chromophores requires a spectral slit width (i.e. the total wavelength range emerging from the monochromator exit slit) to be < 10% of the natural bandwidth of the analyte (Henry, 1985). Thus, because the natural bandwidth of HiCN solutions is 70 nm around 540 nm, spectrophotometers suitable for use with the reference method should have a spectral slit width ≤ 6 nm.

Although the reagent does not absorb light above 480 nm (Fig. 7.2), in practice some diode arrays and other instruments have been identified that show apparent light absorption by the reagent in the 500–600 nm range; the apparent absorbance values were higher for matched quartz glass cuvettes than for optical glass cuvettes (Houwen et al., 1996). It is not clear if the apparent absorption is caused by differences in refractive index between quartz and glass with resulting slight reflective losses at the (quartz) glass–liquid interface, simulating light absorption. Thus, water can be used as blank only if the laboratory has shown that for a particular instrument–cuvette combination the reagent does not absorb light above 480 nm.

The spectrophotometer wavelength scale may be calibrated with the aid of the mercury, hydrogen or deuterium emission spectrum, or with a solution of holmium oxide in perchloric acid (Weidner et al., 1985; Jansen et al., 1986); the absorption scale may be checked using calibrated glass filters, e.g. National Institute of Standards and Technology (previously National Bureau of Standards) SRM 930, or other means which have been certified by a standardizing authority. The absence of stray light must also have been verified, e.g. using sodium nitrite, potassium iodide or specific glass filters (Burnett, 1985).

For many modern spectrophotometers, 'calibration' may resolve itself into merely verifying that the instrument yields an accurate value for A_{HiCN}^{540} of a certified secondary HiCN standard; slight deviations from the expected value may be used to correct measurement results.

Alternative instruments for the routine measurement of c_{tHb} by the HiCN method include:

- direct reading haemoglobinometers with a scale calibrated directly in haemoglobin concentration (g/L; mmol/L);
- photometers requiring the use of standard curves;
- photometers or photoelectric comparators measuring the unknown sample in comparison to a reference solution with known haemoglobin content.

7.1.7 Calculation of C_{tHb} from A_{HiCN}^{540}

HiCN solutions strictly follow Lambert-Beer's law and c_{tHb} is calculated from A_{HiCN}^{540} by means of the following equation:

$$c_{tHb}(g/L) = \frac{A_{HiCN}^{540} \times 16\,114.5 \times F}{11.0 \times d \times 1000}$$

where A_{HiCN}^{540} is the absorbance of the HiCN solution at 540 nm; 16114.5 is the relative molecular mass of the haemoglobin monomer (derived from 64458/4; Braunitzer, 1964); F is the dilution factor used; $11.0 = \varepsilon_{HiCN}^{540}$, the quarter millimolar absorptivity of HiCN (van Kampen and Zijlstra, 1983); d is the lightpath, usually 1.000 cm; and 1000 is the factor to convert mg to g.

For a dilution of 1:251 and 1.000 cm cuvettes:

$$c_{tHb}\,(g/L) = 367.7 \times A_{HiCN}^{540}$$

When a filter photometer is used for the absorbance measurement, c_{tHb} is read from a previously prepared calibration graph or table. A calibration line can be constructed by simply connecting the coordinates of a single calibrator measurement with the origin (Zijlstra and van Kampen, 1962) for photometers with demonstrated linearity.

7.1.8 Expression of results

The International Union of Pure and Applied Chemistry (IUPAC) and the International Federation of Clinical Chemistry (IFCC) recommend that all clinical laboratory results should preferably be reported in amount of substance (unit mole) with the appropriate prefix, per unit of volume, the litre (e.g. mmol/L). ICSH recommends that haemoglobin be reported as mass amount (unit kg), with the appropriate prefix, per unit of volume, the litre (e.g. g/L). ICSH also stated that substance concentration (mmol/L) is acceptable, if desired, but that in such cases the elementary entity on the basis of which the mole is defined must be indicated on the report at all times (i.e. Hb or 4 Hb; Fe or 4 Fe), depending on the use of the haemoglobin monomer or the tetramer (ISCH, 1972, 1973). If expression as substance concentration is desired, the following factors, based on the haemoglobin monomer, should be used:

$$c_{tHb}\,(mmol/L) = c_{tHb}(g/L) \times 0.0621 = c_{tHb}(g/dL) \times 0.621$$
$$c_{tHb}\,(g/dL) = c_{tHb}(mmol/L) \times 1.61$$
$$c_{tHb}\,(g/L) = c_{tHb}(mmol/L) \times 16.1$$

7.1.9 Quality assurance

The original concept of the standardized HiCN method included the supposition that HiCN reference solutions providing a single calibration point would lead to optimal measurement results (Zijlstra and van Kampen, 1962). Interlaboratory trials, however, have shown that incorrect dilution may be an important source of error (van Assendelft and Holtz, 1975) and that haemoglobin control solutions with known c_{tHb} should also be used to check the dilution step. A comprehensive quality assurance programme should therefore include the following:

- use of calibrated (e.g. gravimetric; water, mercury) pipettes and calibrated (e.g. gravimetric; water) class A volumetric glassware;
- spectrophotometer calibration as to wavelength (e.g. Hg, H, D emission; or holmium oxide), absorbance (e.g. certified glass filters, certified liquid absorbance standards, or certified secondary HiCN standards), and checking for linearity and absence of stray light;
- verification of conversion of haemoglobins to HiCN by comparing the light absorption spectrum of the blood–reagent mixtures with the absorption spectrum of pure HiCN solutions (Fig. 7.3) over a suitable wavelength range (e.g. 480–750 nm) and/or the

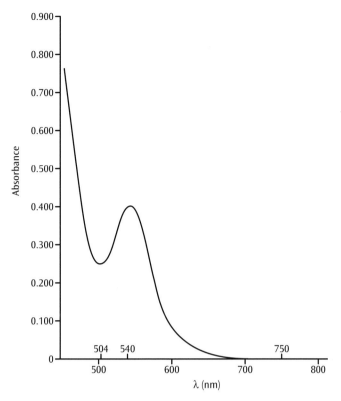

Fig. 7.3 *Light absorption spectrum of international HiCN standard, batch 70600. Recorded with Varian Cary 2290 spectrophotometer, 1.000 cm lightpath, against water as blank.* $A^{750} = 0.000$; $A^{540}/A^{504} = 1.61$.

determination of purity of resultant HiCN solutions by checking A^{750} (≤ 0.003; absence of turbidity) and A^{540}/A^{504} ($\geq 1.59, \leq 1.63$; purity);

- use of haemoglobin solutions with certified value as control material.

7.2 HAEMIGLOBINCYANIDE STANDARDS

HiCN standards can be considered to be the vehicle that transfers $\varepsilon_{HiCN}^{540} = 11.0$ L/mmol/cm to each user of the HiCN method and specifications for such standards have been included in the ICSH recommendations for haemoglobinometry from the very beginning (ICSH, 1967). International HiCN standards have been prepared at the Dutch Institute of Public Health (RIV) from 1965 to 1986, and have been designated International Standard for the Measurement of Haemoglobin in Blood by the World Health Organization (WHO) since 1968 (WHO, 1968).

7.2.1 International HICN Standard

The ICSH International HiCN Standard is used to assign values to secondary HiCN reference solutions or HiCN calibration solutions, and as a reference against which to judge the purity of such HiCN solutions. They were originally manufactured every year, checked for 9–12 months, then issued for a period of 2 years. This ensured that, should an HiCN solution suddenly deteriorate, a second standard would be available for distribution. As stability data accumulated, it was decided to produce a new standard every 3 years, with a 6-year expiration date.

The standards were prepared from washed red cells from human blood tested for the absence of hepatitis and HIV antibodies. The washed cells are haemolysed by toluene and centrifuged free from debris. The haemoglobins are converted to HiCN by adding a calculated amount of haemoglobin solution to a reagent containing $K_3Fe(CN)_6$ (200 mg/L), KCN (50 mg/L) and $NaHCO_3$ (1.0 g/L). The final HiCN solution, with an HiCN concentration of 550–850 mg/L, is filtered (membrane filter, 0.25–0.45 μm mean pore diameter) under pressure for sterilization purposes, and dispensed under aseptic conditions as 10 mL aliquots in sealed, amber borosilicate glass vials (Holtz, 1965).

Each batch of HiCN standard is tested by several haemoglobinometry reference laboratories designated by the board of ICSH. Using an appropriate blank (water or reagent), A^{750}, A^{540} and A^{504} are measured with a calibrated spectrophotometer. The slit width is chosen so that the half intensity bandwidth is ≤ 2 nm. The cuvettes in which the standard is measured are plan-parallel with an inner wall-to-wall distance of 1.000 cm, tolerance 0.5%. The measurements are carried out at 20–25°C. The arithmetic mean and standard error of the measurement results at 540 nm are recorded after erratic results, if any, have been discarded (Dixon, 1953). The HiCN concentration is calculated from the results of at least five of the reference laboratories, using the equation:

$$c_{HiCN} \ (mg/L) = \frac{A^{540}_{HiCN} \times 16\,114.5}{11.0 \times 1.000} = 1465 \times A^{540}_{HiCN}$$

Long-term experience with this procedure has shown that the confidence limits of the final result are well within ±1%.

The purity of HiCN standards is checked by visual inspection of the absorbance curve between 750 and 450 nm (Fig. 7.3); by determining the value of $A^{540}_{HiCN}/A^{504}_{HiCN}$, which must lie between 1.59 and 1.63 (the theoretical value based on ε^{540}_{HiCN} and ε^{504}_{HiCN} is 1.61); and by measuring the absorbance at a wavelength between 730 and 770 nm (e.g. at 750 nm) to check for the absence of turbidity; a value ≤ 0.003 per cm lightpath must be found.

The stability of international HiCN standards is checked by the haemoglobinometry reference laboratories at 3-month intervals before issue of the standards, then at 6-month intervals until the assigned expiration date; the manufacturing laboratory repeats absorbance measurements at regular, more frequent intervals. The standards are stored at 4–6°C and the producer notifies all customers if continued monitoring indicates that a particular batch is no longer acceptable. The sterility of HiCN standards is verified by the manufacturer using current practice of sterility control. The contents of randomly selected vials are inoculated in aerobic and anaerobic media, and are incubated at 22 and at 37°C. Several organisms, especially Gram-negative organisms, are known to be able to grow in a $K_3Fe(CN)_6$/KCN environment, e.g. *Alcaligenes faecalis*, *Paracolobactrum aerogenoides* and *Pseudomonas aeruginosa*. International HiCN standards are labelled with the batch number, the value of the HiCN concentration (mean and standard error), and an expiration date considered well within safe limits. The equivalent haemoglobin concentration of the standard is calculated by multiplying the HiCN concentration by the dilution factor used in the method. For example, 40 μL blood + 10 mL reagent → dilution factor 251×; HiCN concentration of the standard, 592 mg/L: equivalent haemoglobin concentration 251 × 592 = 148.6 g/L. International HiCN standards are made available, for reference use only, to national standardizing committees for haematological methods, or to official government-nominated holders. Where there is no committee or holder, it may be distributed to individuals approved by ICSH. National holders must ensure that an opportunity is given to manufacturers and distributors to use the International HiCN Standard as a reference material, if so desired.

7.2.2 Long-term stability of HICN standards

All batches of international standards issued have been stored at 4–6°C and checked regularly. As data accumulated, the long-term stability was reviewed (van Assendelft *et al.*, 1966, 1967, 1976, 1996; van Kampen and Zijlstra, 1983). Spectrophotometric measurements were made with a Beckman DU, half-intensity bandwidth 1.0, 0.52 and 0.42 nm at 750, 540 and 504 nm, respectively; and/or an Optica CF4 grating spectrophotometer, total bandwidth 0.5, 0.13 and 0.13 nm at 750, 540 and 504 nm, respectively; and/or a Hewlett-Packard 8540A diode array spectrophotometer, total bandwidth 2 nm at all wavelengths of measurement. The measurements were performed against water as blank, with a lightpath of 1.000 cm. The instruments were checked regularly as to wavelength calibration by means of the Hg emission lines at 546.1 and 491.6 nm, as to absorbance calibration at 540 nm with a Corning HT yellow glass filter certified by the National Institute for Standards and Technology (formerly National Bureau of Standards). The absence of stray light was verified at irregular intervals by means of glass and liquid cut-off filters. Table 7.1 summarizes the measurement results at 540 nm and the A^{540}/A^{504} quotients. Measurement results at 750 nm have not been included because values ≤ 0.003 were consistently found, as long as A^{540}/A^{504} remained ≥ 1.59. The first standard, batch 40400, was a pilot preparation and was never issued for distribution. It can be concluded that properly prepared, sterile HiCN solutions, stored at 4°C are generally stable, and show a decrease over time in A^{540}_{HiCN} of no more than 2%, for a period of about 15 years. HiCN solutions may deteriorate progressively after 20 years of storage; the cause and nature of this deterioration are not yet well understood. Very little data are available on the stability of HiCN solutions stored at temperatures other than 4–6°C. Holtz (1965) reported a loss of about 1% per year of A^{540}_{HiCN} for standards stored at 20°C, and about 8% per year when stored at 37°C. van Assendelft *et al.* (1966) reported that HiCN solutions stored at 20°C generally deteriorate after 1–1.5 years. Results from recent accelerated degradation studies indicate no deterioration of HiCN solutions during the first 6 months when stored at 20°C; a decrease of A^{540}_{HiCN} of 0.2–0.5% per month when stored at 37°C; a decrease of 0.5–1% per week when stored at 45°C; and a decrease of up to 3.5% per week when stored at 50°C (van Assendelft *et al.*, 1996).

7.2.3 Alternative source materials

From the viewpoint of biosafety and availability, it could be advantageous to use animal rather than human blood as source material for the production of HiCN standards. It has been shown that measurements of ε^{540}_{HiCN} in various animal species give virtually identical values to those obtained for human blood (Remmer, 1956; Zijlstra and Buursma, 1987; Zijlstra *et al.*, 1994). More recently, 14 bovine specimens were measured using the α,α'-dipyridyl method to determine haemoglobin iron. The results (BCR, 1995), based on 92 individual measurements, gave a value for ε^{540}_{HiCN} only slightly lower than the value of 11.0 L/mmol/cm for human haemiglobincyanide: 10.96 (SEM 0.008). Because the relative molecular mass of bovine haemoglobin is also exactly known – 64 533 for the tetramer (Dayhoff, 1972) – the HiCN concentration of bovine HiCN standards can be calculated according to:

$$c_{HiCN} \text{ (mg/L)} = (A^{540}_{HiCN} \times 64\,533)/(10.96 \times 1.000 \times 4)$$
$$= 1472 \times A^{540}_{HiCN}$$

Table 7.1 *Long-term stability of international haemiglobincyanide (HiCN) standards stored at 4°C*

Batch no.	40400		60400		70400		80400		90400		00400		10400		20400		30400	
	1964		1966		1967		1968		1969		1970		1971		1972		1973	
Age batch (years)	A^{540}	Q	A^{540}	Q	A^{540}	Q	A^{540}	Q	A^{540}	Q	A^{540}	Q	A^{540}	Q	A^{540}	Q	A^{540}	Q
0	0.391	1.61	0.386	1.61	0.405	1.62	0.383	1.60	0.389	1.61	0.395	1.61	0.413	1.61	0.408	1.61	0.403	1.61
0.25			0.387	1.61			0.381	1.61	0.389	1.61	0.395	1.61	0.414	1.60	0.408	1.61	0.402	1.61
0.5			0.387	1.61	0.404	1.62	0.386	1.62	0.388	1.62	0.396	1.61	0.415	1.61	0.408	1.61	0.403	1.62
0.75			0.387	1.61			0.383	1.61										
1	0.389	1.61	0.388	1.61	0.405	1.595			0.388	1.61	0.400	1.62	0.413	1.61	0.408	1.62	0.402	1.61
2–2.5	0.391	1.61	0.387	1.61	0.404	1.62	0.386	1.61	0.390	1.61	0.393	1.60	0.412	1.61	0.404	1.61	0.401	1.61
3–3.5	0.391	1.62	0.388	1.61	0.404	1.61	0.386	1.61	0.387	1.61	0.393	1.61	0.411	1.61	0.407	1.60	0.4035	1.605
5–5.5	0.393	1.61	0.386	1.61	0.404	1.62	0.384	1.61	0.387	1.60	0.393	1.60	0.405	1.61	0.402[a]	1.60		
9–10	0.390	1.60	0.386	1.61	0.404	1.61	0.381	1.61			0.389	1.59	0.405	1.605				
13–15	0.3875	1.59	0.381	1.60	0.405	1.585	0.3865	1.605	0.384	1.59	0.391	1.58					0.400	1.605
16–17	0.3915	1.58	0.380	1.60	0.401	1.595	0.382	1.59	0.386	1.585							0.3965	1.58
18–19	0.382	1.565	0.3805	1.595	0.3995	1.60	0.3805	1.605					0.403	1.595				
20–21	0.380[a]	1.57					0.3795	1.595	0.383[a]	1.60	0.386	1.57					0.3935	1.535
22–25			0.380	1.58	0.3985	1.59	0.378	1.58			0.384[a]	1.56	0.3975	1.535				
26–27			0.372	1.62	0.4015	1.60	0.378	1.595										

| Batch | 40500 | | 50500 | | 60500 | | 70500 | | 80500 | | 90500 | | 20600 | | 40600 | | 70600 | |
| | 1974 | | 1975 | | 1976 | | 1977 | | 1978 | | 1979 | | 1982 | | 1984 | | 1987 | |
Age batch (years)	A^{540}	Q	A^{540}	Q	A^{540}	Q	A^{540}	Q	A^{540}	Q	A^{540}	Q	A^{540}	Q	A^{540}	Q	A^{540}	Q
0	0.3825	1.60	0.379	1.61	0.3925	1.60	0.3945	1.60	0.396	1.60	0.3925	1.61	0.3825	1.60	0.3995	1.60	0.404	1.61
0.25	0.380	1.61	0.381	1.61	0.394	1.61	0.396	1.61	0.393	1.61	0.392	1.61	0.3805	1.61			0.404	1.61
0.5	0.381	1.60	0.3815	1.61	0.392	1.61	0.395	1.61	0.394	1.60	0.3935	1.61			0.402	1.605	0.400	1.595
0.75											0.3925	1.61			0.402	1.605		
1	0.378	1.61	0.3795	1.60	0.3935	1.60	0.395	1.61	0.3935	1.60	0.3925	1.60	0.3815	1.59	0.401	1.61	0.403	1.61
2–2.5			0.380	1.60	0.391	1.61	0.392	1.61	0.393	1.61	0.3915	1.60	0.378	1.61	0.3965	1.605	0.402	1.61
3–4					0.391	1.62			0.3925	1.605	0.3905	1.60	0.3795	1.59	0.398	1.60	0.402	1.60
5–6			0.3795	1.61	0.3875	1.605	0.3915	1.61	0.3935	1.60	0.3865	1.59	0.377	1.60	0.399	1.595	0.4015	1.60
8–11	0.376	1.61	0.3775	1.61	0.393	1.61	0.3925	1.61	0.3955	1.605	0.386	1.595	0.376	1.58	0.3975	1.585	0.400	1.61
11.5–13	0.3775	1.61	0.379	1.605			0.392	1.595	0.3905	1.60			0.3745	1.595	0.391	1.58		
13.5–15			0.376	1.595	0.393	1.58			0.3955	1.59	0.384	1.59	0.372	1.58				
16–19	0.3765	1.595	0.3805	1.595	0.3895	1.59	0.3965	1.605			0.377	1.56						

$Q = A^{540}/A^{504}$

[a] Last ampoule in storage

Preliminary accelerated degradation data indicate that bovine HiCN solutions are at least as stable as, and might even exceed, stability of human HiCN solutions.

7.3 THE ICSH EXPERT PANEL ON HAEMOGLOBINOMETRY

The Expert Panel believes that every standardized method and all standards of biological origin used in the clinical laboratory must not be allowed to become 'static'. Methods as well as standards must be critically evaluated on a continuous basis, while recommendations must be reviewed and, if necessary, amended, and new, thoroughly tested techniques must be used as they become available. This is known as 'dynamic standardization' and is clearly applicable to haemoglobinometry.

REFERENCES

BCR (1995) European Commission, BCR Information, Preparation and certification of a reference material of haemoglobincyanide for standardization of blood haemoglobin measurement, CRM 522. *EUR16101 EN*. Luxembourg: BCR.

Braunitzer, G. (1964) The molecular weight of human haemoglobin. *Bibl. Haematol.* **18**, 59–60.

Braunitzer. G., Gehring-Muller, R., Hilschmann, N. *et al*. (1961) Die Konstitution des normalen adulten Humanhaemoglobins. *Hoppe-Seylers, Z. Physiol. Chem.* **325**, 283–8.

Bull, B.S. and Korpman, R.A. (1982) Intralaboratory quality control using patient's data. In: Cavil, I. (ed.), *Quality Control*. Edinburgh: Churchill Livingstone, 121–50.

Burnett, R.W. (1985) Standards for spectrophotometry. In: Werner, M. (ed.), *Handbook of Clinical Chemistry*, Vol II. Boca Raton, FL: CRC Press, 25–9.

Cannan, R.K. (1958a) Proposal for a certified standard for use in hemoglobinometry. Second and final report. *Am. J. Clin. Pathol.* **30**, 211–13.

Cannan, R.K. (1958b) Haemoglobin as cyanmethaemoglobin in blood. *Clin. Chem.* **4**, 246–51.

Cannan, R.K. (1958c) Haemoglobin standard. *J. Lab. Clin. Med.* **52**, 471–3.

Dayhoff, M.O. (1972) *Atlas of Protein Sequence and Structure*, Vol. 5. Washington, DC: National Biomedical Research Foundation.

deBoroviczeny, Ch.G. (ed.) (1964) Decision of the standardizing committee of the European Society of Haematology concerning haemoglobinometry. *Bibl. Haematol.* **18**, 210–11.

deBoroviczeny, Ch.G., ed. (1965) Recommendations and requirements for haemoglobinometry in human blood. *Bibl. Haematol.* **21**, 213–16.

Dijkhuizen. P., Buursma, A., Gerding, A.M. *et al*. (1977) Sulfhemoglobin. Absorption spectrum millimolar extinction coefficient at 620 nm, and interference with the determination of haemiglobin and haemiglobincyanide. *Clin. Chim. Acta* **78**, 479–87.

Dixon, W.J. (1953) Processing data for outliers. *Biometrics* **9**, 74–89.

Drabkin, D.L and Austin, J.H. (1932) Spectrophotometric Studies I. Spectrophotometric constants for common hemoglobin derivatives in human, dog and rabbit blood. *J. Biol. Chem.* **98**, 719–33.

Drabkin, D.L. and Austin, J.H. (1935/36) Spectrophotometric Studies II. Preparations from washed blood cells; nitric oxide hemoglobin and sulfhemoglobin. *J. Biol. Chem.* **112**, 51–65.

Eilers, R.J. and Crocket, C. (1972) The value of Ringbom curves in hemoglobinometry. In: Izak,G., Lewis, S.M. (eds), *Modern Concepts in Hematology*. New York: Academic Press, 58–65.

Green, P. and Teal, C.F.J. (1959) Modification of the cyanmethemoglobin reagent for analysis of hemoglobin in order to avoid precipitation of globulins. *Am. J. Clin. Pathol.* **32**, 216–21.

Henry, H.L. (1985) Molecular spectrophotometry. In: Werner, M. (ed.), *Handbook of Clinical Chemistry*, Vol II. Boca Raton, FL: CRC Press, 3–23.

Hill, R.J., Konigsberg, W., Guidotti, G. *et al.* (1962) The structure of human haemoglobin I. The separation of the alpha and beta chains and their aminoacid composition. *J. Biol. Chem.* **237**, 1549–54.

Hoek,W., Kamphuis, N. and Gast, R. (1981) Haemiglobincyanide. Molar lineic absorbance and stability constant. *J. Clin. Chem. Clin. Biochem.* **19**,1209–10.

Holtz, A.H. (1965) Some experience with a cyanhaemiglobin solution. *Bibl. Haematol.* **21**, 75–8.

Houwen, B., Hsiao-Liao, N., Kubose-Perry, K.K. *et al.* (1996) The reference method for hemoglobin measurement revisited. *Lab. Haematol.* **2**, 86–93.

ICSH (1966) Report of the Expert Panel on Haemoglobinometry. *Bibl. Haematol.* **24**,194–5.

ICSH (1967) Recommendations for haemoglobinometry in human blood. *Br. J. Haematol.* **13**(Suppl.), 71–5.

ICSH (1972) Recommendations for use of SI in clinical laboratory measurements. *Br. J. Haematol.* **23**, 787.

ICSH (1978) Recommendations for reference method for haemoglobinometry in human blood (ICSH Standard EP 6/2: 1977) and specifications for international haemiglobincyanide reference preparation (ICSH Standard EP 6/3: 1977). *J. Clin. Pathol.* **31**, 139–43.

ICSH (1987) Recommendations for reference method for haemoglobinometry in human blood (ICSH Standard 1986) and specifications for international haemiglobincyanide reference preparation, 3rd edn. *Clin. Lab. Haematol.* **9**, 73–9.

ICSH (1993) Recommendations of the International Council for Standardization in Haematology for ethylenediaminetetraacetic acid anticoagulation of blood for blood cell counting and sizing. *Am. J. Clin. Pathol.* **100**, 371–2.

ICSH (1996) Recommendations for reference method for haemoglobinometry in human blood (ICSH Standard 1995) and specifications for international haemiglobincyanide reference preparation (4th edition). *J. Clin. Pathol.* **49**, 271–4.

ICSH, IFCC, WASP (1973) Recommendations for use of SI in clinical laboratory measurements. *Z. Klin. Chemie Klin. Biochem.* **11**, 93; *Br. J. Haematol.* **23**, 787, 1972.

Itano, H.A. (1972) Molar extinction coefficients of cyanmethemoglobin (hemiglobincyanide) at 540 and 281 nm. In: Izak, G., Lewis, S.M. (eds), *Modern Concepts in Hematology*. New York: Academic Press, 26–8.

Jansen, A.P., van Kampen, E.J., Steigstra, H. *et al.* (1986) Simultaneous spectrophotometric calibration of wavelength and absorbance in an interlaboratory survey using holmium oxide (Ho_2O_3) in perchloric acid as reference, compared with p-nitrophenol and cobaltous sulfate solutions (1978–1984*). J. Clin. Chem. Clin. Biochem.* **24**,141–6.

Liebecq, C. (1946) Libération du fer de l'hémoglobine par les acides. *Comp. Rend. Soc. Biol.* **140**, 1170–5.

Matsubara, T., Okuzono, H. and Tamagawa, S. (1972) Proposal for an improved reagent with hemiglobincyanide method. In: Izak,G., Lewis, S.M. (eds), *Modern Concepts in Hematology*. New York: Academic Press, 29–43.

Matsubara, T., Okuzono, H. and Senba, U. (1979) A modification of van Kampen-Zijlstra's reagent for the hemiglobincyanide method. *Clin. Chim. Acta* **93**, 163–4.

Meyer-Wilmes, J. and Remmer, H. (1956) Die Standardisierung des roten Blutfarbstoffes durch Haemiglobincyanid. I. Mitteilung: Bestimmung der spezifischen Extinktion von Haemiglobincyanid. *Arch. Exp. Path. Pharmakol.* **229**, 441–9.

Morningstar, D.A., Williams, G.Z. and Suutarinen, P. (1966) The millimolar extinction coefficient of cyanmethemoglobin from direct measurement of iron by x-ray emission spectroscopy. *Am. J. Clin. Pathol.* **26**, 603–7.

NCCLS (1994) Reference and Selected Procedures for the Quantitative Determination of Hemoglobin in Blood – Second Edition; Approved Standard. *NCCLS document H15-A2*. Wayne, PA: NCCLS.

Nijveld, H.A.W. (1943) Properties and structure of sulfhemoglobin. *Rec. Trav. Chim. Pays-Bas* **62**, 293–9.

Palmer, W.W. (1918) The colorometric determination of haemoglobin. *J. Biol. Chem.* **33**, 119–22.

Remmer, H.(1956) Die Standardisierung des roten Blutfarbstoffes durch Haemiglobincyanid, II. Mitteilung; Eisengehalt und O_2-Bindungsvermögen von menschlichem Blut. *Arch. Exp. Path. Pharmakol.* **229**, 450–62.

Stadie, W.C. (1920) A method for the determination of methemoglobin in blood. *J. Biol. Chem.* **41**, 237–41.

Sunderman, F.W., MacFabe, R.P., MacFayden, G.F. *et al.* (1953) Symposium on clinical hemoglobinometry. *Am. J. Clin. Pathol.* **23**, 519–98.

Taylor, J.D. and Miller, J.D.M. (1965) A source of error in the cyanmethemoglobin method of determination of hemoglobin concentration in blood containing carbon monoxide. *Am. J. Clin. Pathol.* **43**, 265–71.

Tentori, L., Vivaldi, G. and Salvati, A.M. (1966) The extinction coefficient of human hemiglobincyanide as determined by nitrogen analysis. *Clin. Chim. Acta* **14**, 276–7.

van Assendelft, O.W. (1970) *Spectrophotometry of Haemoglobin Derivatives*. Springfield, IL: Charles C. Thomas.

van Assendelft, O.W. (1971) Photometry and the standardized method for the determination of haemoglobin. *Schweiz. Med. Wochenschr.* **101**, 1649–52.

van Assendelft, O.W. and Holtz, A.H. (1975) Concepts of inter-laboratory trials: an international haematological survey. In: Lewis, S.M., Coster, J.F. (eds), *Quality Control in Haematology*. London: Academic Press, 13–36.

van Assendelft, O.W., Zijlstra, W.G., van Kampen, E.J. and Holtz, A.H. (1966) Stability of haemiglobincyanide reference solutions. *Clin. Chim. Acta* **13**, 521–5.

van Assendelft, O.W., Holtz, A.H., van Kampen, E.J. and Zijlstra, W.G. (1967) Control data of international haemiglobincyanide reference solutions. *Clin. Chim. Acta* **18**, 78–81.

van Assendelft, O.W., Buursma, A., Holtz, A.H. *et al.* (1976) Quality control in haemoglobinometry with special reference to the stability of haemiglobincyanide reference solutions. *Clin. Chim. Acta* **70**, 161–9.

van Assendelft, O.W., Buursma, A. and Zijlstra, W.G. (1996) Stability of haemiglobincyanide standards. *J. Clin. Pathol.* **49**, 275–7.

van Kampen, E.J. and Klouwen, H. (1954) Spectrophotometric determination of carboxyhemoglobin. *Rec. Trav. Chim. Pays-Bas* **73**, 119–24.

van Kampen, E.J. and Zijlstra, W.G. (1961) Standardization of hemoglobinometry. II. The hemiglobincyanide method. *Clin. Chim. Acta* **6**, 538–44.

van Kampen, E.J. and Zijlstra, W.G. (1983) Spectrophotometry of hemoglobin and hemoglobin derivatives. *Adv. Clin. Chem.* **213**, 199–257.

van Oudheusden, A.P.M., van de Heuvel, J.M., van Stekelenberg, G. J. *et al.* (1964) De ijking van de hemoglobinebepaling op basis van ijzer. *Ned. Tijdschr. Geneesk.* **108**, 265–7.

Vanzetti, G. and Franzini, C. (1972) Improved reagents and concentrated reference solutions in hemoglobinometry. In: Izak, G., Lewis, S.M. (eds), *Modern Concepts in Hematology*. New York: Academic Press, 44–53.

Weatherburn, M.V. and Logan, J.E. (1964) The effect of freezing on potassium ferricyanide-potassium cyanide reagent used in the cyanmethemoglobin procedure. *Clin. Chim. Acta* **9**, 581–4.

Weidner, V.R., Mavrodineanu, R., Mielenz, K.D. *et al.* (1985) Spectral transmittance characteristics of holmium oxide in perchloric acid solution. *J. Res. Nat. Bur. Stand.* **90**, 115–25.

World Health Organization (1968) WHO Expert Committee on Biological Standardization, 20th Report. *WHO Technical Report Series No. 385*. Geneva: WHO, 12–3; 86–7.

Zijlstra, W.G. and Buursma, A. (1987) Spectrophotometry of hemoglobin: a comparison of dog and man. *Comp. Biochem. Physiol.* **88B**, 251–5.

Zijlstra, W.G. and van Kampen, E.J. (1960) Standardization of hemoglobinometry. I. The extinction coefficient of hemoglobinometry at 540 nm. *Clin. Chim. Acta* **5**, 719–26.

Zijlstra, W.G. and van Kampen, E.J. (1962) Standardization of hemoglobimonetry III. Preparation and use of a stable hemiglobincyanide standard. *Clin. Chim. Acta* **7**, 96–9.

Zijlstra, W.G, van Assendelft, O.W., Buursma, A. and van Kampen, E.J. (1972) The use of an ion-selective electrode for checking the CN- content of reagent solutions used in the HiCN method. In: Izak, G., Lewis, S.M. (eds), *Modern Concepts in Hematology*. New York: Academic Press, 54–7.

Zijlstra, W.G., Buursma, A. and Meeuwsen-van der Roest, W.P. (1991) Absorption spectra of human fetal and adult oxyhemoglobin, de-oxyhemoglobin, carboxyhemoglobin, and methemoglobin. *Clin. Chem.* **37**, 1633–8.

Zijlstra, W.G., Buursma, A., Falke, H.E. and Catsburg, J.F. (1994) Spectrophotometry of hemoglobin: absorption spectra of rat oxyhemoglobin, deoxyhemoglobin, carboxyhemoglobin, and methemoglobin. *Comp. Biochem. Physiol.* **107B**, 161–6.

Zweens, J., Frankena, H. and Zijlstra, W.G. (1979) Decomposition on freezing of reagents used in the ICSH-recommended method for determination of total hemoglobin in blood; its nature, cause and prevention. *Clin. Chim. Acta* **91**, 337–52.

8

Haemoglobinometry: screening and routine practice[1]

BEREND HOUWEN AND ONNO W. VAN ASSENDELFT

INTRODUCTION

With the availability of a reference method for the determination of the haemoglobin concentration in blood (c_{tHb}) (Ch. 7), the accuracy of different routine laboratory methods and reagent systems for the determination of this analyte can now be scrutinized and evaluated. This has resulted in the availability of accurate and precise methods for routine laboratory practice, as evidenced by various proficiency assessment programmes. It is now possible, for example, to measure reliably the loss or donation of a single unit of blood, or the effectiveness of the transfusion of a single unit. However, although there is little debate that the determination of c_{tHb} forms one of the cornerstones of screening for, and clinical investigation of, anaemia, many screening programmes have continued to use the measurement of relative red cell volume (microhaematocrit method: PCV [packed cell volume; NCCLS, 1993]; haematology analysers: Hct, 'haematocrit') as a primary measure of anaemia. In a number of publications, e.g. the case studies in the *New England Journal of Medicine*, Hct rather than c_{tHb} is used to investigate anaemia; in erythropoietin treatment of renal dialysis patients, Hct, not the more stable c_{tHb} nor the red blood cell count, is considered by many health care providers to be the primary measurement for treatment initiation and monitoring. This can be an important issue because many of the patient specimens are analysed more than 24 hours after blood collection and the actual mean (red) cell volume (MCV), and thus the Hct value, may have changed significantly since collection of the blood specimen. Also, relative red cell volume measurements have certain weaknesses, and determination by the microhaematocrit method may even be biohazardous. A broken glass tube in the microhaematocrit method can create, for instance, significant hazards for laboratory personnel, because of the combination

[1]The use of trade names is for identification only and does not constitute endorsement by the Public Health Service or the US Department of Health and Human Services.

of blood/broken glass, and especially because of potential aerosol formation during centrifugation.

In contrast, haemoglobin concentration remains stable over time: c_{tHb} does not change significantly over periods up to 96 hours when the blood specimens are stored under sterile conditions, preferably at 4°C. Normal red blood cells stored at room temperature (18–25°C), however, show an increase of $\geq$ 15 fL in the MCV, but somewhat less when stored at 4°C. This becomes important when older specimens are analysed and, although the effects of cell volume increase can be decreased by the use of hyperosmolar diluents in haematology analysers, long-term stability of MCV, and thus of Hct, is fraught with difficulties.

Packed cell volume determinations are influenced by how well the red cells are packed. In patients with sickle cell anaemia or hereditary spherocytosis, the microhaematocrit results are extremely unreliable because of poor packing and large increases in plasma trapping. Also, the oxygenation state of haemoglobin in the red cell is already responsible for a 4% change in Hct value, compared with the same specimen in the deoxygenated state (Bryner *et al.*, 1997). Haematology analyser Hct values are subject to the combination of diluent and cell sizing technique used; frequently, 'shape changes' of the red cells affect the Hct measured (Bull *et al.*, 1996).

On the other hand, c_{tHb} is easily cross-calibrated and extremely stable over a wide variety of clinical conditions. The accuracy is threatened mainly by extreme turbidity, e.g. lyse resistance of the red cells, lipaemia, high white blood cell count, high platelet count, although in current haematology analysers this threat is minimal.

Under 'reference conditions' (NCCLS, 1993) (i.e. centrifuge radius > 8.0 cm, relative centrifugal force (RCF) = 10 000–15 000 × g_n at the periphery, soda lime glass type II capillary tubes 1.155 ± 0.085 mm internal diameter without taper, clay seal, microscope stage with vernier scale as reading device, and duplicate determinations which differ < 0.005), a high degree of reproducibility can be attained. Results from the ongoing use of whole blood reference methods for calibration of haematology analysers (ICSH, 1988) in the Loma Linda University School of Medicine are summarized in Table 8.1. The average overall coefficient of variation (CV) increased from 0.395 to 0.62% when the three excluded readings were included in the analysis. Under 'routine conditions' using commercially available 'haematocrit readers', the attainable CVs are significantly larger, as is seen in Table 8.2. We believe that a CV of 1%, as reported in the literature (Henry, 1991), is overly optimistic.

Table 8.1   *Results (L/L) of PCV determination by the microhaematocrit method 'reference conditions' (NCCLS, 1993) for six fresh blood specimens. Average coefficient of variation (CV, %) all measurements = 0.395*

	Specimen					
	1	2	3	4	5	6
Measurement						
#1	0.420	0.422	0.399	0.425	0.452	*
#2	0.425	0.427	0.401	0.422	0.453	0.444
#3	0.422	0.424	0.404	0.421	0.452	0.445
#4	0.423	0.425	0.404	*	0.453	*
Mean	0.4225	0.4245	0.4020	0.4227	0.4525	0.4445
SD	0.0021	0.0021	0.0024	0.0021	0.0006	0.0007
CV (%)	0.49	0.49	0.61	0.49	0.13	0.16

SD, standard deviation.
*Value discarded because deviation > 0.005 from mean.

Table 8.2 *Results (L/L) of PCV determination by a 'routine' microhaematocrit method and of c_{tHb} (g/L) by two automated haematology analysers*

Method/analyser	Microhaematocrit PCV (L/L)	Sysmex K-1000 c_{tHb} (g/L)	Coulter S[Plus] IV c_{tHb} (g/L)
Number of specimens	492	492	492
Mean value	0.357	116	119
Mean paired difference	0.0061	3.0	3.0
SD	0.0071	0.11	0.11
CV(%)	1.17	0.75	0.75

SD, standard deviation; CV, coefficient of variation.

8.1 ROUTINE HAEMOGLOBINOMETRY

The continued use of the relative red cell volume as a primary measure of anaemia may well be a 'left-over' from the situation clinical haemoglobinometry was faced with around the 1950s and, although for the past three decades the haemiglobincyanide (HiCN, cyanmethaemo-globin, methaemoglobincyanide) method has been universally accepted as the most accurate one for the determination of c_{tHb}, some of the older methods remain firmly entrenched in the routine laboratory and for screening for anaemia.

A significant number of blood banks continue to use the semiquantitative copper sulphate ($CuSO_4$) method to screen prospective donors (AABB, 1996). In this method, c_{tHb} of the blood is estimated from its specific gravity (Van Slijke *et al.*, 1950). A drop of blood is brought into contact with a solution of $CuSO_4$ of specific gravity 1.053 or 1.055. The drop becomes encased in a sac of copper proteinate that prevents dispersion of fluid or change in specific gravity of the blood for about 15 seconds. If $c_{tHb} \geq 125$ g/L (specific gravity 1.053 g/mL) or ≥ 135 g/L (specific gravity 1.055 g/mL), the drop will slowly sink; if $c_{tHb} < 125$ g/L or < 135 g/L, respectively, the drop will remain suspended or rise to the surface. In a 1986 study, the copper sulphate method was compared with an oxyhaemoglobin method (Compur M 1000 Miniphotometre, Compur-Electronic GmbH, Munich; Ames Division, Miles Laboratories, Elkhart, IN) using both capillary (skin puncture) and venepuncture specimens to determine eligibility as blood donor on a simple 'yes/no' basis (Ross *et al.*, 1986). For capillary blood sampling from 100 male and 100 female donors, the authors found the percentage of false failures for males to be 1.1%, but for females to be 25.3%. In a follow-up study of 201 additional females with venous sampling, a false failure rate of 28.4% was found. The most likely explanation for the observed male–female difference in testing sensitivity is that female donors tend to lie closer to the cut-off value (125 g/L) for donation acceptability than male donors lie to their cut-off value of 135 g/L. Thus, the likelihood of pass/failure classification errors is significantly increased for female donors.

Many small laboratories, especially in developing countries, continue to use the Sahli acid haematin method (Sahli, 1894). With a Sahli pipette, 20 μL of blood is mixed with 1 mL of 0.1 mol/L hydrochloric acid in a graduated glass tube. After 1 min the resulting solution is diluted with water until the colour visually matches that of a second tube containing a brown-coloured standard. The colour, however, develops gradually, then fades rapidly and errors ranging from 5 to 40% are the rule rather than exception.

Zander *et al.* (1984) described a method to determine c_{tHb} photometrically after conversion of haemoglobin to a haematin/detergent complex which they named haematin-D-575. It has been reported, however, that the results are somewhat dependent on the type of detergent used, that the end-product is prone to minor spectral changes over time, that there is a consistent bias of 2.6% between the method and the HiCN reference method, and that the relationship between the measured absorbance and c_{tHb} is non-linear at both low and high haemoglobin concentrations (van Assendelft and Zijlstra, 1989).

Stott and Lewis (1995) described a new colour scale for estimating c_{tHb} by visual comparison of a blood spot with 10 levels of haemoglobin (30, 40, 50, 60, 70, 80, 90, 100, 120 and 140 g/L) on the scale. The method, an updated version of the Tallqvist (1900) method, is based on new types of absorbent paper that allow a drop of blood to be absorbed as a regular round stain with limited spread, at the same time losing its sheen, within a few seconds. The colour scale against which the bloodstains are visually matched was developed based on computerized analytical spectrophotometry of bloodstains with a range of c_{tHb} from 30 to 140 g/L. The authors claim a precision of ± 5 g/L in estimating c_{tHb}. In an evaluation of the method (Lewis *et al.*, 1998) the presence of anaemia was reliably detected with 91% sensitivity and 86% specificity; serious anaemia, i.e. $c_{tHb} < 80$ g/L, was identified with an efficiency of 89%.

Because of concerns regarding potential risks to laboratory workers when using or disposing of potassium cyanide (KCN) based reagent systems, Vanzetti (1966) proposed measuring c_{tHb} after conversion of haemoglobin to haemiglobin azide (HiN$_3$). This method did not attract much attention, partly because of the potential risk for explosion when using sodium azide, until a new instrument, developed by Leo Diagnostics (Sweden), the HemoCue, became available. The HemoCue makes use of disposable optical measuring cuvettes with a volume of about 10 µL and a short (0.13 mm) light path. Dry reagents – sodium desoxycholate to haemolyse the red cells, sodium nitrite to oxidize haemoglobin to Hi, and sodium azide to convert Hi to Hi$_3$ – are deposited on the inner wall of the cuvette. The blood samples, capillary blood from skin punctures or venepuncture blood, are drawn into the cuvette by capillary action and spontaneously mix with the reagents. Once filled, the cuvette should be kept in a horizontal position and measured, within 10 min, in the HemoCue photometer at 565 and 880 nm. Absorbance measurement at 880 nm allows the instrument to compensate for turbidity caused by, for example, lipids, lipoproteins, or high white cell or platelet counts. The photometer features automatic zero setting between tests, checks the LED light source intensity and the condition of the photocell, and automatically compensates if any deterioration is identified. The factory calibration of the instrument is checked daily with a cuvette containing an optical filter certified by the manufacturer to be equivalent to a given haemoglobin concentration ('red control cuvette'). During an evaluation of 100 instruments and five lots of disposable cuvettes, a systematic error of -3.5% was found, compared with the HiCN reference method; by introducing a revised calibration protocol this bias was reduced to less than -1% (Kwant *et al.*, 1987). The improved calibration protocol consists of (i) accurate determination of c_{tHb} with the HiCN reference method of a fresh, properly anticoagulated blood specimen from an apparently healthy, non-smoking donor; (ii) meticulous calibration of a single HemoCue: 'key instrument'; (iii) calibration of serial instruments with the aid of the 'key instrument'; and (iv) checking each lot of cuvettes for light path and reagent filling by measuring c_{tHb} with the 'key instrument'. Any remaining source of error and imprecision may be ascribed to the blood sampling procedure.

A similar system, HemoSite, has been developed by GDS Diagnostics (Elkhart, IN). The method is based on dry chemistry blood separation technology and allows the use of a first drop of blood from a skin puncture. The sample is applied to the well of a test card consisting of multilayered filtration and reagent membranes. Colour development of the erythrocyte/sodium nitrite–sodium azide mixture takes place in the final layer and is measured with a small reflectance photometer. The manufacturer reports that the precision, expressed as coefficient of variation, is 3.5%; in a comparison of 372 specimens with results obtained with a Coulter haematology analyser, a mean difference of -2 g/L (-0.12 mmol/L; -0.2 g/dL) was found (GDS Diagnostics, personal communication, 1998).

Not only do cyanide-based reagents pose a potential danger to laboratory workers, but there is also the environmental impact, on disposal, of toxic chemicals that may leach into ground water from landfills, and the possible financial burden of adhering to regulations imposed by central or local authorities. Disposal of cyanide waste is theoretically simple: alkaline solutions of sodium or calcium hypochlorite ($NaOCl$, $CaOCl$) will oxidize cyanide to relatively safe cyanate (Broden, 1992) which then decomposes to urea. Alternatively, the laboratory may use a commercial waste handling and disposal company; this, however, may prove to be prohibitively expensive. There has thus been a continuous search for further non-cyanide reagent systems for clinical haemoglobinometry.

Oshiro (Oshiro *et al.*, 1982) was among the first to describe the use of the anionic detergent sodium lauryl sulphate (sodium dodecyl sulphate; $C_{12}H_{25}O_4 \cdot Na$) for the determination of c_{tHb}, naming the end-product measured 'SLS-haemoglobin'. The reaction mechanisms of this method have been studied by Matsubara and Mimura (1990) with a reagent containing, per litre, 0.70 g sodium lauryl sulphate (SLS), 1.0 mL Triton X-100 (a non-ionic detergent), 0.033 mol phosphate buffer, pH 7.35 ± 0.15. One volume of blood is added to 200–250 volumes of reagent and the absorbance of the characteristic peak at 534–536 nm is measured. They hypothesize that the hydrophobic group of SLS disrupts the tertiary structure of the haemoglobin tetramer allowing the haemoglobin-bound O_2, or O_2 dissolved in water, to oxidize the haemoglobin Fe. The hydrophilic group of SLS then combines with Hi to form 'SLS-haemoglobin' ('SLS-Hb'); it is, however, more appropriate to name the end-product haemiglobin SLS (HiSLS). The reagent contains Triton X-100 to protect SLS from precipitating at low temperatures, to promote rapid and complete lysis of the red and white blood cells, and to slow the formation of HiSLS.

Zijlsta *et al.* (unpublished data, 1992) determined that the addition of excess CN^- to an HiSLS solution (250-fold dilution of a whole blood sample) shifts the absorbance maximum from 534 nm to 540–542 nm and results in an absorbance spectrum nearly identical to that of HiCN. The addition of an equal volume of SLS reagent to an HiCN solution (250-fold dilution of a whole blood sample) resulted in a shift of the 540 nm absorbance maximum to 536 nm, with an absorbance spectrum between that of pure HiCN and pure HiSLS. They concluded that excess SLS can partly displace CN^- from HiCN and excess CN^- can displace SLS from HiSLS. The Hi/anion displacement series described previously (van Assendelft, 1970) can thus be extended to read:

$$OH^- < F^- < NO_2^- < N_3^- < SLS < CN^-$$

and the term haemiglobinSLS appears to be the correct term for this compound.

The HiSLS method using an adapted Sysmex K 1000 haematology analyser was compared with the HiCN method for 212 blood specimens. The patient specimens included cord blood, low MCV, haemoglobinopathies, raised plasma bilirubin levels, high white cell and platelet counts, and paraproteinaemia; no significant differences were found between the results obtained with the two methods. Analysis of the results gave a correlation coefficient $r = 0.987$ with an intercept $y = 1.027x - 0.362$ (Houwen, personal communication, 1992).

8.2 HAEMATOLOGY ANALYSERS

The majority of today's laboratories use automated haematology analysers to report a patient's complete blood count (CBC), with a typical analyser capable of processing 60–90 specimens/hour. This had consequences for the determination of c_{tHb}, because a reagent system had to be found that lyses the red cells rapidly and effectively, that prevents background turbidity, or keeps background turbidity minimal, and that converts all haemoglobin derivatives and/or variants to a same end-product that one should be able to measure accurately and reproducibly; all this to be achieved in a short time, typically < 30 seconds. An additional complication for some of the analysers is that white blood cells are kept intact for cell counting and differential counting, thus creating a natural turbid environment in the Hb/WBC channel of the instrument. Automated analysers therefore employ a wide variety of surfactants or other lytic agents and a variety of ligands to achieve a measurable end-product. Examples of such ligands include N,N-dimethyl-laurylamine N-oxide (Bayer), imidazole and imidazole derivatives (Abbott), ethoxylated amine compounds and/or quaternary ammonium salts (Beckman-Coulter), and pyridinium salts (Sysmex). The HiSLS method has also been adapted for use on Sysmex automated haematology analysers with the proprietary reagent SULFOLYSER. Good correlation with the HiCN reference method has been demonstrated by Fujiwara *et al.* (1990) (60 specimens; $r = 0.999$, $y = 1.001x - 0.033$), by Oshiro *et al.* (1990) (120 specimens; $r = 0.998$, $y = 1.025x - 0.332$), and by Saito *et al.* (1990) (100 specimens; $r = 0.998$, $y = 1.004x + 0.007$). Good correlation of the method with automated CN⁻-based methods, using dog, monkey, mouse and rat specimens, has also been reported (Morikawa *et al.*, 1992; Evans and Smith, 1993). Comparability of haematology analyser c_{tHb} results to values obtained with the HiCN reference method remains assured through the analyser calibration process, because the calibrators used generally have assigned c_{tHb} values obtained with the HiCN reference method (ICSH, 1988). Analyser precision is reflected by results from proficiency assessment programmes where, for haemoglobin determination in the healthy reference range, CVs ≤ 1.5% are consistently found. Most manufacturers have thus developed reagent systems that fulfil the needs of the clinical laboratory: adequate accuracy, precision and speed (Tables 8.2 and 8.3). Such accurate and precise measurements allow better screening for anaemia and patient monitoring. Small differences in c_{tHb} for population groups can also be reliably identified. This may be illustrated by results from the National Health and Nutrition Examination Survey (NHANES) for different population groups. The mean haemoglobin level for the non-Hispanic black population (both sexes) lies 5–10 g/L lower than that for the non-Hispanic white population, as is summarized in Table 8.4. A probable cause of this could be a high incidence of a single α gene deletion in black individuals (Reed and Diehl, 1991; Perry *et al.*, 1992).

In conclusion, the determination of c_{tHb} under routine laboratory conditions using either (semi)automated haematology analysers or dedicated 'point-of-care' methods (Table 8.5) provides acceptable accuracy and precision. The determination of c_{tHb} by the copper sulphate

Table 8.3 *Precision, expressed as coefficient of variation (CV, %), of haematological determinations by manual and semi-automated methods (from the literature) and by haematology analysers (manufacturer's specifications)*

Parameter	Manual	Semi-automatic	Multichannel analyser 'High end'	'Low end'	Typical 'low end' performance
Haemoglobin	2.0	NA	≤ 1.0	≤ 1.5	0.79
Haematocrit	1.0	NA	≤ 1.5	≤ 1.5	1.43
White cell count	6.5	4.6	≤ 1.5	≤ 1.5	1.06
Red cell count	NA	2–4.0	≤ 3.0	≤ 3.0	1.45
Platelet count	11.0	4.0	≤ 4.0	≤ 4.0	2.23

Table 8.4   *Mean haemoglobin concentration (g/L) by age and sex for the non-Hispanic black and the non-Hispanic white population, United States 1988–94*

Age group (years)	Number examined		Mean haemoglobin concentration		Standard error of the mean[a]	
	Black	White	Black	White	Black	White
Males						
1–2	275	297	117.2	120.35	0.57	0.53
3–5	419	323	120.1	124.1	0.46	0.5
6–8	229	190	125.3	129.8	0.645	0.66
9–11	267	200	126.7	134.1	0.665	0.64
12–14	184	139	133.1	142.3	0.92	1.04
15–19	298	195	145.3	142.3	0.92	1.04
20–29	463	381	148.5	142.3	0.92	1.04
30–39	461	435	145.7	142.3	0.92	1.04
40–49	336	414	145	142.3	0.92	1.04
50–59	207	410	143.1	142.3	0.92	1.04
60–69	274	493	139	142.3	0.92	1.04
70–79	168	489	135.9	142.3	0.92	1.04
> 80	52	525	128.6	142.3	0.92	1.04
Females						
1–2	265	270	118.3	142.3	0.92	1.04
3–5	433	332	120.7	124.8	0.45	0.51
6–8	220	175	123.7	129.2	0.62	0.725
9–11	252	186	126.5	132.2	0.59	0.76
12–14	220	154	125.4	134.3	0.72	1.04
15–19	326	270	123.2	133.3	0.67	0.74
20–29	589	477	124.2	133	0.55	0.61
30–39	602	572	124.4	134.2	0.6	0.565
40–49	425	457	124.2	133.9	0.8	0.64
50–59	256	473	129	136.1	0.845	0.63
60–69	276	473	128.6	135.3	0.77	0.665
70–79	170	617	127.3	135.3	1.19	0.56
> 80	82	574	119.3	132.7	1.93	0.69

Data are from the National Health and Nutrition Examination Survey (NHANES III), 1988–1994 (to be published).
[a]Standard errors of the mean calculated taking into account sampling weights and complex sample design.

Table 8.5   *Intended use of haemoglobin determinations*

Type of patient	Purpose of testing	Location of testing
In-patient	Monitoring	Central laboratory
Outpatient	Diagnosis	Central or satellite laboratory
Patient at home	Screening	Physician's office laboratory
Self-testing	Monitoring	Point of care

method is clearly outdated. While, for screening purposes, the determination of PCV using (semi)automated haematology analysers shows acceptable precision, with the microhaematocrit method, under routine laboratory conditions, only marginal precision can be attained. In both cases, problems with accuracy may be encountered in various pathological conditions.

REFERENCES

American Association of Blood Banks (AABB) (1996) *Technical Manual*, 12th edn. Bethesda, MD: AABB.

Broden, P.N. (1992) Concerns for the use and disposal of cyanide-containing reagents in the hematology laboratory. *Sysmex J. Int.* **2**, 156–61.

Bryner, M.A., Houwen, B., Westengard, J. and Klein, O. (1997) The spun micro-haematocrit and mean red cell volume are affected by changes in the oxygenation state of red blood cells. *Clin. Lab. Haematol.* **19**, 99–103.

Bull, B.S., Aller, R. and Houwen, B. (1996) MCHC: red cell index or quality control parameter? *Proceedings of the XXVI International Society of Haematology Meeting*; Education Program, ICSH Symposium, Singapore, 40–3.

Evans, G.O. and Smith, D.E.C. (1993) Preliminary studies with an SLS method for haemoglobin determination in three species. *Sysmex J. Int.* **3**, 88–90.

Fujiwara, C., Hamaguchi, Y., Toda, S. and Hayashi, M. (1990) The reagent SULFOLYSER® for hemoglobin measurement by hematology analyzers. *Sysmex J.* **13**, 212–19.

Henry, J.B. (1991) *Clinical Diagnosis and Management by Laboratory Methods*, 18th edn. Philadelphia: Saunders.

ICSH (1988) The assignment of values to fresh blood used for calibrating automated cell counters. *Clin. Lab. Haematol.* **10**, 203–12.

Kwant, G., Oeseburg, B., Zwart, A. and Zijlstra. W.G. (1987) Calibration of a practical hemoglobinometer. *Clin. Lab. Haematol.* **9**, 387–93.

Lewis, S.M., Stott, G.J. and Wynn, K.J. (1998) An inexpensive and reliable new haemoglobin colour scale for assessing anaemia. *J.Clin. Pathol.* **51**, 21–4.

Matsubara, T. and Mimura, T. (1990) Reaction mechanism of SLS-Hb method. *Sysmex J.* **13**, 379–84.

Morikawa, T., Tsjudino, Y. and Hamaguchi, Y. (1992) The application of the SLS-Hb method to animal blood. *Sysmex J. Int.* **2**, 56–65.

NCCLS (1993) Procedure for Determining Packed Cell Volume by the Microhematocrit Method, 2nd edn. *Aproved Standard. H7-A2*. Villanova, PA: NCCLS.

Oshiro, I., Takenaka, T. and Maeda, J. (1982) New method for hemoglobin determination by using sodium lauryl sulfate (SLS). *Clin. Biochem.* **15**, 83–8.

Oshiro, I., Fujii, M., Hatanaka, T. *et al.* (1990) Evaluation of sodium lauryl sulfate (SLS) for hemoglobin determination. Studies of the SLS-Hb method using the automated hematology analyzer 'Sysmex K 1000'. *Sysmex J.* **13**, 220–5.

Perry, G.S., Byers, T., Yip, R. and Margen, S. (1992) Iron nutrition does not account for the hemoglobin differences between blacks and whites. *J. Nutr.* **122**, 1417–24.

Reed, W.W. and Diehl, L.F. (1991) Leukopenia, neutropenia and reduced hemoglobin levels in healthy American blacks. *Arch. Intern. Med.* **151**, 501–5.

Ross, D.G., Gilfillan, A.C., Houston, D.E. and Heaton, W.A.L. (1986) Evaluation of hemoglobin screening methods in prospective blood donors. *Vox Sang.* **50**, 78–80.

Sahli, H. (1894) *Bestimmung des Haemoglobingehaltes des Blutes*. Lehrbuch der Klinischen Untersuchungsmethoden. Leipzig: Deuticke.

Saito, H., Shimizu, Y., Shimazu, C. and Yasuda, K. (1990) Investigation of the reagent SULFOLYSER® for hemoglobin analysis by the SLS-Hb method. *Sysmex J.* **13**, 227–35.

Stott, G.J. and Lewis, S.M. (1995) A simple and reliable method for estimating haemoglobin. *Bull. WHO* **73**, 369–73.

Tallqvist, T.W. (1900) Ein einfaches Verfahren zur directen Schaetzung der Farbstaerke des Blutes. *Z. Klin. Med.* **40**,137–41.

van Assendelft, O.W. (1970), *Spectrophotometry of Haemoglobin Derivatives*. Assen: van Gorcum/Springfield, IL: Charles C. Thomas.

van Assendelft, O.W. and Zijlstra, W.G. (1989) Observations on the alkaline haematin/detergent complex proposed for measuring haemoglobin concentration. *J. Clin. Chem. Clin. Biochem.* **27**, 191–5.

Van Slijke, D.D., Phillips, R.A., Dole, V.P. *et al.* (1950) Calculation of hemoglobin from blood specific gravities. *J. Biol. Chem.* **183**, 349–60.

Vanzetti, G. (1966) An azide-methemoglobin method for hemoglobin determination in blood. *J. Lab. Clin. Med.* **67**, 116–26.

Zander, R., Lang, W. and Wolf, H.U. (1984) Alkaline haematin D-575, a new tool for the determination of haemoglobin as an alternative to the cyanhaemiglobin method. I. Description of the method. *Clin. Chim. Acta.* **136**, 83–93.

3

Haemoglobin A$_2$, F and the abnormal haemoglobins

9

Detection and identification of haemoglobin variants

ONNO W. VAN ASSENDELFT

INTRODUCTION

Largely due to the ease with which quantities of human haemoglobin can be obtained and quantified, these proteins have played a major role in elucidating the processes involved in translating specific deoxyribonucleic (DNA) sequences (i.e. genes) into specific functional proteins.

Haemoglobin is the oxygen (O_2) transport protein found in the red blood cells of vertebrates. Haemoglobin is composed of four globin chains, each associated with an iron-containing prosthetic group, haem, capable of reversibly binding O_2. Typically, haemoglobin molecules comprise two pairs of different globin chains. In normal human haemoglobin, Hb A, these chains have been designated α and β. Thus the formula for the chain composition of Hb A may be written as $\alpha_2\beta_2$. The α- and β-chains are almost equal in length, consisting of 141 and 146 amino acid residues, respectively. They exhibit remarkable homology in amino acid sequence (primary structure) as well as in three-dimensional configuration (tertiary structure). Hb A generally comprises at least 95% of the total haemoglobin present in normal human adult erythrocytes; in addition 1.5–3.5% haemoglobin A_2 and $\leq 1\%$ haemoglobin F, the major haemoglobin of the human fetus, are found in the normal adult erythrocyte. Hb A_2 consists of two α- and two δ-chains ($\alpha_2\delta_2$), with the δ-chain very similar to the β-chain, differing by only 10 amino acid residues. Hb F consists of two α- and two γ-chains ($\alpha_2\gamma_2$), with the γ-chain differing by only 39 amino acid residues from the β-chain. The γ-chain provided the first conclusive evidence of duplicated globin loci, i.e. place or position occupied by genes on chromosomes. The presence of at least two γ-chain loci was demonstrated by finding two types of γ-chains which have either glycine or alanine at position 136 of their amino acid sequence; they are referred to as the $^{G}\gamma$- and $^{A}\gamma$-chain, respectively.

The globin genes, like most other eukaryotic genes, are divided into coding regions (exons) and intervening sequences (introns). The α- and β-like globin genes differ mainly by the presence of a considerably longer second intron in the β-like globin genes. Mutations can occur in any region of a globin gene. The abnormalities resulting from globin gene mutations have been conveniently classified into three major categories: structural variants, thalassaemias and hereditary persistence of fetal haemoglobin (HPFH). Structural haemoglobin variants result from mutations which cause the synthesis of structurally abnormal globin. The thalassaemias result from mutations which cause a defect in the synthesis of one or more globin chains, thus disturbing the normal equimolar synthesis of α- and non-α-chains. The HPFH syndromes result from mutations which cause the persistence of γ-chain synthesis throughout adult life, without an associated thalassaemic phenotype. Some abnormalities, however, have phenotypic features which fall into more than one category.

The majority of haemoglobin structural variants are substitutions of a single amino acid and can be explained, in most cases, by a single base change in the codon which codes for the substituted amino acid. This type of mutation is known as a point mutation. The best known example is haemoglobin S (Hb S) with valine in position 6 of the β-chain instead of the normal glutamic acid. Several haemoglobin structural variants are characterized by two different amino acid substitutions in the same globin chain. An example of such a double amino acid substitution is haemoglobin C Harlem with valine instead of glutamic acid at position 6 of the β-chain and asparagine instead of aspartic acid at position 73. A haemoglobin variant with a shortened β-chain has been described: haemoglobin McKees Rocks. The chain is shortened by two amino acid residues because of a single-base substitution in the codon for the final tyrosine residue causing a chain termination signal. This type of mutation has been called a 'nonsense' mutation.

Mutations in the chain terminator and frameshift mutations have also been described. Because of a single-base substitution in the chain terminator codon, haemoglobin Constant Spring has abnormally long α-chains, with 31 additional amino acid residues at the C-terminal end. Several other variants of this type have been described, all involving the chain termination codon of the α$_2$ gene (Michelson and Orkin, 1980). In haemoglobin Wayne, the α-chain has the normal α-chain amino acid sequence through position 138 followed by a new sequence of eight amino acids at the C-terminal end (Seid-Akhavan *et al.*, 1971). The mechanism of mutation is thought to be deletion of a single base causing a shift in the 'reading frame'. Frameshift mutations have also been described in the β-chain (Bunn *et al.*, 1975; Lehmann *et al.*, 1975). Other variants have been described due to inserted or deleted amino acid residues. Haemoglobin Gun Hill, for example, is a β-chain variant with deletion of five amino acid residues (Bradley *et al.*, 1967), and haemoglobin Grady has three additional amino acids in its α-chain (Huisman *et al.*, 1974). In haemoglobin Lepore, a fusion haemoglobin, the non-α-chain contains δ-globin sequences in the N-terminal portion and β-globin sequences in the C-terminal portion (Baglioni, 1962). Haemoglobin Lepore appears to be the result of non-homologous crossing over between the δ-locus on one chromosome and the β-locus on the other chromosome. In haemoglobin Parchman, the non-α-chain has been shown to have δ-globin sequences in both the C- and N-terminal portions, with β-globin sequences present in an interior segment (Adams *et al.*, 1982).

The clinically important thalassaemias result from a decreased synthesis of either the α-globin chain, α-thalassaemia, or the β-globin chain, β-thalassaemia. Thalassaemias have been described in which synthesis of the δ-chain of Hb A$_2$ or the γ-chain of Hb F is impaired (Ohta *et al.*, 1980; van der Ploeg *et al.*, 1980; Orkin *et al.*, 1981). The primary cause of α-thalassaemia is gene deletion of one or more of the two α$_1$- or two α$_2$-globin genes. The β-thalassaemias may be classified into two types. In β^0-thalassaemia there are no β-globin chains formed by the mutant gene; in β$^+$-thalassaemia there is reduced β-globin chain production. Most β-thalassaemias are not due to gene deletion but result from a variety of mutations.

HPFH refers to a group of conditions in which there is a persistence of fetal haemoglobin synthesis throughout adult life, without an associated thalassaemic phenotype. Thus, in HPFH the synthesis of the γ-chain is able to compensate for the absence of β- and δ-chain synthesis. In a group of related disorders, the βδ-thalassaemias, there is also a complete absence of β- and δ-globin synthesis on the affected chromosomes associated with an increase in γ-chain synthesis; in these cases a thalassaemic phenotype results. Both HPFH and βδ-thalassaemia appear to be largely due to gene deletions (Orkin *et al.*, 1978; Bernards and Flavell, 1980).

At the time of this writing, over 750 variant haemoglobins have been described (Huisman *et al.*, 1997, 1999).

9.1 CLINICAL CLASSIFICATION

The first clinical description of a haemoglobinopathy dates back to 1910 when Herrick described his observation of sickle-shaped erythrocytes in the peripheral blood of a severely anaemic West Indian individual (Herrick, 1910). Hahn and Gillespie (1927) observed, nearly two decades later, that O_2 inhibited the sickling of erythrocytes in sickle cell anaemia and that the defect appeared to reside in the haemoglobin molecule. The genetic basis of sickle cell anaemia was demonstrated by Neel (1949) and by Beet (1949), while Pauling *et al.* (1949) demonstrated that sickle cell anaemia was, in fact, due to a haemoglobin molecule abnormality, and Ingram (1956) demonstrated that sickle cell haemoglobin differed from normal haemoglobin by only a single amino acid substitution. Within a few years, other haemoglobin variants, especially those with relatively high gene frequencies, e.g. haemoglobins C, D and E, were identified.

The majority of haemoglobin variants are not associated with any clinical signs or symptoms. The clinically significant variants may be classified as follows:

- sickling syndromes (sickle cell trait, sickle cell disease);
- unstable haemoglobins (congenital Heinz body anaemia);
- haemoglobins with abnormal O_2 affinity (high affinity, low affinity);
- the M haemoglobins (familial cyanosis);
- structural variants resulting in thalassaemic phenotypes (α-thalassaemic phenotype, β-thalassaemic phenotype).

The majority of haemoglobin variants have been detected because of abnormal electrophoretic behaviour due to amino acid substitutions involving a change of charge. A large portion of clinically significant variants, however, have amino acid substitutions that do not alter the overall charge of the protein and other methods, e.g. citrate agar electrophoresis at acid pH, isoelectric focusing, high-performance liquid chromatography and immunological techniques are necessary for their detection and identification.

9.2 NOMENCLATURE OF HAEMOGLOBIN PHENOTYPES

When more than one haemoglobin type is present, the one in larger concentration is usually listed first. When the haemoglobin present in larger concentration is Hb A, the pattern present is usually that of the heterozygous, trait, condition. For example, Hb AS and Hb AC refer to haemoglobin S and haemoglobin C trait. When two variant haemoglobins are present in approximately equal quantities, the one with the greater clinical significance is listed first, e.g. Hb SC.

Initially, new variants were named by successive letters of the alphabet. However, when haemoglobin Q was identified it became clear that the alphabet would soon be exhausted. Also, some haemoglobins with identical electrophoretic properties were shown to have different structures and investigators started giving newly discovered haemoglobins specific names, many reflecting the geographic origin of the patient or the hospital where they were discovered, e.g. haemoglobin Gun Hill, haemoglobin Constant Spring.

A scientific notation has been developed to denote the affected polypeptide chain, the sequential number (or numbers) of the amino acid(s) involved, the helix number involved, and the nature (substitution, deletion, addition) of the abnormality. Thus, the scientific name for Hb S is $\beta^{6(A3)Glu \rightarrow Val}$ because valine (Val) has been substituted for glutamic acid (Glu) in the sixth sequential amino acid position, which is the third position in the A helical segment, of the β-chain.

9.3 LABORATORY TESTS

Laboratory tests for the detection and identification of haemoglobin variants include:

- a complete blood count with evaluation of red cell morphology;
- haemoglobin electrophoresis on cellulose acetate at pH = 8.4–8.6;
- solubility test to confirm the presence of sickling haemoglobins;
- citrate electrophoresis at acid pH to confirm the identity of haemoglobin variants;
- supravital staining for the presence of Heinz bodies (unstable haemoglobins);
- quantitation of haemoglobins A$_2$ and F.

Tests that are occasionally required are heat denaturation and isopropanol precipitation testing to screen for unstable haemoglobins and globin chain electrophoresis at acid or alkaline pH to differentiate haemoglobins S, D, G and Q, or haemoglobins A$_2$, C, E and O-Arab.

Determination of P$_{50}$ and of 2,3-DPG may be required to screen for abnormal O$_2$ affinity.

9.3.1 Haemoglobin variant detection using cellulose acetate electrophoresis (NCCLS, 1994a)

Normal adult haemoglobin, Hb A, is negatively charged in alkaline buffers and moves toward the positive electrode (anode) during electrophoresis. Most haemoglobin variants are separated from Hb A during electrophoresis because the structural abnormality usually involves changes in electrical charge.

SPECIMEN

Haemolysates, preferably prepared from washed red cells, are the recommended samples. Good electrophoretic separation is generally obtained with a haemoglobin concentration of 20–30 g/L (1.2–1.9 mmol/L).

1   Collect an anticoagulated (acid citrate dextrose [ACD], citrate phosphate dextrose [CPD], ethylenediaminetetra-acetic acid [EDTA], or heparin) venous blood specimen. The specimen may be stored at 4°C for up to 10 days. Note that heparinized blood specimens may form microclots during storage.

2 Centrifuge the specimen at $1500–2000 \times g$ for 5 minutes, remove the plasma and wash the cells one or more times with approximately 10 volumes of isotonic sodium chloride (NaCl) 8.5 g/L (0.145 mol/L) solution.

3 After the final washing and centrifugation, add six volumes of distilled water and 0.5 volume of carbon tetrachloride (CCl_4), chloroform ($CHCl_3$) or toluene (C_7H_8) to the packed red cells and mix to lyse the erythrocytes. These organic solvents are toxic and potentially carcinogenic. Do not pipette by mouth. Use a fume hood.

4 Centrifuge the mixture for 15 minutes at $1500–2000 \times g$ and filter the clear haemoglobin solution through a layer of Whatman No. 1 filter paper, or equivalent. Turbid supernatants may need two layers of filter paper. The resulting solution contains 20–30 g/L (1.2–1.9 mmol/L) haemoglobin.

5 Unwashed erythrocytes packed by sedimentation or centrifugation may be used. Haemolysis is effected by adding six parts of the previously described lysing reagent. If haemolysates are required quickly, or if only a small specimen can be obtained, e.g. from an infant, blood may be collected by skin puncture directly into a haemolysing solution such as saponin (0.1 g/100 mL), or K_2 or Na_2 EDTA, 0.3 g/100 mL (8.9 mmol/L).

(Caution: the organic solvents, as well as freezing/thawing procedures, for the preparation of haemolysates may result in denaturation and precipitation of haemoglobin Bart's, haemoglobin H, or other unstable haemoglobins.)

REAGENTS

Tris hydroxymethyl-aminomethane EDTA/boric acid (TEB) buffer, pH range 8.4–9.2 A 0.084 mol/L buffer with pH 8.4 is obtained when 10.2 g Tris, 0.60 g EDTA and 3.2 g boric acid are diluted to 1.0 L with deionized or distilled water. This buffer may be stored indefinitely at 4°C.

Stain Any suitable, general protein stain may be used. Good results are obtained with, for example, 0.3–0.5% (w/v) Ponceau S in trichloroacetic acid. Mix 300–500 mg Ponceau S with 5 g trichloroacetic acid and dilute to 100 mL with distilled water.

Counterstain A haem-specific counterstain is used to differentiate haem from non-haem proteins. Benzidine and its derivatives may be carcinogenic. Handle with caution. Other haem-specific stains, e.g. o-toluidine dihydrochloride, o-dianisidine (3,3′ dimethoxybenzidine) are reportedly non-carcinogenic but tend to fade with time. Counterstains should be used according to the manufacturer's directions.

Destaining, dehydration and clearing solutions Manufacturers of cellulose acetate provide directions for proper destaining and preservation of their media. Generally, satisfactory results are obtained with acetic acid 3–5% (v/v), methanol 95–100%, or acetic acid in methanol 20% (v/v). Several changes of the reagent are usually required to render the background colourless.

Microporous cellulose acetate This is a readily available, popular electrophoretic support medium, used as either strips or sheets or bonded to a plate. Advantages of cellulose acetate as support medium include minimal preparative work, rapid separation of haemoglobins A, F, S and C, and ease of handling; they may be plasticized and stored as permanent record. Disadvantages include the fact that haemoglobin fractions present in low concentration may not be detectable and that not all haemoglobins, including unstable haemoglobins, separate on cellulose acetate, while hybrid molecules may form in the presence of both an α-chain and a β-chain variant, causing three, even four, major bands. Use of cellulose acetate supported by, or bonded to, a plastic backing is recommended to prevent tearing. Forceps or gloves should be used to prevent contamination.

Applicator An applicator is used to apply 0.5–1.0 μL samples to the surface of the medium. Applicators should be large enough to be easily handled. Parts should be strong enough to withstand rigorous use. Sample amount must be applied uniformly.

Electrophoresis chamber This consists of buffer reservoirs separated by bridges on which the cellulose acetate medium is placed. Either wicks or direct contact of the medium is acceptable for allowing current flow from one reservoir to the other through the cellulose acetate. Electrodes must be strong enough to prevent breakage and well insulated for operator protection.

Power supply This should be constant voltage, direct current (DC), adequately grounded, and capable of delivering up to 450 V. Power supplies should ideally have a timer, 0–60 min, a 'continuous operation' switch, an 'automatic' shut-off, a 'quick disconnect' or manual 'shut-off' switch, and a circuit breaker. The design should incorporate the facility of interrupting the flow of current as soon as the chamber is opened.

PROCEDURE

Instructions of the individual product manufacturers should be followed. The following general steps are appropriate for most systems:

1 Soak wicks, if used, and presoak the cellulose acetate or strip in buffer. Fill chamber with buffer to equal levels in each reservoir.
2 Remove strip or plate from the buffer and blot the medium evenly between two pieces of absorbent paper to remove excess moisture.
3 Apply samples to the cellulose acetate along a line one-third the distance from one edge of the strip or plate. Good results are generally obtained with 0.5–1.0 μL samples. A control sample containing haemoglobins A, F, S and C must be applied to each strip or plate containing unknown samples to compensate for slight current fluctuations, different buffer lots or variations in sample application.
4 Place medium in electrophoresis chamber with the line of sample application closer to the negative pole (cathode). Ensure the cellulose acetate is in contact with the buffer solution.
5 Apply 250–400 V for the required time (see manufacturer's instructions).
6 Turn power off, remove the medium from the chamber and stain (follow manufacturer's directions). If distinct separation with small clear areas between the haemoglobins has not been obtained, it may be necessary to reduce the haemoglobin concentration of the samples and/or adjust the time and voltage of the electrophoresis.
7 Fix, clear and dry the medium (follow manufacturer's directions).

QUALITY CONTROL

A control sample containing haemoglobins A, F, S and C must be included with each strip/plate of unknown samples. With every new lot of cellulose acetate, samples containing a combination of haemoglobins A and F and of haemoglobins S and F should be tested for adequate separation. Distinct separation with a small clear area between these haemoglobins must be obtained (Fig. 9.1).

LIMITATIONS AND SOURCES OF ERROR

Cellulose acetate electrophoresis is used for the detection and preliminary identification of haemoglobin phenotypes on the basis of their differences in electrical charge and their relative proportion. Definitive diagnosis cannot be claimed on the basis of electrophoresis at a single pH; various thalassaemias cannot be positively identified and electrophoresis does not provide accurate quantification of haemoglobins.

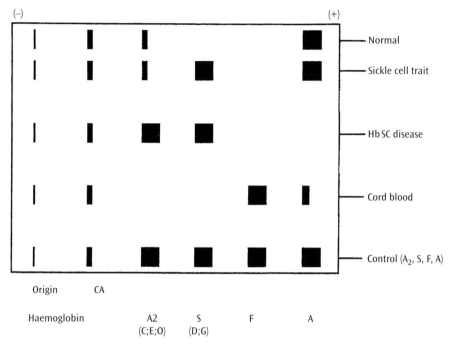

Fig. 9.1 *Diagrammatic presentation of cellulose acetate electrophoresis plate. Note specimen application (origin) at the cathodic side of the plate. CA, carbonic anhydrase.*

Sources of error include:

- cloudy or contaminated buffer;
- improper pH or ionic strength of the buffer;
- dirt, blood or protein contamination of equipment or the cellulose medium plates;
- cloudy or discoloured haemolysates;
- improper presoaking of cellulose acetate plates or strips;
- improper blotting;
- delay in sample application;
- too much or too little sample;
- improper placement of samples on medium or medium in the chamber;
- excessive evaporation during electrophoresis (overheating, too high current, too high buffer concentration, poor vapour seal);
- failure to remove leucocytes from samples, especially in patients with leucocytosis (may result in anomalous band of leucocyte-derived myeloperoxidase with a much faster anodic mobility than any known haemoglobin variant).

The presence of glycohaemoglobin may produce a band slightly anodic to Hb A, especially in poorly controlled diabetics.

Haemolysates that are old, contain red cell stroma or are contaminated may give poor separation, artefacts and/or smearing of haemoglobin bands. Brown discoloration of haemolysates may be due to haemiglobin (methaemoglobin) formation in old or improperly handled specimens. The presence of haemiglobin results in additional minor bands cathodic to the major haemoglobin bands. Addition of a drop of 5% (w/v) potassium cyanide (KCN) to the haemolysate converts haemiglobin to haemiglobincyanide which has the same electrophoretic mobilities as the major oxyhaemoglobin components from which it is derived.

9.3.2 Solubility test to confirm the presence of sickling haemoglobins (NCCLS, 1995)

Erythrocytes that contain a sickling haemoglobin form a characteristic sickle shape in an environment of low oxygen tension. The solubility test may be used to confirm the presence of a sickling haemoglobin after preliminary identification with cellulose acetate electrophoresis. Sickling haemoglobins in the deoxygenated state are relatively insoluble and form a precipitate in a phosphate buffer solution of high molarity, resulting in a turbid solution (Itano, 1953).

SPECIMEN

Collect blood specimens in an anticoagulant, mix well and refrigerate (4–8°C) until tested. Blood stored longer than 3 weeks, or blood from infants less than 6 months old, should not be tested with a solubility test. In these cases the presence of sickling haemoglobins should be confirmed with citrate agar electrophoresis, isoelectric focusing, an immunological test, or a microscopic sickling preparation using a freshly made sodium bisulphite (Na$_2$S$_2$O$_5$) solution (Sneider *et al.*, 1967).

REAGENTS

Phosphate buffer Prepare a stock phosphate buffer solution by dissolving 216 g dipotassium hydrogen phosphate (K$_2$HPO$_4$) anhydrous, in about 60 mL of distilled water. Add 169 g potassium dihydrogen phosphate (KH$_2$PO$_4$) anhydrous and 1 g saponin; mix well and dilute to 1000 mL with distilled or deionized water. The stock buffer may be stored at 4–8°C for about 1 month.

Working solutions On the day of the test, add 5 mg/mL sodium hydrosulphite (Na$_2$S$_2$O$_4$) (dithionite) to the required volume of stock buffer solution.

Glassware Use disposable 12 × 75 mm glass or plastic test tubes free of protein, dust or chemical contaminants.

Reading card or rack Use a reading card or rack with 14- or 18-point black type in straight lines on a white background and about 5 mm apart.

PROCEDURE

Manufacturer's instructions for commercial kits must be followed. The following general steps are appropriate for some kits:

1 Allow the working solution to warm to room temperature (20–25°C) and pipette 2 mL into a labelled disposable test tube.
2 Centrifuge the blood specimen for 5 minutes at 1500–2000 × g, remove plasma and Buffy coat and add 10 μL of packed cells to the working solution. Mix well.
3 After about 5 minutes, hold the tube 2.5 cm in front of the white card with black lines and read the tube for turbidity.

Positive and negative control samples must be included with each group of specimens tested. The blood–reagent mixture should be light red to pink in colour; light orange indicates reagent deterioration.

RESULTS

A very turbid solution indicates a positive test result for sickling haemoglobins; the black type on the white card cannot be seen through the solution. A fine haziness of the solution with the lines or type clearly visible or readable constitutes a negative test.

Haemoglobin S, as well as Hb C-Harlem, Hb S-Travis, Hb C-Ziguinchor, Hb S-Antilles, Hb S-Oman and Hb S-Providence, give a positive test for the presence of a sickling haemoglobin. A positive test does not differentiate between Hb S and Hb AS, Hb SS, HbS/β^+ thalassaemia and other combinations of Hb S and other haemoglobin variants.

LIMITATIONS AND SOURCES OF ERROR

Sources of error include:

- inactive or outdated reagent;
- test on infants less than 6 months old, anaemia, recent transfusion of normal blood, or transfusion of blood with a sickling haemoglobin to an otherwise normal person;
- improper reagent temperature or improper mixing of packed cells with reagent;
- improper interpretation of the reader scale;
- whole blood specimen instead of packed red cells with a false-positive result due to erythrocytosis, hyperglobulinaemia, leucocytosis, or hyperlipidaemia;
- specimens with large number or nucleated red cells, e.g. severe thalassaemia.

9.3.3 Acid citrate agar electrophoresis to confirm identification of variant haemoglobins (Schneider *et al.*, 1974; NCCLS, 1988)

Citrate agar electrophoresis separates haemoglobins on the basis of complex interactions among haemoglobin, agar and agaropectin (small, highly sulphated negatively charged molecules). Agaropectin molecules bind to haemoglobin molecules where charged groups are at the surface; the haemoglobin–agaropectin complex migrates through the supporting agar towards the anode. Thus, separation of haemoglobin variants is determined by the relative affinity for agaropectin of certain haemoglobin molecule surface groups. For example, Hb S and Hb C have charged surface groups that can bind to agaropectin. However, these surface charges are more electropositive on the Hb C molecule than on the Hb S molecule, resulting in a greater affinity between Hb C and agaropectin. Thus Hb C and Hb S are separated from each other on electrophoresis.

Highly purified agar or agarose usually does not provide the desired separations.

SPECIMEN

Haemolysates are prepared as for cellulose acetate electrophoresis (see p. 196). Good electrophoretic separation is generally obtained with a haemoglobin concentration of 5–10 g/L (0.3–0.6 mmol/L) for adult blood samples, 40 g/L (2.4 mmol/L) for neonatal samples (umbilical cord blood).

REAGENTS

Stock citrate buffer 0.5 mol/L Dissolve 147 g sodium citrate ($C_6H_5O_7Na_3{\cdot}2H_2O$) and 4.3 g citric acid ($C_6H_8O_7$) in distilled or deionized water and make up to 1000 mL.

Working citrate buffer 0.05 mol/L Dilute stock buffer 10-fold with distilled or deionized water. Adjust the pH to 6.0 by dropwise addition of a 30 g/100 mL citric acid solution.

Haem-specific stain (e.g. o-dianisidine, o-tolidine) Mix 1 g stain with 25 mL glacial acetic acid, add distilled or deionized water to 100 mL. Before use, mix 10 mL of the stain solution with 5 mL of 3% (v/v) hydrogen peroxide. Simple protein stains, e.g. Ponceau S, are adsorbed to agar and cannot be used. Haem-specific stains are unstable and likely to fade. Alternative staining may be performed with 1% amido black, following manufacturer's directions, and decolorization with acetic acid 5%.

Agar certified suitable for haemoglobin electrophoresis Note that certain lots of agar have been proven to give unsatisfactory results. Therefore each lot of agar must be tested before use. Because many lots of commercially available agar do not provide the desired separation, laboratories have switched to using agarose. Glass or plastic plates are necessary to support the agar; size depends on the needs of the laboratory. Commercially prepared agar plates are available.

Agar plates may be prepared as follows:

1 Add 1.0 g agar to 100 mL working citrate buffer, 0.05 mmol/L.
2 Heat in boiling water bath until a completely clear solution is obtained. Overheating may damage the agar; use of a microwave oven may be an efficient alternative.
3 Place the glass or plastic plates on a level surface and pipette 3.5–4 mL (for 5 × 7.5 cm plates) melted agar, cooled to about 60°C, evenly on the plates. Allow agar to solidify and wrap the plates in plastic (or sealable plastic envelopes).
4 Store at 4–8°C in a tightly covered box containing some moistened cotton wool. Thus stored, the plates will keep for 1 month or more.

Applicator, electrophoresis chamber, wicks and DC power supply See cellulose acetate electrophoresis (p. 198).

PROCEDURE

The following general steps are appropriate for most systems (specific manufacturer's instructions must always be followed):

1 Load applicator with haemolysate as for alkaline cellulose electrophoresis (see p. 196) and apply samples lightly to the surface of the agar plate about 3 cm from the anodic end of the plate; samples may be applied to the middle of the plate. Control samples containing haemoglobins A, F, S and C must be included.
2 Let the plates stand until samples are completely absorbed (usually a few seconds).
3 Adjust the working buffer to pH 6.0–6.2 at room temperature, then cool to 4°C and prepare the electrophoresis chamber with the buffer solution.
4 Drape Whatman No. 3 filter paper wicks on the shoulders of the chamber and place the plates, agar side down, on the wicks. Apply 70–90 V for about 70 minutes (5 × 7.5 cm plates). If the apparatus becomes warm to the touch, place an ice pack on the lid, or surround the chamber with ice, or perform the electrophoresis in a cold room or refrigerated cabinet.
5 Turn power off, remove the plates from the chamber and stain with the haem-specific stain or 1% amido black.
6 Dry the plates in an oven at 100°C for 2–3 hours or allow the agar to slide off the support plate and mount on a card; allow to dry.

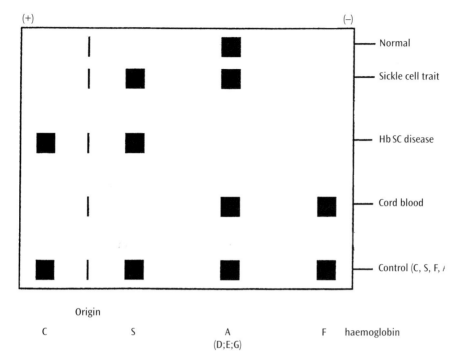

Fig. 9.2 *Diagrammatic presentation of citrate agar electrophoresis plate. Note specimen application (origin) at the anodic side of the plate.*

QUALITY CONTROL

Mobilities of haemoglobins vary to a larger extent than in other methods, with factors such as state and concentration of haemoglobin, small variations in buffer concentration, variations in applied voltage, etc. Simultaneous analysis of control samples is thus imperative. Controls needed include anodically moving Hb S and Hb C, and cathodically moving Hb F and Hb A (Fig. 9.2).

LIMITATIONS AND SOURCES OF ERROR

The combined data of electrophoresis on alkaline cellulose acetate and acid citrate agar provides definitive identification of haemoglobins A, F, S, C, O and several others; it differentiates Hb C, E and O, and distinguishes Hb S from variants that migrate like Hb S on alkaline cellulose acetate electrophoresis.

Sources of error include:

- cloudy or contaminated buffer, or improper pH or ionic strength;
- contamination with dirt, blood, proteins of sample applicator, sample wells or agar plates;
- improperly prepared or deteriorated haemolysates (poor separation, artefacts, and/or smearing of haemoglobin bands);
- delay in applying samples, in applying current, in removing and staining plates;
- applying too much or too little sample;
- improper placement of samples on the plates (to allow haemoglobins to migrate to the cathode, samples must be placed at the midpoint or anodically to the midpoint).

9.3.4 Microcolumn chromatographic determination of haemoglobin A₂ (NCCLS, 1989a)

Column chromatography with mini-columns to quantitatively measure haemoglobin A_2 is simple and precise, does not require much technician time and can be performed on either fresh or stored blood samples (Efvremov et al., 1974; Brosius et al., 1978; Huntsman et al., 1978). In ion exchange chromatography, the charged groups of the ion exchange medium interact with charged groups of the haemoglobin molecules, resulting in separation of different haemoglobin fractions. At pH > 8.5 the majority of haemoglobins bind to the ion exchange medium; at pH = 8.3, Hb A_2 elutes from the column but Hb A remains bound. The Hb A_2 fraction is collected from the column in a flask and the remaining haemoglobins are eluted from the column and collected by passing a buffer of lower pH through the bed of the ion exchange medium. The ratio of the two fractions is then measured spectro-photometrically. Haemoglobins with a charge similar to Hb A_2, e.g. haemoglobins C, E and O, elute with Hb A_2; in this case the method cannot be used quantitatively to determine Hb A_2.

SPECIMEN

Specimens should be collected with 1.5 mg/mL of the sodium or potassium salts of EDTA as anticoagulant. Keep specimen at 4–8°C until testing; do not test blood stored for longer than 10 days.

Separate red cells from plasma by centrifugation at about $1500 \times g$ for 10 minutes. Remove plasma and wash the red cells with 0.145 mol/L (8.5 g/L) NaCl solution. Centrifuge again at $1500 \times g$ and lyse the erythrocytes with 0.4 mL of distilled water per 0.05 mL of washed cells. Mix by shaking and let stand at ambient temperature for about 5 minutes.

REAGENTS

If commercially prepared reagents and prepacked columns are used, follow the manu-facturer's instructions.

Tris/cyanide stock buffer Dissolve 24.22 g trishydroxymethyl-aminomethane and 0.40 g potassium cyanide (KCN) in deionized water and dilute to 4.0 L.

Working buffer A Adjust 3.0 L of the stock buffer to pH = 8.5 with concentrated HCl. Use caution when adding HCl to buffers containing KCN; use a fume hood.

Working buffer B Adjust 500 mL of the stock buffer to pH = 8.3 with concentrated HCl. Use fume hood.

Working buffer C Adjust 500 mL of the stock buffer to pH = 7.0 with concentrated HCl. Use fume hood.

Anion exchange medium Diethylaminoethylcellulose support medium must be used (Huisman et al., 1975; Abraham et al., 1976; Schleider et al., 1977); microgranular DE52 is suitable. Prepare a slurry of DE52 as follows. Place 100 g DE52 into a 600 mL beaker and slowly add buffer A until the beaker is nearly full. Stir for about 10 minutes with a magnetic stirrer and let stand for about 30 minutes. Pour off supernatant, add more buffer, stir, allow to stand and decant the supernatant. Repeat this procedure until the pH of the slurry is within 0.05 pH units of the pH of buffer A. Allow the slurry to settle and decant excess buffer until the fluid volume above the slurry equals about two-thirds of the settled slurry volume. The slurry can be stored in a closed container at 4°C for up to 30 days. Storage at room temperature may promote bacterial contamination. The above amount of slurry yields sufficient ion exchanger for 100–200 mini-columns.

MINI-COLUMNS

Use columns 7–13 cm long with an internal diameter of 0.5–0.8 cm; disposable Pasteur pipettes, for example, are suitable. Prepare the columns on the day of use. Plug the tips with a small amount of cotton wool moistened with buffer A. Allow the slurry to come to room temperature and check the pH. Resuspend the slurry and fill the columns. Allow to drain; the final column height should be 5 cm.

If the internal diameter of the column is 0.5 cm, the column will contain 1 mL ion exchanger. Columns with a diameter of 0.8 cm will require 2.5 mL of exchanger; eluates from these columns contain more haemoglobin and thus give improved sensitivity.

VOLUMETRIC FLASKS

Class A calibrated volumetric flasks, 10 ± 0.03 and 25 ± 0.03 mL, are used to collect the eluates from the columns.

pH METER

A pH meter with an accuracy of ± 0.05 pH units is required to check the pH of the buffers and the slurry. Measuring tris buffers requires the use of calomel or double-junction electrodes.

SPECTROPHOTOMETER

The spectrophotometer must have a bandpass < 10 nm and should be calibrated frequently as to wavelength; linearity of absorbance and absence of stray light should be verified. Cuvettes must have a path length of at least 1.0 cm.

PROCEDURE

Manufacturer's directions for commercial kits must be followed. For reagents and columns prepared in the laboratory the following steps should be followed:

1 Prepare the samples as described (see 'Specimen', above) and set up the mini-columns in racks; allow columns to stand for 20–30 minutes, then carefully remove excess buffer from the top of the columns, leaving a small residual layer of buffer of about 0.05 mL.
2 Apply 0.05 mL haemolysate to the top of the column, being careful not to stir up the exchange medium. Allow the haemolysate to soak into the top of the column. Dilute samples may require application of 0.1 mL.
3 Apply 6 mL of buffer B to the column and collect about 6 mL of the effluent dripping from the bottom of the column into a 10 mL volumetric flask. The final drops of effluent will appear colourless.
4 Dilute the collected effluent to volume with distilled water and label as fraction 1.
5 Apply 6 mL of buffer C to the column and collect the effluent containing the remaining haemoglobin(s) into a 25 mL volumetric flask and dilute to volume with distilled water. Label as fraction 2.
6 Measure the absorbance of the fractions 1 and 2 on the spectrophotometer at 415 nm against buffer C as blank.
7 Calculate the fraction (%) of Hb A_2 in the samples with the following equation: Hb A_2 (%) $= 100 \times \{[\text{abs. fraction 1}]/[\text{abs. fraction 1} + (2.5 \times \text{abs. fraction 2})]\}$, where abs. = the

absorbance at 415 nm; the factor 2.5 corrects for the difference in dilution volumes due to the use of different volumetric flasks.

QUALITY CONTROL

Control samples must be included with each set of unknown samples. Controls may be obtained from commercial sources or prepared in the laboratory from fresh blood specimens or stored haemolysates (Schmidt *et al.*, 1977; Huntsman *et al.*, 1978).

Different lots of ion exchange medium may vary in their affinity for Hb A_2 at any given pH, and the pH of buffer B must therefore be empirically adjusted for each batch of slurry. pH adjustment with a base must be avoided because salts will be formed that strip the haemoglobin from the column.

Prepare a column and apply 0.05 mL haemolysate from a patient known to have Hb S trait. Elute with 10 mL of buffer B followed by 10–15 mL of buffer C. If a small band of haemoglobin (Hb A_2) elutes in the first 6 mL followed by, and well separated from, a major band of haemoglobin (Hb S) that elutes in the next 10–15 mL, leaving about half the haemoglobin still visible in exchange medium bed, the pH of buffer B is satisfactory. If Hb A_2 is not eluted with 10 mL of buffer B, the pH should be lowered by 0.05 pH units. If the remaining haemoglobin moves down the column before buffer C is added, the pH of buffer B is too low.

REFERENCE RANGE

A reference range must be established for each method in each laboratory by determining Hb A_2 levels on at least 20 samples from apparently healthy persons. The usual reference range is 1.5–3.5% Hb A_2. Iron deficiency or α-thalassaemia may lower Hb A_2 values; they may be raised in megaloblastic anaemias. Values of 4–8% are characteristic of β-thalassaemia minor; values in homozygous β-thalassaemia major are variable.

LIMITATIONS AND SOURCES OF ERROR

The method is not specific for haemoglobin A_2. Haemoglobins with a similar electrical charge, e.g. Hb C, Hb E and Hb O, elute with Hb A_2. If a Hb A_2 concentration > 10% is found with this method, it should be assumed that another haemoglobin is present in addition to Hb A_2.

Sources of error include:

- inaccurate pH adjustment of the buffers or the ion exchange medium;
- temperature variations with formation of gas bubbles (it may be necessary to resuspend the slurry);
- overloading or underloading of the column with sample – overloading may cause incomplete separation of Hb A_2; underloading may make visual collection of the A_2 fraction impossible.

9.3.5 Quantitative determination of haemoglobin F with the alkali denaturation method (Betke *et al.*, 1959; NCCLS, 1989b)

Haemoglobin F is more resistant to denaturation by strong alkali than other haemoglobins. A strong base is added to an haemolysate containing a known amount of total haemoglobin and after a specified time the alkali denaturation process is stopped by lowering the pH with ammonium sulphate. This simultaneously precipitates the denatured haemoglobins. The solution is filtered and the remaining, alkali-resistant, haemoglobin is measured.

Hb F is characteristically elevated in adults with, for example, homozygous and heterozygous thalassaemia, homozygous Hb S, Hb S in genetic combination with some other haemoglobin variants (Hb C, Hb D), unstable haemoglobins, and in hereditary persistence of fetal haemoglobin.

Advantages of the alkali denaturation method include the relative ease of performing the test and the acceptable accuracy and precision in the clinically relevant range of 2–40% Hb F (Singer et al., 1951; Garver et al., 1976; ICSH, 1979).

SPECIMEN

Haemolysates, preferably prepared from washed red cells, with a haemoglobin concentration of 80–120 g/L (5–7.5 mmol/L) are the recommended samples.

Collect 5–7 mL venous blood anticoagulated with potassium or sodium EDTA, 1.5 mg/mL blood. Centrifuge the sample at about $1500 \times g$ for about 5 minutes, remove the plasma and wash the packed red cells one or more times with 0.145 mol/L (8.5 g/L) NaCl solution.

After the final washing, add an equal volume of distilled water and 0.5 volume of CCl_4, chloroform, or toluene to lyse the packed cells. These organic solvents are toxic and potentially carcinogenic. Do not pipette by mouth. Use fume hood.

Centrifuge the mixture for 15 minutes at $1500–2000 \times g$, and filter the clear haemoglobin solution through a layer of Whatman No. 1 filter paper. If turbid, filter through two layers. Finally, centrifuge the lysate at $2000 \times g$ for 30 minutes to remove the remaining cell stroma.

If haemolysates are required quickly, or if only a small specimen can be obtained, e.g. from an infant, blood may be collected from a skin puncture directly into a haemolysing solution, e.g. saponin (0.1 g/100 mL), K_2 or Na_2 EDTA (0.3 g/100 mL). (Caution: the organic solvents, as well as freezing/thawing procedures, for the preparation of haemolysates may result in denaturation and precipitation of haemoglobin Bart's, haemoglobin H or other unstable haemoglobins.)

REAGENTS

Modified 'Drabkin's' reagent Dissolve 200 mg ferric potassium cyanide $[K_3Fe(CN)_6]$ and 50 mg potassium cyanide (KCN) in distilled or deionized water and dilute to 1000 mL. The pH of this reagent is about 10; it can be stored for up to 30 days in brown, borosilicate glass bottles; it must not be allowed to freeze.

Sodium hydroxide reagent (1.25 mol/L) Dissolve 5 ± 0.10 g solid NaOH pellets in water and dilute to 100 mL. The reagent can be stored for up to 30 days, but must be discarded if precipitation or turbidity occurs. It may also be prepared by diluting commercially available concentrated NaOH solutions.

Ammonium sulphate solution, saturated Stir 550 g (an excess) $(NH_4)_2SO_4$ into water to make a total volume of 1000 mL. Store in a glass bottle at room temperature (20–25°C). It is stable for up to 3 months. Undissolved crystals should be visible at the bottom at all times.

GLASSWARE

Glassware required includes 17×100 mm test tubes and rack; short stem, 5 cm diameter funnels; volumetric, class A, calibrated flasks 10 ± 0.02, 100 ± 0.08, 1000 mL; pipettes, microlitre 20 ± 0.1 μL, measuring 0.2 ± 0.008 mL, graduated (1/100) 1.0 ± 0.02 mL, and transfer, 1.0, 2.0, 3.0, 4.0, 5.0, 10.0 mL.

SPECTROPHOTOMETER

The spectrophotometer should be capable of isolating a wavelength of 540 ± 2 nm with a half-intensity bandwidth < 20 nm. A filter photometer can be used.

EQUIPMENT, MATERIALS

The method requires two balances, one with a precision ±0.05 mg and another with precision ±50 mg, a centrifuge capable of sustaining up to $2300 \times g$, a vortex mixer, stopwatch, and 7 cm diameter filter paper discs, Whatman No. 1 and No. 42.

PROCEDURE

Perform the procedure at ambient (room) temperature; (20–25°C):

1 Determine the haemoglobin concentration of the haemolysates using an accepted haemiglobincyanide procedure (NCCLS, 1994b).
2 Depending on the haemoglobin concentration, pipette 0.4–0.6 mL of the haemolysates into 10 mL of the modified 'Drabkin's' reagent to make an HiCN solution containing approximately 5 g/L (5 mg/mL; 0.3 mmol/L) (see Table 9.1); mix well.
3 Pipette 3.0 mL of the diluted HiCN solutions into three 17×100 mm tubes; label two tubes 'test', and the third 'total'.
4 Add 0.2 mL of the 1.25 mol/L NaOH solution to each of the 'test' tubes; mix well (vortex mixer).
5 Add 0.2 mL water to the tube labelled 'total'.
6 Exactly 2 minutes after adding the NaOH to the tubes (stopwatch), add 2.0 mL saturated ammonium sulphate to the tubes labelled 'test' and mix well (vortex mixer); also add 2.0 mL to the tube labelled 'total'.
7 After 5 minutes, filter the contents of the 'test' and 'total' tubes through two layers Whatman No. 42 (or No. 1) filter paper folded into the 5 cm funnels. Pipette 1 mL from the filtrate 'total' into 4.0 mL of distilled water.
8 Measure the absorbance of the 'test' filtrates, A$_{fetal}$, and the diluted 'total' filtrate, A$_{total}$, at 540 nm with the spectrophotometer against a blank consisting of 3.0 mL modified 'Drabkin's' reagent + 0.2 mL NaOH (1.25 mol/L) + 2.0 mL saturated ammonium sulphate, filtered through a double layer of Whatman No.42 or No. 1 filter paper.
9 Calculate the fetal haemoglobin fraction using the following equation: Hb F (%) = 100 × $[A_{fetal}/(A_{total} \times 5)] = 20 \times (A_{fetal}/A_{total})$, where 5 indicates the additional dilution factor of the A$_{total}$ filtrate.
10 For Hb F < 5%, the difference in the duplicates should not exceed 0.5% Hb F; for Hb F = 5–15%, the difference should not exceed 1%; and for HbF > 15%, the difference should not exceed 2%.

QUALITY CONTROL

A known normal and a known abnormal haemolysate (ICSH, 1979) should be analysed with each series of patient samples.

Table 9.1 *Haemolysate preparation*

Haemolysate haemoglobin concentration (g/L)	mL haemolysate added to 10 mL modified 'Drabkin's'	Final HiCN concentration (g/L) of HiCN solution
80	0.60	4.6
90	0.55	4.7
100	0.50	4.8
110	0.45	4.7
120	0.40	4.6

REFERENCE RANGE

There is evidence that so-called 'normal values' are technique-dependent (Singer *et al.*, 1951). Thus each laboratory must determine the local reference range using 20–30 specimens from apparently healthy adults. Upper values of both 1 and 2% Hb F have been reported in the literature for normal adults (Singer *et al.*, 1951; Garver *et al.*, 1976; Cooper and Hoagland, 1972).

LIMITATIONS AND SOURCES OF ERROR

Several sources of error may be encountered in the alkali denaturation method, including:

- pipetting errors;
- timing (the 2 minute denaturation time must be strictly adhered to);
- insufficient mixing (a vortex mixer should be used);
- reagent errors – the final concentrations of the NaOH and the saturated ammonium sulphate solutions are critical, and up to 25% of the Hb F present in samples can be lost in the denaturation/precipitation phase;
- use of NaOH older than 30 days;
- turbidity of the final filtrates – if turbid, the filtrates can often be 'cleared' by centrifugation for 10 minutes at $2000 \times g$, followed by filtration using membrane filters with 0.4 μm mean pore diameter;
- filter paper – each new batch must be examined for possible spurious results;
- photometric errors due to incorrect wavelength setting, non-linearity or the presence of stray light.

SMALLER SAMPLE SIZE

If the spectrophotometer is equipped with cuvettes allowing small sample volume (<1.5 mL; semi-micro cuvettes), the required sample and reagent volumes may be decreased. In this case, 5 mL modified 'Drabkin's' reagent may be used, with addition of 0.2 or 0.3 mL haemolysate, 1.5 mL diluted haemolysate, 0.1 mL NaOH and 1.0 mL saturated ammonium sulphate.

9.3.6 Detection and identification of HB variants and quantitation of HB A₂ and HB F using high-performance liquid chromatography

High-performance liquid chromatography (HPLC) is a process that separates components of a mixture more efficiently than normal liquid chromatography, due to technological advances in instrumentation and column design. HPLC instrumentation usually consists of a solvent reservoir, a pump, an injector, a chromatographic column, a detector, a data recorder and a microprocessor.

The pump drives the solvent (the mobile phase) through the injector–column–detector assembly. The pump can generally operate in two different modes:

- isocratic mode – in which the mobile phase composition remains constant throughout the chromatographic run;
- gradient mode – in which the mobile phase is changed stepwise or continuously throughout the chromatographic run.

The most widely used sample injector is the loop injector. In the 'fill' position a sample aliquot is introduced with a syringe into an external loop of the injector, at atmospheric pressure. In the 'inject' mode, the sample loop is rotated into the flowing stream of the mobile phase and the aliquot is flushed into the chromatographic column. Loop injectors are precise, can be used at high pressures, and sample injection can be automated.

The chromatographic column consists of a stainless steel tube which contains the packing, i.e. the stationary phase, and the necessary fittings to connect the column into the chromatography system. Depending on the application, numerous materials may be used as column packing. A wealth of information on columns and column packings is available via 'Chromatography.Net' on the internet (http://www.chromatography.net) (Brady et al., 2000). For the analysis of haemoglobin variants, weak cation- and anion-exchange columns are generally used; and for globin chain analysis, reversed phase columns are used. Column selection, like the selection of all HPLC parameters, should be done in light of the specific application. In neonatal screening applications, columns should be optimized for speed and cost-effectiveness; in adult testing applications optimization for specificity and quantitative accuracy is recommended. Users of HPLC may assemble the various components or purchase available kits commercially. The latter have the advantage that assay parameters have been optimized by the manufacturer. In 'normal phase' HPLC, the functional groups of the stationary phase are polar and the mobile phase consists of non-polar solvents. 'Reversed phase' HPLC requires a non-polar stationary phase with mixtures of solvents used as the mobile phase.

The function of the detector is to detect compounds as they elute from the chromatographic column. The most popular detectors are ultraviolet and visible light photometers, with either fixed or variable wavelength. The output of the detector may be displayed on a strip chart recorder or a printer plotter and shows the chromatogram in an absorbance vs. time format. Under a given set of chromatographic conditions, the time required for a component to pass through a liquid chromatograph, the retention time, is used to identify eluting compounds. The magnitude of the detector response is proportional to the quantity of the compound passing through it. The area or the peak height can be used for quantitation (Fig. 9.3). The incorporation of microprocessors in HPLC instrumentation has resulted in cost-effective data processing and automation of the systems with ease of operation and improved analytical performance.

HPLC has proved to be a useful tool for the detection and presumptive identification of an unknown haemoglobin. HPLC can be used as a primary haemoglobin screening method or as a supplement to electrophoresis, providing different and supplemental structural information. For example, Hb Silver Springs does not separate from Hb A on cellulose acetate or citrate agar electrophoresis, on isoelectric focusing or by globin chain electrophoresis, but was observed using HPLC. Other haemoglobins that are difficult to distinguish from Hb A electrophoretically, e.g. Hb Rainier, Hb Alzette and Hb Puttelange, are also clearly separated with HPLC.

SAMPLE

EDTA anticoagulated blood is used to prepare a haemolysate from washed red cells. Dried blood eluted from filter paper into a haemolysate reagent may also be used (Roa et al., 1996). Some automated HPLC systems use a small amount of whole blood, usually 5 μL, in 1 mL of haemolysate reagent. An appropriate quantity of haemoglobin to be injected onto an HPLC column is 50–250 μg (3.5–15.5 μmol). A general sample preparation procedure is as follows:

1   Wash 100 μL EDTA-anticoagulated blood with 0.150 mol/L (9 g/L) NaCl solution.
2   Add 2–3 volumes of distilled water to the packed cells, mix (vortex mixer) and centrifuge for 5 minutes at $300 \times g$.
3   Add 50 μL of haemolysate to 1 mL of buffer and inject 20 μL onto the column.

REAGENTS

A commonly used two-buffer gradient system is composed of buffer A (10 mmol/L Bis-Tris, 1 mmol/L KCN, pH 6.87) and buffer B (10 mmol/L Bis-Tris, 1 mmol/L KCN, pH 6.57) (Ou and

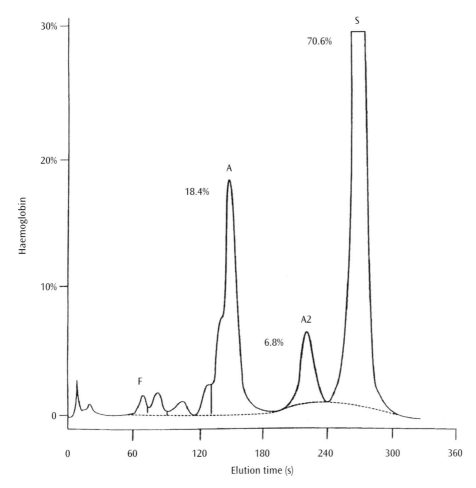

Fig. 9.3 *Example of an high-performance liquid chromatogram (Bio-Rad Laboratories, Inc., Hercules, CA, USA) of a specimen containing haemoglobins A, A₂(increased), F and S. The patient was diagnosed as having sickle-β-thalassaemia (after Shokrani et al., 2000, with permission).*

Rognerud, 1993). The one buffer is weakly eluting, the other strongly eluting. At the beginning of the analysis, the mobile phase contains primarily the weakly eluting component; as the analysis progresses, the elution strength of the mobile phase increases. As the elution strength increases, more strongly retained haemoglobins, e.g. more cationic haemoglobins, elute from the column. Using this gradient system, Riou and Wajcman (1997) determined the characteristic retention times of more than 125 haemoglobin variants.

QUALITY CONTROL

Proper control materials must be run at predetermined intervals. Control materials for quantitative measurements, e.g. Hb A_2 and Hb F, and for qualitative measurement, e.g. haemoglobins A, S and C, may be obtained commercially or prepared from frozen, pooled blood specimens.

CALIBRATION

Use of the most pure haemoglobin materials for calibration and linearity verification is highly desirable. Some are commercially available. ICSH/WHO offers an international reference standard material for Hb A_2 and Hb F (Huntsman *et al.*, 1978; ICSH, 1979). Use of a calibrator for those variants that require accurate quantitation, e.g. Hb A_2 and Hb F, ensures quantitative accuracy under the following conditions:

- *Between injections, within the lifetime of the column.* During the lifetime of a column, the recovery of different haemoglobins may gradually decrease and a percentage value of a sample may be different when a column is first used compared with when the column has been in use for 300–400 analyses. During use, proteins contained in previously injected samples may be irreversibly adsorbed to the column packing.
- *Between columns.* A common calibrator will normalize percentage Hb A_2 or Hb F values between columns. Different columns may have different recovery of different haemoglobins.
- *Between different batches of column packing.* Different batches of a given column packing may have different percentage recovery of different haemoglobins.

LIMITATIONS AND SOURCES OF ERROR

High-performance liquid chromatography, like electrophoresis, provides a presumptive identification, and other methods, e.g. protein sequencing, liquid chromatography/mass spectrometry, tandem mass spectrometry, DNA probes and DNA sequencing, are often necessary for a definitive identification. In some HPLC columns, haemoglobins D, G, and E co-elute with Hb A_2. If levels > 10% HBA_2 are found, additional tests should be performed to detect the presence of those haemoglobins. Some uncommon haemoglobin variants may co-elute with Hb A_2 or Hb F and quantitation of these variants by elution peak area may not be accurate. HPLC, although highly sensitive, is not specific for haemoglobins A_2 and F. For example, some minor components of Hb S may co-elute with Hb A_2 causing falsely elevated values to be measured.

9.3.7 Detection and identification of haemoglobin variants using isoelectric focusing (Basset *et al.*, 1978; Galacteros *et al.*, 1980)

Isoelectric focusing (IEF) is a high-resolution method for separating proteins according to their isoelectric points (pIs), i.e. those points at which the net charges of the molecules are zero. Depending on the net balance of the charged groups, amino groups (ionized as NH_3^+) and carboxyl groups (ionized as COO^-), every form of haemoglobin has a characteristic pH value at which these charges are balanced, i.e. a characteristic pI. A range of pH gradients can be established in a medium such as polyacrylamide or agarose gel by incorporating within the gel a large number of polypeptide fragments called ampholytes. Ampholytes appropriate for haemoglobin analyses by IEF have a pI range of 6–10.

The ampholyte-containing gels are placed in contact with buffered electrolyte solutions, acid at one end, basic at the other end, and subjected to an electric field with the anodic pole at the acidic end, the cathodic pole at the basic end. Each ampholyte moves within this field to focus at its isoelectric position, thus setting up a pH gradient from the anodic/acidic side to the cathodic/basic side of the gel. Haemoglobins applied to the gel move to their respective pIs. The point of application of the sample is not critical; haemoglobins will move from any direction to focus at their pIs as sharp bands. IEF permits considerably sharper resolution of haemoglobin bands and provides a means to identify some haemoglobin variants that do not separate from Hb A, Hb S, or Hb A$_2$ by alkaline electrophoresis. For example Hb A$_1$C, Hb Malmo and Hb Raleigh separate clearly from Hb A; Hb S, Hb D-Punjab and Hb G-Philadelphia separate clearly from each other; Hb C separates clearly from Hb A$_2$; Hb E, however, does not separate clearly from Hb A$_2$ with IEF (Mohammed *et al.*, 1997).

The preparation of polyacrylamide gels for IEF is cumbersome and time-consuming. Also, monoacrylamide is neurotoxic until it has polymerized. Thus gel preparation in clinical laboratories is not recommended and IEF materials should be procured from commercial sources.

Better separation of haemoglobin variants is seen with IEF than with alkaline or acid citrate agar electrophoresis. Haemoglobins give sharply defined bands, and minor haemoglobin bands appear to have greater density and are more easily observed. IEF is a method that is currently widely used for the screening of neonatal specimens for the presence of haemoglobin variants.

Ideally, the IEF positions of haemoglobin variants are defined by their specific pI. However, there are no standards that identify specific pIs. In practice, IEF positions are measured relative to the position of Hb A, with variants anodic to Hb A assigned a positive value in mm and those cathodic to Hb A a negative value in mm. Thus the laboratory is able to develop a map of variant haemoglobins.

SPECIMEN

Whole blood anticoagulated with EDTA, heparin or ACD is acceptable, as are neonatal filter paper blood spots. Specimens are stable for up to 10 days at 4°C.

Mix blood specimen and wash the red cells using 1 mL blood and 10 mL of 0.145 mol/L (8.5 g/L) NaCl solution. Centrifuge for 10 min at 2000 × *g*. Washed cells remaining from cellulose acetate electrophoresis may be used. Dilute 10 µL packed cells with 100 µL elution reagent and mix well (vortex mixer).

REAGENTS

Trichloroacetic acid (10% w/v) Dilute 100 g trichloroacetic acid to 1000 mL.

Sodium acetate buffer (pH 4.7) Dissolve 5.84 g sodium acetate and 2.08 mL glacial acetic acid in distilled or deionized water and dilute to 2000 mL.

When stored at 4°C, the buffer is stable up to 1 year.

O-DIANISIDINE STAIN

Dissolve 20 mg o-dianisidine stain in 50 mL absolute alcohol and 30 mL acetate buffer, pH 4.7. When ready to use, add 0.2 mL hydrogen peroxide, 30% (v/v). The staining reagent is stable for 1 day only.

IEF GEL

Commercially prepared IEF gels are recommended. They should be precast agarose gels containing ampholytes, pH 6.0–8.0, and be accompanied by acid anode solution containing 0.5 mol/L acetic acid, alkaline cathode solution containing 1 mol/L ethanolamine and 0.1% (w/v) KCN, an elution reagent containing < 0.1% cyanide and a small amount of sodium azide. Reagents that contain azide are potentially explosive. Consult institutional safety guidelines for safe disposal.

IEF gels are usually available as 15-lane and 23-lane gels.

MATERIALS, INSTRUMENTS

The following are required: an IEF focusing chamber, a power supply with circuit breaker integral to the unit, electrode wicks, sample application templates and blotting paper.

A known haemoglobin control specimen containing, for example, haemoglobins A, C, S, G-Philadelphia and J-Baltimore or I should be run with each batch of patient samples. Other known haemoglobin variants may be included as needed to match an unknown.

PROCEDURE

Manufacturers' instructions must be followed. Generally the following steps are required:

1 Prepare a label identifying the positions of the samples and the controls. Controls should be applied to lanes 2, 8 and 14 on a 15-lane gel, and to lanes 2, 12 and 22 on a 23-lane gel. Patient specimens should be applied in duplicate with a maximum of six patients on a 15-lane gel, a maximum of 10 patients on a 23-lane gel. Empty lanes should be filled with elution reagent.
2 Remove the IEF gel from the refrigerator and from its packaging. Do not separate from the flexible backing; do not use if the gel is torn or dried out. Allow gels to come to ambient (room) temperature, place on clean flat surface with agarose facing upwards and blot gently with blotting paper.
3 Cool the focusing chamber to 15°C and ensure the chamber is level. Wet the surface with water. Slowly roll the IEF gel onto the grid (15-lane gel with the bottom on line 5, the side on line 7 of the grid; 23-lane gel with the bottom on line 6, the side on line 10). Ensure that there are no air bubbles under the gel and blot excess water from around the edges of the gel.
4 Place the sample template on the IEF gel between lines 2 and 3 on the cathodic end of the chamber. Remove any air bubbles and ensure even contact with the gel. Apply 5 μL haemolysate to the appropriate wells; do not overload. Allow haemolysates to absorb into the gel for 10 minutes. Place sample blotting strip over the wells and remove any excess sample. Remove the template.
5 Apply anode and cathode buffer evenly to the anode and cathode wicks; blot dry with paper towel. Place anode wick with the rough side down on line 4 of the anodic end; place cathode wick with the rough side down on line 4 of the cathodic end. Carefully centre the electrodes over the wicks and connect the leads to the focusing unit. Place cover on the chamber and turn on the power (small gels, 1200 V, 70 minutes; large gels 1400 V, 70 minutes).
6 Turn power supply and cooling unit off; remove cover, lid and wicks. Discard wicks and remove gel from grid. Place gel in staining tray and fix immediately for 10 minutes in trichloroacetic acid, 10% (w/v). Rinse gel for 10 minutes with distilled water in pan on shaker; change water twice, rinse for total of 30 minutes. Stain gel with o-dianisidine and rinse with water for 10 minutes. Dry the gel at room temperature or in a drying oven. Label the dried gel with the label prepared in step 1.
7 Wipe electrodes with distilled water; wipe grid with damp towel and dry.

REPORTING OF RESULTS

Except for common haemoglobin variants, visual inspection only is not sufficient. The mobilities of the various unknowns and controls should be measured with a caliper, in mm, taking the position of Hb A as zero. Haemoglobin bands anodic to Hb A are measured as positive, and bands cathodic to Hb A as negative. Record values on a worksheet.

The laboratory should develop an IEF map showing the expected position (relative to the position of Hb A) of commonly encountered and uncommon haemoglobin variants (Fig. 9.4).

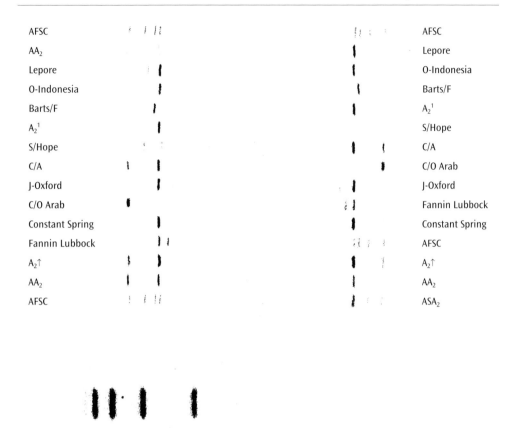

AFSC				AFSC
AA$_2$				Lepore
Lepore				O-Indonesia
O-Indonesia				Barts/F
Barts/F				A$_2$^{1}
A$_2$^{1}				S/Hope
S/Hope				C/A
C/A				C/O Arab
J-Oxford				J-Oxford
C/O Arab				Fannin Lubbock
Constant Spring				Constant Spring
Fannin Lubbock				AFSC
A$_2$↑				A$_2$↑
AA$_2$				AA$_2$
AFSC				ASA$_2$

Fig. 9.4 *Example of a 15-lane isoelectric focusing gel. Note the haemoglobin A, F, S and C-containing control in lane 1 (left and right) and lane 15 (left). The higher magnification insert at the bottom demonstrates the relatively sharply defined haemoglobin bands obtained with IEF. (Courtesy of Dr R. Ellerbrook, Helena Laboratories, Beaumont, TX, USA.)*

9.3.8 Testing for unstable haemoglobins

Over the years more than 100 haemoglobin variants have been identified that exhibit instability either to elevated temperatures (Motulsky and Stomatoyannopoulos, 1968; Huehns, 1970) or to dilute, buffered isopropanol (Carrell, 1972). This instability *in vitro* to mild 'stress' is correlated to instability *in vivo*. Most of these unstable variants have substitutions of polar for non-polar amino acids at the haem contacts within the haem pocket of the haemoglobin molecule. The polar amino acids permit water to enter the haem pocket, destabilizing the haem, allowing it to dissociate from the globin chains and resulting in instability and precipitation of the globin. Many methods to test for haemoglobin instability have been devised; two simple tests that only require visual interpretation of turbidity are widely used. It is, however, necessary to use both tests because some variants that are highly unstable *in vivo* yield negative results with the isopropanol test and positive results with the heat denaturation test. Whenever the Hb F fraction is greater than 5%, a false-positive isopropanol test is usually observed. Thus, in infants, performance of a heat denaturation test is required.

SAMPLE

Whole blood specimens anticoagulated in EDTA, heparin or ACD are acceptable; neonatal filter paper blood spots may be used. Specimens are stable for up to 1 week at 4°C.

Prepare washed red cells by placing 1–2 mL blood into a 15 mL centrifuge tube, add about 12 mL chilled NaCl solution, 0.15 mol/L, mix well and centrifuge for 10 minutes at 2000 × g.

REAGENTS

For the isopropanol test the following reagents are required.

Tris-HCl buffer (0.1 mol/L, pH 7.4) Dissolve 12.1 g trishydroxymethyl-aminomethane completely in about 800 mL of distilled or deionized water. Adjust to pH = 7.4 with HCl and bring to 1000 mL with water. The buffer is stable for up to 1 year when stored at 4°C.

Buffered isopropanol Add 34.0 mL isopropanol, reagent grade (available from commercial sources) to 166.0 mL Tris-HCl buffer, pH 7.4. The solution is stable for up to 1 year when stored at 4°C.

The following are also required: carbon tetrachloride (CCl$_4$), reagent grade, and 0.15 mol/L (9 g/L) NaCl solution. Note that CCl$_4$ is toxic; consult local chemical safety guidelines for proper handling.

A 0.19 mol/L Tris buffer, pH = 8, is required for the heat denaturation test. Dissolve 23.0 g trishydroxymethylaminomethane in about 800 mL of distilled or deionized water. Bring to pH = 8.0 with HCl and dilute to 1000 mL with water. The buffer is stable for up to 1 year when stored at 4°C.

MATERIALS AND EQUIPMENT

- A refrigerated centrifuge
- A 37°C heating block and a water bath
- Pipettes, 100 μL and 1.0 mL
- Test tubes, 10 × 75 mm
- Centrifuge tubes, 15 mL, graduated.

ISOPROPANOL STABILITY TEST

1 Place 0.2 mL washed red cells in a centrifuge tube. Add an equal volume of cold distilled water and one-half the volume of CCl$_4$. Cover the tube and mix thoroughly (vortex mixer) for 2 minutes. Then centrifuge for 30 minutes at 2000 × g in a refrigerated (4°C) centrifuge. Label 10 × 75 mm test tubes 'control' and 'sample'. Pipette 1 mL buffered isopropanol into each tube and let stand at ambient (room) temperature for at least 10 minutes
2 Transfer 0.1 mL of the haemolysates into the tubes and mix well by inversion.
3 Incubate the tubes for 20 minutes in a 37°C heating block.
4 Mix well by inversion and read for the presence of turbidity or precipitation. Re-examine after 2 minutes.

HEAT DENATURATION TEST

1 Label centrifuge tubes 'patient' and 'control, normal' and 'control, abnormal'. Pipette 100 µL washed patient red cells into the tube labelled 'patient', 100 µL 'normal' red cells into the tube labelled 'control, normal', and 100 µL thawed abnormal control into the tube labelled 'control, abnormal'.
2 Add 1 mL Tris buffer, 0.19 mol/L, to each of the tubes and mix. Centrifuge for 30 minutes at $2000 \times g$.
3 Transfer 1 mL of the supernatants from the centrifuged tubes into labelled 12×75 mm tubes.
4 Place the tubes in a water bath at 50°C.
5 After 1 hour, check the tubes for the presence of turbidity or precipitate; the abnormal control must test positive. Replace tubes in the water bath and re-check for turbidity/precipitation after 30 minutes.

QUALITY CONTROL

Normal and abnormal controls must be included in each run of patient specimens. Normal controls may consist of washed red cells from an electrophoretically normal patient or person. Known positive haemolysates should be saved from patients with a positive test result and stored frozen.

REPORTING RESULTS

Normal haemolysates show no turbidity or precipitation and are reported as 'negative'. Unstable haemoglobins show medium to heavy turbidity or precipitation within about 20 minutes and are reported as 'positive'. The end-point may be difficult to interpret, as precipitates may not appear until 1–2 minutes after removal from the heating block. To confirm positivity, shake the tube vigorously and watch for re-formation of precipitates.

LIMITATIONS AND SOURCES OF ERROR

Hb F levels > 5% may give a false-positive isopropanol test. A heat denaturation test should be performed instead.

9.4 THE THALASSAEMIAS (BANK, 1990; COHEN, 1998)

Thalassaemias are disorders in which there is primarily a diminution of haemoglobin formation. They are usually described according to which globin gene is affected.

The widest range in clinical severity is seen with α-thalassaemia, because normally there are four α-globin genes. Deletion of one of these genes (α-thalassaemia-2 trait) often has no clinical or haematological expression, although a small amount of Hb Bart's (γ_4) may be present in the neonate; older children and adults may show mild microcytosis. Deletion of two α-globin genes (homozygous α-thalassaemia-2 or α-thalassaemia-1 trait) usually causes about 5% Hb Bart's in neonatal specimens, microcytosis and mild anaemia in older children and adults. Clinically it is called thalassaemia minor. Deletion of three α-globin genes causes haemoglobin H disease with moderate to severe haemolytic anaemia and microcytosis. Clinically it is called thalassaemia intermedia.

The most severe form of thalassaemia is encountered when all four α-globin genes are absent (homozygous α-thalassaemia-1). This condition is characterized by severe anaemia, congestive heart failure, liver and other organ decompensation in the fetus, and death, usually in the second trimester. Clinically it is called Hb Bart's hydrops fetalis. Some α-chain variants are also associated with α-thalassaemia because they are usually caused by a chromosome that lacks the normal complement of two α-globin genes. Those most frequently encountered are Hb G-Philadelphia, Hb Hasharon, Hb Mahidol and Hb Constant Spring, which are common in South-east Asia.

In most cases of β-thalassaemia trait, there is little or no anaemia. Hb A$_2$ quantitation is useful in identifying β-thalassaemia trait in which Hb A$_2$ is commonly increased. Hb A$_2$ quantitation fails, however, to identify some cases of β-thalassaemia trait or the rare γδβ thalassaemias due to deletion of an entire chromosome. In homozygous β-thalassaemia or compound heterozygotes for different thalassaemia β-thalassaemia mutations, there may be severe anaemia, growth retardation and bone malformation. Some haemoglobin variants are expressed with a thalassaemic phenotype, e.g. Hb Lepore and Hb E.

Clinically heterozygosity for β-thalassaemia mutations usually results in thalassaemia minor, although some mutations may cause thalassaemia intermedia. Homozygosity for the more severe β^0-thalassaemia causes severe and life-threatening anaemia associated with skeletal and facial malformations and growth retardation, clear features of thalassaemia major.

The most useful tests for the laboratory diagnosis of thalassaemias include:

- complete blood count, including reticulocyte count
- evaluation of red cell morphology
- cellulose acetate electrophoresis
- quantitation of Hb A$_2$ and Hb F
- evaluation of iron status
- globin chain synthesis
- DNA analysis.

9.5 NEONATAL SCREENING

Since the publication of a report of a randomized trial that demonstrated reduced morbidity and mortality of infants suffering from sickle cell anaemia when treated prophylactically with penicillin (Gaston *et al.*, 1986), screening for sickling disorders joined screening for phenyl-ketonuria and hypothyroidism. The screening methods used aim to detect and identify haemoglobin variants and the absence of normal adult Hb A. Methods used must be sufficiently sensitive to detect low levels of normal and abnormal haemoglobins and very small quantities of Hb A in cord blood specimens, capillary specimens, or dried filter paper blood spots. The most useful tests are cellulose acetate electrophoresis, which is cheap but labour-intensive, isoelectric focusing, HPLC, solubility testing for sickling haemoglobins, and specific immunological antibody testing. For any genetic screening programme, one should clearly establish the aims and purpose, the level of accuracy of the screening test and the predictive power, the value of knowledge gained for the individuals being screened, potential social implications, availability of therapeutic measures for the diagnosed condition, and the resource requirements (Chapman, 1999).

9.6 CONCLUSIONS

Haemoglobin variants cannot be identified definitively by a single laboratory test. Results of two or more laboratory tests must be integrated with appropriate clinical data, a complete blood count with red cell indices and morphology, family studies and ethnic background. The most informative screening test is cellulose acetate electrophoresis. Citrate agar electrophoresis is especially useful to distinguish Hb S from Hb D and Hb G and to distinguish Hb C from Hb O-Arab and Hb C-Harlem. Sickling haemoglobins migrate near the Hb S position and can be confirmed by solubility testing.

Quantitative tests for Hb A_2 and Hb F are useful for distinguishing among the thalassaemias. Abnormal erythrocyte morphology may be seen in many haemoglobinopathies. Hypochromia and microcytosis are seen in most thalassaemias and are associated with some haemoglobin variants such as Hb E and Hb Lepore. Target cells may be seen with many haemoglobinopathies. Sickled erythrocytes are common in sickle cell disease, sickle cell/β-thalassaemia, and Hb S + Hb C disease. An elevated reticulocyte count is often associated with unstable haemoglobins. These should be suspected in individuals with a history of haemolytic anaemia and may be confirmed by precipitation tests. Better separation of haemoglobin variants is seen with isoelectric focusing than with alkaline or acid citrate agar electrophoresis. HPLC is a useful tool for the detection and presumptive identification of unknown haemoglobins and lends itself to automation.

Rule-based expert systems have been developed to assist in the diagnosis of haemoglobin disorders by various investigators. An example of such a rule-based system that processes laboratory data, i.e. results of electrophoresis, quantitation of haemoglobins A_2 and F, and the results of solubility testing, was published by Nguyen *et al.* (1996).

The major sources of error in detecting and identifying haemoglobin variants are failure to obtain correct laboratory findings and failure to interpret laboratory data correctly. To avoid laboratory errors, quality control guidelines must be instituted and all procedures must be carefully monitored. Controls must be included with all electrophoresis runs. Equipment must be well maintained and for quantitative tests the laboratory must establish its own reference range(s).

REFERENCES

Abraham, E.C., Reese, A., Stallings M. and Huisman, T.H.J. (1976) Separation of human hemoglobins by DEAE-cellulose chromatography using glycine-KCN-NaCl developers. *Hemoglobin* **1**, 27–44.

Adams, J.G., Morrison, W.T. and Steiberg, M.H. (1982) Hb Parchman: a double crossover within a single human gene. *Science* **218**, 291–3.

Baglioni, C. (1962) The fusion of two polypeptide chains in hemoglobin Lepore and its interpretation as a genetic deletion. *Proc. Natl Acad. Sci. USA* **48**, 1880–6

Bank, A., ed. (1990) Sixth Cooley's Anemia Symposium. *Ann. NY Acad. Sci.* **612**, 1–126.

Basset, P., Beuzard, Y., Garel, M.C. and Rosa, J. (1978) Isoelectric focusing of human hemoglobin: its application to screening, to characterization of 70 variants, and to the study of modified fractions of normal hemoglobins. *Blood* **51**, 971–81.

Beet, E.A. (1949) The genetics of the sickle-cell trait in a Bantu tribe. *Ann. Eugen.* **14**, 279–84.

Bernards, R. and Flavell, R.A. (1980) Physical mapping of the globin gene deletion in hereditary persistence of fetal hemoglobin (HPFH). *Nucleic Acids Res.* **8**, 1521–34.

Betke, K., Marti, H.R. and Schlicht, I. (1959) Estimation of small percentages of foetal hemoglobin by alkali denaturation. *Nature* **184**, 1877–8.

Bradley, T.B., Wohl, R.C. and Rieder, R.F. (1967) Hemoglobin Gun Hill: deletion of five amino acid residues and impaired hemoglobin binding. *Science* **157**, 1581–3.

Brady, T., Romac, M.K. and Young, D. (2000) Selecting the right chromatography column: the starting point for chromatographic research. *Am. Lab.* **32**, 27–31.

Brosius, E.M., Wright, J.M., Baine, R.M. and Schmidt, R.M. (1978) Microchromatographic methods for HbA$_2$ compared. *Clin. Chem.* **24**, 2196–9.

Bunn, H.F., Schmidt, G.J., Haney, D.N. and Dluhy, R.G. (1975) Hemoglobin Cranston, an unstable variant having an elongated β-chain due to nonhomologous crossover between two normal β-chain genes. *Proc. Natl Acad. Sci. USA* **72**, 3609–13.

Carrell, R.W. and Kay, R. (1972) A simple method for the detection of unstable haemoglobins. *Br. J. Haematol.* **23**, 615–19.

Chapman, C.S. (1999) Neonatal screening for haemoglobinopathies. *Clin. Lab. Haematol.* **21**, 229–34.

Cohen, A.R., ed. (1998) Cooley's Anemia, seventh symposium. *Ann. NY Acad. Sci.* **850**, 1–376.

Cooper, H.A. and Hoagland, H.C. (1972) Fetal hemoglobin. *Mayo Clin. Proc.* **47**, 401–13.

Efvremov, G.D., Huisman, T.H.J., Bowman, K. *et al.* (1974) Microchromatography of hemoglobins. II. A rapid method for the determination of hemoglobin A$_2$. *J. Lab. Clin. Med.* **83**, 657–61.

Galacteros, F., Kleman, K., Caburi-Martin, J. *et al.* (1980) Cord blood screening for haemoglobin abnormalities by thin layer isoelectric focusing. *Blood* **56**, 1068–71.

Garver, F.A., Jones, C.S., Baker, M.H. *et al.* (1976) Specific radioimmunochemical identification and quantitation of hemoglobins A$_2$ and F. *Am. J. Hematol.* **1**, 459–69.

Gaston, M.H., Verter, J.I., Woods, G. *et al.* (1986) Prophylaxis with oral penicillin in children with sickle cell anemia. A randomised trial. *New Eng. J. Med.* **314**, 1593–9.

Hahn, E.V. and Gillespie, E.G. (1927) Sickle-cell anemia. Report of a case greatly improved by splenectomy. Experimental study of sickle-cell formation. *Arch. Intern. Med.* **30**, 233–40.

Herrick, J.B. (1910) Peculiar elongated and sickle-shaped red blood corpuscles in a case of severe anemia. *Arch. Intern. Med.* **6**, 517–21.

Huehns, E.R. (1970) Disease due to abnormalities of hemoglobin structure. *Ann. Rev. Med.* **21**, 157–78.

Huisman, T.H.J., Wilson, J.B., Gravely, M. and Hubbard, M. (1974) Hemoglobin Grady: the first example of a variant with elongated chains due to an insertion of residues. *Proc. Natl Acad. Sci. USA* **71**, 3270–3.

Huisman, T.H.J., Schroeder, W.A., Brodie, A.R. *et al.* (1975) Microchromatography of hemoglobins. III. A simplified procedure for the determination of hemoglobin A$_2$. *J. Lab. Clin. Med.* **80**, 700–2.

Huisman, T.H.J., Carver, M.F.H. and Baysal, E. (1997) *A Syllabus of Thalassemia Mutations*. Augusta, GA: The Sickle Cell Anemia Foundation.

Huisman, T.H.J., Carver, M.F.H. and Efremov, G.D. (1999) *A Syllabus of Human Hemoglobin Variants*, 2nd edn. Augusta, GA: The Sickle Cell Anemia Foundation.

Huntsman, R.G., Carrell, R.W. and White, J.M. (1978) ICSH recommendations for selected methods for quantitative estimation of Hb A$_2$ and for Hb A$_2$ reference preparation. *Br. J. Haematol.* **38**, 573–8.

ICSH (1979) Recommendations for fetal hemoglobin reference preparations and fetal hemoglobin determination by the alkali denaturation method. *Br. J. Haematol.* **42**, 133–6.

Ingram, V.M. (1956) A specific chemical difference between the globins of normal human and sickle cell anemia haemoglobin. *Nature* **178**, 792–3.

Itano, H.A. (1953) Solubilities of naturally occurring mixtures of human hemoglobin. *Arch. Biochem. Biophys.* **47**, 148–52.

Lehmann, H., Casey, R., Lang, A. *et al.* (1975) Haemoglobin Tak: a β-chain elongation. *Br. J. Haematol.* **31**, 119–23.

Michelson, A.M. and Orkin, S.H. (1980) The 3´ untranslated regions of the duplicated human alpha globin genes are unexpectedly divergent. *Cell* **22**, 371–7.

Mohammed, A.A., Okorududu, A.O., Bissell, M.G. *et al.* (1997) Clinical application of capillary isoelectric focusing on fused silica capillary for determination of Hb variants. *Clin. Chem.* **43**, 1798–804.

Motulsky, A.G. and Stamatoyannopoulos, G. (1968) Drugs, anesthesia, and abnormal hemoglobins. *Ann. NY Acad. Sci.* **151**, 807–21.

NCCLS (1988) Citrate agar electrophoresis for confirming the identification of variant hemoglobins; tentative guideline. *Document H23-T*. Villanova, PA: NCCLS.

NCCLS (1989a) Chromatographic (microcolumn) determination of hemoglobin a_2; Approved Standard. *Document H9-A*. Villanova, PA: NCCLS.

NCCLS (1989b) Quantitative measurement of fetal hemoglobin by the alkali denaturation method; Approved Guideline. *Document H13-A*. Villanova, PA: NCCLS.

NCCLS (1994a) Detection of abnormal hemoglobin using cellulose acetate electrophoresis, 2nd edn; Approved Standard. *Document H8-A2*. Villanova, PA: NCCLS.

NCCLS (1994b) Reference and selected procedures for the quantitative determination of hemoglobin in blood, 2nd edn; Approved Standard. *Document H15-A2*. Villanova, PA: NCCLS.

NCCLS (1995) Solubility test to confirm the presence of sickling hemoglobins, 2nd edn; Approved Standard. *Document H10-A2*. Villanova, PA: NCCLS.

Neel, J.V. (1949) The inheritance of sickle-cell anemia. *Science* **110**, 64–6.

Nguyen, A.N.D., Hatwell, E. and Milam, J.D. (1996) A rule-based expert system for laboratory diagnosis of hemoglobin disorders. *Arch. Pathol. Lab. Med.* **120**, 817–27.

Ohta, Y., Yasokawa, M., Saito, S. *et al.* (1980) Homozygous δ-thalassemia in Japan. *Hemoglobin* **4**, 417–23.

Orkin, S.H., Alter, B.P., Altay, C. *et al.* (1978) Application of endonuclease mapping to the analysis and prenatal diagnosis of thalassemias caused by gene deletion. *New Engl. J. Med.* **299**, 166–70.

Orkin, S.H., Goff, S.C. and Nathan, D.G. (1981) Heterogeneity of DNA deletion in γδβ-thalassemia. *J. Clin. Invest.* **67**, 878–84.

Ou, C.N. and Rognerud, C.L. (1993) Rapid analysis of hemoglobin variants by cation exchange HPLC. *Clin. Chem.* **39**, 820–4.

Pauling, L., Itano, H.A., Singer, S.J. and Wells, I.C. (1949) Sickle-cell anemia, a molecular disease. *Science* **110**, 543–5.

Riou, J. and Wajcman, H. (1997) Cation exchange HPLC evaluated for presumptive identification of hemoglobin variants. *Clin. Chem.* **43**, 34–9.

Roa, D., Turner, E.A. and Aguinaga, M.dP. (1996) Effect of the environment on the detection of hemoglobin variants from dried blood filter paper specimens by HPLC. *Ann. Clin. Lab. Sci.* **23**, 433–8.

Schleider, C.T.H., Mayson, S.M. and Huisman, T.H.J. (1977) Further modification of the microchromatographic determination of hemoglobin A_2. *Hemoglobin* **1**, 503–4.

Schmidt, R.M., Brosius, E.M. and Wright, J.M. (1977) Preparation and use of a quality control hemolysate for microchromatographic determinations of Hb A2. *Am. J. Clin. Pathol.* **67**, 215–18.

Schneider, R.G., Hosty, T.S., Tomloin, G. and Atkins, R. (1974) Identification of hemoglobins and hemoglobinopathies by electrophoresis on cellulose acetate plates impregnated with citrate agar. *Clin. Chem.* **20**, 74–7.

Seid-Akhavan, M., Winter, W.P., Abramson, R.K. and Rucknagel, D.L. (1971) Hemoglobin Wayne: a frameshift mutation detected in human hemoglobin α-chains. *Proc. Natl Acad. Sci. USA* **73**, 882–4.

Singer, K., Chernoff, A.I. and Singer, L. (1951) Studies on abnormal hemoglobins. I. Their demonstration in sickle cell anemia and other hematologic disorders by means of alkali denaturation. *Blood* **6**, 413–27.

Shokrani, M., Terrell, F., Turner, E.A. and del Pilar Asguinaga, M. (2000) Chromatographic measurements of hemoglobin A_2 in blood samples that contain sickle hemoglobin. *Ann. Clin. Lab. Sci.* **30**, 191–4.

van der Ploeg, L.H.T., Konings, A., Oort, M. *et al.* (1980) γ-β-Thalassemia studies showing that deletion of the γ and δ-genes influences β-globin gene expression in man. *Nature* **283**, 637–42.

4

Erythrocyte sedimentation

10

Measuring the erythrocyte sedimentation rate

JOHN A. KOEPKE

INTRODUCTION

The erythrocyte sedimentation rate (ESR; also known as the sedimentation rate) is one of most widely used laboratory tests, particularly in the outpatient setting (Hardison, 1968). This test, first conceived by the Swedish physician Fahraeus (1921) to follow patients' illnesses, has continued to serve as a sensitive screening test for the presence of disease (Pincherle and Shanks, 1967; Zacharski and Kyle, 1967).

ESRs have been measured in physician's offices for many years. The advantages of performing patient tests in the office include lower cost and readily available test results upon which the physician can act immediately. The sedimentation rate fits into this context rather well for new patients in that it is a useful procedure serving as a 'sickness index' in conjunction with the patient's history and physical examination (Fincher and Page, 1986). The ESR can help to determine the possible presence as well as the severity of the patient's illness during an initial office visit. For patients already diagnosed and under treatment, the test may be used to monitor the progression or regression of the patient's illness, again concurrent with the visit to the physician's office. If therapy requires to be modified, the physician can do so on the same visit.

A comprehensive review of the implications of sedimentation rate methodology by Bull (1981) pointed out how the test results would vary depending upon the various methods. Methods used at that time were judged to be less than ideal. In recent years the sedimentation rate test itself has been the subject of efforts to improve the technical as well as the bio-hazardous aspects of the testing procedure. These technical advances have undoubtedly improved the reliability of the test results. For example, there are 'micro' methods and devices to help read the blood cell meniscus. Other innovations such as filling the tubes without exposure to the blood have been designed to control biohazards. A number of disposable ESR systems are now marketed (Table 10.1). Some of these modifications were successful while others were less helpful.

There have also been a number of sedimentation rate methods which have shortened the testing time to just a few minutes. One early rapid method held the tube at a 45° angle (Washburn *et al.*, 1956). The zeta sedimentation method was the first automated device which did the test rapidly (4 minutes) on a capillary tube filled with anticoagulated blood. Unfortunately, this device is no longer marketed. The automated systems are noted in Table 10.1.

This proliferation of methods led to the need for a reliable reference method against which to compare the newly designed equipment and newer methods such as the zeta sedimentation rate (ZSR) or the HemoCue B-ESR. An early independent study carefully compared the Wintrobe, Westergren and ZSR methods with a candidate reference method (Moseley and Bull, 1982). Subsequently, both the National Committee for Clinical Laboratory Standards (1993) and the International Council for Standardization in Haematology (1993) have published methods for evaluating the standardization and performance of this test (see Section 10.2.3).

Table 10.1 *Technical innovations for ESR testing*

Name	Manufacturer	Evaluation
Manual methods		
Dispette 2®	Guest	Niejadlik and Engelhardt (1977)
ESrT®	Labdi KB	
SediRate®	Globe	
Seditainer®	Becton Dickinson	Bridgen and Page (1993), Hurd and Knight (1986), Patton *et al.* (1989), Short *et al.* (1990)
Automated and semi-automated methods		
B-ESR®	HemoCue	Brunborn and Martensson (1995)
Sedimatic 8®ª and 100®	AnalysInstrument AB	Kallner (1991), Wendland *et al.* (1994)
StaRRsed®	Mechatronics R & R	
Test 1®	Sire Analytic Systems	Plebani *et al.* (1998)
Mini-Ves® and Ves-Matic 20®	Diesse	Bridgen and Page (1993), Koepke *et al.* (1990), Wendland *et al.* (1994)

ªAlso marketed as the ESR-8® by Streck Laboratories, Inc.

10.1 BIOCHEMICAL AND MECHANICAL FACTORS AFFECTING RED CELL SEDIMENTATION IN PLASMA

The concept of measuring the rate of fall of red cells in their native plasma is straightforward. Long ago it was noted that in many disorders the red cells in a test tube sedimented at a faster rate. Three innovative investigators published methods to quantitate this phenomenon, each using a unique vessel to hold the anticoagulated blood column. Westergren (1926) used a 200 mm pipette, marked along its length with a millimetre scale so that the fall of the red cells could be read directly. Wintrobe and Landsberg (1935) used a 100 mm 'test tube' which was also marked along its length with a millimetre scale. Cutler (1940) used a calibrated test tube with an internal diameter somewhat larger than the Wintrobe tube.

The observed red cell sedimenting phenomenon is, in reality, an interaction of the red cells with the blood plasma. Changes in either one or both of these components can affect the sedimentation rate, making interpretation problematic at times. As the red cells rouleaux/ aggregate in the suspending plasma, the aggregates fall. Being heavier than the plasma, the red cell clumps cause a countercurrent or upward flow of the plasma in the tube or pipette as the red cells fall. The 'sum' of these two opposing forces constitutes the sedimentation rate.

Three phases of sedimentation have been delineated, i.e. the lag, decantation and packing phases (Fig. 10.1). While usually all three phases occur within the hour of testing, very low or very high sedimentation rates may obscure one or more of the phases. In fact, the character of this sigmoid curve was used in the past as a special test to monitor tuberculosis therapy. More recently, this concept has been the subject of clinical research to determine if differing time/sedimentation curves might provide useful clues in certain illnesses.

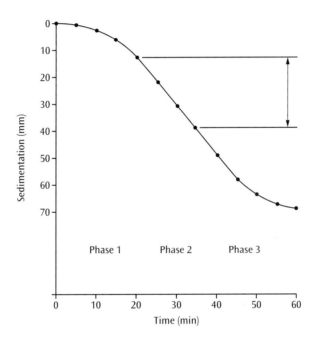

Fig. 10.1 *The three characteristic phases of erythrocyte sedimentation. It is important to note that the elapsed time for the individual phases may vary significantly with specimens having very low or very high sedimentation rates (see text).*

Certain plasma proteins (e.g. immunoglobulins and fibrinogen which are increased in many diseases) promote the aggregation of the red cells and thus accelerate erythrocyte sedimentation (Bain, 1983). Box 10.1 lists these so-called acute-phase proteins which accelerate the ESR and Box 10.2 lists the various clinical conditions in which the concentration of such proteins may be elevated. It is quite evident that the ESR is seen as a useful yet simple objective means to screen for a large number of clinical disorders.

Changes in red cells (both number and/or morphology) also affect the rate of sedimentation. Anaemia ordinarily accelerates the sedimentation rate. This led to the development of

Box 10.1   Plasma protein changes which increase the erythrocyte sedimentation rate

Increased acute-phase proteins
   C-reactive protein
   Fibrinogen
   Haptoglobin
   Caeruloplasmin
   Alpha-1-acid glycoprotein
   Alpha-1-antitrypsin
Increased immunoglobulins
Decreased albumin

Box 10.2   Conditions associated with acute-phase protein increases

Acute tissue damage, e.g. acute myocardial infarction
Chronic inflammation, e.g. pulmonary tuberculosis
Chronic infection, e.g. urinary tract infection
Collagen-vascular diseases, e.g. rheumatoid arthritis
Malignancy
Pregnancy, after first trimester

correction charts which sought to obviate the effect of anaemia (Wintrobe and Landsberg, 1935). This correction method became less popular for a number of reasons, chief of which may be the development of a number of commercial methods which frequently employ the Westergren technique. Methods to 'correct' the Wintrobe results for anaemia have for the most part been almost completely abandoned (Hardison, 1968).

Erythrocyte shape changes can also affect the sedimentation rate. For example, red cells containing sickle haemoglobin may sickle *in vivo* or *in vitro* if the degree of oxygenation of the blood is decreased and the resulting sedimentation rate is decreased (Jan *et al.*, 1981). Target cells in thalassaemia act almost like parachutes, impeding the red cell sedimentation despite the presence of anaemia which ordinarily increases the sedimentation rate. So it is possible for a red cell change such as sickling or target cell formation to obscure an increased ESR due to acute-phase reactants.

10.2 TESTING VARIABLES

10.2.1 Specimen requirements

In his original studies, Westergren (1926) used sodium citrate, the then current anticoagulant for blood specimens. This citrate solution was used in the original dilution, i.e. four volumes of blood to one volume of citrate anticoagulant. Subsequent studies by Gambino *et al.* (1965), and others, have shown that another anticoagulant, EDTA, can also be used and that the required dilution with physiological saline can be made in the laboratory without affecting the sedimentation rate. (NB: it is important *never* to use the 9:1 citrate tube commonly used for coagulation testing.)

So, presently, the more convenient specimen is whole blood collected in EDTA anti-coagulant. The same specimen can be used for the blood count as well as the sedimentation rate if both tests have been requested, thus avoiding the collection of a second specimen. If the ESR is not done immediately, it should be performed within 4 hours if the specimen is held at room temperature, or it can be kept at refrigerator temperature for up to 12 hours and still yield reliable results (Gambino *et al.*, 1965). Specimens must be brought to room temperature and also be well mixed (eight complete inversions of the tube) before testing. If specimens are kept for longer periods, appropriate studies should validate such practice.

10.2.2 Methodology

Two sedimentation rate methods have been most commonly used, i.e. the Westergren method and the Wintrobe method. Careful comparisons of these two methods indicates a greater sensitivity for the Wintrobe method in lower sedimentation rate ranges, but a greater sensitivity of the Westergren method in the higher ranges (Bull, 1981).

Almost all currently marketed systems (Table 10.1) are selected methods (see below) in which the variables are better controlled and the technical aspects of the testing are made more convenient as well as being less biohazardous. In addition, the standardization has improved the reliability of the testing.

To measure a sedimentation rate, a blood specimen diluted with either saline or citrate solution is used to fill the Westergren pipette. This tube, with an internal diameter of at least 2.55 mm, holds a 200 mm column of blood vertically. Plastic has been shown to be equivalent to glass pipettes (Roddie and Pollock, 1987). After 1 hour, the meniscus at the top of the sedimenting red cells is noted and recorded as the sedimentation rate, i.e. the distance (in mm) that the red cell meniscus has fallen in 1 hour. Occasionally the interface may be indistinct. A 'best guess' might be used for the reading, but a repeat test on a new specimen would be preferable. Avoidance of vibration, direct sunlight or other interferences is necessary (Table 10.2).

Some systems, e.g. the Diesse Ves-Matic (Diesse Diagnostica Senese, Italy), use reaction vessels different from the Westergren pipette. In such cases, comparative studies have validated the comparability with standard methods (Koepke *et al.*, 1990).

Table 10.2 *Testing variables which can affect the erythrocyte sedimentation rate (ESR)*

Variable	Frequent ESR effect
Ambient temperature	
Elevated (> 25°C)	Elevated (Manley,1957)
Decreased (< 18°C)	Decreased (Manley, 1957)
Delays in testing (> 4 to < 24 hours)	None, if specimen is refrigerated, brought to ambient temperature and well mixed (Gambino *et al.*, 1965)
Tubes, pipettes	
Non-vertical	Increased
Narrow (< 2.55 mm)	Imprecision
Vibration	Increased
Elevated specimen PCV	Variable
Undiluted sample	Imprecision

PCV, packed cell volume.

10.2.3 Method calibration and evaluation

As noted earlier, two standardization groups published their recommendations for the ESR determination (ICSH, 1993; NCCLS, 1993). To help understand these detailed presentations, one must be acquainted with the hierarchy of levels of testing. Three levels were defined (ICSH, 1993):

- *Reference method.* The use of a 200 mm open-ended Westergren pipette filled with undiluted blood with a packed cell volume (PCV) of 0.35 or less which has been collected in EDTA.
- *Standardized method.* The use of a 200 mm glass or plastic Westergren-type pipette with an internal diameter of at least 2.55 mm using undiluted blood with a PCV of 0.35 or less collected in EDTA. The ICSH (1993) proposal developed the concept of a reference or standardized method which uses undiluted bloods with PCVs of 0.35 or less. This was done in order to avoid the potential for any errors when diluting the blood specimen prior to testing. It can be seen that differences between the reference and selected methods are insignificant.
- *Selected method.* Also known as the working or routine method, this uses methods that minimize biohazardous risks. Disposable pipettes, tubes or containers are acceptable even if the classic Westergren pipette is not used. It is incumbent upon the manufacturer and/or user to ensure that the results are consistent with the standardized method.

In addition, detailed methods for comparing the selected, working or routine methods against the standardized method are also outlined. Thomas *et al.* (1993) performed a comprehensive study which validated the performance of the chosen Westergren method. The ICSH Expert Panel was especially concerned with biohazards and therefore sought methods or systems with less potential for exposure to blood specimens than the use of re-usable Westergren pipettes. A perusal of the commercial working methods will indicate that most now use disposable plastic or glass pipettes or other disposable reaction vessels and diluters.

The NCCLS method (1993) presented details for the selected, i.e. Westergren, method which uses a 4:1 dilution of blood collected in EDTA. This method is similar to the one proposed by the ICSH (see above). In addition, a short protocol for the evaluation of the laboratory working method is given. Finally, several methods for the quality control of the testing are proposed. Calculation of acceptable limits for duplication and the development of 'Levey–Jennings' plots of such differences are suggested. The use of commercial controls is not included since such materials were not yet marketed.

10.3 REFERENCE RANGES

The interpretation of the erythrocyte sedimentation has been fraught with problems originating from a number of sources. First of all, methodology is variable, e.g. Westergren, Wintrobe, Cutler and others, which do not yield numerically similar results and therefore have different reference ranges. Recall that the zeta sedimentation rate, which was scientifically quite sound, was especially unpopular with clinicians primarily because the results required an entirely new set of reference ranges. In addition, lack of standardization of specimen preparation (diluted vs. undiluted) and equipment (e.g. variation in internal diameter of pipettes) has led to non-harmonious results (see Section 10.4.1). There has been a trend for laboratories to move towards the Westergren method, probably due to the availability of disposable equipment and reliable instrumentation which use this method (Table 10.3).

Table 10.3   *Reference values for the Westergren ESR*[a]

Age (years)	Female Mean	Female Upper limit	Male Mean	Male Upper limit
18–30	5	11	3	9
31–40	6	12	3	10
41–50	6	13	5	11
51–60	9	13	6	12
> 60	9	20	5	14

[a]Data modified from Lentner (1984) and Lewis (1980).
ESRs (in mm in 1 hour) rounded to the nearest whole number.

In an effort to achieve the maximum diagnostic efficiency when interpreting the results of the ESR test, special attention should also be given to the gender and age of the patient. Therefore both the NCCLS (1993) and ICSH (1993) ESR documents suggest that reference ranges be established locally by gender and decade. It has been appreciated for many years that females have higher sedimentation rates than males, presumably due to both increased plasma fibrinogen concentrations associated with menstrual cycles and the normally lower red blood cell counts. Also sedimentation rates slowly increase with age (Caswell *et al.*, 1993). In addition to the diseases noted in Box 10.2, there are variations associated with pregnancy and with smoking.

Penev *et al.* (1996) measured ESRs twice monthly for six consecutive months in 52 clinically healthy adults between the ages of 20 and 50 in order to study the long-term biological variation of this test. As expected, the male subjects had lower sedimentation rates (median 3.8 mm in 1 hour) with smaller variabilities ($\pm$ 1.2 mm in 1 hour), whereas the females subjects had both higher mean values (9.7 mm in 1 hour) and greater variability ($\pm$ 3.2 mm in 1 hour). These investigators stated critical changes to be > 3.1 mm in 1 hour for males but > 8.1 mm in 1 hour for females.

It may not be appreciated that there is an apparent increase in the upper limit of normal of from 2 to 13 mm in one hour in the reference ranges of black individuals. These increases are thought to be actual racial differences which are independent of age, gender, red cell count and certain chronic diseases (Gillum, 1993).

10.4 QUALITY ASSURANCE CONSIDERATIONS

In the United States the sedimentation rate tests performed in physicians' office laboratories are one of the laboratory tests that has been 'waived', i.e. excused, from the requirements of the Clinical Laboratory Improvement Amendments of 1988 (CLIA, 1988). The waived status indicates that the test has been judged to be a simple procedure which has an insignificant risk of erroneous results. Therefore the regulatory requirements of CLIA '88 (such as quality control and proficiency testing) were not imposed. However the regulations indicate that if control materials become available, they should be used.

Accurate ESR testing is based primarily upon the selection of a reliable method and then meticulous adherence to the various steps of the procedure, including careful timing of the final reading. A very important consideration is meticulous attention to the details of the test procedure itself. Table 10.2 lists some of the more common variables which can affect the testing process. In the author's experience, one of the more common causes for problems is failure to make the required dilution of the blood specimen. This frequently results in inconsistent results, particularly in specimens with higher PCVs.

In the NCCLS ESR standard, several suggested quality control methods, including periodic duplicate testing, are proposed (NCCLS, 1993). However some of these are not well suited for office laboratories, primarily due to the need for larger numbers of tests in order to generate useful quality control charts.

A number of commercial controls are now marketed (e.g. Accu-Sed, HiChem, Brea, CA; ESR-Chex, Streck, Omaha, NE; Hema-Trol, Hycor, Irvine, CA; SED-Control R&R Lukens, Albuquerque, NM; and Sed-Check, Polymedco, Cortlandt Manor, NY). These controls include both normal and elevated sedimentation rate specimens. Stability in unopened containers is stated to be 5–6 months. However, after the vials are opened, a 2-week storage time is recommended.

10.4.1 Interlaboratory proficiency testing programmes

With the development of stable control materials, it became feasible to incorporate ESRs in interlaboratory proficiency testing programmes. Since 1998 the College of American Pathologists survey programme has included this analyte. Two samples are included in the kits which are sent out three times a year to over 4000 participating laboratories.

Perusal of the participant summary of results indicates the about 77% of the participants use a 'Westergren' method which more or less corresponds with the ICSH/NCCLS guidelines for this procedure. But about 15% of these did not dilute the survey specimens before testing. About 3% of the laboratories still use the Wintrobe method as compared with 74% almost 30 years ago (Koepke, 1971). Finally, 35% of the participants used one of the automated ESR methods (CAP, 2001).

The precision of the manual methods within the reference range in health, expressed as coefficient of variation (CV), ranged from around 9 to 34%. Surprisingly, the automated methods had greater variability, ranging up to 32%. The greater variability of the automated methods may conceivably be due to faulty programming of these instruments. In the abnormal range, the CVs ranged from 9% to about 19% for the manual methods, while the precision of the automated methods was similar.

10.5 CLINICAL USEFULNESS AND INTERPRETATION

10.5.1 Disease detection

Given the knowledge of the factors which affect the sedimentation of red cells in diluted plasma, clinical conditions which affect these factors will result in abnormal ESRs (Kenny *et al.*, 1981). Markedly elevated sedimentation rates were found in about 1% of patients studied by Lluberas-Acosta and Schumacher (1996). Infection, followed by malignant tumours and renal disease, has also been associated with marked elevations (Liljestrand and Oldhagen, 1955).

A more recent study of more than 1000 outpatients indicated that while infection may be the most common cause of markedly elevated sedimentation rates, a variety of other illnesses are also accompanied by elevated sedimentation rates (Fincher and Page, 1986). Other causes are listed in Box 10.2. The degree of abnormality of the sedimentation rate seems to reflect the severity of acute inflammatory disease, i.e. pelvic inflammatory disease in one carefully done study (Miettinen *et al.*, 1993).

10.5.2 Disease monitoring

This laboratory test, although non-specific, has also proven to be quite useful in monitoring the progression and response to therapy of certain diseases, particularly those associated with immune responses. For many years physicians have monitored temporal arteritis patients with sedimentation rate tests. Patients with rheumatoid arthritis are also frequently checked with sedimentation rates (Bull *et al.*, 1989). Other chronic conditions can also be followed with periodic ESRs. In following patients with chronic renal disease, the sedimentation rate changes are apparently due to alterations in fibrinogen concentration as well as constituents of uraemic plasma independent of the degree of anaemia (Shusterman *et al.*, 1985). One study, which compared the C-reactive protein (CRP) with ESR, concluded that ESR is the preferable test for monitoring disease (Pearlman *et al.*, 1998).

10.5.3 Disease prognosis

Studies linking the ESR with short- and long-term disease prognosis have also been published. A recent study of ischaemic stroke patients indicates that an elevated sedimentation rate on admission to the hospital is associated with clinical deterioration during the first 24 hours after the onset of the stroke, perhaps serving as an indirect marker of thrombus formation (Chamorro *et al.*, 1995). Interestingly, patients with congestive heart failure who had higher sedimentation rates had better haemodynamic and clinical benefits following therapy. They also had better 1- and 2-year survivals (Haber *et al.*, 1991). In patients with renal cell carcinoma, but without metastases, a high sedimentation rate indicated a poor prognosis (Hannisdal *et al.*, 1989). However, the authors caution that the ESR should not be used as a screening test for early renal cell carcinoma. Another interesting study which monitored patients with early-stage Hodgkin's disease showed that the sedimentation rate could identify a group of patients at high risk for relapse and subsequent death (Henry-Amar *et al.*, 1991).

10.6 ALTERNATIVE METHODS TO SCREEN FOR DISEASE

Two other procedures, CRP measurement and whole blood or plasma viscosity, have been advanced as alternatives to the ESR as measures of acute-phase proteins. A number of studies have been carried out to compare these methods (Ball, 1978; ICSH, 1988; Pearlman *et al.*, 1998; Stuart and Lewis, 1988). The conclusions indicate that CRP is more sensitive to the inflammatory response to tissue damage in the first 24 hours after such damage takes place (ICSH, 1984). Thereafter, the testing responses appear to be similar.

10.6.1 Viscosity

Both whole blood and plasma have been used to measure viscosity, but it has been recommended that plasma collected in EDTA anticoagulant is the specimen of choice. Centrifuged specimens are stable for up to 6 hours if left undisturbed. If the specimen will not reach the laboratory within 6 hours, the plasma should be separated before transportation; the plasma can be stored for up to 24 hours and refrigeration is not required (ICSH, 1984).

The Harkness viscometer was formerly used to measure viscosity. But it was a rather complex apparatus consisting of a capillary section, a plasma specimen reservoir and a mercury pressure and timing section. All these components are placed in a 37°C water bath during the testing (ICSH, 1984). Other much simpler and less cumbersome methods were subsequently developed, including rotational viscometers which measure the shear rates of plasma. Capillary viscometers have also been promoted for this measurement.

As noted above, the apparent advantage of viscosity measurements over the ESR include the 'portability' of the specimens. However, the wide availability of disposable ESR systems and also the availability of reading devices and even totally automated methods have made the ESR the method of choice to screen for and/or to monitor disease.

10.6.2 C-reactive protein

Within the last several years, CRP has been touted as a sensitive indicator of early (< 24 hour) acute disease. Earlier measurements of CRP used manual methods such as the semi-qualitative latex agglutination and capillary precipitation methods. The more recent introduction of qualitative biochemical methods has significantly improved the accuracy and precision of this measurement (Tracy, 1998).

Taking advantage of these newer methods, several reports have indicated that the CRP is predictive of 'cardiovascular disease events' such as unstable angina (Liuzzo et al., 1996), impending cardiac rupture after myocardial infarction (Ueda et al., 1996), or peripheral vascular disease (Ridker et al., 1998). Other reports have indicated clinically useful sensitivity and specificity in acute abdominal disease (Chi et al., 1996), or acute pelvic inflammation (Miettinen et al., 1993). The rapid turnaround of CRP results has made this test especially useful in the care of patients presenting with acute signs and symptoms of significant disease.

10.7 SUMMARY AND CONCLUSIONS

The ESR test is perceived as a simple and straightforward procedure with little chance of error. However, with the recent development of a large number of commercial methods, the need for a reference or standardized method against which to compare these methods is clear. It has become apparent that a number of factors can significantly degrade the quality of ESR results. With the development of comparative methods and interlaboratory surveys, the various kits in the marketplace can now be evaluated. Such scrutiny can only help to improve the technology and therefore the quality of ESR testing.

There has been a move toward the Westergren method for ESR testing. A number of commercial methods are now marketed which have been shown to compare satisfactorily with reference/standardized methods. Methods which can yield results in shorter periods of time can be expressed in terms equivalent to the hour-long Westergren procedure. The choice of a reliable method is of primary importance. Subsequent quality control requires meticulous attention to the details of the testing itself, particularly if a manual method is being used. The automated methods have, by their very design, ensured for the most part more precise and accurate ESR testing.

Finally, the CRP may have a useful, but limited, place in the diagnosis of patients presenting with acute disease.

REFERENCES

Bain, B.J. (1983) Some influences on the ESR and the fibrinogen level in healthy subjects. *Clin. Lab. Haematol.* **5**, 45–54.

Ball, W. (1978) ESR vs. C-reactive protein. *Lab. Med.* **8**, 23–7.

Bridgen, M.L. and Page, N.E. (1993) Three closed-tube methods for determining erythrocyte sedimentation rate. *Lab. Med.* **24,** 97–102.

Brunborn, L. and Martensson, B. (1995) Jamforelse mellan venosa och kapillara bloprovid kliniskt kemiska analyser och utyardering av en ny metod for blodsanka. Vardhogskolan i Malmo, Lund, April, 1–15.

Bull, B.S. (1981) Clinical and laboratory implications of present ESR methodology. *Clin. Lab. Haematol.* **3,** 283–98.

Bull, B.S., Westengard, J.C., Farr, M. *et al.* (1989) Efficacy of tests used to monitor rheumatoid arthritis. *Lancet* **ii**, 965–7.

College of American Pathologists (2001) *CAP Participant Summary Report, ESR Survey.* Northfield, IL: College of American Pathologists.

Caswell, M., Pike, L.A., Bull, B.S. and Stuart, J.(1993) Effect of patient age on tests of acute-phase response. *Arch. Pathol. Lab. Med.* **117,** 906–10.

Chamorro, A., Vila, N. and Ascaso, C. (1995) Early prediction of stroke severity: role of the erythrocyte sedimentation rate. *Stroke* **26**, 573–6.

Chi, C., Shiesh, S., Chen, K. *et al.* (1996) C-reactive protein for the evaluation of acute abdominal pain. *Am. J. Emerg. Med.* **14,** 254–6.

Cutler, J.W. (1940) Standardized technique for sedimentation rate. *J. Lab. Clin. Med.* **26,** 242–6.

Fahraeus, R. (1921) The suspension stability of the blood. *Acta Med. Scand.* **55**, 1–7.

Fincher, R.E. and Page M.I. (1986) Clinical significance of extreme elevation of the erythrocyte sedimentation rate. *Arch. Intern. Med.* **146**, 1581–3.

Gambino, S.R., DiRe, J.J., Monteleone, M. and Budd, D.C. (1965) The Westergren sedimentation rate using K3EDTA. *Am. J. Clin. Pathol.* **44**, 173–80.

Gillum, R.F. (1993) A racial difference in erythrocyte sedimentation. *J. Natl Med. Assoc.* **85**, 47–50.

Haber, H.L., Leavy, J.A. and Kessler, P.D. (1991) The erythrocyte sedimentation rate in congestive heart failure. *N. Engl. J. Med.* **324,** 353–8.

Hannisdal, E., Bostad, L. and Grottum, K.A. (1991) Erythrocyte sedimentation rate as a prognostic factor in renal cell carcinoma. *Eur. J. Surg. Onc.* **15**, 333–6.

Hardison, C.S. (1968) The sedimentation rate. *J. Am. Med. Assoc.* **204,** 165.

Henry-Amar, M., Frieman, S., Hayat, M. *et al.* (1991) Erythrocyte sedimentation predicts early relapse and survival in early-stage Hodgkin's disease. *Ann. Intern. Med.* **114**, 361–5.

Hurd, C. and Knight, T. (1986) Laboratory evaluation of the Seditainer ESR system. *Med. Tech. Sci.* 74–6.

ICSH (1984) Recommendation for a selected method for the measurement of plasma viscosity. *J. Clin. Pathol.* **37,** 1147–52.

ICSH (1988) Guidelines on selection of laboratory tests for monitoring the acute phase response. *J. Clin. Pathol.* **41,** 1203–12.

ICSH (1993) Recommendations for measurement of erythrocyte sedimentation rate. *J. Clin. Pathol.* **46**, 198–203.

Jan, K.-M., Usami, S. and Smith, J.A. (1981) Influence of oxygen tension and hematocrit reading on ESRs of sickle cells. *Arch. Intern. Med.* **141,** 1815–18.

Kallner, A. (1991) On the temporary development of erythrocyte sedimentation rate using sealed vacuum tubes. *Am. J. Hematol.* **37**, 186–9.

Kenny, M.W., Worthington, D.J., Stuart, J. *et al.* (1981) Efficiency of haematological screening tests for detecting disease. *Clin. Lab. Haematol.* **3**, 299–305.

Koepke, J.A. (1971) Survey of sedimentation rate methodology. *Lab. Med.* **2**, 36.

Koepke, J.A., Caracappo, P. and Johnson, L. (1990) The evolution of erythrocyte sedimentation rate methodology. *LabMedica* **7**, 46–8.

Lentner, C. (ed.) (1984) *Geigy Scientific Tables*, 8th edn. Basle: Ciba-Geigy, Vol. 3, 1962–4.

Lewis, S.M. (1980) Erythrocyte sedimentation rate and plasma viscosity. *Association of Clinical Pathologists Broadsheet* **94**.

Liljestrand, A. and Olhagen, B. (1955) Persistently high erythrocyte sedimentation rate: diagnostic and prognostic aspects. *Acta Med. Scan.* **151**, 425–39.

Lluberas-Acosta, G. and Schumacher, H.R. (1996) Markedly elevated erythrocyte sedimentation rates: consideration of clinical implications in a hospital population. *Br. J. Clin. Pract.* **50**, 138–43.

Liuzzo, G., Biasucci, L.M., Rebuzzi, A.G. *et al.* (1996) Plasma protein acute-phase response in unstable angina is not induced by ischemic injury. *Circulation* **94**, 2373–80.

Manley, R.W. (1957) The effect of room temperature on erythrocyte sedimentation rate and its correction. *J. Clin. Pathol.* **10**, 354–6.

Miettinen, A.K., Heinonen, P.K., Laippala, P. *et al.* (1993) Test performance of erythrocyte sedimentation rate and C-reactive protein in assessing the severity of acute pelvic inflammatory disease. *Am. J. Obstet. Gynecol.* **169**, 1143–9.

Moseley, D.L. and Bull, B.S. (1982) A comparison of the Wintrobe, the Westergren and the ZSR erythrocyte sedimentation rate (ESR) methods to a candidate reference method. *Clin. Lab. Haematol.* **4**, 169–78.

National Committee for Clinical Laboratory Standards (1993) Methods for the erythrocyte sedimentation (ESR) test, 3rd edn. Approved Standard. *Document H2-A3*. Villanova, PA: NCCLS.

Patton, W.N., Meyer, P.J. and Stuart, J. (1989) Evaluation of sealed vacuum extraction method (Seditainer) for measurement of erythrocyte sedimentation rate. *J. Clin. Pathol.* **42**, 313–17.

Pearlman, E.S., Tan, S., Rafael, J. and Saran, A. (1998) Can C-reactive protein replace the erythrocyte sedimentation rate? *S. Am. J. Clin. Pathol.* **109**, 470 (Abstract).

Penev, M.N., Doukova-Peneva, P. and Kalinov, K.J. (1996) Study on long-term biological variability of erythrocyte sedimentation rate. *Scand. J. Lab. Invest.* **56**, 285–8.

Pincherle, G. and Shanks, J. (1967) Value of the erythrocyte sedimentation rate as a screening test. *Br. J. Prev. Soc. Med.* **21**, 133–8.

Plebani, M., de Tani, A. and San Zari, M. (1998) Test 1 automated system: a new method for measuring the erythrocyte sedimentation rate. *Am. J. Clin. Pathol.* **110**, 334–40.

Ridker, P.M., Cushman, M., Stampfer, M.J. *et al.* (1998) Plasma concentration of C-reactive protein and risk of developing peripheral vascular disease. *Circulation* **97**, 425–8.

Roddie, A.M.S. and Pollock, A. (1987) Plastic ESR tubes: does static electricity affect the results? *Clin. Lab. Haematol.* **9**, 175–80.

Short, R., Holliday, J. and Concannon, A. (1990) Investigating safer ESR methodology. *Austr. J. Med. Lab. Sci.* **11**, 66–8.

Shusterman, N., Kimmel, P.L., Kiechle, F.L. *et al.* (1985) Factors influencing erythrocyte sedimentation in patients with chronic renal failure. *Arch. Intern. Med.* **145**, 1796–9.

Stuart, J. and Lewis, S.M. (1988) Monitoring the acute phase response – alternative test to measuring erythrocyte sedimentation rate. *Br. Med. J.* **297**, 1143–4.

Thomas, R.D., Westengard, J.C., Hay, K.L. and Bull, B.S. (1993) Calibration and validation for erythrocyte sedimentation tests. Role of the International Committee on Standardization in Hematology reference procedure. *Arch. Pathol. Lab. Med.* **117**, 719–23.

Tracy, R.P. (1998) C-reactive protein and cardiovascular disease. *Clin. Lab. News* (Aug), 14–16.

Ueda, S., Ikeda, U., Iamamoto, K. *et al.* (1996) C-reactive protein as a predictor of cardiac rupture after acute myocardial infarction. *Am. Heart J.* **131**, 857–60.

Washburn, A.H. and Meyers, A.J. (1956) The sedimentation of erythrocytes at an angle of 45 degrees. *J. Lab. Clin. Med.* **49**, 318–30.

Wendland B., Kreofsky, T.J. and Hanson, C.A. (1994) Erythrocyte sedimentation rate: a laboratory comparison of two automated instruments with the standard Westergren method (Abstract). *Am. J. Clin. Pathol.* **101**, 67.

Westergren, A. (1926) The technique of the red cell sedimentation reaction. *Am. Rev. Tuberculosis* **14**, 94–101.

Wintrobe, M.M. and Landsberg, J.W. (1935) A standardized technique for the blood sedimentation test. *Am. J. Med. Sci.* **189**, 102–15.

Zacharski, L.R. and Kyle, R.A. (1967) Significance of extreme elevation of erythrocyte sedimentation rate. *J. Am. Med. Assoc.* **202**, 264–6.

5

Haematopoietic factors

11

The measurement of ferritin

MARK WORWOOD

INTRODUCTION

The storage iron protein ferritin is found in both prokaryotes and eukaryotes. It consists of a protein shell of molecular mass approximately 500 kDa composed of 24 subunits. The protein shell encloses a core of ferric-hydroxy-phosphate which can hold up to 4000 atoms of iron. Proteins with a similar overall structure are found throughout the plant and animal kingdom as well as in bacteria, although bacterial ferritin appears to have evolved separately with no amino acid sequence homology with animal ferritins. Bacterial ferritin (from *E. coli*) contains haem (about one per two subunits) as well as the core of non-haem iron. Ferritin is ancient in evolutionary terms and also has a long biochemical history. Since it was first isolated by Laufberger (1937), two main interests have dominated ferritin research: its structure and the mechanism of iron uptake and release. Recently, the molecular biology of ferritin has come to the fore and it has become a paradigm for studies of the regulation of synthesis at the level of translation. A detailed review of structure and function was carried out by Harrison and Arosio (1996).

11.1 GENETICS

A range of isoferritins is found in various human tissues. These are composed of combinations of two types of subunit, H and L (Arosio *et al.*, 1978). The expressed gene for the H-subunit is on chromosome 11 at 11q13 (Worwood *et al.*, 1985) and that for the L-subunit is on chromosome 19 at 19q13-ter. There are, however, multiple copies of the ferritin genes. The other H sequences (about 15 copies) on a number of chromosomes appear to be processed pseudogenes (i.e. without introns) with no evidence for expression (Costanzo *et al.*, 1986). The same applies to the other 'L' sequences found on chromosomes 19, 21 and X (Santoro *et al.*, 1986). For the expressed L-gene in the rat, there are three introns located between exons coding for the four major α-helical regions of the peptide sequences (Leibold and Munro, 1987). Human H (Costanzo *et al.*, 1986) and L (Santoro *et al.*, 1986) genes have a similar structure, although the introns differ in size and sequence. The mRNA for the human ferritin genes contains about 1.1 kb. The H-subunit is slightly larger than the L-subunit (178 and 174 amino acids, respectively), but on electrophoresis in polyacrylamide gels under denaturing conditions the apparent differences in relative molecular mass are rather greater (21 and 19 kDa, respectively). Human H and L sequences are only 55% homologous, whereas the homology between L-subunits and H-subunits from different species is of the order of 85% (Harrison and Arosio, 1996).

11.2 STRUCTURE

A ferritin subunit has five helices (A–E) and a long inter-helical loop L (Fig. 11.1). The loop L and the N-terminal residues are on the outside of the assembled molecule of 24 subunits. The C-terminal residues are within the shell. H and L chains adopt the same conformation within the molecule. A description of the three-dimensional structure of apoferritin will be found in the recent review by Harrison and Arosio (1996).

In human tissues (Worwood, 1990) H-rich isoferritins (pI 4.5–5.0) are found in heart muscle, red blood cells, lymphocytes, monocytes, also in HeLa cells and other, but not all, cultured cells. L-rich isoferritins are more basic (pI 5.0–5.7) and are found in liver, spleen and placenta. The pI of ferritin is not significantly affected by its iron content, which varies from tissue to tissue and with the tissue iron content.

Ferritin is purified from tissues by taking advantage of its ability to withstand a temperature of 75°C, by the high density of the iron-rich molecule (which allows concentration by ultra-centrifugation) and by crystallization in the presence of cadmium sulphate. However, it should be noted that, whereas ultracentrifugation tends to concentrate molecules rich in H-subunits, crystallization from cadmium sulphate solution tends to give a lower overall recovery and selects molecules rich in L-subunits (ICSH, 1984).

11.3 HAEMOSIDERIN

Ferritin is a soluble protein but is degraded to insoluble haemosiderin which accumulates in lysosomes. Both ferritin and haemosiderin provide a store of iron which is available for protein and haem synthesis. Normally much of the storage iron in the body (about 1 g in men and less in premenstrual women and children) is present as ferritin, but in iron overload the proportion present as haemosiderin increases. Purified preparations of ferritin always contain

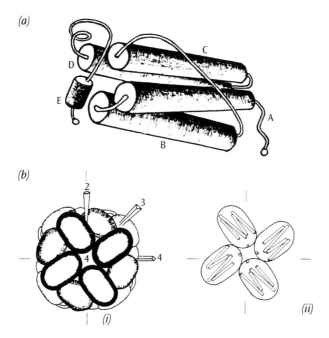

Fig. 11.1 *(a) Schematic drawing of a ferritin subunit showing the five helices A–E and the long inter-helix loop. The loop and the N-terminal residues (A) lie on the outside of the protein shell. Helix E runs from outside to inside. (b) The subunit arrangement in an apoferritin molecule viewed down a fourfold axis: (i) complete 24-subunit molecule showing symmetry axes; (ii) subunits related to a fourfold axis. The iron core occupies the inside of the protein shell. [From Banyard, S.H., Stammers, D.K. and Harrison, P.M. (1976) Electron density map of apoferritin at 2.8 Å resolution.* Nature **271**, *282–4, with permission.]*

a small proportion of molecules in the form of dimers, trimers and other oligomers (Williams and Harrison, 1968). These may be intermediates in the formation of haemosiderin. Andrews *et al.* (1987) isolated a soluble ferritin from iron-loaded rat liver lysosomes which contained a peptide of molecular mass 17.3 kDa which may be a precursor of insoluble haemosiderin. Although haemosiderin iron shows considerable chemical similarity to ferritin iron, there are significant differences between haemosiderins from primary and secondary iron-overloaded livers (Harrison and Arosio, 1996). Peptides extracted from preparations of haemosiderin have been found to react with antibodies to ferritin (Richter, 1984; Weir *et al.*, 1984).

11.4 REGULATION OF FERRITIN SYNTHESIS AND BREAKDOWN

Ferritin synthesis is induced by iron administration. Drysdale and Munro (1966) showed that the initial response of apoferritin synthesis to the administration of iron was by regulation of translation rather than transcription. This requires movement of stored mRNA from the ribonucleoprotein fraction (RNP) to the polysomes (Zahringer *et al.*, 1975), followed by an increased rate of translation of ferritin subunits. This response is the same for H- and L-subunits. However, after iron administration there is an eventual increase in the rate of transcription of the L-subunit gene. This causes the increased ratio of L- to H-subunits in ferritin synthesized after iron administration (White and Munro, 1988). The translational control mechanism has now been defined (Klausner *et al.*, 1993).

The 5′ untranslated region of the ferritin mRNA contains a sequence which forms a 'stem-loop' structure. This has been termed an 'iron response element' (IRE) (Fig. 11.2). Similar cytoplasmic proteins (IRP-1 and IRP-2) bind to the IRE in the absence of iron but are inactivated (IRP-1) or degraded (IRP-2) when iron supply increases (Hentze and Kuhn, 1996). Binding to mRNA prevents ferritin synthesis, but in the absence of binding, polysomes form and translation proceeds. IRP-1 is the iron-sulphur protein, aconitase, encoded by a gene on chromosome 9 (and functioning as a cytosolic aconitase in its iron-replete state). A model involving conformation changes which permit RNA binding has been proposed (Klausner *et al.*, 1993).

A related mechanism operates in reverse for the transferrin receptor. Here there are stem-loop sequences in the 3′ untranslated region and protein binding prevents degradation of mRNA. Hence iron deficiency enhances transferrin receptor synthesis. Translational regulation has also been described for erythroid ALA synthase and aconitase.

Although ferritin is generally considered to be an intracellular protein and most of the mRNA in the liver is associated with free ribosomes, there is evidence of synthesis of ferritin on membrane-bound polysomes (Campbell *et al.*, 1989). This finding may be of special relevance to the origin of plasma ferritin (see later).

The way in which ferritin is degraded remains largely a mystery. Studies on rat liver (Drysdale and Munro, 1966) indicated that the half-life of a ferritin molecule was about 72 hours and was extended by iron administration. The relationship between ferritin breakdown and formation of haemosiderin is unclear, as is the fate of the iron core after degradation of the protein shell.

11.5 FUNCTIONS RELATED TO IRON STORAGE

The major function of ferritin is clearly that of providing a store of iron which may be used for haem synthesis when required. *In vitro*, iron uptake requires an oxidizing agent and iron release a reducing agent (reviewed by Harrison and Arosio, 1996). Differences in the rate of iron uptake between apoferritins with varying proportions of H- and L-subunits were described by Wagstaff *et al.* (1978) who showed that H-rich isoferritins had the highest rate of iron uptake. Such isoferritins are found in cells which either have a high requirement of iron for haem synthesis (nucleated red cells, cardiac muscle) or do not appear to be involved in iron storage (e.g. lymphocytes). In the tissues where iron is stored, such as liver and spleen, the ferritin contains mostly L-subunits. Recent studies with recombinant H_{24} and L_{24} molecules have demonstrated that the ferroxidase activity of ferritin is a property of the H-subunit and that L_{24} molecules have little ability to catalyse iron uptake (Harrison and Arosio, 1996). The maturation of monocytes to macrophages *in vitro* is associated with loss of the more acidic isoferritins (Worrall and Worwood, 1991). Iron storage therefore seems to require ferritin rich in L-subunits.

11.6 CARCINO-FETAL FERRITINS

There has been considerable interest in specific 'carcino-fetal' ferritins (i.e. ferritins peculiar to fetal or malignant cells). This term originated in a paper by Alpert *et al.* (1973) who used it to describe the more acidic ferritins found in rat fetal liver and in some neoplastic tissues. It is now accepted that the variation in isoelectric point in ferritin molecules from various tissues

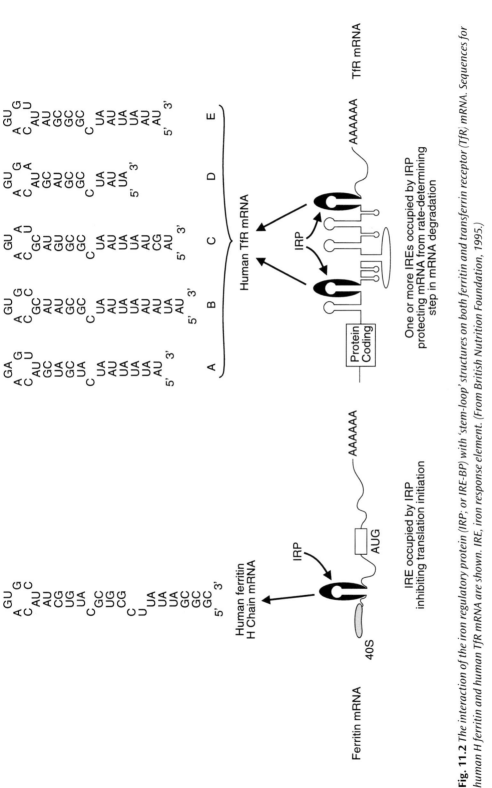

Fig. 11.2 *The interaction of the iron regulatory protein (IRP; or IRE-BP) with 'stem-loop' structures on both ferritin and transferrin receptor (TfR) mRNA. Sequences for human H ferritin and human TfR mRNA are shown. IRE, iron response element. (From British Nutrition Foundation, 1995.)*

is effectively explained in terms of the two-subunit model of Arosio *et al.* (1978). Furthermore, the wide distribution of 'acidic' isoferritins in human tissues denies the validity of the 'carcino-fetal' ferritin hypothesis. Later Moroz *et al.* (1985) took up the search for a carcino-fetal ferritin. They chose human placental ferritin (PLF) as a possible source of unique, antigenic ferritin structures which might be described as onco-fetal ferritin. They described the production and characterization of a monoclonal antibody (H9) which bound to placental but not liver or spleen ferritin. Furthermore, they showed that the protein recognized by this antibody was not composed of the H- and L-subunits found in liver and spleen but was made up of a single subunit of relative molecular mass 43 kDa (for a review see Moroz and Bessler, 1989). However, others have not observed this subunit in human placental ferritin (Konijn *et al.*, 1985).

The placental-specific monoclonal antibody detected the 43 kDa subunit in cultured cells derived from a breast tumour, but not normal breast epithelium or monocytes from normal subjects. The K562 human leukaemia cell was also shown to express a larger mRNA than H ferritin mRNA (corresponding to the 43 kDa peptide), with expression declining during differentiation of the cells. Furthermore, this species of mRNA was found in Con-A-activated T-cells but not in T-cells which have not been so activated (Moroz *et al.*, 1989).

11.7 EFFECT OF FERRITIN ON T-LYMPHOCYTES

Earlier studies of Moroz *et al.* (1977) showed that lymphocytes isolated from patients with breast cancer or Hodgkin's disease have ferritin bound to the cell membrane. This ferritin, which could be removed by incubation with Levamisole or fetal calf serum, inhibited the formation of sheep red blood cell rosettes. This ferritin was shown to be acidic and to bind the specific placental monoclonal antibody (M-H9).

Acidic isoferritins have also been shown to have an immunosuppressive effect in other *in vitro* systems (Moroz and Bessler, 1989): reactivity in mixed lymphocyte culture, blastogenic response to mitogens, T-lymphocyte transformation by phytohaemagglutinin and concanavalin A.

The percentage of ferritin-bearing lymphocytes has been measured in order to investigate this as a marker for early breast cancer. However, there did not appear to be a simple relationship between the percentage of lymphocytes with surface ferritin and the histopathological type of a tumour (benign, premalignant, stage I, II, III or IV). Determination of placental type isoferritin concentrations in serum has also been reported for patients with Hodgkin's disease, non-Hodgkin's lymphoma, myeloma and chronic lymphocytic leukaemia. Higher values were found in patients with Hodgkin's disease and non-Hodgkin's lymphoma compared with patients with myeloma, or chronic lymphocytic leukaemia and normal subjects. However, the specificity of the assay for particular tumours has not been established and similar changes in concentration are seen if serum ferritin is determined with antibodies to spleen or liver ferritin.

The changes in serum levels during pregnancy have led Maymon and Moroz (1996) to propose that PLF is also an immunoregulatory cytokine playing an important role in the development of the immunosuppression of pregnancy which prevents maternal rejection of the implanted conceptus. Low levels of PLF in pregnancy may indicate abnormal gestation. How plasma levels relate to conventional serum ferritin concentrations is not clear and the structural relationship between PLF and other isoferritins containing H- and L-subunits has not been established.

11.8 FERRITIN AS A REGULATOR OF ERYTHROPOIESIS

The first indication of a role of ferritin in the regulation of haemopoiesis not apparently related to iron storage was provided by Broxmeyer *et al.* (1981), who showed that the protein responsible for a 'leukaemia-associated inhibitory activity' (LIA) was an acidic isoferritin. This protein fraction, and an acidic isoferritin preparation from the spleen of a patient with chronic myeloid leukaemia, suppressed colony formation *in vitro* for CFU-GM, BFU-E and CFU-GEMM progenitor cells from the marrows of normal donors but was ineffective in marrow or blood from patients with acute leukaemia, myelodysplasia and some other haematological disorders. The link between LIA and acidic or 'H-subunit-rich' isoferritins was established by comparison with the purified ferritin preparation described above and by the use of polyclonal and monoclonal antibodies to ferritin to reverse the inhibitory effects.

Sala *et al.* (1986) were unable to confirm the effects described by Broxmeyer *et al.* using purified preparations of H-subunit-rich ferritins. The original ferritin preparation from the spleen of a patient with chronic myeloid leukaemia was acidic (pI approx. 4.7) and able to bind to concanavalin A, suggesting that it was a glycoprotein. Later analysis of this preparation showed that the ferritin content determined immunologically was only a fraction of the assigned protein concentration (Sala *et al.*, 1986). The original preparation showed inhibitory activity at concentrations as low as 10^{-18} mol/L. However, more recent studies with recombinant H_{24} molecules which are not glycosylated (Broxmeyer *et al.*, 1986) have activity at higher concentrations of 10^{-10}–10^{-11} mol/L. Either glycosylation is essential for activity or molecules containing both H- and L-subunits are required.

In vitro ferritin acts on progenitors which are in the DNA synthesis (S) phase of the cell cycle (reviewed by Broxmeyer, 1992). Acidic isoferritins appear to have a direct action on progenitor cells as inhibition is apparent even with highly purified progenitors.

In normal bone marrow, the cells which release acidic isoferritins appear to be mononuclear phagocytes – monocytes and macrophages. Monocytes are more likely to be the source of acidic isoferritins, as macrophages appear to synthesize ferritin containing more L-subunits (see above). Further proof of the biological significance of the inhibitory activity of acidic isoferritin comes from studies in which recombinant human H_{24} ferritin was injected into mice causing reduction of proliferative rates of CFU-GM, BFU-E and CFU-GEMM in both marrow and spleen in a dose-dependent, time-related and reversible way. Recombinant human L ferritin did not produce these effects.

A number of questions about the mode of action of acidic isoferritins remain:

- *Are the effects purely local?* Concentrations of acidic isoferritin in serum, determined with monoclonal antibodies to H-rich isoferritin, are low (below the limit of detection of about 1 µg/L or 2×10^{-12} mol/L). This applies to serum from patients with cancer as well as from normal subjects (see later). Furthermore, there is evidence of specific binding proteins in human serum which bind ferritin molecules containing H-subunits (Covell *et al.*, 1984; Bellotti *et al.*, 1987) and presumably cause rapid elimination of such molecules from the circulation. Inhibitory activity in bone marrow may therefore require release from cells in close proximity to the target cells.
- *Is the inhibitory action related to ferritin receptors on progenitor cells?* Receptors for H-rich isoferritins have been described in studies of a number of haematopoietic cell lines (Covell and Cook, 1988; Fargion *et al.*, 1988). Receptors for L-rich isoferritins have so far only been identified on hepatocytes (Adams *et al.*, 1988).
- *Is the inhibition dependent on iron?* Recombinant H-ferritins lacking ferroxidase activity lack myelosuppressive activity (Broxmeyer, 1992) and Broxmeyer has suggested that by

catalysing the conversion of ferrous to ferric iron, H-ferritin might prevent the uptake of transferrin iron by cells. It is possible that it is the iron carried by the ferritin which is important, as uptake of iron as well as its release (Gutteridge *et al.*, 1983; Henley and Worwood, 1991) may cause hydroxyl ion formation and free radical generation.

11.9 FERRITIN IN INFLAMMATION, INFECTION AND OTHER CHRONIC DISORDERS

Inflammation, infection, surgery and malignancy are often associated with anaemia. As well as anaemia, there may be low serum Fe concentration and evidence of increased levels of storage Fe in the bone marrow (Konijn and Hershko, 1989). Inflammation leads to the release of interleukin 1β (IL-1β) and other cytokines. IL-1β stimulates ferritin synthesis (Rogers, 1996). The stimulation of apoferritin synthesis traps Fe in phagocytic cells. This leads to a reduced supply of Fe to the bone marrow.

11.10 PLASMA (SERUM) FERRITIN

Interest in plasma ferritin began in the 1940s when ferritin was first detected by assaying vasodepressor activity in a rat meso-appendix preparation (Shorr, 1956). In 1956, Reissman and Dietrich assayed ferritin directly by precipitation with a rabbit anti-human ferritin, followed by measurement of the amount of iron in the precipitate. Ferritin iron was detectable in serum from patients with hepatic necrosis, but not normal sera or in serum from patients with iron overload but without hepatic necrosis. However, the introduction of a sensitive immunoradiometric assay (Addison *et al.*, 1972) revealed not only the presence of ferritin in normal serum but also a striking relationship between serum ferritin concentration and the amount of storage iron in the body (Walters *et al.*, 1973). This relationship is the reason for the widespread use of the serum ferritin assay in the diagnosis of iron deficiency or overload.

11.10.1 Clinical use – relationship with storage iron levels

As a detailed review is available (Worwood, 1982) the clinical use of the assay will only be summarized here. In non-anaemic adults, serum ferritin concentrations are within the range 15–300 µg/L (Table 11.1). Mean values are lower in women before the menopause than in men, reflecting the lower iron stores caused by the iron losses of menstruation and childbirth. Concentrations in infants, children and adolescents are summarized in Table 11.2. The changes in serum ferritin concentration during development from birth to old age reflect changes in the level of storage iron in the tissue (Worwood, 1982).

In patients with iron deficiency anaemia, serum ferritin concentrations are almost always less than 15 µg/L. Conversely, serum ferritin concentrations are high in patients with iron overload. It should be noted that when screening for inherited (or idiopathic) haemochromatosis, it is essential to measure the percentage saturation of transferrin, as this rises early in the development of iron overload, often before a significant rise in serum ferritin concentration occurs (Edwards and Kushner, 1993). Unfortunately a simple relationship between tissue iron concentration and serum ferritin concentration is rarely found in hospital patients, as there are other causes of ferritinaemia apart from raised iron stores.

Table 11.1   *Serum ferritin concentrations (µg/L) in adults*

Age (years)	Men			Women		
	No.	Mean	5–95%	No.	Mean	5–95%
18–24	107	80	15–223	96	30	5–73
25–34	211	108	21–291	226	38	5–95
35–44	202	120	21–328	221	38	5–108
45–54	166	139	21–395	177	60	5–217
55–64	140	143	22–349	162	74	12–199
65–74	127	140	12–374	138	91	7–321
75+	80	110	10–309	99	77	6–209
Total	1033	121	16–328	1119	56	5–170

Source: White *et al.* (1993). Subjects being treated with drugs for iron deficiency (*n* = 26) were included.
For other surveys of populations in North America and Europe, see Cook *et al.* (1976), Finch *et al.* (1977), Jacobs and Worwood (1975), Milman *et al.* (1986), Valberg *et al.* (1976) and Custer *et al.* (1995).

11.10.2 Liver damage

The high concentration of ferritin in the liver means that damage leads to release of ferritin into the circulation. In the presence of liver damage it is safe to assume that a serum ferritin concentration in the normal range rules out any elevation of storage iron levels. However, confirmation that iron overload is the cause of an elevated serum ferritin concentration will require careful consideration of the clinical history and liver function tests.

11.10.3 Inflammation and infection

In hospital patients, anaemia is often secondary to infection, inflammation or malignancy. The serum iron concentration is usually low but the transferrin concentration (or total iron binding capacity) will be either normal or depressed. The diversion of iron from circulating haemoglobin to tissue ferritin and haemosiderin means that serum ferritin will generally be higher than in normal subjects, but a low serum ferritin concentration is a reliable indicator of depleted iron stores.

Distinguishing between patients with the anaemia of chronic disease who have no storage Fe and those who have apparently adequate amounts of storage Fe has been a problem for many years. Many clinical studies have demonstrated that patients with the anaemia of chronic disease, with no stainable Fe in the bone marrow, may have serum ferritin concentrations considerably in excess of 15 µg/L, and there has been much debate (Witte, 1991) about the practical application of the serum ferritin assay in this situation. Values of less than 15 µg/L indicate the absence of storage Fe and values of greater than 100 µg/L indicate the presence of storage Fe. It is the 'grey' area from 15 to 100 µg/L which is difficult to interpret. Although it would seem logical to combine the assay of serum ferritin with a measure of disease severity such as the erythrocyte sedimentation rate or C-reactive protein, this approach does not appear to be significantly better than measuring serum ferritin concentration on its own (Coenen *et al.*, 1991). Ferguson *et al.* (1992) have suggested that in patients with chronic disease, only those with an absence of storage Fe have raised levels of the serum transferrin receptor, and this has now been confirmed (Punnonen *et al.*, 1997). Various algorithms involving measurement of serum ferritin concentration, transferrin saturation, mean cell volume (MCV) and mean cell haemoglobin (MCH) have been proposed. In general, these

Table 11.2 *Serum ferritin concentrations (µg/L) in infants, children and adolescents*

No. of children	Age	Population	Selection	Mean	Range	Reference
46	0.5 months	Helsinki	Non–anaemic	238	90–628	Saarinen and Siimes (1978)
46	1 month	Helsinki	Non–anaemic	240	144–399	Saarinen and Siimes (1978)
47	2 months	Helsinki	Non–anaemic	194	87–430	Saarinen and Siimes (1978)
40	4 months	Helsinki	Non–anaemic	91	37–223	Saarinen and Siimes (1978)
514	0.5–15 years	San Francisco	Non–anaemic	30[a]	7–142	Siimes *et al.* (1974)
323	5–11 years	Washington	Low income families	21[a]	10–45[d]	Cook *et al.* (1976)
117	5–9 years	Nutrition Canada Survey	Random	15[b]	2–107[e]	Valberg *et al.* (1976)
335	6–11 years	Denmark	Random, urban	29[a]	12–67[c]	Milman and Kaas Ibsen (1984)
251 12–18 years						
126 male	12–18 years	Washington	Low income families	23[a]	10–63[d]	Cook *et al.* (1976)
125 female				21[a]	6–48[d]	
204 10–19 years						
98 male	10–19 years	Nutrition Canada Survey	Random	18[b]	3–125[e]	Valberg *et al.* (1976)
106 female				17[b]	2–116[e]	
574 12–17 years						
269 male	12–17 years	Denmark	Random, urban	28[a]	11–68[c]	Milman and Ibsen (1984)
305 female				25[a]	6–65[c]	

[a]Median.
[b]Geometric mean.
[c]5–95% interval in median values for ages 6–11 months.
[d]10–90 percentile.
[e]Confidence interval.
[f]There were no significant differences.

appear to offer little improvement on a simple determination of serum ferritin concentration (see Mulherin *et al.*, 1996). This may be because there is direct inhibition of erythropoiesis by IL-1β as well as the effect of the reduced plasma iron concentration resulting from stimulation of apoferritin synthesis.

11.10.4 Serum ferritin and malignancy

High concentrations of ferritin are seen in most patients with pancreatic carcinoma, lung cancer, hepatoma and neuroblastoma, although in most cases of cancer of the oesophagus, stomach and colon, serum ferritin concentrations are within the normal range. In breast cancer, concentrations are usually raised in patients with metastatic disease, but the assay has not proved to be useful in predicting development of metastasis. Patients presenting with acute leukaemia generally have elevated serum ferritin concentrations, but patients with chronic leukaemia do not necessarily have elevated concentrations. In Hodgkin's disease, concentrations increase with the stage of disease but are not related to the histological type of disease.

The concept of carcino-fetal ferritin has been discussed and a logical extension of the concept is to search for changes in the immunological properties of serum ferritin in order to detect malignant disease or monitor the effect of therapy. A number of assays using acidic isoferritins from HeLa cells (Hazard and Drysdale, 1977; Jones and Worwood, 1978; Hann *et al.*, 1988) or heart ferritin (Jones and Worwood, 1978; Niitsu *et al.*, 1980) have been described and applied to serum from patients with cancer. The results have been inconsistent but later studies using monoclonal antibody (Cavanna *et al.*, 1983) confirm some of the studies with polyclonal antisera and indicate that concentrations of H-rich isoferritin in serum are very low compared with L-rich isoferritins even in patients with cancer. It is likely that high concentrations of ferritin in the serum in malignancy are due to increases in the level of storage iron, to liver damage or to inflammation, as well as direct release from the tumour. Whatever the cause, the result is an elevation of L-rich isoferrritin concentration in the serum rather than accumulation of 'tumour-specific' isoferritins.

11.11 BIOCHEMISTRY AND PHYSIOLOGY OF PLASMA FERRITIN

Immunologically, plasma ferritin resembles liver or spleen ferritin and is recognized by polyclonal or monoclonal antibodies raised against these ferritins (see above). In patients with iron overload, plasma ferritin has a relatively low iron content (0.02–0.07 μg Fe/μg protein in purified preparations [Worwood *et al.*, 1976; Cragg *et al.*, 1981] or a mean of 0.06 μg Fe/μg protein by immunoprecipitation) (Pootrakul *et al.*, 1988). Purified horse serum ferritin had an iron content of < 0.01 μg Fe/μg protein (Linder *et al.*, 1996). In the liver and spleen of patients with iron overload, the iron content of ferritin is > 0.2 μg Fe/μg protein. Despite these findings, several recent papers have indicated that serum ferritin has a much higher iron content. ten Kate *et al.* (1997) purified ferritin by immunochemical precipitation and measured the iron content by atomic absorption spectrophotometry. They found a mean iron saturation of ferritin of 24% in normal serum (0.13 μg Fe/μg protein). They point out that the extensive purification used in earlier studies would lead to loss of iron, although this is unlikely, unless reducing agents were present in the buffers used. Herbert *et al.* (1997) claim that measurement of serum ferritin iron by a similar procedure provides an accurate assessment of the whole range of human body iron status unconfounded by inflammation. Recently, Nielsen *et al.* (2000) employed the method of ten Cate *et al.* (1997) to determine the iron content of serum ferritin from patients with iron overload and tissue damage. The iron saturation was about 5% and they found that the assay of ferritin iron was of little benefit in the diagnosis of iron overload. It must be pointed out that liver damage leads to the release of iron-rich ferritin (Reissmann and Dietrich, 1956). Another consideration is that in a normal subject with a serum iron concentration of 20 µmol/L and a serum ferritin concentration of 100 µg/L (25% saturation of iron) the ferritin iron concentration is only 1% of the transferrin iron concentration. Clearly, specific antibodies and effective washing of the immuno-precipitate would be essential.

Yamanishi et al. (1996) concluded that ferritin iron may interfere with the ICSH recom-mended method for serum iron determination. Their results indicate ferritin iron concen-trations from 0.02 to 0.04 µg Fe/µg ferritin protein in serum samples with ferritin concentrations greater than 2000 µg/L. These results do not support the high values found by ten Cate et al. (1997).

On isoelectric focusing, both native and purified serum ferritin contain a wide range of isoferritins covering the pI range found in human tissues (McKeering et al., 1976; Worwood et al., 1976), yet on anion exchange chromatography, serum ferritin is apparently a relatively basic isoferritin (Worwood et al., 1976). The reason for this discrepancy and the heterogeneity on isoelectric focusing appears to be glycosylation. In normal serum, about 60% of ferritin binds to concanavalin A (Worwood et al., 1979) whereas tissue ferritins do not bind. Incubation with neuraminidase converts the acidic ferritins of serum to the more basic isoferritins, but the pI of acidic heart ferritin is unaffected (Cragg et al., 1980). A carbohydrate containing G-subunit in addition to the H- and L-subunits has also been identified in purified preparations of serum ferritin (Cragg et al., 1981; Santambrogio et al.,1987).

These findings suggest that some ferritin may enter the circulation by secretion (Campbell et al., 1989) rather than release from damaged cells (Fig. 11.3). Secreted ferritin may originate from phagocytic cells degrading haemoglobin. When there is tissue damage, direct release of cytosolic ferritin through damaged cell membranes becomes important. In patients with ferritinaemia resulting from necrosis of the liver, the plasma ferritin shows reduced binding to concanavalin A.

Another explanation for the differences between plasma and tissue ferritins may be differential clearance from the circulation. $[^{131}I]$-labelled plasma ferritin was removed only slowly ($T_{1/2} < 24$ hours) from the plasma after intravenous injection into normal subjects (Worwood et al., 1982), but $[^{131}I]$-labelled spleen ferritin was cleared very rapidly ($T_{1/2} \sim 9$ minutes) (Cragg et al., 1983). Such rapid clearance may be due to interaction with ferritin receptors on hepatocytes (Adams et al., 1988) which appear to have a higher affinity for liver ferritin than serum ferritin, at least in the rat. Rapid clearance may also be initiated by inter-action with ferritin-binding proteins in the plasma (Covell et al., 1984; Belloti et al., 1987; Santambrogio et al., 1989). Many isoferritins may be released into the plasma but those which normally accumulate are L_{24} molecules and glycosylated molecules which are rich in L-subunits and again contain little iron. The L_{24} molecules take up iron slowly in vitro and have been termed 'natural apoferritin' by Arosio et al. (1977) and may accumulate because clearance by receptors or interaction with binding proteins requires at least some H-subunits. The glycosylated protein may have little opportunity to acquire iron during secretion (see Fig. 11.3).

11.12 EXCEEDINGLY HIGH SERUM FERRITIN CONCENTRATIONS

The factors controlling plasma ferritin concentrations are synthesis, release from cells and

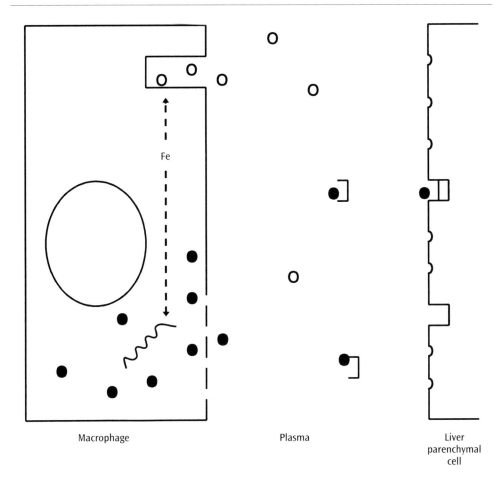

Fig. 11.3 *Cytosolic ferritin (•) is released directly from damaged cell membranes into plasma or secreted (top) after synthesis on membrane-bound polysomes and glycosylation (o). In the circulation, non-glycosylated ferritin may interact with ferritin-binding proteins followed by removal of the complex from the circulation. Many cells also carry ferritin receptors presumably for both secreted ferritin and cytosolic ferritin (see text). Injection of spleen ferritin into the circulation in humans is followed by rapid uptake by the liver.*

clearance from the plasma. There are no instances yet known where very high ferritin concentrations are due to abnormalities in ferritin clearance, but abnormalities in both synthesis and release occur.

In iron overload, serum ferritin concentrations are unlikely to exceed 4000 µg/L in the absence of concomitant liver damage (Worwood, 1980) but the stimulation of synthesis by a combination of iron and cytokines can lead to ferritin concentrations > 20 000 µg/L in adult-onset Still's disease (Ota *et al.*, 1987). In the reactive haemophagocytic syndrome there is inappropriate activation of monocytes leading to haemophagocytosis and cytokine release. Ferritin concentrations of up to 400 000 µg/L have been reported in children (Esumi *et al.*, 1988) and adults (Koduri *et al.*, 1995).

Patients with AIDS may also have the reactive haemophagocytosis syndrome and high concentrations may also occur in AIDS patients with disseminated histoplasmosis (Kirn *et al.*, 1995a,b). Tissue damage has already been discussed in connection with liver necrosis and also leads to ferritin concentrations in excess of 50 000 µg/L (Prieto *et al.*, 1975).

11.13 HIGH SERUM FERRITIN CONCENTRATIONS AND CONGENITAL CATARACT

An interesting cause of elevated ferritin concentration in the absence of iron overload is that associated with inherited cataract formation. In has now been demonstrated that there is a mutation in the 'stem loop' structure of the ferritin L-subunit which leads to synthesis of the 'L' subunit of ferritin in the tissues which is no longer regulated by iron concentration (Beaumont et al., 1995; Cazzola et al., 1997). This causes elevated serum ferritin concentrations (~ 1000 µg/L) in the absence of iron overload.

11.14 RED CELL FERRITIN AND ITS DIAGNOSTIC USE

The ferritin in the circulating erythrocyte is but a tiny residue of that in its nucleated precursors in the bone marrow. Normal erythroblasts contain ferritin which is immunologically more similar to heart than liver ferritin (i.e. ferritin rich in H-subunits) and mean concentrations are about 10 fg ferritin protein/cell (Hodgetts et al., 1986). Concentrations decline throughout maturation and only about 10 ag/cell (10^{-18} g/cell) remains in the erythrocyte (measured with antibodies to L-ferritin), with somewhat higher levels detected with antibodies to H-type ferritin (Cazzola et al., 1983; Peters et al., 1983). Red cell ferritin concentrations have generally been measured with antibodies to L-ferritin and reflect the iron supply to the erythroid marrow. Concentrations tend to vary inversely with red cell protoporphyrin levels (Cazzola et al., 1983). Thus, in patients with rheumatoid arthritis and anaemia, low concentrations are found in those with microcytosis and low serum iron concentrations regardless of the serum ferritin levels (Davidson et al., 1984). Red cell ferritin levels do not therefore necessarily indicate levels of storage iron. Red cell ferritin levels may be useful in the differential diagnosis of hereditary haemochromatosis from alcoholic liver disease (van der Weyden et al., 1983) and possibly in distinguishing heterozygotes for haemochromatosis from normal subjects (Cazzola et al., 1983). Van der Weyden et al. (1983) found that the mean red cell ferritin content in patients with untreated inherited haemochromatosis was about 70 times the normal mean and fell during phlebotomy. In some patients, levels were still elevated after phlebotomy even when serum ferritin concentrations were within the normal range. This was shown to reflect liver parenchymal cell iron concentrations which were still elevated. Van der Weyden et al. (1983) showed that the ratio of red cell ferritin (ag/cell) to serum ferritin (µg/L) was about 0.5 in hereditary haemochromatosis but only 0.03 in patients with alcoholic cirrhosis, thus clearly separating the two conditions. There may also be advantages over the assay of serum ferritin in determining iron stores in patients with liver damage, as red cell ferritin levels should not be greatly influenced by the release of ferritin from damaged liver cells. However, high levels of red cell ferritin are also found in thalassaemia (Piperno et al., 1984; van der Weyden et al., 1989), megaloblastic anaemia (van der Weyden and Fong, 1984) and myelodysplastic syndromes (Peters et al., 1983), presumably indicating a disturbance of erythroid iron metabolism in these conditions.

Despite these specific, diagnostic advantages (Cazzola and Ascari, 1986) the assay of red cell ferritin has seen little routine application. This is because it is necessary to have fresh blood in order to prepare red cells free of white cells (which have much higher ferritin levels).

11.15 ASSAY OF SERUM FERRITIN

The first reliable method was an immunoradiometric assay (Addison *et al.*, 1972) in which excess radiolabelled antibody reacts with ferritin and the excess antibody is removed with an immunoadsorbent. This assay was replaced by the two-site immunoradiometric assay (Miles *et al.*, 1974). Since then the principle of the two-site immunoradiometric assay has been extended to include enzyme, fluorescent or chemiluminescent labels. Many commercial kits are available. Ferritin is one of the options in the latest generation of automated immunoassay analysers (both batch and random access). A simple two-site enzyme-linked assay is described here and later some criteria for evaluating commercial analysers will be given.

11.16 AN ENZYME IMMUNOASSAY FOR FERRITIN

The technique is based on well-known principles (Flowers *et al.*, 1986) and is one developed by the International Committee for Standardization in Haematology, Expert Panel on Iron (Worwood *et al.*, 1991). Some information on the preparation of ferritin and antibodies to ferritin is included below but such reagents are now available commercially.

11.16.1 Ferritin

Ferritin is most readily prepared from iron-loaded, human liver or spleen obtained at operation (spleen) or postmortem. The agreement of the patient or the patient's relatives must be obtained. Evidence of lack of infection with HIV or hepatitis virus is essential. Tissue should be obtained as soon as possible after death and may be stored at 20°C for 1 year. Ferritin is purified by methods which exploit its stability at 75°C followed by chromatography and either ultracentrifugation or precipitation from cadmium sulphate solution. Purity should be assessed by polyacrylamide gel electrophoresis and the protein content determined. Human ferritin may be stored in solution at 4°C, at 1–4 mg protein/mL, in the presence of sodium azide as a preservative, for up to 5 years. Purified ferritin solutions must not be frozen as this causes denaturation. Full details of these methods are given in Worwood (1980).

11.16.2 Antibodies to human ferritin

High affinity antibodies to human liver or spleen ferritin are suitable (Worwood, 1980). Polyclonal antibodies may be raised in rabbits or sheep by conventional methods and the titre checked by precipitation with human ferritin. An IgG-enriched fraction of antiserum obtained by precipitation with sodium sulphate is required for labelling with enzyme. Monoclonal antibodies which are specific for 'L' subunit-rich ferritin (liver or spleen ferritin) are also suitable and may be prepared by standard methods. Store antibody preparations in water at 10 mg protein/mL at 20°C. [Suitable rabbit antihuman ferritin antibodies (including a preparation labelled with horseradish peroxidase) may be obtained from Dako Ltd, High Wycombe, Bucks, UK.]

11.16.3 Conjugation of antiferritin IgG preparation to horseradish peroxidase

This is carried out by standard methods (see, for example, Wilson and Nakane, 1978). The conjugate should be stored in glycerol solution (30%) at 4°C.

11.16.4 Assay reagents

Buffer A Phosphate-buffered saline, pH 7.2, containing 0.05% Tween 20. A 10 times concentrated (1.5 mol/L) stock solution is prepared by dissolving sodium chloride, 80 g; potassium chloride, 2 g; anhydrous disodium phosphate, 11.5 g and anhydrous potassium phosphate (KH_2PO_4) in l L of water. This may be stored at room temperature. Buffer A is prepared adding 0.5 mL of Tween 20 and may be stored at 4°C for up to 2 weeks.

Buffer B This is prepared by dissolving 0.5 g of bovine serum albumin fraction V (BSA) in 100 mL of buffer A and may be stored at 4°C for 1 week.

Buffer C Carbonate buffer, 0.05 mol/L, pH 9.6, is prepared by dissolving sodium carbonate, 1.59 g, and sodium bicarbonate, 2.93 g, in 1 L of water and may be stored at room temperature for one month.

Buffer D Citrate phosphate buffer, 0.15 mol/L, pH 5.0. Citric acid monohydrate (21 g) is dissolved in 1 L of water and stored at 4°C. Anhydrous disodium phosphate (28.4 g) is dissolved in 1 L of water and stored at room temperature. Buffer D is prepared on the day of assay by mixing 49 mL of citric acid solution with 51 mL of phosphate solution.

Substrate solution This is prepared immediately before use by adding 9 µL of hydrogen peroxide, 30%, to 25 mL of buffer and mixing well. Add one 10 mg tablet of o-phenylenediamine dihydrochloride (Sigma) and mix. The powdered reagent should be avoided, as it may be carcinogenic. Twenty-five millilitres is sufficient for one plate.

11.16.5 Preparation and storage of a standard ferritin solution

Dilute a solution of human ferritin to approximately 200 µg/mL in water. Measure the protein concentration as described by Worwood (1980) after diluting further to 20–50 µg/mL. Then dilute the ferritin solution (approx. 200 µg/mL) to a concentration of 10 µg/mL in 0.05 mol/L sodium barbitone solution containing 0.1 mol/L NaCl, 0.02% NaN_3, bovine serum albumin (5 g/L) and adjusted to pH 8.0 with 5 mol/L HCl. Deliver 200 µL into small plastic tubes, cap tightly and store at 4°C for up to 1 year. For use, dilute in buffer B to 200 µg/L, then prepare a range of standard solutions between 0.2 and 20 µg/L. Calibrate this working standard against the third WHO standard for the assay of serum ferritin (reagent 94/578, recombinant human ferritin). [Available from National Institute for Biological Standards and Control (NIBSC), South Mimms, Herts EN6 3QG, UK.]

11.16.6 Coating of plates

Ninety-six-well microtitre plates for immunoassay are required (e.g. Immuno Plate II, Nunc or Immulon-II, Dynatech Laboratories; plate seals are also available). Coat the plates by adding to each well 200 µL of antiferritin IgG preparation diluted to 2 µg/mL in buffer C. Seal the plate and leave overnight at 4°C. On the following day, empty the wells by sharply inverting the plate and drain by tapping briefly on paper and towels and standing upside down on the towels. Block unreacted sites by adding 200 µL of 0.5% (w/v) bovine serum albumin in buffer C. After 30 minutes at room temperature, wash each plate three times by filling each well with buffer A (using a syringe and needle) and emptying and draining as described above.

11.16.7 Samples

Collect venous blood and separate the serum. Samples may be stored at 4°C for 1 week or for 2 years at −20°C. Plasma is also suitable, collected in heparin or EDTA, in this assay but not in all systems. For assay, dilute 50 µL of serum to 1 mL with buffer B. Further dilutions may be made in the same buffer if required.

11.16.8 Assay procedure

The use of a multi-channel pipette for rapid addition of solutions is recommended. Standards and sera, in duplicate, should be added to each plate within 20 minutes. Automation of the dilution, addition and washing steps is desirable and standard microtitre plate systems are suitable.

Add 200 µL of standard solution or diluted serum to each well. Cover the plate and leave at room temperature on a draught-free bench away from direct sunlight for 2 hours. Empty the wells by sharply inverting the plate and dry by draining on paper towels. Wash three times by filling each well with buffer A using a syringe and needle, leaving for 1 minute at room temperature and draining as described above.

Dilute the conjugate in 1% bovine serum albumin in buffer A. The optimal dilution (of the order of 10 000 times) must be ascertained. Add 200 µL of diluted horseradish peroxidase conjugate to each well and leave the covered plate for a further 1 hour at room temperature. Wash three times with buffer A. Add 200 µL of substrate solution to each well. Incubate the plate for 30 minutes in the dark. Stop the reaction by adding 50 µL of 5 mol/L sulphuric acid to each well. Read the absorbance at 492 nm within 30 minutes using an automatic plate reader.

11.16.9 Calculation of results

Calculate the mean absorbance for each point on the standard curve and plot against ferritin concentration using semilogarithmic paper. Read concentrations for the test sera from this curve. If using a computer program for result calculation, the log-logit plot provides a linear dose–response. For serum ferritin concentrations > 200 µg/L, re-assay at a dilution of 100 times or greater. Control sera should be included in each assay.

11.16.10 Pitfalls

There are a number of theoretical and practical problems associated with the assay of serum ferritin. In theory, there may be problems because ferritin consists of a family of isoferritins which differ in subunit composition and in isoelectric point and it is possible to generate specific antibodies which recognize particular isoferritins (see above). In practice, this has not been a problem because in general the ferritin found circulating in the plasma is similar to the L-rich ferritin found in liver or spleen (see earlier). A more practical concern is the very wide range of ferritin concentrations which can be encountered in serum. In hospital patients, ferritin concentrations range from < 1 μg/L in some patients with iron deficiency anaemia to in excess of 100 000 μg/L in patients with necrosis of the liver. The early two site immuno-radiometric assays suffered from a problem called the 'high-dose hook' effect. In this situation, very high ferritin concentrations could give readings in the lower part of the standard curve. In order to ensure that results were not artefactually low due to the high-dose hook effect, it was necessary to assay at two dilutions and to show that increasing the dilution reduced the apparent ferritin concentration.

Interference by non-ferritin proteins in serum may occur with any method, but particularly with labelled antibody assays. Serum proteins may inhibit the binding of ferritin to the solid phase when compared with the binding in buffer solution alone. Such an effect may be avoided by diluting the standards in a buffer containing a suitable serum or by diluting serum samples as much as possible. For example, for two-site immunoradiometric assays, the sample may be diluted 20 times with buffer while the standards are prepared in 5% normal rabbit serum (if antibodies have been raised in rabbits) in buffer. Further dilutions of the sera are carried out with this solution. Some methods give low recoveries of ferritin from plasma collected in EDTA and the use of the plasma samples should therefore be investigated carefully.

Another problem has been that of anti-animal antibodies found in some human serum. These can interfere with the assay of serum ferritin, giving spuriously high ferritin concentrations (Boscato and Stuart, 1988).

11.16.11 Standardization

The serum ferritin assay is often applied to epidemiological surveys in which the iron status of populations is examined. For such assays to be comparable, it is important that there is a common standard and that the assays are calibrated against this. The first WHO standard for the assay of serum ferritin was introduced in 1990 (reagent 80/602), and was replaced by the second international standard in 1993 (reagent 80/578). A third international standard, which is a recombinant ferritin, is just being made available (reagent 94/572). The introduction of an international standard has led to considerable improvements in the standardization of ferritin assay (ICSH, 1984), but there are still differences in reference ranges (Dawson *et al.*, 1992) and problems with comparisons with longitudinal studies (Looker *et al.*, 1991). Discrepancies remain in the definition of normal ranges. Some manufacturers define a normal range as the ferritin concentrations found in unselected, apparently normal subjects. However, a proportion of the normal population have almost no storage iron without being anaemic, particularly young women, and a smaller proportion will be anaemic. The 'normal range' in young females will thus include ferritin concentrations found in iron deficiency. This confusion between 'normality' and iron deficiency causes difficulties in interpretation of ferritin concentrations (Ellis *et al.*, 1997).

Most current commercial assay systems are free from problems of protein interference or high-dose hook effects and are well standardized (Ellis *et al.*, 1997; Worwood and Ellis, 2000), but these points should be investigated before adopting a system for routine use in the clinical laboratory.

REFERENCES

Adams, P.C., Powell, L.W. and Halliday, J.W. (1988) Isolation of a human hepatic ferritin receptor. *Hepatology* **8**, 719–21.

Addison, G.M., Beamish, M.R., Hales, C.N. *et al.* (1972) An immunoradiometric assay for ferritin in the serum of normal subjects and patients with iron deficiency and iron overload. *J. Clin. Pathol.* **25**, 326–29.

Alpert, E., Coston, R.L. and Drysdale, J.W. (1973) Carcino-foetal human liver ferritins. *Nature* **242**, 194–6.

Andrews, S.C., Treffry, A. and Harrison, P.M. (1987) Siderosomal ferritin. The missing link between ferritin and haemosiderin? *Biochem. J.* **245**, 439–46.

Arosio, P., Yokota, M. and Drysdale, J.W. (1977) Characterization of serum ferritin in iron overload: possible identity to natural apoferritin. *Br. J. Haematol.* **36**, 199–207.

Arosio, P., Adelman, T.G. and Drysdale, J.W. (1978) On ferritin heterogeneity. Further evidence for heteropolymers. *J. Biol. Chem.* **253**, 4451–8.

Beaumont, C., Leneuve, P., Devaux, I. *et al.* (1995) Mutation in iron responsive element of the L ferritin mRNA in a family with dominant hyperferritinaemia and cataract. *Nature Genet.* **11**, 444–6.

Bellotti, V., Arosio, P., Cazzola, M. *et al.* (1987) Characteristics of a ferritin-binding protein present in human serum. *Br. J. Haematol.* **65**, 489–93.

Boscati, I.M. and Stuart, M.C. (1988) Heterophyllic antibodies: a problem for all immunoassays. *Clin. Chem.* **34**, 27–33.

Broxmeyer, H.E. (1992) H-ferritin: a regulatory cytokine that down-modulates cell proliferation. *J. Lab. Clin. Med.* **120**, 367–70.

Broxmeyer, H.E., Bognacki, J., Dorner, M.H. and de Sousa, M. (1981) Identification of leukemia-associated inhibitory activity as acidic isoferritins. A regulatory role for acidic isoferritins in the production of granulocytes and macrophages. *J. Exp. Med.* **153**, 1426–44.

Broxmeyer, H.E., Lu, L., Bicknell, D.C. *et al.* (1986) The influence of purified recombinant human heavy-subunit and light-subunit ferritins on colony formation in vitro by granulocyte-macrophage and erythroid progenitor cells. *Blood* **68**, 1257–63.

Campbell, C.H., Ismail, R. and Linder, M.C. (1989) Ferritin mRNA is found on bound as well as on free polyribosomes in rat heart. *Arch. Biochem. Biophys.* **273**, 89–98.

Cavanna, F., Ruggeri, G., Iacobello, C. *et al.* (1983) Development of a monoclonal antibody against human heart ferritin and its application in an immunoradiometric assay. *Clin. Chim. Acta* **134**, 347–56.

Cazzola, M. and Ascari, E. (1986) Annotation. Red cell ferritin as a diagnostic tool. *Br. J. Haematol.* **62**, 209–13.

Cazzola, M., Dezza, L., Bergamaschi, G. *et al.* (1983) Biologic and clinical significance of red cell ferritin. *Blood* **62**, 1078–87.

Cazzola, M., Bergamaschi, G., Tonon, L. *et al.* (1997) Hereditary hyperferritinemia-cataract syndrome: relationship between phenotypes and specific mutations in the iron-responsive element of ferritin light-chain mRNA. *Blood* **90**, 814–21.

Coenen, J.L., van Dieijen-Visser, M.P., van Pelt, J. *et al.* (1991) Measurements of serum ferritin used to predict concentrations of iron in bone marrow in anemia of chronic disease. *Clin. Chem.* **37**, 560–3.

Cook, J.D., Finch C.A. and Smith, N.J. (1976) Evaluation of the iron status of a population. *Blood* **48**, 449–55.

Costanzo, F., Colombo, M., Staempfli, S. *et al.* (1986) Structure of gene and pseudogenes of human apoferritin H. *Nucl. Acids Res.* **14**, 721–36.

Covell, A.M. and Cook, J.D. (1988) Interaction of acidic isoferritins with human promyelocytic HL60 cells. *Br. J. Haematol.* **69**, 559–63.

Covell, A.M., Jacobs, A. and Worwood, M. (1984) Interaction of ferritin with serum: implications for ferritin turnover. *Clin. Chim. Acta* **139**, 75–84.

Cragg, S.J., Wagstaff, M. and Worwood, M. (1980) Sialic acid and the microheterogeneity of human serum ferritin. *Clin. Sci.* **58**, 259–62.

Cragg, S.J., Wagstaff, M. and Worwood, M. (1981) Detection of a glycosylated subunit in human serum ferritin. *Biochem. J.* **199**, 565–71.

Cragg, S.J., Covell, A.M., Burch, A. *et al.* (1983) Turnover of ^{131}I-human spleen ferritin in plasma. *Br. J. Haematol.* **55**, 83–92.

Custer, E.M., Finch, C.A., Sobel, R.E. and Zettner, A. (1995) Population norms for serum ferritin. *J. Lab. Clin. Med.* **126**, 88–94.

Davidson, A., van der Weyden, M.B., Fong, H. *et al.* (1984) Red cell ferritin content: a re-evaluation of indices for iron deficiency in the anaemia of rheumatoid arthritis. *Br. Med. J.* **289**, 648–50.

Dawson, D.W., Fish, D.I. and Shackleton, P. (1992) The accuracy and clinical interpretation of serum ferritin assays. *Clin. Lab. Haematol.* **14**, 47–52.

Drysdale, J.W. and Munro, H.N. (1966) Regulation of synthesis and turnover of ferritin in rat liver. *J. Biol. Chem.* **241**, 3630–7.

Edwards, C.Q. and Kushner, J.P. (1993) Screening for hemochromatosis. *N. Engl. J. Med.* **328**, 1616–20.

Ellis, R., Henley, R. and Worwood, M. (1997). Three commercial automated ferritin assays. *MDA Evaluation Report MDA/97/41.* London: Medical Devices Agency, National Health Services.

Esumi, N., Ikushima, S., Hibi, S. *et al.* (1988) High serum ferritin level as a marker of malignant histiocytosis and virus-associated hemophagocytic syndrome. *Cancer* **61**, 2071–6.

Fargion, S., Arosio, P., Fracanzani, A.L. *et al.* (1988) Characteristics and expression of binding sites specific for ferritin H-chain on human cell lines. *Blood* **71**, 753–7.

Ferguson, B.J., Skikne, B.S., Simpson, K.M. *et al.* (1992) Serum transferrin receptor distinguishes the anemia of chronic disease from iron deficiency anemia. *J. Lab. Clin. Med.* **119**, 385–90.

Finch, C.A., Cook, J.D., Lanne, R.F. and Culala, M. (1977) Effect of blood donation on iron stores as evaluated by serum ferritin. *Blood* **50**, 441–7.

Flowers, C.A., Kuizon, M., Beard, J.L. *et al.* (1986) A serum ferritin assay for prevalence studies of iron deficiency. *Am. J. Hematol.* **23**, 141–51.

Gutteridge, J.M., Halliwell, B., Treffry, A. *et al.* (1983) Effect of ferritin-containing fractions with different iron loading on lipid peroxidation. *Biochem. J.* **209**, 557–60.

Hann, H.W., Stahlhut, M.W. and Evans, A.E. (1988) Basic and acidic isoferritins in the sera of patients with neuroblastoma. *Cancer* **62**, 1179–82.

Harrison, P.M. (1986) The structure and function of ferritin. *Biochem. Educ.* **14**, 153–62.

Harrison, P.M. and Arosio, P. (1996) Ferritins: molecular properties, iron storage function and cellular regulation. *Biochim. Biophys. Bioenergetics* **1275**, 161–203.

Hazard, J.T. and Drysdale, J.W. (1977) Ferritinaemia in cancer. *Nature* **265**, 755–6.

Henley, R. and Worwood, M. (1991) Luminol peroxidation catalyzed by human isoferritins. *Arch. Biochem. Biophys.* **286**, 238–43.

Hentze, M.W. and Kuhn, L.C. (1996) Molecular control of vertebrate iron metabolism: mRNA-based regulatory circuits operated by iron, nitric oxide and oxidative stress. *Proc. Natl Acad. Sci. (USA)* **93**, 8175–82.

Herbert, V., Jayatilleke, E., Shwa, S. *et al.* (1997) Serum ferritin iron, a new test, measures human body iron stores unconfounded by inflammation. *Stem Cells* **15**, 291–6.

Hodgetts, J., Peters, S.W., Hoy, T.G. and Jacobs, A. (1986) The ferritin content of normoblasts and megaloblasts from human bone marrow. *Clin. Sci.* **70**, 47–51.

ICSH (1984) Preparation, characterization and storage of human ferritin for use as a standard for the assay of serum ferritin. International Committee for Standardization in Haematology (Expert Panel on Iron). *Clin. Lab. Haematol.* **6**, 177–91.

Jacobs, A and Worwood, M. (1975) Ferritin in serum. Clinical and biological implications. *N. Engl. J. Med.* **292**, 951–6.

Jones, B.M. and Worwood, M. (1978) An immunoradiometric assay for the acidic ferritin of human heart: application to human tissues, cells and serum. *Clin. Chim. Acta* **85**, 81–8.

Kirn, D.H., Fredericks, D., Mccutchan, J.A. *et al.* (1995a) Marked elevation of the serum ferritin is highly specific for disseminated histoplasmosis in AIDS. *AIDS* **9**, 1204–5.

Kirn, D.H., Fredericks, D., Mccutchan, J.A. *et al.* (1995b) Serum ferritin levels correlate with disease activity in patients with AIDS and disseminated histoplasmosis. *Clin. Infect. Dis.* **21**, 1048–9.

Klausner, R.D., Rouault, T.A. and Harford, J.B. (1993) Regulating the fate of mRNA: the control of cellular iron metabolism. *Cell* **72**, 19–28.

Koduri, P.R., Carandang, G., Demarais, P. and Patel, A.R. (1995) Hyperferritinemia in reactive hemophagocytic syndrome report of four adult cases. *Am. J. Hematol.* **49**, 247–9.

Konijn, A.M. and Hershko, C. (1989) The anaemia of inflammation and chronic disease. In: de Sousa, M. and Brock, J.H. (eds), *Iron and Immunity, Cancer and Inflammation*. Chichester: John Wiley, 111–43.

Konijn, A.M., Tal, R., Levy, R. and Matzner, Y. (1985) Isolation and fractionation of ferritin from human term placenta – a source for human isoferritins. *Analyt. Biochem.* **144**, 423–8.

Laufberger, M. (1937) Sur la cristallisation de la ferritine. *Bull. Soc. Chim. Biol.* **19**, 1575–82.

Leibold, E.A. and Munro, H.N. (1987) Characterization and evolution of the expressed rat ferritin light subunit gene and its pseudogene family. Conservation of sequences within noncoding regions of ferritin genes. *J. Biol. Chem.* **262**, 7335–41.

Linder, M.C., Schaffer, K.J., Hazeghazam, M. *et al.* (1996) Serum ferritin: Does it differ from tissue ferritin? *J. Gastroenterol. Hepatol.* **11**, 1033–6.

Looker, A.C., Gunter, E.W., Cook, J.D. *et al.* (1991) Comparing serum ferritin values from different population surveys. Vital & Health Statistics - Series 2: *Data Evaluation & Methods Research* 1–19.

Maymon, R. and Moroz, C. (1996) Placental isoferritin: a new biomarker from conception to delivery. *Br. J. Obstet. Gynaec.* **103**, 301–5.

McKeering, L.V., Halliday, J.W., Caffin, J.A. *et al.* (1976) Immunological detection of isoferritins in normal human serum and tissue. *Clin. Chim. Acta* **67**, 189–97.

Miles, L.E., Lipschitz, D.A., Bieber, C.P. and Cook, J.D. (1974) Measurement of serum ferritin by a 2-site immunoradiometric assay. *Analyt. Biochem.* **61**, 209–24.

Milman, N. and Kaas Ibsen, K. (1984) Serum ferritin in Danish children and adolescents. *Scand. J. Haematol.* **33**, 260–6.

Milman, N, Andersen, H.C. and Strandberg Pedersen, N. (1986) Serum ferritin and iron status in 'healthy' elderly individuals. *Scand. J. Clin. Lab. Invest.* **46**, 19–26.

Moroz, C. and Bessler, H. (1989) Ferritin as a marker of malignancy. In: de Sousa, M. and Brock, J.H. (eds), *Iron in Immunity Cancer and Inflammation*. Chichester: John Wiley, 283–99.

Moroz, C., Lahat, N., Biniaminov, M. and Ramot, B. (1977) Ferritin on the surface of lymphocytes in Hodgkin's disease patients. A possible blocking substance removed by levamisole. *Clin. Exp. Immunol.* **29**, 30–5.

Moroz, C., Kupfer, B., Twig, S. and Parhami-Seren, B. (1985) Preparation and characterization of monoclonal antibodies specific to placenta ferritin. *Clin. Chim. Acta* **148**, 111–18.

Moroz, C., Shterman, N., Kupfer, B. *et al.* (1989) T-cell mitogenesis stimulates the synthesis of a mRNA species coding for a 43-kDa peptide reactive with CM-H-9, a monoclonal antibody specific for placental isoferritin. *Proc. Nat. Acad. Sci. USA* **86**, 3282–5.

Mulherin, D., Skelly, M., Saunders, A. *et al.* (1996) The diagnosis of iron deficiency in patients with rheumatoid arthritis and anemia: an algorithm using simple laboratory measures. *J. Rheum.* **23**, 237–40.

Nielsen, P., Gunther, U., Durken, M. *et al.* (2000) Serum ferritin iron in iron overload and liver damage: correlation to body iron stores and diagnostic relevance. *J. Lab. Clin. Med.* **135**, 413–18.

Niitsu, Y., Goto, Y., Kohgo, Y. *et al.* (1980) Evaluation of heart isoferritin assay for diagnosis of cancer. In: Albertini, A. (ed.), *Radioimmunoassay of Hormones, Proteins and Enzymes*. Amsterdam: Excerpta Medica, 256–66.

Ota, T., Higashi, S., Suzuki, H. and Eto, S. (1987) Increased serum ferritin levels in adult Still's disease [letter]. *Lancet* **1**, 562–3.

Peters, S.W., Jacobs, A. and Fitzsimons, E. (1983) Erythrocyte ferritin in normal subjects and patients with abnormal iron metabolism. *Br. J. Haematol.* **53**, 211–16.

Piperno, A., Taddei, M.T., Sampietro, M. *et al.* (1984) Erythrocyte ferritin in thalassaemia syndromes. *Acta Haematol.* **71**, 251–6.

Pootrakul, P., Josephson, B., Huebers, H.A. and Finch, C.A. (1988) Quantitation of ferritin iron in plasma, an explanation for non-transferrin iron. *Blood* **71**, 1120–3.

Prieto, J., Barry, M. and Sherlock, S. (1975) Serum ferritin in patients with iron overload and with acute and chronic liver diseases. *Gastroenterology* **68**, 525–33.

Punnonen, K., Irjala, K. and Rajamaki, A. (1997) Serum transferrin receptor and its ratio to serum ferritin in the diagnosis of iron deficiency. *Blood* **89**, 1052–7.

Reissmann, K.R. and Dietrich, M.R. (1956). On the presence of ferritin in the peripheral blood of patients with hepatocellular disease. *J. Clin. Invest.* **35**, 588–95.

Richter, G.W. (1984) Studies of iron overload. Rat liver siderosome ferritin. *Lab. Invest.* **50**, 26–35.

Rogers, J.T. (1996) Ferritin translation by interleukin-1 and interleukin-6: the role of sequences upstream of the start codons of the heavy and light subunit genes. *Blood* **87**, 2525–37.

Saarinnen, U.M. and Siimes, M.A. (1978) Serum ferritin in assessment of iron nutrition in healthy infants. *Acta Paediatr. Scand.* **67**, 741–51.

Sala, G., Worwood, M. and Jacobs, A. (1986) The effect of isoferritins on granulopoiesis. *Blood* **67**, 436–43.

Santambrogio, P. and Massover, W.H. (1989) Rabbit serum alpha-2–macroglobulin binds to liver ferritin: association causes a heterogeneity of ferritin molecules. *Br. J. Haematol.* **71**, 281–90.

Santambrogio, P., Cozzi, A., Levi, S. and Arosio, P. (1987) Human serum ferritin G-peptide is recognized by anti-L ferritin subunit antibodies and concanavalin-A. *Br. J. Haematol.* **65**, 235–7.

Santoro, C., Marone, M., Ferrone, I. *et al.* (1986) Cloning of the gene coding for human L apo-ferritin. *Nucl. Acids Res.* **14**, 2863–76.

Shorr, E. (1956) Intermediary metabolism and biological activities of ferritin. *Harvey Lectures. Series 50.* New York: Academic Press, 112–53.

Siimes, M.A., Addiego, J.E. Jr, and Dallman, P.R. (1974) Ferritin in serum: diagnosis of iron deficiency and iron overload in infants and children. *Blood* **43**, 581–90.

ten Kate, J., Wolthuis, A., Westerhuis, B. and Vandeursen, C. (1997) The iron content of serum ferritin: physiological importance and diagnostic value. *Eur. J. Clin. Chem. Clin. Biochem.* **35**, 53–6.

Valberg, L.S., Sorbie, L., Ludwig,T. and Pelletier, D. (1976) Serum ferritin and the iron status of Canadians. *Can. Med. Assoc. J.* **114**, 417–21.

van der Weyden, M.B. and Fong, H. (1984) Red cell basic ferritin content of patients with megaloblastic anaemia due to vitamin B12 or folate deficiency. *Scand. J. Haematol.* **33**, 373–7.

van der Weyden, M.B., Fong, H., Salem, H.H. *et al.* (1983) Erythrocyte ferritin content in idiopathic haemochromatosis and alcoholic liver disease with iron overload. *Br. Med. J.* **286**, 752.

van der Weyden, M.B., Fong, H., Hallam, L.J. and Harrison, C. (1989) Red cell ferritin and iron overload in heterozygous ß-thalassemia. *Am. J. Hematol.* **30**, 201–5.

Wagstaff, M., Worwood, M. and Jacobs, A. (1978) Properties of human tissue isoferritins. *Biochem. J.* **173**, 969–77.

Walters, G.O., Miller, F.M. and Worwood, M. (1973) Serum ferritin concentration and iron stores in normal subjects. *J. Clin. Pathol.* **26**, 770–2.

Weir, M.P., Gibson, J.F. and Peters, T.J. (1984) Haemosiderin and tissue damage. *Cell Biochem. Func.* **2**, 186–94.

White, K. and Munro, H.N. (1988) Induction of ferritin subunit synthesis by iron is regulated at both the transcriptional and translational levels. *J. Biol. Chem.* **263**, 8938–42.

White, A., Nicolaas, G., Foster K. *et al.* (1993) *Health Survey for England 1991.* London: HMSO.

Williams, M.A. and Harrison, P.M. (1968) Electron-microscopic and chemical studies of oligomers in horse ferritin. *Biochem. J.* **110**, 265–80.

Wilson, M.B. and Nakane, P.K. (1978) Recent developments in the periodate method of conjugating horseradish peroxidase (HRPO) to antibodies. In: Knapp, W., Holubar, K., Wick, G. (eds), *Immunofluorescence and Related Staining Techniques.* New York: Elsevier, 215–24.

Witte, D.L. (1991) Can serum ferritin be effectively interpreted in the presence of the acute-phase response? *Clin. Chem.* **37**, 484–5.

Worrall, M. and Worwood, M. (1991) Immunological properties of ferritin during in vitro maturation of human monocytes. *Eur. J. Haematol.* **47**, 223–8.

Worwood, M. (1980) In: Cook, J.D. (ed.) *Ferritin in Iron*. New York: Churchill Livingstone, 59–80.

Worwood, M. (1982) Ferritin in human tissues and serum. *Clin. Haematol.* **11**, 275–307.

Worwood, M. (1990) Ferritin. *Blood Rev.* **4**, 259–69.

Worwood, M. and Ellis, R. (2000) *AutoDelfia Serum Ferritin Assay*. MDA 00032. London: Medical Devices Agency, National Health Service.

Worwood, M., Dawkins, S., Wagstaff, M. and Jacobs, A. (1976) The purification and properties of ferritin from human serum. *Biochem. J.* **157**, 97–103.

Worwood, M., Cragg, S.J., Wagstaff, M. and Jacobs, A. (1979) Binding of human serum ferritin to concanavalin A. *Clin. Sci.* **56**, 83–7.

Worwood, M., Cragg, S.J., Jacobs, A. *et al.* (1980) Binding of serum ferritin to concanavalin A: patients with homozygous beta thalassaemia and transfusional iron overload. *Br. J. Haematol.* **46**, 409–16.

Worwood, M., Cragg, S.J., Williams, A.M. *et al.* (1982) The clearance of ^{131}I-human plasma ferritin in man. *Blood* **60**, 827–33.

Worwood, M., Brook, J.D., Cragg, S.J. *et al.* (1985) Assignment of human ferritin genes to chromosomes 11 and 19q13.3-19qter. *Hum. Genet.* **69**, 371–4.

Worwood, M., Thorpe, S.J., Heath, A. *et al.* (1991) Stable lyophilized reagents for the serum ferritin assay. *Clin. Lab. Haematol.* **13**, 297–305.

Yamanishi, H., Iyama, S., Fushimi, R. and Amino, N. (1996) Interference of ferritin in measurement of serum iron concentrations: comparison by five methods. *Clin. Chem.* **42**, 331–2.

Zahringer, J., Konijn, A.M., Baliga, B.S. and Munro, H.N. (1975) Mechanism of iron induction of ferritin synthesis. *Biochem. Biophys. Res. Commun.* **65**, 583–90.

12

The measurement of serum vitamin B$_{12}$, serum folate and red cell folate

SUNITHA N. WICKRAMASINGHE AND KATAYOUN REZVANI

INTRODUCTION

Measurements of the concentrations of vitamin B$_{12}$ (B$_{12}$, cobalamin) and folate in serum and of folate in red cells remain first-line investigations in the assessment of B$_{12}$ and folate status. Such measurements are required in investigating subjects with macrocytosis with or without anaemia, gastrointestinal diseases, various neurological or psychiatric symptoms and sub-optimal diets. Other investigations useful in evaluating B$_{12}$ and folate status include the deoxyuridine suppression test (dUST) performed on bone marrow cells, measurement of serum methylmalonic acid (MMA) and homocysteine (HCYS) levels and various B$_{12}$ absorption tests. B$_{12}$ and folate were initially measured using microbiological assays, but in most laboratories these have now been replaced by assays based on competitive protein binding. The only criterion by which any assay method for B$_{12}$ or folate can be judged is whether the assay provides an accurate and precise measure of the concentration of the analyte without interference from other substances that may be present in the biological material being investigated. Two different questions that are of considerable importance to the practising clinician relate to the sensitivity and specificity of these measurements in detecting clinically relevant deficiency states that are benefited by treatment. With any of the many available methods for assaying B$_{12}$ or folate, it is important that recommended methodological details are strictly adhered to and that method-specific 95% reference limits for healthy subjects are used. The latter is important as different reference ranges may be obtained with different assay kits. Furthermore, as the normal ranges quoted by the manufacturers of some assay kits have been incorrect, such ranges should be independently verified before their adoption.

12.1 MICROBIOLOGICAL ASSAYS

12.1.1 Vitamin B$_{12}$

Microbiological assays for B$_{12}$ are based on the fact that certain microorganisms require B$_{12}$ as a growth factor. The amount of B$_{12}$ in a serum extract can be calculated from the extent of growth caused when the extract is added to a culture of such a microorganism in medium free of any B$_{12}$ but containing an excess of all other substances necessary for optimal growth. Using cultures containing graded amounts of added cyanocobalamin in the medium, a standard curve is prepared relating added cyanocobalamin to growth (measured turbidimetrically), and the amount of cyanocobalamin corresponding to the extent of growth caused by the serum extract is determined from this curve. No other chemicals present in the serum extract should be able to modify the growth of the organism. Shorb (1948) used *Lactobacillus lactis Dorner* as the assay organism in early studies leading to the isolation of B$_{12}$. However, this organism proved too difficult for routine use, and others which were more reliable in their behaviour were soon introduced. These were *Lactobacillus leichmannii* (Skeggs et al., 1948; Hoffman *et al.*, 1949), *Euglena gracilis* (Hutner et al., 1949; Ross, 1950; Ross et al., 1957), *Ochromonas malhamensis* (Ford, 1953; Hutner et al., 1953) and a cobalamin/methionine auxotrophic mutant of *Escherichia coli* (Davis and Mingioli, 1950; Burkholder, 1951). Assays based on *Ochromonas malhamensis* are considered to be the most specific, as the growth of this organism is supported by cobalamins but not to any significant extent by other corrins, whereas that of the other three organisms is supported both by cobalamins and by certain other corrins. Most workers have used either *L. leichmannii* or *E. gracilis* for the microbiological assay of B$_{12}$ and we will therefore restrict our comments to assays based on these two organisms. The three major disadvantages of most microbiological assays are that:

- they involve the use of sterile techniques and therefore require specially trained personnel;
- they are time-consuming;
- they are subject to the vagaries of a complex living organism.

LACTOBACILLUS LEICHMANNII ASSAY

In the assays based on *L. leichmannii* (NCIB 8117, ATCC 7830 or ATCC 4797), the first step is to extract the B$_{12}$ from the serum and to convert the extracted B$_{12}$ to cyanocobalamin. This is achieved by denaturing the serum transcobalamins by heating to 100°C for 20 minutes in acetate buffer (pH 4.4–4.9; final concentration 30–150 mmol/L sodium acetate) (Beck, 1983). Assayable B$_{12}$ is lower at final buffer concentrations below 30 mmol/L sodium acetate and is higher in the presence than in the absence of cyanide. In addition, the extent of this cyanide effect may differ in different serum samples, which may be one source of inaccuracy in this assay. The *L. leichmannii* assay is not influenced by cobalamin analogues.

Like any other microbiological assay, the *L. leichmannii* assay is prone to fail occasionally (Chanarin, 1969). For example, significant growth may sometimes occur in tubes without added B$_{12}$, indicating contamination of a reagent, usually the distilled water, with B$_{12}$. Contamination of the assay organism with other bacteria may also be responsible for assay failure characterized by overgrowth. Occasionally, the assay may fail because of a 'declining' assay organism which results in slow growth and a flat standard curve. In addition, certain drugs, such as penicillin, amoxycillin, erythromcyin, co-trimoxazole, carbenicillin, lincomycin, chloramphenicol, cephalothin, rifampicin and folate antagonists, inhibit the growth of *Lactobacillus leichmannii* and sera from patients receiving such drugs give falsely low B_{12} results.

The coefficient of variation (CV) for the between-run imprecision in the *L. leichmannii* assay has been reported to vary between 9.4 and 13.8% (Matthews, 1962; Spray, 1962). In one study, the 95% reference range obtained with sera from 100 healthy volunteers was 181–746 ng/L (mean, 368 ng/L) (Bain *et al.*, 1982).

Kelleher *et al.* (1987) reported that the use of colistin-sulphate-resistant strains of *L. leichmannii* enables serum B_{12} to be assayed without aseptic precautions. However, the new assay demonstrated an increased tendency to be affected by antibiotics when compared with a traditional technique. In a subsequent study, Kelleher *et al.* (1990) showed that pre-treatment of sera with β-lactamase markedly reduced the frequency of antibiotic interference in the assay, as this enzyme inactivates the penicillins (ampicillin, amoxycillin and flucloxacillin), augmentin and the third-generation cephalosporins – cefotaxime, ceftizoxime and ceftazidime. Such pretreatment would prevent delays caused by having to repeat assays. Recently, a miniaturized microbiological assay has been described based on colistin-sulphate-resistant organisms (NCIB 12519) and β-lactamase pretreated sera (Kelleher and O'Broin, 1991). This assay is performed in 96-well microtitre plates and is considerably quicker than the conventional assays largely because of the speed at which modern automated microtitre plate readers operate compared with the slow reading of individual tubes on a spectrophotometer. The within-run and between-run imprecision in this microtitre plate assay were excellent with CVs in the range 1.9–4.3% and 1.2–3.5%, respectively, and the recovery of added cyanocobalamin was 95–102%. Results obtained by this assay correlated well with those obtained by a conventional *L. leichmannii* assay ($n = 90$, $r = 0.98$, slope = 1.06, intercept = −7.26 ng/L).

EUGLENA GRACILIS ASSAY

The growth of *E. gracilis* is equally influenced by hydroxocobalamin and cyanocobalamin and, consequently, the inclusion of cyanide during the extraction of B_{12} from serum is unnecessary. As serum inhibits growth, standards must include a small volume of serum so that the serum-induced inhibition is similar to that caused by the test samples (Anderson, 1964). The growth of *E. gracilis* is also inhibited by low concentrations of sulphonamides and this should be prevented by the addition of para-aminobenzoic acid to the medium. Whereas the period of incubation with the test material is 18–20 hours (37°C) in the assay based on *L. leichmannii*, it is 3–5 days (optimum temperature 27–29°C) in *Euglena* assays employing the faster growing strain *E. gracilis* var. 'z' (ATCC 12716). In addition, since the growth of *E. gracilis* is influenced by slight variations in lighting and temperature, assays based on this organism require specially constructed illuminated water baths or incubators. For these reasons, few laboratories have continued to use the *Euglena* assay. Nevertheless, the sensitivity of the *Euglena* assay is greater than that of the *L. leichmannii* assay; a growth response can be obtained with *Euglena* with as little as 1 ng added B_{12} per litre. The *Euglena* assay is unaffected by anti-biotics and antimetabolites at concentrations that may usually be found in patient sera.

When serum was present in the standards, the CVs for within-run and between-run imprecision were, respectively, 3.7 and 3.1–10% (combined CV = 5.1%) (Anderson, 1964). In another study, the CVs for within-run and between-run imprecision of the Euglena assay were 2.4–5 and 6.7–7.8%, respectively (Anderson and Sourial, 1983). Results obtained by this assay correlate well with those obtained by competitive protein-binding assays based on purified intrinsic factor. In one study, the 95% reference range for 196 normal subjects was 230–826 ng/L (170–610 pmol/L) (Anderson and Sourial, 1983).

12.1.2 Folate

Folate can be measured in the serum or in red cells using *Lactobacillus casei* or *Streptococcus faecalis*, the growth of which is dependent on a supply of pre-formed folate (Baker *et al.*, 1959; Herbert, 1961; Waters and Mollin, 1961; Hoffbrand *et al.*, 1966). *L. casei* has been used more frequently than *Strep. faecalis*. The folate in serum is almost entirely in the form 5-methyl-tetrahydrofolate monoglutamate which undergoes spontaneous oxidative degradation *in vitro*. If samples are to be stored frozen prior to assay, this degradation must be prevented by the addition of dry ascorbate to the serum. Folates in red cells are present as polyglutamates which must be converted to monoglutamates before assay (Hoffbrand *et al.*, 1966). This is usually achieved via the action of the conjugase enzyme normally present in plasma, by adding one part of whole blood to nine parts of 1% (w/v) ascorbic acid in distilled water. The ascorbate has a dual effect – first it protects the folate from oxidation and secondly it provides an optimal pH (4.5) for the action of the conjugase. Serum samples for assay must be completely free of haemolysed or intact red cells, as red cells contain considerably more folate than serum.

LACTOBACILLUS CASEI ASSAY

Lactobacillus casei (NCIB 8081 or ATCC 7469) shows a growth response to a wide variety of folates including pteroylglutamic acid (PGA), 10-formyltetrahydrofolate (10-formyl-THF) and 5-methyl-THF (Shane *et al.*, 1980) and the *L. casei* folate assay is usually standardized against PGA. The difficulties encountered with the *L. casei* assay for folate are similar to those encountered with the *L. leichmannii* assay for B$_{12}$. The assay is time-consuming and the period of incubation with the test material is 18–20 hours (37°C). Problems may occur due to contamination with folate of the apparatus or a reagent, especially the distilled water. The latter should be glass-distilled rather than prepared by ion-exchange columns since these may harbour folate-producing bacteria. Overgrowth may sometimes occur due to contamination of the assay organism with other bacteria and the assay may occasionally fail due to a 'declining' assay organism. Finally, samples from patients receiving certain antibiotics give falsely low folate results due to an antibiotic-mediated inhibition of the growth of *L. casei*. Such antibiotics include penicillin, amoxycillin, chloramphenicol, tetracyclines, lincomyin, erythromycin, streptomycin and methicillin (Reizenstein, 1965; Beard and Allen, 1967). Methotrexate also inhibits bacterial growth.

The CV for the between-run imprecision in the *L. casei* assay for serum folate has been reported to be in the range 11–16.8%, and that for red cell folate in the range 12.4–15% (Hoffbrand *et al.*, 1966).

The requirement for sterile techniques in the microbiological assays for serum and red cell folate can be overcome by using a chloramphenicol-resistant strain of *L. casei* (NCIB 10463), and a miniaturized assay based on this organism has been developed for performance on microtitre plates (O'Broin and Kelleher, 1992). The reported within-run and between-run imprecision of this assay was excellent, with coefficients of variation of 2.05–3.7% and 2.7–4.9%, respectively, for serum folate and 4.7–5.1% and 3.1–6.6%, respectively, for whole blood folate. In quality assurance programmes, the mean values for red cell folate determined with chloramphenicol-resistant *L. casei* have been slightly higher than those determined with non-resistant strains (Dawson *et al.*, 1987).

12.2 ASSAYS BASED ON COMPETITIVE PROTEIN BINDING

The first competitive protein-binding assays for serum B_{12} were reported in 1961 (Barakat and Ekins, 1961; Rothenberg, 1961) and for serum and red cell folate between 1971 and 1976 (Waxman *et al.*, 1971; Rothenberg *et al.*, 1972, 1974; Dunn and Foster, 1973; Tajuddin and Gardyna, 1973; Longo and Herbert, 1976). Over the past 25 years, microbiological assays for B_{12} and folate have been gradually replaced by assays based on competitive protein binding. This is because the latter are technically simple, do not require sterile conditions and are un-affected by antibiotics, antimetabolites or other drugs that may be present in the serum. In addition, they are rapid, with total incubation periods of not more than 1–2 hours. With most non-automated competitive protein-binding assays, the total time taken to assay one batch of 40 samples is 4–5 hours. Competitive protein-binding assays employing radiolabelled vitamin B_{12} or folate are often referred to as radioassays.

Several kits for the assay of serum B_{12} and serum and red cell folate have been produced by various companies over the last two decades; some of these have been discontinued over this period and some have been modified. For example, in 1992, Bio-Rad reviewed the normal ranges for their B_{12} and folate assays and re-validated their product. In 1993, the standard-ization procedures for the Bio-Rad assays were reviewed and spectrophotometrically verified PGA standards were introduced; the upgraded product was named Quantaphase II. The frequency of the usage of various methods in diagnostic laboratories has changed markedly with time. In 1997, about 68% of UK laboratories used fully automated methods, with about 45% using the Abbott IM_x assays, 14% the Chiron Diagnostics ACS:180 assays and 7% the Bayer Immuno 1 assays. The remaining UK laboratories used methods that are not fully auto-mated ('non-automated' assays), such as Bio-Rad Quantaphase (10%), ICN Simultrac-SNB (7.5%), ICN Charcoal [^{57}Co-B_{12} or ^{125}I-folate] (5%) and ICN Simultrac-S (3%). Bio-Rad assays are globally the most frequently used non-automated B_{12} and folate assay methods.

12.2.1 Serum B_{12}

The B_{12} in serum consists mainly of methylcobalamin, together with some adenosylcobalamin, hydroxocobalamin and cyanocobalamin. In the competitive protein-binding assays for serum B_{12}, the various cobalamins are extracted from their binding proteins (transcobalamins) either by boiling in an alkaline buffer (pH 9.2–9.4) in the presence of cyanide or, without boiling, by treatment with a more alkaline buffer (pH about 13) containing cyanide. The pH used at the boiling step is higher than that of 4.4–4.9 used at the same step in the *L. leichmannii* assay because the binding of B_{12} to intrinsic factor (IF) is inhibited at a very acid pH and also because an alkaline pH is required if folate is to be assayed simultaneously. The cyanide converts the released B_{12} to cyanocobalamin. A known quantity of labelled cyanocobalamin, usually ^{57}Co-cyanocoblamin, is then added and an aliquot of the mixture reacted with a protein that specifically binds B_{12}. The non-radioactive cyanocobalamin derived from the serum competes with the labelled cyanocobalamin for the B_{12} binding sites on the binding protein so that there is an inverse relationship between the amount of B_{12} in the serum and the amount of radio-activity bound to the binding protein. The assay is calibrated using solutions containing various concentrations of non-radioactive cyanocobalamin. In order to avoid the limitations associated with the use of a radiolabelled compound (including short shelf-life and disposal problems), ^{57}Co-cyanocobalamin has been replaced in some commercially available assays by acridinium-ester-coupled cyanocobalamin, B_{12}-alkaline phosphatase conjugate or Europium-labelled B_{12}. In addition, one company has developed a non-isotopic assay based on the CEDIA principle (see p. 297). An important factor limiting the sensitivity of assays employing ^{57}Co-cyanocobalamin is the use of a relatively low specific activity compound. However, the sensitivity of current assays based on non-radioactive derivatives of cyanocobalamin is no better than that of radioassays, presumably (at least partly) because the affinity of such derivatives for IF is less than that of cyanocobalamin.

The binding agents used have been porcine (IF) (Rothenberg, 1961; Lau *et al.*, 1965; Friedner *et al.*, 1969; Raven *et al.*, 1969) or various sources of R binder (haptocorrin) such as pooled normal serum, chronic myeloid leukaemia serum, chick serum and saliva (Matthews *et al.*, 1967; Rothenberg, 1968; Carmel and Coltman, 1969; Green *et al.*, 1974). The intrinsic factor preparations employed in several assay methods have been impure, with 51–85% haptocorrin (gastric R binder) (Kolhouse *et al.*, 1978). Assays based on haptocorrin or impure IF give higher results than those based on pure IF (Green *et al.*, 1974; Kubasik *et al.*, 1980; Chen *et al.*, 1981), apparently because IF binds cyanocobalamin almost exclusively whereas haptocorrin binds both cyanocobalamin and other biologically inactive cobalamin-like molecules (Chanarin and Muir, 1982). Kolhouse *et al.* (1978) found that assays based on porcine or human R binder failed to detect four or five out of 21 (20%) clinically proven cases of B$_{12}$ deficiency and attributed this to the ability of R binders to bind cobinamide. Consequently, all current competitive protein-binding assays use as the binding protein either purified IF or impure IF with the contaminating gastric R binder blocked with an excess of cobinamide. However, Herbert *et al.* (1984) found that the comparative rank order of results was similar regardless of whether the binder used was IF plus R binder, IF plus R binder plus cobinamide, highly purified porcine IF or salivary R binder, and emphasized that all methods allow reliable clinical conclusions provided method-specific normal ranges are used.

A number of approaches have been used to separate the bound B$_{12}$ from the unbound B$_{12}$. These include removal of the unbound B$_{12}$ by:

- adsorption with haemoglobin- or albumin-coated or uncoated charcoal followed by centrifugation (Ekins and Sgherzi, 1965; Lau *et al.*, 1965; Liu and Sullivan, 1972);
- dialysis (Barakat and Ekins, 1963);
- ultrafiltration (Friedner *et al.*, 1969).

Other methods devised for removing the bound B$_{12}$ are based on using solid phase intrinsic factor, i.e. intrinsic factor linked to material such as Sepharose, Sephadex, cellulose, polymer beads, glass beads or paramagnetic particles, followed by centrifugation or magnetic separation (Kakei and Glass, 1962; Mantzos *et al.*, 1967).

NON-AUTOMATED METHODS

The essential features of some of the commercially available non-automated methods (kits) for the assay of B$_{12}$ are summarized in Table 12.1 and for the simultaneous assay of B$_{12}$ and folate in Table 12.2.

The 'no boil' kits have the obvious advantage of eliminating a cumbersome, time-consuming step that is a source of variability in results. However, with the 'no boil' approach, the pH has to be carefully re-adjusted to around 9.3 after the extraction step. If a 'no boil' method results in incomplete denaturation of transcobalamins, as might happen with sera from patients with chronic granulocytic leukaemia which have very high transcobalamin I (TCI) levels, some of the radiolabelled B$_{12}$ will bind to the TCI. Consequently, spuriously low results may be expected from systems employing charcoal separation since the bound counts will increase, and spuriously high results may be expected from systems employing IF bound to a solid phase as the counts bound to IF will decrease (Zucker *et al.*, 1981). It has also been pointed out that boiling not only extracts B$_{12}$ by denaturing transcobalamins but also inactivates other interfering substances such as blocking IF antibodies present in a proportion of

Table 12.1 *Characteristics of some commercially available kits for the assay of serum B$_{12}$*

Kit	Extraction of cobalamin	Identity of labelled cobalamin	Binding protein	Separation of bound from unbound cobalamin
Vitamin B$_{12}$ [^{57}Co]/charcoal radioassay (ICN)[a]	DTT, KCN, 100°C for 15 min, pH 9.3	^{57}Co-cyanocobalamin (added before extraction)	Porcine IF, R binders blocked with B$_{12}$ analogues	Dextran-coated charcoal/centrifugation/supernatant counted
Quantaphase II B$_{12}$ radioassay (Bio-Rad)	DTT, KCN, 100°C for 20 min, pH 9.35	^{57}Co-cyanocobalamin (added before extraction)	Purified porcine IF bound to polymer beads	Centrifugation/pellet counted
Magic Lite (Ciba Corning)	DTT, KCN, alkaline buffer	Acridinium ester-labelled B$_{12}$ (added during reaction of analyte with binding protein)	Purified porcine IF covalently bound to paramagnetic particles	Magnetic separation/pellet used for analysis

[a]Formerly, the Becton Dickinson B$_{12}$ [^{57}Co] radioassay.

Table 12.2 *Characteristics of some commercially available kits for the simultaneous assay of B_{12} and folate*

Kit	Extraction of vitamin	Identity of labelled vitamins	Binding proteins	Separation of bound from unbound vitamin
Simultrac B$_{12}$ [^{57}Co]/Folate [^{125}I] radioassay (ICN)	DTT, KCN, 100°C for 15 min, pH 9.3	^{57}Co-cyanocobalamin, ^{125}I-PGA	Porcine IF (R binders blocked with B$_{12}$ analogues) and purified bovine milk FBP	Dextran-coated charcoal/ centrifugation
Simultrac®-S B$_{12}$ [^{57}Co]/ Folate [^{125}I] radioassay (ICN)	DTT, KCN, 100°C for 15 min, pH 9.3	^{57}Co-cyanocobalamin, ^{125}I-PGA	Purified porcine IF and purified bovine milk FBP covalently linked to a solid phase	Centrifugation
Simultrac®-SNB B$_{12}$ [^{57}Co]/ Folate [^{125}I] radioassay (ICN)	DTT, KCN, alkaline buffer (pH 12–13)	^{57}Co-cyanocobalamin, ^{125}I-PGA	Purified porcine IF and purified bovine milk FBP covalently linked to a solid phase	Centrifugation
Quantaphase II B$_{12}$/Folate radioassay (Bio-Rad)	DTT, KCN, 100°C for 20 min, pH 9.35	^{57}Co-cyanocobalamin, ^{125}I-PGA	Purified porcine IF and bovine milk FBP bound to polymer beads	Centrifugation
Magic B$_{12}$ [^{57}Co] FOL [^{125}I] (Ciba Corning)	DTT, KCN, > 95°C for 15 min	^{57}Co-cyanocobalamin, ^{125}I-PGA	Purified porcine IF and bovine milk FBP covalently bound to microscopic iron particles	Magnetic separation
Magic B$_{12}$ [^{57}Co] FOL [^{125}I] (NB) (Ciba Corning)	DTT, KCN, alkaline buffer (pH 12–13)	^{57}Co-cyanocobalamin, ^{125}I-PGA	Purified porcine IF and bovine milk FBP covalently bound to microscopic iron particles	Magnetic separation

pernicious anaemia sera. According to some investigators, the original 'no boil' procedures did not completely denature anti-IF antibodies and sera containing such antibodies therefore gave spuriously high B_{12} values with these kits (Zucker et al., 1981; Allen, 1982; El Shami and Durham, 1983; Higgins and Wu, 1983). In the study by Zucker et al. (1981), two 'no boil' kits failed to give subnormal results with two out of 12 and seven out of 12 pernicious anaemia sera containing anti-IF antibodies. Fish and Dawson (1983) have questioned whether this was really due to the anti-IF antibodies since eight out of 12 pernicious anaemia sera without anti-IF antibodies studied by Zucker et al. (1981) also gave incorrect results with one of the 'no boil' assays. In their own study, Fish and Dawson (1983) found that 11 pernicious anaemia sera containing a potent blocking antibody to IF gave appropriately low values with six 'no boil' kits. It has to be pointed out that the biochemical basis of the differences in the results obtained with several of the currently available kits has not been fully researched and the proposed explanations are often speculative.

Bain et al. (1982) evaluated the performance of the Becton Dickinson Vitamin B_{12} [^{57}Co] radioassay kit (ICN ^{57}Co/charcoal), which employs a boiling step, impure IF with R proteins blocked by vitamin B_{12} analogues and dextran-coated charcoal. They found that the precision and linearity of this assay were good and that sera from 20 patients with B_{12}-responsive disorders gave subnormal results both by this radioassay and by the L. leichmannii assay. The average value for serum B_{12} in 100 healthy adults determined by this radioassay was not significantly different from that determined in parallel by the L. leichmannii method. According to the manufacturers, B_{12} results obtained on 132 serum samples by the SimulTRAC-S kit (employing purified IF) correlated very well with the results by the E. gracilis assay ($r = 0.97$, slope = 1.23, intercept = 0.22 ng/L). Similarly, results obtained by the SimulTRAC-SNB kit (which also uses purified IF) showed a good correlation with the results by the Euglena method ($n = 132$, $r = 0.96$, slope = 1.1, intercept = 0.32 ng/L).

Wentworth et al. (1994) compared the Magic Lite assay, which does not involve a boiling step, with an in-house B_{12} radioassay method in which the B_{12} was released by boiling at acid pH and the binding protein was crude IF treated with an excess of cobinamide to block contaminating R binders. Within-run and between-run imprecision of the Magic Lite assay were acceptable and both assays discriminated between normal and abnormal samples equally well. However, the results with the Magic Lite assay were considerably lower than those of the in-house assay in samples with low B_{12} levels and slightly higher in samples with B_{12} values > 592 ng/L. Lower values with Magic Lite at low B_{12} levels are also evident in the correlation between the B_{12} concentrations obtained by the Simultrac-S Boil B_{12}/folate radioassay (ICN) and the Magic Lite assay illustrated in the manufacturer's technical information sheets ($n = 100$, $r = 0.959$, slope = 1.016, intercept = −41 ng/L). The explanation for this is uncertain. In another study, Arnaud et al. (1994) analysed the B_{12} concentrations in 146 serum samples arriving in a diagnostic laboratory using a L. leichmannii assay (ATCC 7830), and three commercially available assays that did not include a boiling step, namely Magic B_{12} FOL (NB), SimulTRAC-SNB and Magic Lite. Median (range) B_{12} concentrations (ng/L) obtained by these four assays were, respectively, 428 (20–1743) (L. leichmannii method), 479 (47–3121), 513 (50–2728) and 479 (34–4683), and these differences were statistically significant. Thus, all three of these competitive binding assays gave higher results than the microbiological assay. Values for between-run imprecision of the four methods were similar with CVs of 7.1–9.9% with the microbiological assay, 10.2–10.6% with the Magic B_{12} FOL (NB) kit, 7–10.3% with the SimulTRAC-SNB kit and 7.9–10.3% with the Magic Lite kit. Regression coefficients for the correlation with the results of the microbiological assay were 0.92 for the Magic B_{12} FOL (NB) kit, 0.90 for the SimulTRAC-SNB kit and 0.88 for the Magic Lite kit. Better regression coefficients (0.95–0.96) were obtained for the correlation between the Magic Lite and Magic B_{12} FOL (NB) or SimulTRAC-SNB kits and between the SimulTRAC-SNB and Magic B_{12} FOL (NB) kit.

12.2.2 Folate

As mentioned previously, most of the folate in the serum consists of 5-methyltetrahydro-folate (methyl-THF) monoglutamate. About one-third of this folate is loosely bound to albumin and some is bound to a specific folate-binding serum protein. The procedures used to extract the bound folate are the same as those in the competitive protein-binding assays for B$_{12}$, i.e. either boiling at a pH of 9.2–9.4 or treatment with a buffer of pH about 13. As in the case of the microbiological assays, oxidative degradation of folate must be prevented and this is achieved by the use of ascorbic acid during the preparation of haemolysates and of dithiothreitol (DTT) during the extraction procedure. In addition, the various folate poly-glutamates found in red cells have to be converted to monoglutamates via the action of serum folate-conjugase prior to assay by a competitive protein-binding method. The folate monoglutamates in serum or those derived from red cells are mixed with a labelled folate compound such as ^{125}I-pteroylglutamic acid (^{125}I-PGA) (usually), ^{3}H-PGA (Rothenberg et al., 1972, 1974; Schreiber and Waxman, 1974) or ^{75}Se-selenofolate (Johnson et al., 1977; Johnson and Rose, 1978), and an aliquot of the mixture reacted with a specific folate-binding protein. The binding protein usually employed is affinity purified folate-binding protein (FBP) from bovine milk. In some assay methods, the radiolabelled PGA has been replaced by a folate-dimethyl acridinium ester conjugate or a folate-alkaline phosphatase conjugate. Since most of the folate in serum is methyl-THF, in the ideal competitive protein-binding assay for serum folate one would wish to use this compound both as the labelled tracer and as the calibrator. Early assays did use this approach but ran into difficulties because of the instability of methyl-THF. Following the report by Givas and Gutcho (1975) that both methyl-THF and PGA have nearly the same affinity for the milk folate-binding protein at a pH of 9.3, labelled PGA was used as tracer and PGA was used as the calibrator in assays for both serum folate and red cell folate. However, whereas the use of labelled PGA in assays of serum folate can by justified as outlined above, its use in assays of red cell folate may be less satisfactory as recent studies have indicated that, after deconjugation, red-cell-derived folate monoglutamates largely consist not of methyl-THF but of other unidentified folate compounds, including formyl-folates (Lucock et al., 1996). Conceivably, what is being assayed is a mixture of folates with or without hydrogen atoms at positions 5, 6, 7 and 8 and with their one-carbon group at different stages of oxidation. These folate monoglutamates may have different affinities for the binding protein (Shane et al., 1980). Such considerations imply that the accuracy of currently available assays for serum folate, and especially for red cell folate, is questionable.

NON-AUTOMATED METHODS

The important characteristics of some of the commercially available non-automated methods (kits) for the assay of folate are given in Table 12.3 (for simultaneous assay of folate and B$_{12}$, see Table 12.2).

The manufacturers of most kits for the assay of serum and red cell folate quote satisfactory values for recovery of added analyte and for within-run and between-run imprecision. However, there have been few published hospital-based evaluations of the analytical perform-ance of such kits and of the biological/clinical relevance of the data obtained. In one study, the Becton Dickinson Radioassay Kit (^{125}I) (ICN ^{125}I/charcoal) for the assay of red cell folate was found to be acceptable with regard to precision and to give red cell folate levels below the reference range in 24 of 25 folate-deficient patients (Bain et al., 1984). By contrast, the specificity of the assay in detecting clinically relevant folate deficiency appeared to be less satisfactory, as eight of 45 macrocytic patients giving a normal deoxyuridine-suppressed value,

Table 12.3 *Characteristics of some commercially available kits for the measurement of folate concentrations*

Kit	Extraction of folate	Identity of labelled folate	Binding protein	Separation of bound from unbound folate
Folate [125I]/charcoal radioassay (ICN)[a]	DTT, 100°C for 15 min, pH 9.3	125I-PGA (added before extraction)	Purified bovine milk FBP	Dextran-coated charcoal/ centrifugation/supernatant counted
Quantaphase II folate radioassay (Bio-Rad)	DTT, 100°C for 20 min, pH 9.35	125I-PGA (added before extraction)	Purified bovine milk FBP bound to polymer beads	Centrifugation/pellet counted
Magic Lite (Ciba Corning)	DTT, NaOH	Folate-dimethyl acridinium ester conjugate (added during reaction of analyte with binding protein)	Purified bovine milk FBP bound to paramagnetic particles	Magnetic separation/pellet used for analysis

[a]Formerly, the Becton Dickinson Folate [125I] radioassay.

and four of 50 other patients who were considered unlikely to be folate-deficient, had sub-normal red cell folate levels. It seems unlikely, however, that the Becton Dickinson Radioassay is any worse in this respect than microbiological assays but this was not established. Other important observations from this study were that: (i) the relationship between the red cell folate level and the packed cell volume (PCV) was not linear but curvilinear, with higher values at low PCVs; and (ii) the measured red cell folate continued to fall beyond the recommended 90-minute pre-assay incubation of the lysate, up to 5 hours, emphasizing the need to comply strictly with the manufacturer's instructions. In addition, the 95% reference range of 199–795 µg/L obtained by Bain *et al.* (1984), which was based on samples from 200 healthy adults, differed considerably from that stated by the manufacturer, underlining the importance of verifying quoted normal ranges.

An unsatisfactory degree of interlaboratory variation in red cell folate results obtained by radioassay has been reported in quality assurance programmes conducted both in Britain and Australia, with average CVs of 30.4% (Dawson *et al.*, 1987) and 39.3% (Brown et al., 1990). Interestingly, the CVs for serum folate determined by the same methods (using the same reagents) were lower, being 18.7 and 25%, respectively. Brown *et al.* (1990) investigated the high interlaboratory variation in red cell folate radioassay results and identified a number of possible contributory factors. As could be predicted from earlier data (Bain *et al.*, 1984), the dilution of the haemolysate was one such factor and kits that recommended the highest dilution gave the highest mean red cell folate values. The use of a folate-poor lysate as the diluent was shown to eliminate this problem. A second factor identified by these authors was the frequent failure to correct for the contribution made by serum folate in calculating the red cell folate concentration. At serum folate concentrations of 5–9 µg/L, this omission could overestimate red cell folate by 15–25%. A third factor is failure strictly to adhere to instructions provided by the manufacturer. Brown *et al.* (1990) also found that (i) when active DTT is present in the assay system, higher red cell folate levels are found than when inactive (old) DTT or no DTT is present; (ii) 'boil' methods tended to give higher values than 'no boil' methods; and (iii) previously frozen lysates gave higher red cell folate levels than freshly prepared lysates.

The complete conversion of folate polyglutamates to folate monoglutamates is an important step in measuring red cell folate by a competitive protein-binding assay. This is because folate polyglutamates have a greater affinity for FBP than folate monoglutamates (Shane *et al.*, 1980); for example, in one study, folate triglutamates and heptaglutamates had, respectively, 2.9 and 5.6 times the affinity of the monoglutamate for the FBP at pH 9.3 (Gutcho, 1978). The optimum pH for the conversion to monoglutamates via the action of folate conjugase is around 4.2. The use in some kits of sodium ascorbate rather than ascorbic acid during the preparation of the haemolysate may result in pH values considerably higher than 4.2, incomplete deconjugation of polyglutamates and an increase in apparent folate levels in radioassays (Dawson *et al.*, 1987). However, in one study, no significant differences were observed with lysates prepared without ascorbate and with 0.2–1% sodium ascorbate (Brown *et al.*, 1990).

Oxidation or photodecomposition of folate during storage may lower the folate level. Nevertheless, some studies have shown that EDTA or heparinized blood can be stored at 4°C without added ascorbate for up to 7 days with no loss of red cell folate activity as determined by a competitive protein-binding assay (Schreiber and Waxman, 1974; Mortensen, 1978; Wickramasinghe *et al.*, 1996). By contrast, one group found that folate activity in heparinized blood is preserved at 4°C only if ascorbic acid is added (Rothenberg *et al.*, 1974). Folate activity, measured by the Abbott IM$_x$ folate assay (see below), is stable for up to 7 days as claimed by the manufacturers, if lysates containing ascorbic acid are frozen at −20°C immediately after their preparation (Wickramasinghe *et al.*, 1996).

12.2.3 Fully automated B₁₂ and folate assays

There are now a few fully automated B_{12} and folate assays based on competitive protein binding and these include the Abbott IM_x assay, the Bayer Immuno I assay and the automated chemiluminescence system – ACS 180 VB_{12} assay and folate assay (Chiron Diagnostics). These have the advantage of reducing imprecision due to procedures such as manual pipetting. Their essential features are summarized in Table 12.4. Fully automated assays based on the cloned enzyme donor immunoassay (CEDIA) principle are also available from Boehringer-Mannheim – namely, the CEDIA vitamin B_{12} (no boil) and folate (no boil) assays. Another fully automated assay system for serum B_{12}, serum folate and red cell folate which has recently become available is the Elecsys (Boehringer Mannheim/Roche). The relatively recently introduced AutoDELFIA™ kits for the assay of serum B_{12} and serum and red cell folate (Wallac) are automatically performed on microtitre plates and use Europium-labelled B_{12} and folate as the labelled analytes.

ABBOTT IM$_x$ ASSAYS

The Abbott IM_x assay for serum B_{12} is based on microparticle enzyme immunoassay technology (Kuemmerie *et al.*, 1992). The steps involved are:

1 extraction of B_{12} from serum using a reagent containing α-monothioglycerol and cobinamide;
2 reaction of the extracted B_{12} with microparticles coated with porcine intrinsic factor (IF) purified by vitamin B_{12}-agarose affinity chromatography;
3 transfer of a measured volume of the incubation mixture containing microparticles with B_{12}–IF complexes to a glass matrix to which the microparticles bind;
4 washing the matrix to remove unbound material and addition of B_{12}-akaline phosphatase conjugate which binds to free B_{12}-binding sites on the IF coating the particles;
5 washing the matrix to remove unbound conjugate and addition of 4-methylumbelliferyl phosphate, the substrate for alkaline phosphatase;
6 measurement of the rate of generation of fluorescent product.

The measured rate is inversely proportional to the serum B_{12} concentration. The recovery of added B_{12} in this assay has been reported to be good, being between 83 and 122% (average 100%), and the CV for total assay imprecision to be 6.6–7.9% (Kuemmerie *et al.*, 1992).

The Abbott IM_x assay for serum and red cell folate is based on ion capture technology. The steps involved in this assay are:

1 addition of dithiothreitol and KOH to the sample followed by the capture reagent consisting of affinity-purified bovine milk FBP combined with a monoclonal anti-FBP antibody covalently coupled to carboxymethylamylose (a polyanion);
2 transfer of a measured volume of the reaction mixture containing polyanion–antibody–FBP–folate complexes to a positively charged glass-fibre matrix which electrostatically captures the polyanion complexes;
3 washing the matrix followed by addition of a pteroic acid–alkaline phosphatase conjugate which binds to unoccupied folate-binding sites on the FBP;
4 washing the matrix to remove unbound conjugate and addition of 4-methylumbelliferyl phosphate;
5 measurement of the fluorescent product generated.

Since the folate in the test sample is incubated with the FBP before adding the labelled folate, the binding of the labelled folate is by a non-competitive reaction. Solutions

Table 12.4 *Characteristics of some fully automated methods for the assay of vitamin B_{12} or folate concentrations*

Method	Extraction of vitamin	Identity of labelled vitamin	Binding protein	Separation of bound from unbound vitamin
Abbott IM_x B_{12} assay	α-monothioglycerol, NAOH, KCN	B_{12}–alkaline phosphatase conjugate (added after binding of microparticles to matrix)	Purified porcine IF-coated microparticles	Binding of microparticles to glass-fibre matrix
ACS:180 V B_{12} assay (Chiron Diagnostics)	DTT, NaOH, KCN	Acridinium ester-labelled B_{12} (added during reaction of analyte with binding protein)	Purified porcine IF covalently bound to paramagnetic particles	Magnetic separation
Technicon Immuno 1® System–B_{12} assay (Bayer)	DTT, NaOH, KCN	B_{12}–alkaline phosphatase conjugate (added during reaction of analyte with binding protein)	Fluorescein-conjugated porcine IF	Anti-fluorescein antibody bound to magnetic particles
Abbott IM_x Folate assay	DTT, KOH	Pteroic acid–alkaline phosphatase conjugate (added after binding of capture reagent to positively charged glass-fibre matrix)	Purified bovine milk FBP combined with a monoclonal anti-FBP antibody covalently coupled with carboxymethyl-amylose (capture reagent)	Positively charged glass-fibre matrix
Technicon Immuno 1® System–Folate assay (Bayer)	DTT, NaOH, KCN	Folate–alkaline phosphatase conjugate (added during reaction of analyte with binding protein)	Fluorescein-conjugated bovine milk FBP	Anti-fluorescein antibody bound to magnetic particles
ACS:180 Folate assay (Chiron Diagnostics)	DTT, NaOH	Folate–dimethylacridinium ester conjugate (added during reaction of analyte with binding protein)	Purified bovine milk FBP immobilized on paramagnetic particles	Magnetic separation

containing PGA are used to calibrate the assay, and these solutions are calibrated against 5-methyl-THF.

In a recent study (Wickramasinghe *et al.*, 1996), the accuracy of serum B_{12} assayed by the IM_X method was investigated using the 1st International Reference Reagent for human serum vitamin B_{12} and was found to be very good. The CVs for the within-run and between-run imprecision in the Abbott IM_X assay for B_{12} were found to be 2.6–5.1 and 1.8–5.1%, respectively, in the serum B_{12} range 90–785 ng/L. The corresponding figures for the Abbott IM_X serum folate assay were 2.5 and 3.0%, respectively. The CV for the within-run imprecision in the Abbott IM_X red cell folate assay ranged from 3 to 5.8% for three samples with red cell folate levels of 87–353 µg/L. The results of the IM_X assays correlated well with those of the Becton Dickinson radioassays for B_{12} and red cell folate (ICN B_{12} [^{57}Co]/charcoal radioassay and ICN Folate [^{125}I]/charcoal radioassay). When discrepant results were found by the two methods, a retrospective analysis revealed that the serum B_{12} and red cell folate levels measured by the IM_X method appeared to be more frequently consistent with clinical details and serum homocysteine levels than those measured by the radioassay.

BAYER IMMUNO 1 ASSAYS

These have been developed for use with the fully automated, Technicon Immuno 1 random access analyser. In the B_{12} assay, the B_{12} is released from serum binders using reagents containing DTT, NaOH and KCN, and the released B_{12} is reacted with fluorescein-conjugated porcine intrinsic factor. Vitamin B_{12}–calf alkaline phosphatase conjugate is added next and the reaction mixture subjected to a further incubation. Immunomagnetic particles linked with mouse monoclonal antibody to fluorescein are then used to bind the fluorescein–IF conjugates after which the particles are immobilized in a magnetic field, washed and incubated with para-nitrophenyl phosphate (pNPP). The alkaline phosphatase in the IF–fluorescein–antibody–particle complexes converts the pNPP to para-nitrophenoxide, the generation of which is measured by its absorbance at 405 nm. The CVs for within-run and between-run imprecision were 1–7.3 and 1.5–12%, respectively, with three serum pools containing 169–1274 ng/L, and the recovery of vitamin B_{12} added to the serum was 96 ± 6%. Serum B_{12} results obtained by this method correlated well with those obtained by the Bio-Rad Quantaphase Radioassay kit ($n = 140$, $r = 0.96$, slope = 0.88, intercept = 22 ng/L) and the Abbott IM_X method ($n = 149$, $r = 0.97$, slope = 0.91, intercept = −8 ng/L).

The steps in the Technicon Immuno 1 assay for folates are:

1 release of folate from endogenous folate binders using reagents containing DTT, NaOH and KCN;
2 reaction of released folate with fluorescein-conjugated folate-binding protein;
3 incubation with folate–calf alkaline phosphatase conjugate;
4 incubation with immunomagnetic particles linked with mouse monoclonal antibody to fluorescein;
5 washing of particles followed by addition of para-nitrophenyl phosphate;
6 measurement of the generation of para-nitrophenoxide.

The performance characteristics reported by the manufacturers are a CV for total assay imprecision of 11.6, 9.4, 7.6, 5 and 5.3% for serum folate levels of 1.5, 2.6, 3.0, 5.7 and 14.1 µg/L, respectively, and good correlation of results with the Bio-Rad Quantaphase method ($n = 80$, $r = −0.93$) and the Ciba-Corning ACS:180 assay ($n = 97$, $r = 0.93$).

A red cell folate assay can be performed on 50 µL of whole blood subjected to lysis in a 90-minute preparation step using the same procedure as for serum folate. Results are available 88 minutes after the lysate is placed in the analyser and 120 tests can be performed per hour.

According to the manufacturer's information, the CV for total assay imprecision for samples with red cell folates of 158, 260, 335 and 432 µg/L were 9, 7, 6.7 and 6%, respectively, and the results of the Technicon Immuno 1 red cell folate assay correlated well with those of the Bio-Rad Quantaphase II assay (n = 151, r = 0.95, slope = 1.09, intercept = −37.5 µg/L) and the Ciba-Corning ACS:180 assay (n = 150, r = 0.926, slope = 0.93, intercept = − 85 µg/L).

AUTOMATED CHEMILUMINESCENCE SYSTEM ASSAYS

These have been developed for use on the Ciba Corning Diagnostics Corp. ACS:180™ fully automated random access analyser. In the ACS:180V B$_{12}$ assay (Chiron Diagnostics), an aliquot of the serum is dispensed into a cuvette and the B$_{12}$ is released from its binders using a reagent containing sodium hydroxide and potassium cyanide. Purified hog intrinsic factor covalently bound to paramagnetic particles is then added and after incubation at 37°C for 5 minutes, acridinium-ester-labelled vitamin B$_{12}$ is added and the mixture incubated for a further 2.5 minutes. The particles are then separated and washed, the chemiluminescent reaction is initiated by oxidation of the bound acridinium-ester-labelled compound with alkaline hydrogen peroxide and the light emitted measured. According to the manufacturer's literature, the serum B$_{12}$ results obtained by this method correlated well with results obtained by the Bio-Rad method (n = 196, r = 0.979 slope = 0.86, intercept = 60 ng/L for samples with B$_{12}$ levels < 2000 ng/L). The CV for total assay imprecision with serum samples containing 1147, 661, 204 and 169 ng B$_{12}$/L were, respectively, 3.44, 3.24, 4.79 and 6.28%. In the ACS:180 B$_{12}$ assay, the total incubation time is 10.5 minutes and the first result is available in 15 minutes.

In the automated chemiluminescence system for serum folate (ACS:180 folate assay), folate is released from endogenous binders using DTT and NaOH and incubated first with FBP-coated paramagnetic particles and then with a folate–acridinium ester conjugate. After separating and washing the particles, the chemiluminescence reaction is initiated. Red cell folate may be assayed by this method using a 1:21 dilution of whole blood with a reagent containing 0.2% ascorbic acid. The technical information provided by the manufacturer indicates that serum and red cell folate values obtained by this method correlated well with those obtained by the Bio-Rad method (for serum folate: n = 212, r = 0.97, slope = 0.87, intercept = 1.11 µg/L; for red cell folate: n = 100, r = 0.94, slope = 0.81, intercept = 35.8 µg/L). Recovery of 5-methyl-THF added to serum was 95.1–105.5% (average 100%) and the CV for total assay imprecision was 3.4–8.7% over the serum folate range 2.89–21.82 µg/L. The ACS:180 folate assay has a total incubation time of 7.5 minutes and the first result is available in 15 minutes.

CEDIA® VITAMIN B$_{12}$ (NO BOIL) AND FOLATE (NO BOIL) ASSAYS

These assay systems supplied by Boehringer Mannheim (BM) are intended for use on automated clinical analysers such as the BM/Hitachi 911 analyser or the Cobas-Mira analyser (Van der Weide et al., 1992). Unlike in other CEDIA systems, the antibody is replaced by IF in the case of the B$_{12}$ assay and FBP in the case of the folate assay.

CEDIA assays employ two enzymatically inactive fragments of the bacterial enzyme β-galactosidase (an enzyme acceptor fragment and an enzyme donor fragment) prepared by recombinant DNA technology. When mixed together, these fragments combine spontaneously to form the active enzyme. After the initial extraction step (alkaline pH), the cyanocobalamin or folate derived from serum competes with cyanocobalamin or folate conjugated to enzyme donor fragments for a limiting amount of porcine IF or FBP, respectively. Binding of the analyte–enzyme–donor–fragment conjugate to IF or FBP prevents the conjugated enzyme donor fragments from re-associating with the enzyme-acceptor fragments in the reaction mixture. The concentration of B_{12} or folate in the sample is proportional to the amount of active enzyme formed which is quantified spectrophotometrically by the extent of enzyme-induced hydrolysis of chlorophenol red-β-D-galactopyranoside in the case of the B_{12} assay and o-nitrophenyl-β-D-galactopyranoside in the case of the folate assay.

According to the manufacturer's data sheet, in the CEDIA serum vitamin B_{12} assay (using the BM/Hitachi 199 analyser), cross-reactivity with cobinamide is less than 0.75%, the recovery of B_{12} added as serum is 94–103%, the CVs for within-run imprecision are 3.5–6.5% and the CVs for between-run imprecision are 5.0–10.6%. Comparison of results obtained from 129 samples by the CEDIA method with those obtained by the Bio-Rad Quantaphase II method gave a correlation coefficient of 0.98 (slope = 0.95, intercept = −32.9 ng/L). In the CEDIA serum folate assay, the recovery of folate added as serum was 99–109%, the CVs for within-run imprecision were 2.4–14.7% and the CVs for between-run imprecision were 3.8–14.2%. Comparison with the Bio-Rad Quantaphase II folate method gave a correlation coefficient of 0.96 ($n = 83$, slope = 0.95, intercept = 0.03 μg/L). In another study using the Cobas-Mira analyser, within-run CVs were 3.7–11% for the B_{12} assay and 1.2–10.7% for the serum folate assay, and between-run CVs were 9.5–11.9% for the B_{12} assay and 6.1–18.5% for the serum folate assay. Results of the CEDIA assays correlated well with a 'boil' radioassay from Becton Dickinson, with regression coefficients of 0.98 for the B_{12} assay ($n = 51$, slope = 0.90, intercept = 74 ng/L) and 0.97 for the folate assay ($n = 57$, slope = 1.45, intercept = 0.79 μg/L) (Van der Weide et al., 1992).

ELECSYS ASSAYS

In the Elecsys serum B_{12} and serum and red cell folate assay, bound B_{12}/folate is released from an aliquot of the serum sample or haemolysate by treatment with alkaline reagents which denature binding proteins. The treated samples are then incubated with ruthenium-labelled IF/ruthenium-labelled FBP, which reacts with B_{12}/folate to form a complex, the quantity of which is proportional to the concentration of the analyte. Streptavidin-coated microparticles and biotin-labelled B_{12}/folate are then added, which results in the attachment of the biotin-labelled compounds to the unbound sites of the ruthenium-labelled IF/FBP, and the formation of a ruthenium-labelled IF–B_{12}–biotin complex or a ruthenium-labelled FBP–folate–biotin complex. These complexes are bound to the solid phase as a result of the reaction between biotin and streptavidin. Following transfer to a measuring cell, the microparticles are magnetically captured onto an electrode and unbound material removed. A voltage is then applied to the electrode and the resulting ruthenium complex-based chemiluminescence measured by a photomultiplier.

The first result appears after 5 minutes and subsequent results become available every 60 seconds. The performance characteristics reported by the manufacturers include good CVs for within-run and total imprecision and regression of 0.98 for correlation with serum B_{12} levels measured by Bio-Rad or Abbott IM_x methods and of 0.97 for correlation with serum folate levels measured by these two methods. Red cell folate values obtained by the Elecsys method correlated well with those determined by the Bio-Rad ($r = 0.84$), ACS:180 ($r = 0.79$) and IM_x ($r = 0.85$) methods.

AUTODELFIA™ B_{12} AND FOLATE ASSAYS

In the AutoDELFIA assays (Wallac), anti-IF or anti-FBP antibody is reacted with microtitre plates coated with anti-mouse IgG. Europium-labelled B_{12} or folate, porcine IF or FBP and cyanocobalamin or folates derived from the sample (by treatment with DTT, NaOH, KCN and cobinamide) are then added. The IF or FBP combines with the bound anti-IF or anti-FBP antibody, and labelled and unlabelled B$_{12}$ or folate compete for binding sites on IF or FBP. Europium ions are then released from the bound B$_{12}$ or folate by the addition of a special reagent and a fluorescent chelate is produced. The fluorescence is measured and is inversely proportional to the quantity of analyte in the sample.

The performance characteristics for the B$_{12}$ assay reported by the manufacturer are good, with CVs for within-run imprecision of 3.2–8.2% and for between-run imprecision of 2.5–6.3% (serum B$_{12}$ 149–1069 ng/L) and a mean recovery of added B$_{12}$ of 96% (range 79–111). For the red cell folate assay, the CVs for within-run imprecision were 1.5–1.7% and for between-run imprecision 4.9–8.2% (red cell folate 101–185 µg/L). The total assay running time is about 2 hours. Correlations with results from B$_{12}$ and folate assays based on other methods are not presented.

12.3 RADIOIMMUNOASSAYS FOR SERUM B$_{12}$

Rothenberg et al. (1984) and O'Sullivan et al. (1992) have described radioimmunoassays for serum B$_{12}$ based on antibodies raised in rabbits against a carboxylic acid derivative of cyanocobalamin coupled to human serum albumin. In the method reported by O'Sullivan et al. (1992), test sera were autoclaved in acetate cyanide buffer to destroy the B$_{12}$-binding capacity of serum, release TC-bound B$_{12}$ and convert the released B$_{12}$ to cyanocobalamin prior to reaction with the specific antibody. The radiolabelled compound used was high specific activity [57]Co-cyanocobalamin. Magnetizable particles coated with donkey anti-rabbit gamma globulin were used to separate bound from free vitamin B$_{12}$. The results of this radio-immunoassay correlated well with those of the L. leichmannii assay and there was 100% recovery of added B$_{12}$.

12.4 HIGH-PERFORMANCE LIQUID CHROMATOGRAPHY

High-performance liquid chromatography (HPLC) allows the separate identification and quantitation of the different forms of functional cobalamins (Binder et al., 1982) as well as various cobalamin analogues (Frenkel et al., 1979). Nevertheless, this approach has not been developed for the assay of cobalamins in serum samples. By contrast, an HPLC-based method has been described for the assay of 5-methyl-THF in plasma (Lucock et al., 1989).

12.5 CORRELATION OF DU-SUPPRESSED VALUES AND METABOLITE MEASUREMENTS WITH SERUM B$_{12}$, SERUM FOLATE AND RED CELL FOLATE LEVELS

Two other approaches have now been well established for the detection of B$_{12}$ or folate deficiency. The first is the deoxyuridine suppression test (dUST) on bone marrow cells, which provides information on the efficiency of methylation of deoxyuridylate which is dependent on 5,10-methylenetetrahydrofolate and, indirectly, on methylcobalamin (Wickramasinghe and Matthews, 1988). The second is the measurement of serum methylmalonic acid (MMA) which is high in B$_{12}$ but not in folate deficiency, or the measurement of serum homocysteine (HCYS) which is high in either B$_{12}$ or folate deficiency. The concentrations of these metabolites fall to within the normal range in patients treated with the deficient vitamin (Allen et al.,

1990). It has been estimated that about 98% of clear-cut clinically confirmed cases of B_{12} deficiency have elevated MMA levels and about 96% have elevated HCYS levels (Savage *et al.*, 1994). Raised HCYS levels are, however, seen in conditions other than B_{12} or folate deficiency, such as alcoholism, pyridoxine deficiency, impaired renal function and in heterozygotes for homocystinuria (Green, 1995). The percentage of clear-cut cases of folate deficiency without renal failure showing raised HCYS and MMA levels, were, respectively, 91 and < 1% (Savage *et al.*, 1994).

It is now known that of patients with cobalamin-responsive disorders, about 25–38% lack macrocytosis (Carmel, 1990; Stabler *et al.*, 1990), 44% lack anaemia (Stabler *et al.*, 1990) and some even lack subnormal serum B_{12} levels. In one study, the serum B_{12} levels measured by a radioassay employing purified IF (Quantaphase, Bio-Rad) were within the normal range in 12 of 419 (2.9%) consecutive patients seen between 1975 and 1988, and nine of 173 consecutive patients (5.2%) seen between 1984 and 1988 who had clinically proven B_{12} deficiency (Lindenbaum *et al.*, 1990). The 12 cases with normal serum B_{12} levels had elevated serum MMA and HCYS concentrations.

On the other hand, the use of metabolite assays has revealed that a substantial number of patients with low serum B_{12} or low red cell folate levels do not suffer from biochemical disturbances known to result from B_{12} or folate deficiency. For example, in one study involving all samples submitted for the assay of serum B_{12} (*E. gracilis* method) and red cell folate (*L. casei* method), only 25% of 151 samples with low serum B_{12} (with or without low red cell folate) and only 27% of 130 samples with low red cell folate and normal serum B_{12} had evidence of tissue deficiency as judged by increased serum HCYS levels (Curtis *et al.*, 1994). In another study, 31 of 42 (74%) consecutive patients with low serum B_{12} (measured by a 'no-boil' kit employing purified IF) had elevated serum MMA levels and the remaining 26% had no evidence of tissue cobalamin deficiency (Moelby *et al.*, 1990). The significance of these unexplained low serum B_{12} and red cell folate levels remains to be determined. At least some of them may be indicative of a stage of negative B_{12} or folate balance at which there is little or no impairment of the activities of homocysteine methyltransferase or methylmalonyl-CoA mutase. In addition, some unexplained low serum B_{12} levels may be due to the presence of low TCI concentrations.

As has already been mentioned, whereas serum MMA is highly specific for B_{12} deficiency, serum HCYS is considerably less specific for either B_{12} or folate deficiency. Nevertheless, these metabolite assays are more sensitive indicators of B_{12} and folate status than serum B_{12} or red cell folate levels, detecting both frank and clinically inapparent degrees of deficiency. The evidence for this is as follows. First, during haematological relapse in inadequately treated B_{12} deficiency, metabolite levels increase before the serum B_{12} becomes subnormal (Lindenbaum *et al.*,1990). Secondly, in elderly subjects, the proportion of B_{12}-deficient individuals as judged by high metabolite values was much greater than that judged by low serum B_{12} levels (Joosten *et al.*, 1993). Thus in 64 healthy elderly subjects, the percentages of cases with low serum B_{12}, low serum folate, high serum HCYS and high serum MMA levels were, respectively, 6, 5, 30 and 23. The corresponding values in 286 hospitalized elderly patients were, respectively, 5, 19, 51 and 39. In the latter group there was also a statistically significant weak inverse correlation between serum B_{12} and serum MMA or serum HCYS levels, and between serum folate and serum HCYS levels. A statistically significant weak inverse correlation has also been reported between serum B_{12} and total serum HCYS and between serum folate and total serum HCYS but not between serum B_{12} and serum MMA in healthy subjects (Jacobsen *et al.*, 1994), suggesting that the B_{12} or folate status of some healthy subjects may not be optimal.

In a study of 50 patients with low serum B_{12} concentrations and few or no features of tissue B_{12} deficiency, Carmel *et al.* (1996) found that 68% gave increased dU-suppressed values (without additives), 50% had raised serum HCYS levels, 40% had raised serum MMA levels and 60% had either a raised serum MMA or a raised serum HCYS level. The data suggested that the dU-suppressed value was somewhat more sensitive than the metabolite assays in detecting early B$_{12}$ deficiency.

12.6 ASSAY OF HOLOTRANSCOBALAMIN II

Most of the B$_{12}$ in the serum is bound to TCI which is not involved in cellular uptake of B$_{12}$. Only 6–20% is bound to transcobalamin II (TCII), the B$_{12}$-binding protein involved in delivery of B$_{12}$ to cells. It would therefore be expected that the concentration of TCII-bound B$_{12}$ (holo-TCII) would be a better measure than total serum B$_{12}$ of the ability of serum to supply cells with B$_{12}$. Attempts have therefore been made to measure holo-TCII levels in serum. One method for doing so involves adsorption of the holo-TCII from an aliquot of the serum using a slurry containing Quso G32 or G761 (PQ Corporation, Valley Forge, PA, USA), a microfine precipitate of silica. The B$_{12}$ concentrations in untreated and adsorbed serum are measured by a competitive protein-binding assay and the difference is taken as the holo-TCII concentration (Das *et al.*, 1991). Using synthetic amorphous precipitated silica (Sipernat 283 LS; PQ Corporation), instead of Quso, Wickramasinghe and Fida (1993) found that the total serum B$_{12}$ levels correlated more weakly with holo-TCII levels measured in this way ($r = 0.72$) than with holo-haptocorrin concentrations ($r = 0.97$). The correlation between holohaptocorrin and holo-TCII concentrations was even weaker ($r = 0.576$), underlining the theoretical importance of measuring holo-TCII levels. However, in one study, the value of serum holo-TCII measurements in the differential diagnosis of macrocytosis was found to be limited and this was attributed partly to factors other than B$_{12}$ status (e.g. erythroid hyperplasia) affecting holo-TCII levels and partly to methodological problems (Wickramasinghe and Ratnayaka, 1996). The methodological problems are:

- the lower limit for the sensitivity of most currently used methods for measuring Cbl is around 60 ng/L and holo-TCII assays involving samples of untreated or adsorbed sera giving a B$_{12}$ value below 60 ng/L will be unreliable;
- treatment with silica only removes about 90% of the holo-TCII;
- there is some dilution of the silica-adsorbed sera from the water in the silica slurry and the extent of this dilution is difficult to assess accurately;
- the reproducibility of holo-TCII measurements is relatively poor, with a CV of 18% for between-run imprecision.

The latter is at least partly due to the fact that holo-TCII levels are calculated as a difference between two assay results each with its own imprecision.

Vu *et al.* (1993) found that assays using different lots of Quso gel gave unacceptable differences in holo-TCII results, and therefore used acid-washed and buffered microfine glass powder (ground and screened through 325 mesh) instead of Quso to absorb the TCII. They also spun an aliquot of the glass slurry in a microcentrifuge and removed the supernatant before mixing the pellet with the plasma; this would have the effect of markedly reducing the dilution of the sample that occurred with the original Quso method and early modifications of it. The CVs for the within-run and between-run imprecision with this modified method were satisfactory for serum samples with a total B$_{12}$ of 497–747 ng/L, being 8.7–9.3 and 6.0–10.7%, respectively. Another modification of the method of Das *et al.* (1991) has been reported by Benhayoun *et al.* (1993), who absorbed the TCII using Heparin Sepharose instead of Quso.

Methodological differences markedly influence the 95% reference limits obtained for holo-TCII levels in healthy subjects, which were 12.9–544.7 ng/L ($n = 50$) in one of the studies (Wickramasinghe and Ratnayake, 1996) and 84–140 ng/L ($n = 10$) in another (Vu *et al.*, 1993).

12.7 INTERNATIONAL REFERENCE REAGENTS

International Reference Reagents for serum B_{12} and red cell folate are now available and provide useful tools in the development and evaluation of assay techniques and the development of quality control material. They may be obtained from the National Institute of Biological Standards and Control (NIBSC), Potters Bar, Herts, UK.

In 1992 the World Health Organization (WHO) established the 1st International Reference Reagent (IRR) (formerly the 1st British Standard) for human serum vitamin B_{12} (81/563). This consists of pooled human serum that was stored in the dark at $-40°C$ until distribution in 1 mL aliquots into non-actinic neutral glass ampoules followed by freeze-drying. The ampoules are stored at or below $-20°C$ in the dark. Individual blood donations were negative for hepatitis B and the final product did not contain antibody to HIV. The freeze-dried pooled serum was assayed in seven laboratories using a turbidimetric *Euglena* assay based on a single strain of the organism and calibrated against cyanocobalamin standards used routinely in the participating laboratories. The agreed potency of the IRR was 320 pg of vitamin B_{12} per ampoule.

The 1st International Standard for Whole Blood Folate (NIBSC code: 95/528) became available in 1996. This standard was prepared using whole blood from two donors each of whom was negative for HBsAg, anti-HIV and anti-HCV. The pooled blood was mixed with 0.05% (w/v) ascorbic acid solution in the ratio 1 volume of blood to 10 volumes of the ascorbic acid solution, dispensed into ampoules, freeze-dried and subjected to secondary desiccation. Using microbiological assays and radioassays that were calibrated against in-house standards, this material was evaluated by 13 laboratories in five countries and assigned a folate content of 13 ng/ampoule. However, the obvious drawback of this initial approach is that the assigned value is a consensus of results obtained with different assay methods.

12.8 CONCLUSION

Microbiological assays for B_{12} and folate have been progressively replaced by assays based on competitive protein binding. The precision of most competitive protein-binding assays is good and, recently, precision has been further improved by the introduction of fully automated assay techniques. However, uncertainty still remains regarding the accuracy of such assays for folate and especially for red cell folate. It is likely that the major difficulty in assaying red cell folate accurately is that even when deconjugation of the folate polyglutamates in red cells is complete, the sample to be assayed contains several forms of folate monoglutamate, some of which may not have the same affinity for the FBP as PGA. One theoretical solution to this may be to convert all folate monoglutamates to a single form of folate prior to assay, and to use a labelled version of this form of folate during the competitive binding step, but whether this is feasible remains to be seen. Further progress in the accurate analysis of serum and red cell folate is urgently needed in view of recent epidemiological evidence suggesting that folate deficiency is implicated in the aetiology of neural tube defects, causes uracil misincorporation into human DNA and chromosome breakage (Blount *et al.*, 1997) and is a risk factor for certain forms of cancer and, by virtue of its effect of elevating serum homocysteine levels, also for coronary artery disease and stroke.

The absence of 'gold standard' methods of assay (Herbert *et al.*, 1984) and completely reliable reference material continue to be important obstacles in evaluating new approaches to the measurement of B_{12} and folate. In the current circumstances, it is of paramount importance that investigators use method-specific reference ranges established in diagnostic laboratories and that new assay methods are validated by assay of sera from patients with clinically confirmed deficiency states. Since the range of vitamin B$_{12}$ and folate concentrations observed in patients deficient in these vitamins overlaps with the reference range for healthy individuals, manufacturers of several assay kits now quote 'indeterminate' ranges. However, this approach does not help the clinician to identify those subjects with a vitamin level within the 95% reference range who may benefit from folate or B$_{12}$ therapy or supplementation.

Results from quality assurance schemes indicate that the average interlaboratory all-methods CVs for serum B$_{12}$, serum folate and red cell folate are, respectively, about 10, 20 and 35%. Analysis of data circulated by the UK NEQAS scheme suggests that at least some fully automated competitive protein-binding assays give better interlaboratory CVs for folate measurements than assays that are not fully automated. For example, the interlaboratory CVs for serum folate and red cell folate assayed by the Abbott IM$_x$ method have been around 12 and 17%, respectively. Clearly, additional research is needed to understand the basis of the wide interlaboratory variation in folate assay results by most current methods.

REFERENCES

Allen, R.H. (1982) More on no-boil assay. *Ligand Q.* **5**, 48–9.

Allen, R.H., Stabler, S.P., Savage, D.G. and Lindenbaum, J. (1990) Diagnosis of cobalamin deficiency I: usefulness of serum methylmalonic acid and total homocysteine concentrations. *Am. J. Haematol.* **34**, 90–8.

Anderson, B.B. (1964) Investigations into the Euglena method for the assay of the vitamin B$_{12}$ in serum. *J. Clin. Pathol.* **17**, 14–26.

Anderson, B. B. and Sourial, N.A. (1983) The assay of serum cobalamin by Euglena gracilis. In: Hall, C.A. (ed.), *The Cobalamins. Methods in Haematology*, Vol. 10. Edinburgh: Churchill Livingstone, 51–64.

Arnaud, J., Cotisson, A., Meffre, G. *et al.* (1994) Comparison of three commercial kits and a microbiological assay for the determination of vitamin B$_{12}$ in serum. *Scand. J. Clin. Lab. Invest.* **54**, 235–40.

Bain, B., Broom, G.N., Woodside, J. *et al.* (1982) Assessment of a radioisotopic assay for vitamin B$_{12}$ using an intrinsic factor preparation with R proteins blocked by vitamin B$_{12}$ analogues. *J. Clin. Pathol.* **35**, 1110–13.

Bain, B.J., Wickramasinghe, S.N., Broom, G.N. *et al.* (1984) Assessment of the value of a competitive protein binding assay of folic acid in the detection of folic acid deficiency. *J. Clin. Pathol.* **37**, 888–94.

Baker, H., Herbert, V., Frank, O. *et al.* (1959) A microbiological method for detecting folic acid deficiency in man. *Clin. Chem.* **5**, 275–80.

Barakat, R.M. and Ekins, R.P. (1961) Assay of vitamin B$_{12}$ in blood. *Lancet* **1**, 25–6.

Barakat, R.M. and Ekins, R.P. (1963) An isotopic method for the determination of vitamin B$_{12}$ levels in blood. *Blood* **21**, 70–9.

Beard, M.E.J. and Allen, D.M. (1967) Effect of antimicrobial agents on the *Lactobacillus casei* folate assay. *Am. J. Clin. Pathol.* **48**, 401–4.

Beck, W.S. (1983) The assay of serum cobalamin by Lactobacillus leichmannii and the interpretation of serum cobalamin levels. In: Hall, C.A. (ed.), *The Cobalamins. Methods in Haematology*, Vol. 10, Edinburgh: Churchill Livingstone, 31–50.

Benhayoun, S., Adjalla, C., Nicolas, J.P. *et al.* (1993) Method for the direct specific measurement of vitamin B$_{12}$ bound to transcobalamin II in plasma. *Acta Haematol.* **89**, 195–9.

Binder, M., Kilhouse, J.F., Van Horne, K.C. and Allen, R.H. (1982) High-pressure liquid chromatography of cobalamin and cobalamin analogs. *Anal. Biochem.* **125**, 253–8.

Blount, B.C., Mack, M.M., Wehr, C.M. *et al*. (1997) Folate deficiency causes uracil misincorporation into human DNA and chromosome breakage: implications for cancer and neuronal damage. *Proc. Natl Acad. Sci. USA* **94**, 3290–5.

Brown, R.D., Jun, R., Hughes, W. *et al*. (1990) Red cell folate assays: some answers to current problems with radioassay variability. *Pathology* **22**, 82–7.

Burkholder, P.R. (1951) Determination of vitamin B$_{12}$ with a mutant strain of Escherichia Coli. *Science* **114**, 459–60.

Carmel, R. (1990) Subtle and atypical cobalamin deficiency states. *Am. J. Hematol.* **34**, 108–14.

Carmel, R., Rasmussen, K., Jacobsen, D.W. and Green, R. (1996) Comparison of the deoxyuridine suppression test with serum levels of methylmalonic acid and homocysteine in mild cobalamin deficiency. *Br. J. Haematol.* **93**, 311–18.

Carmel, R. and Coltman, C.A. Jr. (1969) Radioassay for serum vitamin B$_{12}$ with the use of saliva as the vitamin B$_{12}$ binder. *J. Lab. Clin. Med.* **74**, 967–75.

Chanarin, I. (1969) *The Megaloblastic Anaemias*, 1st edn. Oxford: Blackwell Scientific Publications, 204.

Chanarin, I. and Muir, M. (1982) Demonstration of vitamin B$_{12}$ analogues in human sera not detected by microbiological assay. *Br. J. Haematol.* **51**, 171–3.

Chen, I.W., Silberstein, E.B., Maxon, H.R. *et al*. (1981) Clinical significance of serum vitamin B$_{12}$ measured by radioassay using pure intrinsic factor. *J. Nucl. Med.* **22**, 447–51.

Curtis, D., Sparrow, R., Brennan, L. and Van Der Weyden, M.B. (1994) Elevated serum homocysteine as a predictor for vitamin B$_{12}$ or folate deficiency. *Eur. J. Haematol.* **52**, 227–32.

Das, K.C., Manusselis, C. and Herbert, V. (1991) Determination of vitamin B$_{12}$ (cobalamin) in serum and erythrocytes by radioassay, and of holo-transcobalamin II (holo-TCII) and holo-haptocorrin (holo-TCI and III) in serum by adsorbing holo-TCII on microfine silica. *J. Nutr. Biochem.* **2**, 455–63.

Davis, B.D. and Mingioli, E.S. (1950) Mutants of Escherichia coli requiring methionine or vitamin B$_{12}$. *J. Bact.* **60**, 17–28.

Dawson, D.W., Fish, D.I., Frew, I.D.O. *et al*. (1987) Laboratory diagnosis of megaloblastic anaemia: current methods assessed by external quality assurance trials. *J. Clin. Pathol.* **40**, 393–7.

Dunn, R.T. and Foster, L.B. (1973) Radioassay of serum folate. *Clin. Chem.* **19**, 1101–5.

Ekins, R.P. and Sgherzi, A.M. (1965) The microassay of vitamin B$_{12}$ in human plasma by the saturation assay technique. In: *Radiochemical Methods of Analysis*, vol. 2. Vienna: International Atomic Energy Agency, 239.

El Shami, A.S. and Durham, A.P. (1983) More on vitamin B$_{12}$ results as measured with "boil" and "no boil" kits. *Clin. Chem.* **29**, 2115–16.

Fish, D.I. and Dawson, D.W. (1983) Comparison of methods used in commercial kits for the assay of serum vitamin B$_{12}$. *Clin. Lab. Haematol.* **5**, 271–7,

Ford, J.E. (1953) The microbiological assay of 'vitamin B$_{12}$'. The specificity of the requirement of Ochromonas malhamensis for cyanocobalamin. *Br. J. Nutr.* **7**, 299–306.

Frenkel, E.P., Kitchens, R.L. and Prough, R. (1979) High-performance liquid chromatographic separation of cobalamins. *J. Chromatogr.* **174**, 393–400.

Friedner, S., Josephson, B. and Levin, K. (1969) Vitamin B$_{12}$ determination by means of radioisotope dilution and ultrafiltration. *Clin. Chim. Acta* **24**, 171–9.

Givas, J.K. and Gutcho, S. (1975) pH dependence of the binding of folates to milk binder in radioassay of folates. *Clin. Chem.* **21**, 427–8.

Green, R. (1995) Metabolite assays in cobalamin and folate deficiency. *Bailliére's Clin. Haematol.* **8**, 533–66.

Green, R., Newmark, P.A., Musso, A.M. and Mollin, D.L. (1974) The use of chicken serum for measurement of serum vitamin B$_{12}$ concentration by radioisotope dilution: description of method and comparison with microbiological assay results. *Br. J. Haematol.* **27**, 507–26.

Gutcho, S. (1978) Source of error in determination of erythrocyte folate by competitive binding radioassay–comments. *Clin. Chem.* **24**, 388–9.

Herbert, V. (1961) The assay and nature of folic acid activity in human serum. *J. Clin. Invest.* **40**, 81.

Herbert, V., Colman, N., Palat, D. *et al.* (1984) Is there a 'gold standard' for human serum vitamin B$_{12}$ assay? *J. Lab. Clin. Med.* **104**, 829–41.

Higgins, T. and Wu, A. (1983) Differences in vitamin B$_{12}$ results as measured with boil and no boil kits. *Clin. Chem.* **29**, 587–8.

Hoffbrand, A.V., Newcombe, B.F.A. and Mollin, D.L. (1966) Method of assay of red cell folate activity and the value of the assay as a test for folate deficiency. *J. Clin. Pathol.* **19**, 17–28.

Hoffmann, C.E., Stockstad, E.L.R., Hutchings, B.L. *et al.* (1949) The microbiological assay of vitamin B$_{12}$ with Lactobacillus leichmannii. *J. Biol. Chem.* **181**, 635–44.

Hutner, S.H., Provasoli, L. and Filfus, J. (1953) Nutrition of some phagotrophic fresh-water chrysomonads. *Ann. NY Acad. Sci.* **56**, 852–62.

Hutner, S.H., Provasoli, L., Stokstad, E.L.R. *et al.* (1949) Assay of anti-pernicious anemia factor with *Euglena. Proc. Soc. Exp. Biol. Med.* **70**, 118–20.

Jacobsen, D.W., Gatautis, V.J., Green, R. *et al.* (1994) Rapid HPLC determination of total homocysteine and other thiols in serum and plasma: sex differences and correlation with cobalamin and folate concentrations in healthy subjects. *Clin. Chem.* **40**, 873–81.

Johnson, I. and Rose, M. (1978) Measurement of red cell folate with ^{75}Se-selenofolate radioassay. *J. Clin. Pathol.* **31**, 47–9.

Johnson, I., Guildford, H. and Rose, M. (1977) Measurement of serum folate: experience with ^{75}Se-selenofolate radioassay. *J. Clin. Pathol.* **30**, 645–8.

Joosten, E., van den Berg, A., Riezler, R. *et al.* (1993) Metabolic evidence that deficiencies of vitamin B-12 (cobalamin), folate, and vitamin B-6 occur commonly in elderly people. *Am. J. Clin. Nutr.* **58**, 468–76.

Kakei, M. and Glass, B.G.J. (1962) Separation of bound and free vitamin B$_{12}$ on Sephadex G-25 column. *Proc. Soc. Exp. Biol. Med.* **3**, 270–4.

Kelleher, B.P. and O'Broin, S.D. (1991) Microbiological assay for vitamin B$_{12}$ performed in 96-well microtitre plates. *J. Clin. Pathol.* **44**, 592–5.

Kelleher, B.P., Walshe, K.G., Scott, J.M. and O'Broin, S.D. (1987) Microbiological assay for vitamin B$_{12}$ with use of a colistin-sulphate-resistant organism. *Clin. Chem.* **33**, 52–4.

Kelleher, B.P., Scott, J.M. and O'Broin, S.D. (1990) Use of beta-lactamase to hydrolyse interfering antibiotics in vitamin B$_{12}$ microbiological assay using Lactobacillus leichmannii. *Clin. Lab. Haematol.* **12**, 87–95.

Kolhouse, J.F., Kondo, H., Allen, N.C. *et al.* (1978) Cobalamin analogues are present in human plasma and can mask cobalamin deficiency because current radioisotope dilution assays are not specific for true cobalamin. *N. Engl. J. Med.* **299**, 785–92.

Kubasik, N.P., Ricotta, M. and Sine, H.E. (1980) Commercially-supplied binders for plasma cobalamin (vitamin B12) analysis – "purified" intrinsic factor, "cobinamide" – blocked R-protein binder, and non-purified intrinsic factor-R-protein binder – compared to microbiological assay. *Clin. Chem.* **26**, 598–600.

Kuemmerie, S.C., Boltinghouse, G.L., Delby, S.M. *et al.* (1992) Automated assay of vitamin B-12 by the Abbott IMx® analyzer. *Clin. Chem.* **38**, 2073–7.

Lau, K.S., Gottlieb, C., Wasserman, L.R. and Herbert, V. (1965) Measurement of serum vitamin B$_{12}$ level using radioisotope dilution and coated charcoal. *Blood* **26**, 202–14.

Lindenbaum, J., Savage, D.G., Stabler, S.P. and Allen, R.H. (1990) Diagnosis of cobalamin deficiency: II. Relative sensitivities of serum cobalamin, methylmalonic acid, and total homocysteine concentrations. *Am. J. Hematol.* **34**, 99–107.

Liu, Y.K. and Sulllivan, L.W. (1972) An improved radioisotope dilution assay for serum vitamin B$_{12}$ using hemoglobin-coated charcoal. *Blood* **39**, 426–32.

Longo, D.L. and Herbert, V. (1976) Radioassay for serum and red cell folate. *J. Lab. Clin. Med.* **87**, 138–51.

Lucock, M.D., Hartley, R. and Smithells, R.W. (1989) A rapid and specific HPLC-electrochemical method for the determination of endogenous 5-methyltetrahydrofolic acid in plasma using solid phase sample preparation with internal standardization. *Biomed. Chromat.* **3**, 58–63.

Lucock, M.D., Daskalakis, I., Schorah, C.J. *et al.* (1996) Analysis and biochemistry of blood folate. *Biochem. Mol. Med.* **58**, 93–112.

Mantzos, J., Gfytaki, H. and Alevizou, V. (1967) Isotopic determination of serum vitamin B_{12} level using Sephadex G-25. *Nuklearmedizin* **6**, 311–20.

Matthews, D.M. (1962) Observations on the estimation of serum vitamin B_{12} using Lactobacillus leichmannii. *Clin. Sci.* **22**, 101–11.

Matthews, D.M., Gunasegaram, R. and Linnell, J.C. (1967) Results with radioisotopic assay for serum B_{12} using serum binding agents. *J. Clin. Pathol.* **20**, 683–6.

Moelby, L., Rasmussen, K., Jensen, M.K. and Pedersen, K.O. (1990) The relationship between clinically confirmed cobalamin deficiency and serum methylmalonic acid. *J. Intern. Med.* **228**, 373–8.

Mortensen, E. (1978) Effect of storage on the apparent concentration of folate in erythrocytes, as measured by competitive protein binding radioassay. *Clin. Chem.* **24**, 663–8.

O'Broin, S. and Kelleher, B. (1992) Microbiological assay on microtitre plates of folate in serum and red cells. *J. Clin. Pathol.* **45**, 344–7.

O'Sullivan, J.J., Leeming, R.J., Lynch, S.S. and Pollock, A. (1992) Radioimmunoassay that measures serum vitamin B_{12}. *J. Clin. Pathol.* **45**, 328–31.

Raven, J.L., Robson, M.B., Walker, P.R. and Barkhan, P. (1969) Improved method for measuring vitamin B_{12} in serum using intrinsic factor, $^{57}CoB_{12}$ and coated charcoal. *J. Clin. Pathol.* **22**, 205–11.

Reizenstein, P.E. (1965) Errors and artefacts in serum folic-acid assays. *Acta Med. Scand.* **178**, 133–9.

Ross, G.I.M. (1950) Vitamin B_{12} assay in body fluids. *Nature* **166**, 270–1.

Ross, G.I.M., Hutner, S.H. and Bach, M.K. (1957) An improved *Euglena* method of vitamin B_{12} assay. In: Heinrich, H.C. (ed.), *Vitamin B_{12} und Intrinsic Factor* I. (Europaisches Symposion, Hamburg, 1956.) Stuttgart: Enke, 305–10.

Rothenberg, S.P. (1961) Assay of serum vitamin B_{12} concentration using ^{57}Co-B_{12} and intrinsic factor. *Proc. Soc. Exp. Biol. Med.* **108**, 45–8.

Rothenberg, S.P. (1968) A radioassay for serum B_{12} using unsaturated transcobalamin I as the B_{12} binding protein. *Blood* **31**, 44–54.

Rothenberg, S.P., da Costa, M. and Rosenberg, Z. (1972) A radioassay for serum folate: use of a two-phase sequential-incubation, ligand-binding system. *N. Engl. J. Med.* **286**, 1335–9.

Rothenberg, S.P., da Costa, M., Lawson, J. and Rosenberg. Z. (1974) The determination of erythrocyte folate concentrations using a two phase ligand binding radioassay. *Blood* **43**, 437–43.

Rothenberg, S.P., Marcoullis, G.P., Schwarz, S. and Lader, E. (1984) Measurement of cyanocobalamin in serum by a specific radioimmunoassay. *J. Lab. Clin. Med.* **103**, 959–72.

Savage, D.G., Lindenbaum, J., Stabler, S.P. and Allen, R.H. (1994) Sensitivity of serum methyl-malonic acid and total homocysteine determinations for diagnosing cobalamin and folate deficiencies. *Am. J. Med.* **96**, 239–46.

Schreiber, C. and Waxman, S. (1974) Measurement of red cell folate levels by ^{3}H-PteGlu radioassay. *Br. J. Haematol.* **27**, 551–8.

Shane, B., Tamura, T. and Stokstad, R. (1980) Folate assay: a comparison of radioassay and microbiological methods. *Clin. Chim. Acta* **100**, 13–19.

Shorb, M.S. (1948) Activity of vitamin B_{12} for the growth of Lactobacillus lactis. *Science* **107**, 397–8.

Skeggs, H.R., Huff, J.W., Wright, L.D. and Bosshardt, D.K. (1948) The use of Lactobacillus leichmannii in the microbiological assay of the 'animal protein factor'. *J. Biol. Chem.* **176**, 1459–60.

Spray, G.H. (1962) The estimation and significance of the level of vitamin B_{12} in serum. *Postgrad. Med. J.* **38**, 35–40.

Stabler, S.P., Allen, R.H., Savage, D.G. and Lindenbaum, J. (1990). Clinical spectrum and diagnosis of cobalamin deficiency. *Blood* **76**, 871–81.

Tajuddin, M. and Gardyna, H.A. (1973) Radioassay of serum folate, with use of a serum blank and non-dialysed milk as folate binder. *Clin. Chem.* **19**, 125–9.

Van der Weide, J., Homan, H.C., Cozijnsen-van Rheenen, E. *et al.* (1992) Nonisotopic binding assay for measuring vitamin B$_{12}$ and folate in serum. *Clin. Chem.* **38**, 766–8.

Vu, T., Amin, J., Ramos, M. *et al.* (1993) New assay for the rapid determination of plasma holotranscobalamin II levels: preliminary evaluation in cancer patients. *Am. J. Hematol.* **42**, 202–11.

Waters, A.H. and Mollin, D.L. (1961) Studies on the folic acid activity of human serum. *J. Clin. Pathol.* **14**, 335–44.

Waxman, S., Schreiber, C. and Herbert, V. (1971) Radioisotopic assay for measurement of serum folate levels. *Blood* **38**, 219–28.

Wentworth, S., McBride, J.A. and Walker, W.H.C. (1994) Chemiluminescence receptor assay for measuring vitamin B$_{12}$ in serum evaluated. *Clin. Chem.* **40**, 537–40.

Wickramasinghe, S.N. and Fida, S. (1993) Correlations between holo-transcobalmin II, holo-haptocorrin and total B$_{12}$ in serum samples from healthy subjects and patients. *J. Clin. Pathol.* **46**, 537–9.

Wickramasinghe, S.N. and Matthews, J.H. (1988) Deoxyuridine suppression: biochemical basis and diagnostic applications. *Blood Rev.* **2**, 168–77.

Wickramasinghe, S.N. and Ratnayaka, I.D. (1996) Limited value of serum holo-transcobalamin II measurements in the differential diagnosis of macrocytosis. *J. Clin. Pathol.* **49**, 755–8.

Wickramasinghe, S.N., Ratnayaka, I.D. and Hussein, H.A. (1996) Evaluation of the Abbott IM$_x$* systems for the assay of serum B$_{12}$, red cell folate and serum folate. *MDA Evaluation Report MDA/96/70.* Norwich: HMSO.

Zucker, R.M., Podell, E.R. and Allen, R.H. (1981) Multiple problems with current no-boil assays for serum cobalamin. *Ligand Q.* **4**, 52–8 and 59–63.

6

Coagulation testing

With respect to the polymers contained within heparin preparations, there are three important size classes: < 5 saccharide units, 5–17 saccharide units and >17 saccharide units. There is a requirement for a pentasaccharide to potentiate the action of AT (Choay et al., 1981). Polymers less than 5 units in length have no anticoagulant activity. For inhibition of thrombin, heparin must bind both to the enzyme and to AT. Fractions with fewer than 18 saccharide units are unable to bind thrombin and AT simultaneously (Casu et al., 1981) and therefore do not catalyse inhibition of thrombin. Simultaneous binding of enzyme and heparin is not required for neutralization of activated factor X (Casu et al., 1981). Fragments with 5–17 (or a greater number) of saccharides are therefore able to catalyse inhibition of activated factor X (Lane et al., 1984). These relationships are shown schematically in Figure 13.1.

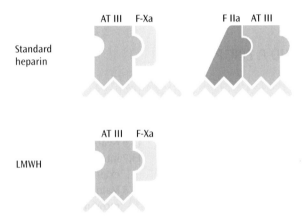

Fig. 13.1 *Inhibition of activated factor X (Xa) and thrombin (IIa) by antithrombin (AT) and heparin polymers of different lengths as found in standard (unfractionated) heparin and low-molecular-weight heparin (LMWH).*

Heparin – Mode of Action

Approximately one-third of heparins binds to AT and the remainder are thought to have minimal anticoagulant effect (Lam et al., 1976). A second plasma co-factor, heparin co-factor II (HCII), can bind the fractions with low affinity for AT and has some anticoagulant action (Tollefsen et al., 1982).

The complex of heparin with AT is able to inactivate a number of coagulation enzymes, including factor IIa (thrombin), factor VIIa, factor Xa, factor XIIa, factor XIa and factor IXa, although the most important effects relate to the inhibition of factors IIa or Xa. The heparin effect on the enzymes of the coagulation cascade is shown in Figure 13.2. Since many low-molecular-weight heparins contain few heparin fragments sufficiently large to inhibit thrombin, the anticoagulant actions of LMWH are exerted mainly through neutralization of factor Xa, as described above.

Another recently characterized inhibitor of coagulation, tissue factor pathway inhibitor (TFPI), may be involved in the anticoagulant and antithrombotic actions of heparin. The action of this inhibitor of factor Xa is enhanced by heparin, at least in purified systems (Broze et al., 1988), and injection of heparin results in a several-fold increase in TFPI activity in the blood (Sandset et al., 1988). Several studies have subsequently concluded that TFPI contributes to the antithrombotic activity of unfractionated and low-molecular-weight heparin (Lindahl et al., 1991).

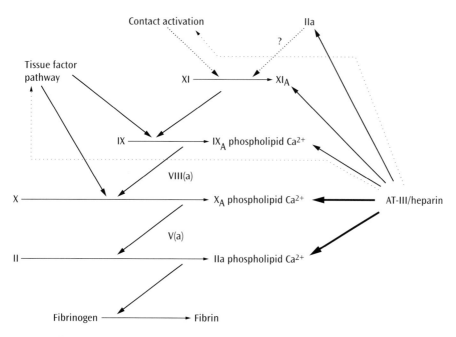

Fig. 13.2 *The effect of heparin–antithrombin (AT) complex on enzymes of the coagulation cascade.*

Clinical use of heparin

Heparin is widely used in the treatment of established thromboembolic disease, and prophylactically to prevent thrombosis and embolism. Accepted indications for treatment include deep vein thrombosis (DVT), pulmonary embolism, myocardial infarction (MI), unstable angina pectoris and acute peripheral arterial occlusion. Reviews have been published in relation to the clinical use of unfractionated heparin (Hirsh, 1991) and the increasing use of LMWH in the treatment and prophylaxis of venous thrombosis (Hull and Pineo, 1994; Barrowcliffe, 1995) and acute coronary disease (Armstrong, 1997). The clinical use of heparin is beyond the scope of this chapter and the reader is referred to the above-mentioned reviews.

Heparin-induced thrombocytopenia

One of the most important potential side-effects of heparin therapy is heparin-induced thrombocytopenia (HIT). Moderate early reductions (within 1–2 days) in the platelet count occur in as many as 10% of all patients receiving heparin, with the count often returning to normal during therapy (Greinacher, 1995). The clinically severe reduction in platelet count often referred to as HIT, which may be associated with catastrophic thrombotic complications, threatening life and limb, appears between the fourth and 20th day after initiation of therapy in first exposure patients (Kelton, 1986). HIT should be suspected if reductions to 50% of the initial platelet count occur after several days of heparin therapy (Greinacher, 1995).

Alternative therapy with LMWH (dalteparin) was shown to be successful in seven patients, with a positive HIT test employing standard heparin, but a negative HIT test employing dalteparin (Ramakrishna *et al.*, 1995). In a study of 230 patients with HIT, the heparinoid, danaparoid (Orgaran, Organon International, The Netherlands), was considered a suitable alternative to unfractionated heparin since only 10% of plasmas giving positive HIT test results with UF were also positive with Orgaran (Magnani, 1993).

Since continued UF heparin therapy is contraindicated if HIT occurs, and alternatives are available, patients receiving heparin should have regular platelet counts (two to three times per week) performed in addition to dosage monitoring, particularly where therapy is prolonged.

13.1 PRE-ANALYTICAL VARIABLES

13.1.1 Sample collection and processing for activated partial thromboplastin time determinations

A number of different blood sample collection systems are available for coagulation tests, including those used for heparin monitoring. Evacuated collection systems are increasingly used in the USA, Europe and elsewhere. Collection tubes may vary in relation to the types of stopper, tube composition (plastic or glass) and siliconization, and in addition there are proprietary differences between manufacturers. Whilst trisodium citrate is the anticoagulant most commonly used, there is some variation in the formulation employed. Many collection tubes appropriately employ buffered anticoagulant to help maintain the pH and therefore the stability of pH-dependent tests such as activated partial thromboplastin time (APTT). There is evidence that use of 0.109 mol/L trisodium citrate (3.2%) or 0.129 mol/L trisodium citrate (3.8%) can influence APTTs of patients receiving intravenous (i.v.) unfractionated heparin (Adcock et al., 1997), results being longer in samples collected into 0.129 mol/L citrate. Within an individual laboratory, if there is a change in the collection system employed, it is important to compare matched old and new tubes collected from a minimum of 25 patients receiving heparin in addition to a group of at least 25 healthy normal subjects to identify any possible impact on heparin monitoring.

It is now well known that after blood has been collected, the heparin present may be partially neutralized as a consequence of any delay before analysis. This is caused by release of platelet factor 4 (PF4) from platelets within the sample (Rucinski et al., 1979). PF4 binds to and neutralizes heparin. Samples from heparinized patients can be collected into an anti-coagulant cocktail which inhibits platelet release, thereby avoiding PF4-mediated neutralization of heparin. It has been demonstrated that collection of blood into citrate, theophylline, adenosine, dypyridamole mixture (CTAD) can greatly reduce the neutralization of heparin activity in blood (Contant et al., 1983), and for this reason Van den Besselaar et al. (1987) recommended the use of CTAD for heparin monitoring samples. Using this cocktail sample storage at room temperature was satisfactory. These authors recommended minimum centrifugation of $940 \times g$ for 30 minutes or $2200 \times g$ for 10 minutes (Van den Besselaar et al., 1987).

There is evidence that the volume of blood within a particular vial size can markedly influence the APTT for heparin monitoring, even when the ratio of anticoagulant to blood (1:9) is maintained (Ray, 1991). This relates to the volume of air within the collection tube. Thus, the air bubble of 4.7 mL within samples containing 2 mL of blood caused greater mixing, release of PF4 and neutralization of heparin than the 1.7 mL air bubble in samples containing 5 mL of blood. There is evidence that this effect is abolished if CTAD is used as the anticoagulant (Ray et al., 1993). Thus for heparin monitoring, it is inappropriate to use sample containers which contain a large air volume unless CTAD is used as the anticoagulant.

If the APTT is used for heparin monitoring, it is important to perform the measurement within 5–6 hours if CTAD is used as anticoagulant. At present, citrate is the most commonly used anticoagulant for heparin dosage monitoring. With these samples the analysis should be performed within 2 hours of collection. Testing more than 2 hours after collection may lead to important underestimation of *in vivo* heparin effects.

13.1.2 Heparin assays – sample collection and processing

The system of sample collection and processing can influence results of heparin assays. Platelet factor 4 secreted during blood collection (into citrate) from heparinized patients can result in underestimation (by 11%) of the heparin concentration as determined by a chromogenic anti-Xa assay (Levine *et al.*, 1984). As with the APTT, it is therefore important to perform heparin assay determinations as soon as possible after sample collection.

Most commercial heparin assays involve inhibition of added activated factor X (Xa) and determination of residual Xa activity using chromogenic substrates (Teien *et al.*, 1976) or a clotting technique (Yin *et al.*, 1973). For both types of assay, freezing and thawing of plasma before testing may affect the result obtained. This effect was demonstrated by van den Besselaar *et al.* (1990), who noted a small (11%) but significant reduction in anti-Xa activity after freeze/thaw of plasmas for samples centrifuged at low or high speed. This small loss of activity would not be expected to influence patient management.

13.1.3 Timing of sample collection in relation to therapy

The timing of blood sample collection for heparin monitoring will depend on the method by which the drug is administered. If heparin is given by i.v. infusion, the sample should be collected after equilibrium has been reached (Samama, 1995a; Olson *et al.*, 1998), normally 4–6 hours after initiation of the infusion. A similar lag phase should pass prior to sampling following a dose adjustment. When unfractionated heparin is given by subcutaneous injection, the maximal response of the APTT occurs after 4–6 hours (Hull *et al.*, 1982). Samples should therefore be collected at the mid-interval between injections if given twice daily. These blood collection times have been successfully used in clinical trials (Hull *et al.*, 1986).

There has been some debate about the importance of adequate initial doses of UF heparin, as evidenced by therapeutic APTT within 24 hours, and the risk of recurrent thrombo-embolism. Anand *et al.* (1996) performed a pooled analysis of several studies and could find no convincing evidence that the risk of recurrence was critically related to achieving therapeutic APTT results within 24–48 hours. In contrast, a pooled analysis of three studies by Hull *et al.* (1997) suggested that venous thromboembolism was four times more likely in patients for whom therapeutic APTT was not achieved at 24 hours compared with subjects whose APTT exceeded the therapeutic threshold by 24 hours.

13.2 MONITORING HEPARIN – ACTIVATED PARTIAL THROMBOPLASTIN TIME

13.2.1 Reagent responsiveness to heparin effect

The most widely used test for heparin monitoring is the APTT. In a study of thrombo-prophylaxis, Basu *et al.* (1972) concluded that the risk of venous thromboembolism was reduced when APTT ratios (patient:control) were greater than 1.5 and they suggested a therapeutic range of 1.5–2.5. The same range was shown to be effective by Hull *et al.* (1992)

and this range remains in widespread use. There is evidence that the correlation between heparin concentration and APTT result is improved if a ratio is used rather than reporting the APTT in seconds (van den Besselaar *et al.*, 1990). In this study the ratio was obtained by dividing the patient APTT by the same patient APTT after removal of heparin with ECTEOLA-Cellulose, a resin which binds heparin. Such an approach may not be appropriate for routine use in view of the additional time and expense. A practical alternative is to divide the patient's APTT by the mean normal APTT, although this is likely to yield a poorer correlation with heparin concentration since it does not take account of the patient's APTT in the absence of heparin (Kitchen and Preston, 1996).

A number of studies have identified differences in the responsiveness of different APTT reagents to heparin (van den Besselaar *et al.*, 1990; Kitchen and Preston, 1996; Kitchen *et al.*, 1996), although caution is required in the interpretation of some studies since the response of plasma to which heparin has been added *in vitro* is quite different from that obtained using *ex vivo* samples from patients receiving heparin (Banez *et al.*, 1980).

Using a manual technique, Kitchen and Preston (1996) demonstrated marked differences in the heparin sensitivity of six APTT reagents commonly used in the UK. APTTs were also determined using the Automated Coagulation Laboratory (ACL) coagulometer (Instrumentation Laboratory, Warrington, UK) for two of the six reagents. The ratios of patient to mean normal APTT were calculated for each method. Results are shown in Table 13.1. Clearly the differences between results with different reagents were sufficient to influence patient management. This is further illustrated by APTT ratios in three individual patient samples shown in Table 13.2. As a consequence, the fixed therapeutic range of 1.5–2.5 does not apply to all reagents. The ranking of APTT ratios with different reagents was not constant for all samples, indicating that components other than heparin within the test plasmas can influence the relationship between APTTs with different reagents. If a centre changes APTT reagent, there are important implications for patient management. A method for reagent evaluation that will identify if two reagents are sufficiently similar for clinical purposes has been suggested (Olson *et al.*, 1998).

There is evidence of variation between APTT reagents in respect of sensitivity to the levels of clotting factors (Hoffman and Meulendijk, 1978), particularly factor VIII:C. Since factor

Table 13.1 *Ratios of patient to mean normal activated partial thromboplastin time (APTT) in patients (n = 30) receiving heparin (with INRs < 1.3). Mean results obtained with different techniques are ranked in order of heparin responsiveness (from least to most responsive). (Reproduced by kind permission from Kitchen and Preston, 1996)*

Reagent	End-point detection	APTT ratio Observed range	Mean	Reagent activator	Activation time
B	Manual	1.00–3.62	1.80	Kaolin	3
DK	Manual	1.00–4.75	1.94	Kaolin	2
DB	Manual	0.90–4.17	2.13	Kaolin	2
MS	Manual	1.04–4.28	2.18	Kaolin	10
ML	Manual	0.97–6.21	2.46	Not stated	5
IL	Manual	1.06 to > 7.00	2.66	Micronized silica	5
IL	Automated	1.08 to > 7.00	2.73	Micronized silica	5
ML	Automated	0.91 to > 7.00	3.34	Not stated	5

B, Boehringer; DK, Diagen KPS; DB, Diagen Bell & Alton; MS, Manchester Standard; ML, Manchester Low Opacity; IL, Instrumentation Laboratory.

Table 13.2   *Activated partial thromboplastin time (APTT) ratios obtained with different techniques in three different patients (receiving i.v. unfractionated heparin). (Reproduced by kind permission from Kitchen and Preston, 1996)*

Reagent	End-point detection	APTT ratio		
		Patient 1	Patient 2	Patient 3
B	Manual	1.2	1.5	3.2
DK	Manual	1.2	1.7	2.8
DB	Manual	1.3	1.6	3.7
MS	Manual	1.4	1.9	3.4
ML	Manual	1.4	2.8	5.5
IL	Manual	1.7	2.6	4.5
IL	Automated	2.0	2.6	5.1
ML	Automated	1.9	3.6	> 7.0
Heparin level by protamine titration (U/mL)		0.15	0.40	0.55

B, Boehringer; DK, Diagen KPS; DB, Diagen Bell & Alton; MS, Manchester Standard; ML, Manchester Low Opacity; IL, Instrumentation Laboratory.

VIII is an acute-phase reactant, levels are likely to vary markedly in a group of patients with thromboembolic disease and may have contributed to the difference in responsiveness of the reagents (Levine *et al.*, 1994).

Methodological differences which might contribute to the differences between reagents (in Table 13.1) in respect of heparin responsiveness include the use of different activators and activation times and the different lipid profiles of APTT reagents. Using high-performance thin layer chromatography densitometry (Cartwright and Higgins, 1995) to analyse phospholipid content of seven APTT reagents we observed a 25-fold variation (8–205 µg/mL) in total phospholipid concentration in the final APTT reaction mixture (Kitchen *et al.*, 1999a). The range of final concentration of two important phospholipids, phosphatidyl choline and phosphatidyl serine, was found to be 2.7–109 and 0–22 µg/mL, respectively. The lipid profiles of seven different APTT reagents are shown in Figure 13.3. Since phospholipids influence results (Stevenson *et al.*, 1986; van den Besselaar *et al.*, 1993) it is not surprising that reagent sensitivity varies so widely. There is also evidence that different activation regimes with the same phospholipid reagent are associated with marked differences in heparin responsiveness (Barrowcliffe and Gray, 1981). Thus there are a number of reasons why APTT reagents have different heparin responsiveness and it has been recommended that manufacturers should provide data on this (Olson *et al.*, 1998).

13.2.2 Reagent specific therapeutic ranges

The recommended therapeutic range of 1.5–2.5 is based largely on studies in which the equivalent heparin level was 0.2–0.4 U/mL, measured by the protamine titration assay (Hirsh, 1991). The view that a heparin level of 0.2 U/mL (by protamine titration) is an appropriate lower limit for effective therapy is supported by clinical studies (Hull *et al.*, 1986; Levine *et al.*, 1994). The evidence for an increased risk of bleeding when a heparin level of 0.4 U/ml is exceeded is less well established (Hull *et al.*, 1992). Nevertheless one approach to the problem of variation between reagents with respect to heparin sensitivity is for a laboratory to establish a therapeutic range for the APTT reagent in use which corresponds to a heparin concentration of 0.2–0.4 U/mL by protamine titration (Hirsh, 1991). Since the relationship between heparin

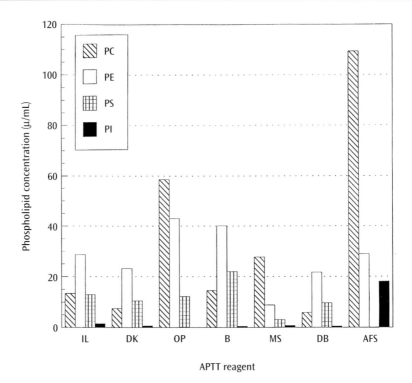

Fig. 13.3 *Phospholipid profile of activated partial thromboplastin time (APTT) reagents. APTT reagents: IL, Instrumentation Laboratory; DK, Diagen KPS; OP, Organon Teknika Platelin LS; B, Boehringer; MS, Manchester Standard; DB, Diagen Bell and Alton; AFS, actin FS. Phospholipids: PC, phosphatidyl choline; PE, phosphatidyl ethanolamine; PS, phosphatidyl serine; PI, phosphatidyl inositol.*

concentration and APTT is different according to whether heparin is added to plasma *in vitro* or *ex vivo*, protamine titration must be performed using samples from patients receiving heparin. The sample size needed to standardize an APTT therapeutic range has not been clearly defined (Rosborough, 1997).

The relationship between APTT ratios (as determined using six reagents) and heparin level by protamine titration is shown in Figure 13.4, and the range of ratios equivalent to 0.2–0.4 U/mL by protamine titration is shown in Table 13.3. There was relatively poor correlation between heparin concentration and APTT ratios (Table 13.3). There was a high degree of discordance between the therapeutic information provided by the APTT ratio and the heparin assay, where one technique suggested that the patient was within the therapeutic range and the other suggested the patient was outside the therapeutic range. These are important difficulties related to the use of the APTT for monitoring heparin dosage.

When heparin and warfarin are administered simultaneously, caution is necessary in interpreting the APTT ratio since the APTT may be influenced by both drugs. It should also be noted that variations between heparin sensitivity of different lots or batches of reagent produced by the same manufacturer can occur (Shojania *et al.*, 1988; Brill-Edwards *et al.*, 1993). Different methods for taking this into account have been described (Rosborough, 1998).

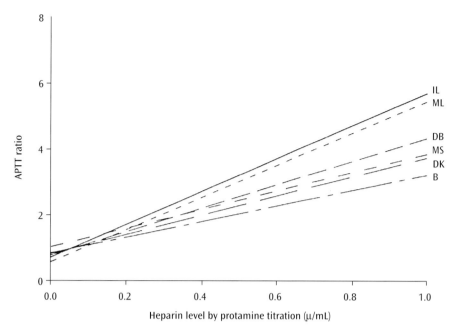

Fig. 13.4 *Relationship between heparin levels by protamine titration and activated partial thromboplastin time (APTT) ratios are determined using six different reagents and manual technique. All patients had international normalized ratios (INRs) < 1.3. Regression lines are shown. IL, Instrumentation Laboratory; ML, Manchester Low Opacity; DB, Diagen Bell and Alton; MS, Manchester Standard; DK, Diagen KPS; B, Boehringer. (Reproduced by kind permission from Kitchen and Preston, 1996.)*

13.2.3 Coagulometer effects on APTT for heparin dosage monitoring

The results of APTTs determined for heparin dosage monitoring can be influenced by the method of end-point detection (D'Angelo *et al.*, 1990). We have demonstrated that use of one particular coagulometer (ACL) with one reagent was not associated with differences between APTT ratio when compared with manual end-point detection (Kitchen and Preston, 1996), whereas with the same instrument a significant increase in APTT ratios was obtained using another reagent (manual mean APTT ratio 2.5, compared with ACL mean 3.3). A locally established therapeutic range for heparin should therefore take account of both reagent and instrument.

13.2.4 An International Sensitivity Index/International Normalized Ratio system for heparin dosage monitoring

The problems of different prothrombin time reagent sensitivity in respect of the defect induced by oral anticoagulants have been largely solved by the adoption of the International Sensitivity Index (ISI)/International Normalized Ratio (INR) system as recommended by WHO (1983). Several studies have therefore examined the possible use of a similar system to standardize laboratory control of heparin therapy by APTT. In a large multicentre study, use of a single sensitivity index for a reagent employed in different laboratories was not advised (Van der Velde and Poller, 1995) and two other studies (Reid *et al.*, 1994; Kitchen and Preston, 1995) also indicated that the ISI/INR system is an inappropriate model for standardization of heparin dosage monitoring using the APTT.

Table 13.3 *Relationship between activated partial thromboplastin time (APTT) ratios and heparin level by protamine titration. (Reproduced by kind permission from Kitchen and Preston, 1996)*

Reagant/end-point detection	Correlation with heparin assay (*r*)	APTT ratio corresponding to 0.2–0.4 U/mL heparin	Heparin level corresponding to APTT ratio of 1.5–2.5
B – manual	0.47	1.61–1.93	0.13–0.76
DR – manual	0.44	1.71–2.13	0.09–0.58
DB – manual	0.62	1.77–2.45	0.12–0.41
MS – manual	0.44	1.39–2.31	0.01–0.49
ML – manual	0.57	2.20–2.99	0.06–0.32
IL – manual	0.53	2.20–2.99	0.02–0.27
IL – ACL	0.51	2.25–3.07	0.02–0.26
ML – ACL	0.59	2.60–3.94	0.04–0.18

B, Boehringer; DK, Diagen KPS; DB, Diagen Bell & Alton; MS, Manchester Standard; ML, Manchester Low Opacity; IL, Instrumentation Laboratory; ACL, Automated Coagulation Laboratory.

13.3 HEPARIN ASSAYS DURING UNFRACTIONATED HEPARIN THERAPY

13.3.1 Advantages of heparin assay over APTT

Whilst the APTT remains the most commonly used test for monitoring unfractionated heparin therapy, the correlation between APTT and heparin level is poor. This is a reflection of the lack of specificity of APTT for the heparin effect. In addition, there are a number of occasions when the APTT may be inappropriate for heparin monitoring.

Situations in which APTT may be within the target range for heparin therapy in the presence of suboptimal heparin concentrations are shown in Table 13.4. Conditions in which excessive doses of heparin may be required to prolong APTT into the target therapeutic range are shown in Table 13.5. In some of these cases the heparin assay is more appropriate as an index of the antithrombic effect of heparin.

An important study by Levine *et al.* (1994) compared the results of a heparin assay with APTT for dosage monitoring in patients requiring large (>35 000 IU) daily dosages of heparin. Patients were randomized into two equal groups, one of which was monitored by APTT, and

Table 13.4 *Situations in which activated partial thromboplastin time (APTT) may appear therapeutic in the presence of suboptimal heparin combinations*

Situation	Comments
Combined heparin and oral anticoagulants	APTT prolonged by reduction of IX, X, II
Lupus anticoagulant	Inhibition of phospholipid-dependent reactions prolongs APTT
Isolated clotting factor deficiency	Reduction of factor II, V, VII, VIII, IX, XI or XII (factor XII being most common in routine practice) prolongs APTT
Combined thrombolytic and heparin therapy	Reduction of fibrinogen and factors V and VIII prolongs APTT

Table 13.5 *Situations in which activated partial thromboplastin time (APTT) may appear sub-therapeutic in the presence of adequate heparin concentration*

Situation	Comments
Elevated FVIII	Particularly related to acute-phase reaction in thrombotic patients, leading to markedly short baseline APTT
Elevated fibrinogen	As above, although effect relatively minor compared with FVIII
Increased platelet factor 4 (PF4)	Heparin is neutralized by PF4 released *in vitro*
Decreased AT-III	Insufficient AT-III available to bind heparin
Pregnancy	Elevated levels of several clotting factors including FVIII

the other by a chromogenic anti-Xa assay. For both techniques, therapeutic ranges were equivalent to 0.2–0.4 U/mL heparin by protamine titration, considered to be the reference therapeutic range. Patients in the APTT-monitored group required significantly more heparin in the first day after randomization. The APTTs of the anti-Xa-monitored group were shorter than the APTT-monitored group and were often sub-therapeutic. Importantly, the smaller dose of heparin given to the anti-Xa monitored group appeared to be adequate since the rate of recurrence of thromboembolism was similar in the two groups. There were four bleeding events in patients monitored by APTT (receiving more heparin) and one event in the anti-Xa monitored group. The authors concluded that monitoring with anti-Xa was safe and effective in patients whose APTT remains sub-therapeutic despite large daily doses of heparin. More studies which include clinical outcome assessment are required to confirm that anti-Xa assays can be successfully employed in the majority of heparinized patients.

13.3.2 Heparin assay techniques

The evidence that heparin levels of 0.2–0.4 U/mL by protamine titration assay represent an appropriate therapeutic range is reviewed above. This assay is described in detail elsewhere (Kitchen and Preston, 1996) but is not widely available. Many other types of heparin assay have been described employing a range of different principles. Anti-factor Xa assays have been widely evaluated since they are more specific for heparin than APTT. These measure the ability of heparin-accelerated AT to inhibit activated factor X added to plasma or dilutions of plasma. Residual enzyme is then measured by its clotting activity (Yin *et al.*, 1973) or amidolytically by a chromogenic substrate (Teien *et al.*, 1976). Peptide substrates in the chromogenic substrate are cleaved by factor Xa, releasing the chromogenic group para-nitroaniline (pNA) from linkage to a 3–4 amino acid chain (Fig. 13.5). Cleavage is associated with increase in yellow colour measured at 405 nm. In this assay the strength of colour is inversely proportional to heparin activity. In the clotting assay, a proportion of added factor Xa is neutralized by heparin/antithrombin. The plasma is then clotted with a recalcification mixture containing clotting factors, phospholipid and calcium, the clotting time being directly proportional to heparin concentration (high heparin leading to lower residual Xa and subsequently longer clotting times).

Other types of heparin assay employ fluorescent substrates (Mitchell *et al.*, 1978), neutralization of thrombin (van den Besselaar *et al.*, 1990) or polyanion sensors (Ma *et al.*, 1993).

Results of heparin assays may differ according to the technique employed. It has been reported that heparin levels of 0.2–0.4 U/mL by protamine titration equate to 0.35–0.67 U/mL by anti-Xa assays (Levine *et al.*, 1994). We recently compared results of eight commercially available anti-Xa assays and the heparin assay by protamine titration in samples from 43 patients receiving i.v. porcine mucosal heparin (Kitchen *et al.*, 2000). Results are shown in Table 13.6.

Some anti-Xa assay techniques involve the addition of exogenous antithrombin III to the plasma. The results of this type of assay do not reflect the overall *in vivo* anticoagulant effect *in vivo* and therefore may be clinically less relevant (Holm *et al.*, 1987). Heparin therapy usually produces a decrease in circulating antithrombin which is independent of initial dose. This effect is initially detectable after 1 day. Antithrombin levels fall by approximately 30% after 2–4 days of heparin therapy and then return to normal 2–3 days after cessation of therapy (Marciniak and Gockerman, 1977; Holm *et al.*, 1985). The reduction is a consequence of shortened half-life (Collen *et al.*, 1977) and may lead to suboptimal therapy at plasma levels below 0.6 U/mL AT (Bick, 1984).

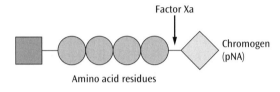

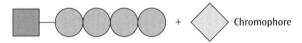

Fig. 13.5 *Structure of synthetic peptide substrates used in anti-Xa assays. (Reproduced from* Heparin: Chromogenix Monograph Series, *1995, by kind permission of Chromogenix AB, Sweden.)*

Table 13.6 *Results of heparin assays in patients (n = 43) receiving unfractionated heparin therapy*

Assay	Company	Principle	Mean level (U/mL)	Anti Xa levels equivalent to 0.2-0.4 U/mL by protamine titration
Protamine titration		Protamine heparin neutralization	0.31	–
Diagen	Diagnostic Reagents, Thame, UK	Clotting anti-Xa	0.41[a]	0.27–0.52
Heptest	Sigma, Poole, UK	Clotting anti-Xa	0.40[a]	0.32–0.47
Staclot	Shield Diagnostic, Dundee, UK	Clotting anti-Xa	0.42[a]	0.33–0.45
Chromostrate	Organon Teknika	Chromogenic anti-Xa	0.32	0.24–0.39
Coacute	Quadratech, UK	Chromogenic anti-Xa	0.32	0.25–0.38
Coatest	Quadratech, UK	Chromogenic anti-Xa	0.40[b]	0.28–0.49
IL	Instrumentation Laboratory, Warrington, UK	Chromogenic anti-Xa	0.36	0.26–0.44
Stachrom	Shield Diagnostics, Dundee, UK	Chromogenic anti-Xa	0.40[b]	0.29–0.49

[a]Significantly greater than results with protamine titration (*P* < 0.01).
[b]Significantly greater than results with protamine titration (*P* < 0.05).

13.3.3 Unfractionated heparin standards

When determining heparin levels in plasma, it is necessary to construct a reference or calibration curve. This typically involves the addition of heparin to pooled normal plasma at a range of concentrations to include the range likely to be encountered in test samples for conventional therapy. The heparin being used for patient treatment has been used in this way (Yin *et al.*, 1973). However, the heparin of choice is a World Health Organization (WHO) International Standard (IS) for unfractionated heparin (Thomas *et al.*, 1984), presently available from the UK National Institute for Biological Standards and Control (NIBSC, Blanche Lane, South Mimms, Potters Bar, Herts, UK).

After reconstitution, the IS can be diluted in saline to a suitable lower concentration and stored deep frozen in aliquots for subsequent use over a further 12 months.

13.4 OTHER TESTS FOR MONITORING UNFRACTIONATED HEPARIN

Tests other than APTT and direct measurement of heparin activity in plasma are used for heparin monitoring. One such test is the recalcification clotting time of platelet-rich plasma, sometimes referred to as the Howell test, which is said to be less sensitive and accurate than the APTT (Samama, 1995a). Another is the thrombin time, which has been used for heparin monitoring and was found to be more closely related to plasma heparin concentration than one APTT method (Bounameaux *et al.*, 1980), a finding which was confirmed in a later study employing a concentrated thrombin reagent (Ray *et al.*, 1996). One problem with this test is that the sensitivity of the thrombin time to increasing concentrations of heparin is not linear (Ray *et al.*, 1996). In particular, the sample may become incoagulable at doses of heparin not far above the therapeutic range, making differentiation between moderate and excessive over-dosage difficult.

13.5 MONITORING LOW-MOLECULAR-WEIGHT HEPARIN THERAPY

There is an increasing body of evidence that low-molecular-weight heparins (LMWHs) are at least as effective as unfractionated (UF) heparin in preventing and treating deep vein thrombosis (Hull and Pineo, 1994). The necessity for laboratory monitoring is not yet established. However, since the interpatient variability in dosage requirements is much lower for LMWH (Handeland *et al.*, 1990) than for UF heparin and since the half-life of LMWH (unlike UF) is essentially independent of dose (Boneu *et al.*, 1987), it is unlikely that laboratory monitoring of LMWH will need to be as frequent as for UF, although different LMWH preparations should not be considered as identical drugs (Fareed *et al.*, 1996).

A guidelines document published on behalf of the College of American Pathologists (Laposta *et al.*, 1998) recommends that clinically stable patients receiving LMWH pre- or postoperatively for prophylaxis of venous thromboembolism, or uncomplicated patients treated for venous thromboembolism by a weight-adjusted, fixed-dose regimen do not require laboratory monitoring. There is, however, a growing view that in some cases monitoring may provide useful information. This might be the case in patients in whom pharmacokinetic characteristics are unpredictable, e.g. in obese patients, in paediatric patients, or where renal insufficiency occurs. Laboratory monitoring may be helpful in those receiving prolonged therapy, including pregnancy, and in any patients with complications or with high risk of complications such as haemorrhage or recurrent thrombosis.

LMWHs have less effect on AT-mediated inhibition of thrombin than UF, since they contain fewer of the large chains necessary to catalyse this reaction (see 'Structure of heparin', p. 293). For this reason, LMWHs prolong APTT (or thrombin time) weakly compared with UF, an effect which is correlated to their anti-Xa/anti-IIa ratio (Boneu et al., 1991). Indeed, after administration of LMWH, the longer chains supporting inhibition of IIa are cleared twice as quickly as the shorter chains supporting only anti-Xa activity (Bendetoweiz et al., 1994).

If laboratory monitoring is deemed necessary, the test of choice is the anti-Xa activity assay, even though the relationship between anti-Xa and efficacy or risk of haemorrhage is not established. In one review, Samama (1995b) suggested optimum anti-Xa ranges as follows: prophylaxis for a moderate risk 0.10–0.25 U/mL; prophylaxis for a high risk, 0.20–0.50 U/mL; prophylaxis for established deep vein thrombosis, 0.50 to 1.0-1.2 U/mL. In the guidelines document published on behalf of CAP (Laposta et al., 1998), a target anti-Xa activity of 0.5–1.1 IU/mL was recommended for samples collected 4 hours after subcutaneous injection from patients receiving twice-daily dosing therapy. It is important that the sample is collected 4 hours after the drug is injected if these ranges are to be employed.

There is evidence that some clotting-based anti-Xa assays (Boneu et al., 1991) may underestimate anti-Xa activity relative to chromogenic assays and other studies evaluating anti-Xa results during LMWH therapy have been published (Sie et al., 1987; Houbouyan et al., 1996).

There is evidence that the WHO International Standard for UF heparin is unsuitable as a standard for LMWH assays (Barrowcliffe et al., 1985) and the heparin of choice for calibration of anti-Xa assays for monitoring LMWH therapy should be the 1st WHO International Standard for LMWH (Barrowcliffe et al., 1988), presently available from the NIBSC. Aliquots of reconstituted material can be stored deep frozen for at least 1 year.

We have compared results of five chromogenic and three clotting anti-Xa assays in samples from patients receiving enoxaparin or dalteparin for prophylaxis or treatment of venous thromboembolic disease and patients receiving danaparoid as an alternative to UF heparin in the presence of heparin-induced thrombocytopenia (Kitchen et al., 1999b). Assays of danaparoid were calibrated using the preparation adopted for patient treatment since the composition of this material is different for the IS for LMWH and it has not been established whether this standard is suitable for assays of this material. Results are shown in Table 13.7. There were statistically significant differences ($P < 0.05$) between results of assays in patients receiving all three preparations. Results of the Heptest clotting assay were significantly lower than results obtained by some other clotting and chromogenic assays by approximately 50% in dalteparin therapy and 100% in enoxaparin therapy (Kitchen et al., 1999b). It has been suggested that the chromogenic method should be the assay of choice (Laposta et al., 1998)

Table 13.7 *Results of anti-Xa assay in samples from patients receiving enoxaparin/Clexane dalteparin/Fragmin or danaparoid/Organan*

| Assay | Principle | Mean anti-Xa (IU/mL) | | |
		Patients receiving enoxaparin ($n = 13$)	Patients receiving dalteparin ($n = 25$)	Patients receiving danaparoid ($n = 20$)
Diagen	Clotting	0.58	0.57	0.36
Heptest	Clotting	0.28	0.43	0.30
Staclot	Clotting	0.64	0.69	0.36
Chromostrate	Chromogenic	0.45	0.49	0.47
Coacute	Chromogenic	0.42	0.55	0.65
Coatest	Chromogenic	0.49	0.54	0.48
IL	Chromogenic	0.60	0.62	0.57
Stachrom	Chromogenic	0.59	0.51	0.62

because of the influence of anti-IIa activity on some clotting assays, although not all clotting techniques are affected in this way (Dignac *et al.*, 1993; Kitchen *et al.*, 1999b). In danaparoid therapy anti-Xa results with all three clotting assays were lower than results with all five chromogenic assays.

The target anti-Xa ranges for LMWH therapy are largely based on chromogenic techniques. Caution should be exercised if monitoring employs other types of assay, particularly in danaparoid therapy.

13.6 NEAR-PATIENT TESTING (NPT)

The *in vitro* changes discussed above pose a problem when delays occur between sample collection and analysis in a central laboratory. Several instruments have now been developed which allow heparin monitoring to be performed at the patient's bedside. Some of these are designed for higher dose heparinization during coronary angioplasty or cardiothoracic surgery, whereas others have been developed for monitoring patients treated with heparin for thromboembolic disease. Most have the advantage of providing results from whole blood, removing the requirement for centrifugation of samples. Many require native blood (without anticoagulant) collected by fingerstick, whereas others required anticoagulated blood.

In two studies employing the Thrombolytic Assessment System (TAS, Cardiovascular Systems, Raleigh, USA) near-patient APTTs correlated well with conventional APTT methods (Rose *et al.*, 1993; Linder *et al.*, 1996). This was also the case (Werner *et al.*, 1994) for near-patient APTTs determined with the Biotrak 512/Coag U Chek Plus instrument (Boehringer Mannheim, Germany).

British Committee for Standardization in Haematology (BCSH) guidelines for near-patient testing in haematology (including monitoring of heparin therapy) have been published (England *et al.*, 1995). These recommend that if APTTs are determined using a NPT system, APTTs should also be determined with the conventional APTT technique in local use in samples, to include a full range of heparin levels encountered in normal clinical practice prior to adoption of the NPT system. Where possible, anti-Xa activity should also be determined on these samples. The guidelines recommend that the professional head of the central laboratory should take responsibility for all aspects of the NPT service with joint ownership of results. Standard operating procedures should be written by an appropriate senior member of the central laboratory staff, who may also take responsibility for internal quality control matters. The advantages and limitations of NPT or point-of-care testing in coagulation have been reviewed (Macik, 1995).

13.7 INTERNAL QUALITY CONTROL (IQC) AND EXTERNAL QUALITY ASSESSMENT (EQA)

Provision of reliable laboratory results which are reproducible and consistent from day to day is important in relation to APTT, heparin assay and other tests for monitoring heparin therapy. Adequate IQC procedures should involve continued and immediate checks to ensure that test results are reliable enough to be reported and to assist clinicians in the management of patients.

A suitable control material should be similar in properties to the test material and be stable over its period of use. This may be difficult for IQC of heparin dosage monitoring. For APTT, both a normal and an abnormal control material should be available. A normal QC sample should be tested with each group of test samples. An abnormal control should be included at least once per day or shift or when uncertainty exists about the quality of test results. All vials or aliquots of the IQC material must be practically identical so that any variation between results does not reflect inter-vial variation. Results obtained at different times will not be identical but will vary according to the precision of the test system. For IQC, acceptable target ranges of results are required. These are often provided by manufacturers of commercial control materials, but for APTT, target limits must take account of both reagent and method of end-point detection. One approach suitable for local use is to test the IQC material on 20 different occasions when the method is believed to be adequately controlled and to calculate the mean and standard deviation of these results. Any future control values which lie within 2 standard deviations above or below the mean are then considered acceptable. Results outside this range indicate that the QC material has deteriorated or been handled incorrectly, or that the method is not properly controlled. Medium- or long-term drift in test results, e.g. as a consequence of instrument deterioration or change in the case of automated analyses, can be detected by maintaining a cumulative record of all IQC results, e.g. on a chart as in Figure 13.6.

External quality assessment (EQA) is the process by which a laboratory's results are scrutinized objectively by an outside agency to identify the level of between-laboratory comparability of test results. EQA of heparin dosage monitoring is available to participants of the College of American Pathologists (CAP) EQA scheme (Gawoski *et al.*, 1987), the UK NEQAS for Blood Coagulation (Kitchen *et al.*, 1996), or the WHO International External Quality Assessment Scheme (IEQAS). Samples for distribution through the CAP have traditionally been prepared by addition of heparin to normal plasma (Gawoski *et al.*, 1987). This was also the case for samples distributed through UK NEQAS and IEQAS prior to October 1993, after which time samples have been prepared by pooling plasma from patients receiving heparin (Kitchen *et al.*, 1996). The heparin sensitivity of APTT reagents to heparin in *ex vivo* samples is substantially different from that observed in samples to which heparin has been added *in vitro* (Table 13.8). This is not surprising as there are several differences between heparinized

Table 13.8 *Ranking of activated partial thromboplastin time (APTT) reagents by response to heparin for samples to which heparin had been added* in vitro *and samples from patients receiving heparin. (Reproduced by kind permission of BMJ Publishing Group from Kitchen* et al.*, 1996)*

NEQAS samples prepared by the in vitro addition of heparin to normal plasma (mean result of four NEQAS surveys)		NEQAS samples prepared by pooling samples from patients receiving heparin (mean result of two NEQAS surveys)	
Reagent	Mean APTT ratio	Reagent	Mean APTT ratio
ML	3.43	OP	2.06
A	2.63	IL	2.0
DB	2.45	ML	1.94
M	2.36	OA	1.90
OP	2.33	M	1.70
IL	2.27	A	1.65
OA	2.15	DB	1.57
B	2.14	DK	1.49
DK	2.02	B	1.33

APTT ratios are mean results obtained in different centres employing the same reagent. All reagents were used in at least 10 centres.
ML, Manchester Low Opacity; A, actin FS; DB, Diagen Bell & Alton; M, Manchester; OP, Organon Teknika Platelin LS; IL, Instrumentation Laboratory; OA, Organon Teknika Auto APTT; B, Boehringer; DK, Diagen KPS.

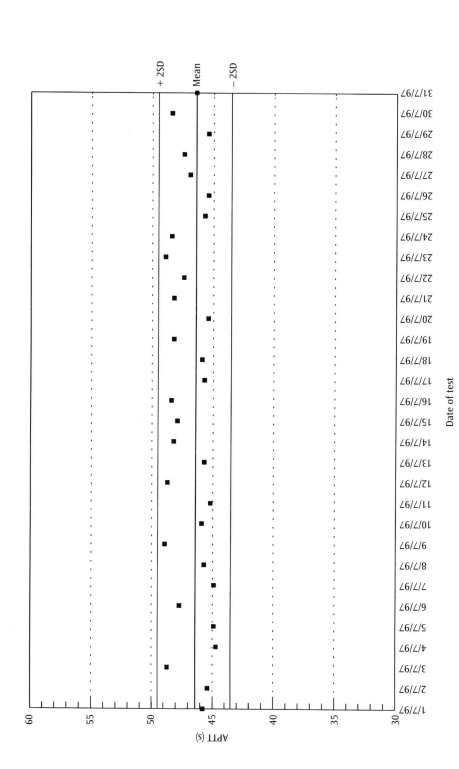

Fig. 13.6 *Cumulative record of activated partial thromboplastin time (APTT) results of an internal quality control sample. Solid lines indicate the mean and ± 2 standard deviations (SD) of 20 APTT determinations performed on different days.*

normal plasma and samples from heparinized patients, particularly with respect to clotting factor concentrations. The levels of factor VIII:C and fibrinogen were more than twofold greater in pooled *ex vivo* samples compared with normal plasma samples heparinized *in vitro*, the levels of other clotting factors being similar (Kitchen *et al.*, 1996). Samples prepared by *in vitro* addition of heparin to normal plasma can clearly be misleading.

The importance of reagent differences in heparin sensitivity is emphasized by the clinical conclusions based on results of one UK NEQAS survey (using *ex vivo* samples) in which 94% of users of one reagent considered the heparin dosage to be inadequate, whereas 90% of users of another reagent regarded it as adequate. The range of results obtained on the same sample, and grouped according to the reagent in local use, is shown in Table 13.9.

Within the UK NEQAS for Blood Coagulation, participants are invited to determine heparin levels in pooled samples from patients receiving i.v. UF heparin. Heparin assay results from lyophilized aliquots of the one sample analysed in 39 centres were in the range 0.21–1.10 U/mL, with a coefficient of variation (CV) of 50%. As for APTT results there is a wide range of results on the same sample analysed in different centres. EQA has an important role in highlighting these differences and the need for further improvements in standardization of tests for heparin dosage monitoring.

Table 13.9 *Activated partial thromboplastin time (APTT) ratios obtained by UK NEQAS (Blood Coagulation) participants for the same sample analysed in different centres. Results are grouped according to APTT reagent in local use*

APTT reagent	Number of users	Median APTT ratio[a]	Coefficient of variation (%)	Range of results
Boehringer Mannheim	17	1.46	11.6	1.08–1.68
Dade Actin FS	25	1.69	15.0	0.85–2.12
Diagen B & A	12	1.53	12.5	1.35–2.02
Diagen KPS	48	1.47	8.8	1.28–1.90
Instrumentation Lab F/D	204	1.67	7.2	1.40–2.11
Manchester	12	1.80	10.6	1.60–2.15
Manchester Low	10	1.92	22.3	1.59–2.70
Organon Teknika Auto	17	1.70	7.0	1.50–2.02
Organon Teknika Platelin LS	23	1.96	9.0	1.49–2.26

Only reagents used in > 10 centres are shown and results include all methods of end-point detection.
[a]Test: midpoint of local normal range

13.8 MAIN COMMENTS AND RECOMMENDATIONS

13.8.1 Blood sample

1   The anticoagulant of choice for unfractionated heparin dosage monitoring is CTAD.
2   If citrate is used as anticoagulant, tests should be completed within 2 hours of sample collection.
3   Freeze and thaw of plasma samples prior to APTT determinations should be avoided.
4   Samples should be collected 4–6 hours after initiation of infusion, dose adjustment or injection.

13.8.2 APTT for monitoring unfractionated heparin therapy

1 Reagents and techniques vary markedly in responsiveness and sensitivity to heparin.
2 Coagulometers can influence heparin responsiveness of some reagents.
3 The therapeutic range for APTT corresponding to 0.2–0.4 U/mL heparin by protamine titration should be established locally for the technique in use, and must employ samples from heparinized patients.
4 Heparin responsiveness can vary between lots (batches) of APTT reagent from the same manufacturer.
5 *In vitro* addition of heparin to normal plasma prior to APTT determinations can give misleading information in relation to heparin responsiveness and should be avoided.
6 The correlation between APTT results by most techniques and heparin concentration is poor, reflecting the lack of specificity of APTT for heparin effect.
7 The heparin level can be used for heparin monitoring where APTT is invalid.
8 Regular platelet counts should be performed to identify HIT, particularly when UF heparin therapy is prolonged.

13.8.3 Heparin assays

1 Results of anti-Xa assays are often greater than heparin levels by protamine titration.
2 In UF heparin therapy, anti-Xa assay results are similar by different techniques when assays are calibrated with the WHO International Standard for UF heparin.
3 The material of choice for calibration of anti-Xa assays in heparin therapy is the WHO International Standard for UF heparin.
4 LMWH therapy may require laboratory monitoring in selected circumstances.
5 The method of choice for monitoring LMWH is the anti-Xa assay and it should be noted that results by some clotting-based assays are substantially lower than results by some chromogenic assays.

REFERENCES

Abildgaard, U. (1968) Highly purified antithrombin 3 with heparin cofactor activity prepared by disc electrophoresis. *Scand. J. Clin. Lab. Invest.* **21**, 89–91.

Adcock, D.M., Kressin, D.C. and Marlar, R.A. (1997) Effect of 3.2% and 3.8% sodium citrate concentrations on routine coagulation testing. *Am. J. Clin. Pathol.* **107**, 105–10.

Anand, S., Ginsberg, J., Kearon, C., Gent, M. *et al.* (1996) The relation between the APTT response and recurrence in patients with venous thrombosis treated with continuos intravenous heparin. *Arch. Int. Med.* **156,** 1677–81.

Armstrong, P.W. (1997) Heparin in acute coronary disease – requiem for a heavyweight? *N. Engl. J. Med.* **337**, 492–4.

Banez, E.I., Triplett, D.A. and Koepke, J. (1980) Laboratory monitoring of heparin therapy – the effect of different salts of heparin on the APTT. *Am. J. Clin. Pathol.* **74**, 569–74.

Barrowcliffe, T.W. (1995) Low molecular weight heparin. *Br. J. Haematol.* **90**, 1–7.

Barrowcliffe, T.W. and Gray, E. (1981) Studies of phospholipid reagents used in coagulation II: factors influencing their sensitivity to heparin. *Thromb. Haemost.* **46**, 634–7.

Barrowcliffe, T.W., Curtis, A.D., Tomlinson, T.P. *et al.* (1985) Standardisation of low molecular weight heparin: A collaborative study. *Thromb. Haemost.* **54**, 675–9.

Barrowcliffe, T.W., Curtis, A.D., Johnson, E.A. and Thomas, D.P. (1988) An international standard for low molecular weight heparin. *Thromb. Haemost.* **60**, 1–7.

Basu, D., Gallus, A., Hirsh, J. and Cade, J. (1972) A prospective study of the value of monitoring heparin treatment with the APTT. *N. Engl. J. Med.* **287**, 324–7.

Bendetoweiz, A., Beguin, S., Caplain, H. and Hemker, H.C. (1994) Pharmacokinetics and pharmacodynamics of low molecular weight heparin (Enoxaparin) after subcutaneous injection; comparison with unfractionated heparin. *Thromb. Haemost.* **71**, 305–13.

Bick, R.L. (1984) Role of antithrombin III in clinical management of pulmonary embolism. *Am. J. Med.* **77**, 78.

Boneu, B., Buchanan, M.R., Caronoke, C. *et al.* (1987) The disappearance of a low molecular weight heparin fraction (CY216) differs from standard heparin in rabbits. *Thromb. Res.* **46**, 845–53.

Boneu, B., Faruel-Bille, V., Pierrejean, D. and Gabaig, A.M. (1991) Limitations of the chronometric assays to determine plasma antifactor Xa activity during low molecular weight heparin therapy. *Nouv. Rev. Fr. Haematol.* **33**, 287–91.

Bounameaux, H., Marbet, G.A., Lammle, B. *et al.* (1980) Monitoring of heparin treatment. Comparison of thrombin time, activated partial thromboplastin time and plasma heparin concentration, and analysis of behaviour of antithrombin III. *Am. J. Clin. Pathol.* **74**, 68–73.

Brill-Edwards, P., Ginsberg, J.S., Johnston, M. and Hirsh, J. (1993) Establishing a therapeutic range for heparin. *Ann. Int. Med.* **119**, 104–9.

Broze, G.J., Warren, L.A., Novotny, W.F. *et al.* (1988) The lipoprotein associated coagulation inhibitor that inhibits the factor VIIa-tissue factor complex also inhibits factor Xa: insight into its possible mechanism of action. *Blood* **71**, 335–43.

Cartwright, I.J. and Higgins, J.A. (1995) Intracellular events in the assembly of very-low-density-lipoprotein lipids with apolipoprotein B in isolated rabbit hepatocytes. *Biochem. J.* **310**, 897–907.

Casu, B., Oreste, P., Torri, G. *et al.* (1981) The structure of heparin oligosaccharide fragments with high anti-factor Xa activity containing the minimal antithrombin III bonding sequence: chemical and 13C nuclear magnetic resonance studies. *Biochem. J.* **197**, 599–609.

Choay, J., Lormeau, J.C., Petitou, M. *et al.* (1981) Structural studies on a biologically active hexasaccharide obtained from heparin. *Ann. NY Acad. Sci.* **370**, 644–9.

Collen, D., Schetz, J., de Cock, F. *et al.* (1977) Metabolism of antithrombin III (heparin cofactor) in man: effects of venous thrombosis and of heparin administrations. *Eur. J. Clin. Invest.* **7**, 27–35.

Contant, G., Gouault-Heilmann, M. and Martinoli, J.L. (1983) Heparin inactivation during blood storage: its prevention by blood collection in citric acid, theophylline, adenosine, and dipyridamole – C.T.A.D. mixture. *Thromb. Res.* **31**, 365–74.

D'Angelo, A., Seveso, M.P., D'Angelo, S.V. *et al.* (1990) Effect of clot-detection methods and reagents on APTT – implications in heparin monitoring by APTT. *Am. J. Clin. Pathol.* **94**, 297–306.

Dignac, M., Gabaig, A.M., Cambus, J.P. and Boneu, B. (1993) A new chronometric assay to determine plasma antifactor Xa activity which is insensitive to the antithrombin activity of low molecular weight heparin. *Nouv. Rev. Fr. Hematol.* **35**, 545–9.

England, J.M., Hyde, K., Lewis, S.M. *et al.* (1995) Guidelines for near patient testing in Haematology. *Clin. Lab. Haematol.* **17**, 301–10.

Fareed, J., Jeske, W., Hoppensteadt, M.S. *et al.* (1996) Are the available low molecular weight heparin preparations the same? *Sem. Thromb. Haemostas.* **22**(Supp 1), 77–91.

Gawoski, J.M., Arkin, C.F., Bovill, T. *et al.* (1987) The effects of heparin on the APTT of College of American Pathologists survey specimens. Responsiveness, precision, and sample effects. *Arch. Pathol. Lab. Med.* **111**, 785–90.

Greinacher, A. (1995) Heparin associated thrombocytopaenia. *Excerpta Medica*: *Vessels* **1**, 17–20.

Handeland, G.F., Abildgaard, U., Holm, H.A. and Arnesen, K.A. (1990) Dose adjusted heparin treatment of deep venous thrombosis: a comparison of unfractionated and low molecular weight heparin. *Eur. J. Clin. Pharm.* **39**, 107–12.

Hirsh, J. (1991) Heparin. *N. Engl. J. Med.* **324**, 1565–74.

Hoffman, J.J.M.L. and Meulendijk, P.N. (1978) Comparison of reagents for determining the APTT. *Thromb. Haemost.* **39**, 640–5.

Holm, H.A., Kalvanes, S. and Abildgaard, U. (1985) Changes in plasma antithrombin (heparin cofactor activity) during intravenous heparin therapy: observations in 198 patients with deep venous thrombosis. *Scand. J. Haematol.* **35**, 564–9.

Holm, H.A., Abildgaard, U., Larsen, M.L. and Kalvenes, S. (1987) Monitoring of heparin therapy: should heparin assays also reflect the patients' antithrombin concentration? *Thromb. Res.* **46**, 669–75.

Houbouyan, L., Boutiere, B., Contant, G. *et al.* (1996) Validation protocol of analytical haemostasis systems: measurement of anti Xa activity of low molecular weight heparins. *Clin. Chem.* **42**, 1223–30.

Hull, R.D. and Pineo, G.F. (1994) Low molecular weight heparin treatment of venous thromboembolism. *Prog. Card. Dis.* **37**, 71–4.

Hull, R., Delamore, T., Carter, C. *et al.* (1982) Adjusted subcutaneous heparin versus warfarin sodium in the long term treatment of venous thrombosis. *N. Engl. J. Med.* **307**, 1676–81.

Hull, R.D., Raskob, G.E., Hirsh, J. *et al.* (1986) Continuous intravenous heparin compared with intermittent subcutaneous heparin in the initial treatment of proximal vein thrombosis. *N. Engl. J. Med.* **315**, 1109–14.

Hull, R.D., Raskob, G.E., Rosenbloom, D. *et al.* (1992) Optimal therapeutic level of heparin therapy in patients with venous thrombosis. *Arch. Intern. Med.* **152**, 1589–95.

Hull, R.D., Raskob, G.E., Brant, R.F. *et al.* (1997) Relation between the time to achieve the lower limit of the APTT therapeutic range and recurrent venous thromboembolism during heparin treatment for deep vein thrombosis. *Arch. Int. Med.* **157**, 2562–8.

Kelton, J.G. (1986) Heparin induced thrombocytopaenia. *Haemostasis* **16**, 173–86.

Kitchen, S. and Preston, F.E. (1995) The INR/ISI system is an inappropriate model for heparin monitoring by the APTT. *Br. J. Haematol.* **89**, 50.

Kitchen, S. and Preston, F.E. (1996) The therapeutic range for heparin therapy: relationship between six APTT reagents and two heparin assays. *Thromb. Haemost.* **75**, 734–9.

Kitchen, S., Jennings, I., Woods, T.A.L. and Preston, F.E. (1996) Wide variability in the sensitivity of APPT reagents for monitoring heparin dosage. *J. Clin. Pathol.* **49**, 10–4.

Kitchen, S., Cartwright, I., Woods, T.A.L. *et al.* (1999a) Lipid composition of seven APTT reagents in relation to heparin sensitivity. *Br. J. Haematol.* **106**, 801–8.

Kitchen, S., Iampietro, R., Woolley, A.M. and Preston, F.E. (1999b) Anti Xa monitoring during treatment of LMWH or danaparoid: Inter-assay variability. *Thromb. Haemost.* **82**, 1289–93.

Kitchen, S., Theaker, J., Philips, J.K. and Preston, F.E. (2000) Comparison of anti Xa assays and the heparin assay by protamine titration. *Blood Coag. Fibrinol.* **11**, 137–44.

Lam, L.H., Silbert, J.E. and Rosenberg, R.D. (1976) The separation of active and inactive form of heparin. *Biochem. Biophys. Res. Commun.* **69**, 570–7.

Lane, D.A., Dewton, J., Flynn, A.M. *et al.* (1984) Anticoagulant activities of heparin oligosaccharides and their neutralisation by platelet factor 4. *Biochem. J.* **218**, 725–32.

Laposta, M., Green, D., Van Cott, E.M. *et al.* (1998) The clinical use and laboratory monitoring of LMWH, Danaparoid, Hirudin, and related compounds, and Agatroban. *Arch. Pathol. Lab. Med.* **122**, 799–807.

Levine, M.N., Hirsh, J., Gent, M. *et al.* (1994) A randomised trial comparing APTT with heparin assay in patients with acute venous thromboembolism requiring large daily doses of heparin. *Arch. Int. Med.* **154**, 49–56.

Levine, S.P., Sorenson, R.R., Varns, M.A. *et al.* (1984) The effect of PF4 on assays of plasma heparin. *Br. J. Haematol.* **57**, 585–96.

Lindahl, U., Backsrom, G., Hook, M. *et al.* (1979) Structure of the antithrombin-binding site in heparin. *Proc. Natl Acad. Sci. USA* **76**, 3198–202.

Lindahl, A.K., Abildgaard, U. and Staalesen, R. (1991) The anticoagulant effect in heparinised blood and plasma resulting from interactions with extrinsic pathway inhibitor. *Thromb. Res.* **64**, 155–68.

Linder, R., Grip, L., Olason, E. and Blomback, M. (1996) Bedside heparin monitoring by the APTT measured with a dry reagent. *Clin. Chem.* **42**, 1488–9.

Ma, S., Yang, V.C., Fu, B. and Meyerhoff, M.E. (1993) Electrochemical sensor for heparin: further characterisation and bioanalytical applications. *Anal. Chem.* **65**, 2078–84.

Macik, B.G. (1995) Designing a point-of-care program for coagulation testing. *Arch. Pathol. Lab. Med.* **119**, 929–38.

Magnani, H.N. (1993) Heparin induced thrombocytopaenia: an overview of 230 patients treated with orgaran (Org 10172). *Thromb. Haemost.* **70**, 554–61.

Marciniak, E. and Gockerman, J.P. (1977) Heparin-induced decrease in circulating antithrombin III. *Lancet* **ii**, 581–4.

McClean, J. (1916) The thromboplastic action of cephalin. *Am. J. Physiol.* **41**, 250–7.

Mitchell, G.A., Gargiulo, R.J., Husbeby, R.M. *et al.* (1978) Synthetic peptide substrate for thrombin: introduction of the fluorophore aminoosopthalic acid, dimethyl ester. *Thromb. Res.* **13**, 47–52.

Olson, J.D., Arkin, C.F., Brandt, J.T. *et al.* (1998) Laboratory monitoring of unfractionated heparin. *Arch. Pathol. Lab. Med.* **122,** 782–98.

Ramakrishna, R., Manoharan, A., Kwan, Y.L. and Kyle, P.W. (1995) Heparin-induced thrombocytopaenia: cross-reactivity between standard heparin, low molecular weight heparin, dalteparin (Fragmin) and heparinoid, danaparoid (Organ). *Br. J. Haematol.* **91**, 736–8.

Ray, M.J. (1991) An artefact related to the ratio of sample volume to the blood collection vial size which affects the APTTs of specimens taken to monitor heparin therapy. *Thromb. Haemost.* **66**, 387–8.

Ray, M.J., Carroll, P.A., Just, S.J.E. and Hawson, G.A.T. (1993) A low volume specimen container suitable for monitoring the APTT of heparinised patients. *Blood Coag. Fibrinol.* **4**, 805–7.

Ray, M.J., Perrin, E.J., Smith, I.R. and Hawson, G.A.T. (1996) A proposed model to monitor heparin therapy using the concentrated thrombin time which allows standardisation of reagents and improved estimation of heparin concentrations. *Blood Coag. Fibrinol.* **7**, 515–21.

Reid, S.V., Haddon, M.E. and Denson, K.W.E. (1994) An attempt to standardise the APTT for heparin monitoring using the PT ISI/INR system of calibration: results of a 13 centre study. *Thromb. Res.* **74**, 515–22.

Rosborough, T.K. (1997) Comparison of anti Xa heparin activity and APTT in 2773 plasma samples from unfractionated – heparin treated patients. *Am. J. Clin. Pathol.* **108**, 662–8.

Rosborough, T.K. (1998) Comparing different lots of APTT reagent: analysis of two methods. *Am. J. Clin. Pathol.* **110**, 173–7.

Rose, V.L., Dermott, S.C., Murray, B.F. *et al.* (1993) Decentralised testing for prothrombin time and APTT using a dry chemistry portable analyser. *Arch. Pathol. Lab. Med.* **117**, 611–17.

Rosenberg, R.D. and Lam, L. (1979) Correlation between structure and function of heparin. *Proc. Natl Acad. Sci. USA* **76**, 1218–22.

Rucinski, B., Niewiarowski, S., James, P. *et al.* (1979) Anti-heparin protein secreted by human platelets: purification, characterisation and radioimmunoassay. *Blood* **53**, 47–62.

Samama, M.M. (1995a) Laboratory monitoring of unfractionated heparin treatment. *Clin. Lab. Med.* **15**, 109–17.

Samama, M.M. (1995b) Contemporary laboratory monitoring of low molecular weight heparins. *Clin. Lab. Med.* **15**, 119–23.

Sandset, P.M., Abildgaard, U. and Larsen. M.L. (1988) Heparin induces release of extrinsic pathway inhibitor (EPI). *Thromb. Res.* **50**, 803–13.

Shojania, A.M., Tetreault, J. and Turnbull, G. (1988) The variations between heparin sensitivity of different lots of APTT reagents produced by the same manufacturer. *Am. J. Clin. Pathol.* **89**, 19–23.

Sie, P., Aillaud, M.F., De Prost, D. *et al.* (1987) Measurement of low molecular weight heparin ex vivo activities in clinical laboratories using various anti Xa assays: interlaboratory agreement and requirement for an agreed low molecular weight heparin standard. *Thromb. Haemost.* **58**, 879–83.

Stevenson, K.V., Easton, A.C., Curry, A. *et al.* (1986) The reliability of APTT methods and the relationship to lipid composition and ultrastructure. *Thromb. Haemost.* **55**, 250–8.

Teien, A.N., Lie, M. and Abildgaard, U. (1976) Assay of heparin in plasma using a chromogenic substrate for activated factor X. *Thromb. Res.* **8**, 413–16.

Thomas, D.P., Curtis, A.D. and Barrowcliffe, T.W. (1984) A collaborative study designed to establish the 4th international standard for heparin. *Thromb. Haemost.* **52**, 148–53.

Tollefsen, D.M., Majerus, D.W., Blank, M.K. *et al.* (1982) Heparin cofactor II: purification and properties of a heparin dependent inhibitor of thrombin in human plasma. *J. Biol. Chem.* **257**, 2162–9.

Van den Besselaar, A.M.H., Meeuwisse-Braun, J., Jansen-Gruter, R. and Bertina, R.M. (1987) Monitoring heparin therapy by the APTT – the effect of pre-analytical conditions. *Thromb. Haemost.* **57**, 226–31.

Van den Besselaar, A.M.H.P., Meeuwisse-Braun, J. and Bertina, R.M. (1990) Monitoring heparin therapy: relationships between the APTT and heparin assays based on ex-vivo samples. *Thromb. Haemost.* **63**, 16–23.

Van den Besselaar, A.M.H.P., Neuteboom, J. and Bertina, R.M. (1993) Effect of synthetic phospholipid on the response of the APTT to heparin. *Blood Coag. Fibrinol.* **4**, 895–903.

Van der Velde, E.A. and Poller, L. (1995) The APTT monitoring of heparin – the ISTH/ICSH collaborative study. *Thromb. Haemost.* **73**, 73–91.

Werner, M., Gallagher, J.V., Ballo, M.S. and Karcher, D.S. (1994) Effect of analytical uncertainty of conventional and point-of-care assays of APTT on clinical decisions in heparin therapy. *Am. J. Clin. Pathol.* **102**, 237–41.

WHO Expert Committee on Biological Standards (1983) Requirements for thromboplastins and plasma used to control oral anticoagulant therapy. Thirty Third report. *WHO Tech. Report Series No. 33* **687**, 81–105.

Yin, E.T. and Wessler, S. (1973) Plasma heparin: a unique, practical, submicrogram-sensitive assay. *J. Lab. Clin. Med.* **81**, 298–310.

14

Coagulation instrumentation: hospital laboratory to the home[1]

ANNETTE SCHLUETER AND JOHN D. OLSON

INTRODUCTION

The relationship between the presence of a bleeding diathesis and the rate of blood clotting *in vitro* has been recognized for centuries. In the early part of the 1900s, the skin bleeding time was introduced for the evaluation of a haemorrhagic tendency. In the 1920s the whole blood clotting time was described. In the latter part of the 1920s, a procedure for evaluation of coagulation, exploiting increased viscosity of the specimen during coagulation, was described. This methodology, in the form of the thromboelastograph, is still used in some laboratories and in many operating rooms to evaluate haemorrhage in rapidly bleeding patients (Anonymous, 1995). As development of coagulation testing evolved with the development of the prothrombin time (PT) in 1935 (Quick *et al.*, 1935) and the partial thromboplastin time (APTT) in 1953 (Langdell *et al.*, 1953), interest in the use of the laboratory to detect and evaluate patients with haemorrhagic disorders has grown. The initial tests were performed by manual methods by tilting or rolling test tubes with a trained observer looking for gel or fibrin strand formation in the specimen. These manual methods became burdensome and somewhat impractical as the popularity of the tests grew substantially during the 1950s and 1960s. The first mechanical coagulation testing device (Fibrometer®, B.B.L.) became available in the latter part of the 1950s (Barnett *et al.*, 1966). During the 1950s and 1960s there was also an explosion of information on the mechanism of plasma coagulation with a concomitant increase in demand both for screening and more specialized assays of newly described

[1]The authors would like to thank Tina Swartzendruber for her assistance in preparing this manuscript.

coagulation factors. Instrument manufacturers, with an interest in the clinical laboratory, rapidly developed new instruments which were designed to measure the coagulation end-point (Davey *et al.*, 1972; Sibley and Singer, 1972; Bostick *et al.*, 1975). The end-point is, of course, dependent on the formation of the enzyme thrombin, the subsequent generation of fibrin monomer and its polymerization to fibrin. The polymerization process produces changes in the specimen which can be detected by a variety of optical methods, by methods sensitive to change in viscosity, or by methods which detect the formation of fibrin strands mechanically. In addition to developing clever methods for detecting the end-point of the coagulation reaction, instruments have become more automated with the development of positive displacement pipetting of specimens and reagents, use of simple as well as complex robotics for specimen preparation and handling, and the use of computers for specimen recognition, data reduction, result reporting and various internal instrument controls. Newer immunological methods (spectrophotometric) enable these more highly developed instruments to expand their test menus to assays of a variety of haemostatic proteins.

Below are described some of the methods used for end-point detection in current instruments. Applications for these instruments both in the hospital laboratory and at points of care are discussed, as are some of the issues regarding the variations in haemostasis test results attributable to the measurement system.

14.1 PRE-ANALYTICAL ISSUES INFLUENCING INSTRUMENT FUNCTION

14.1.1 Specimen collection

Specimens for coagulation testing are collected by venepuncture or capillary incision (finger-stick or heelstick). The specimens may or may not be anticoagulated depending on the procedure used. In addition, separation of plasma may be necessary.

All instruments using optical methodology for end-point detection require preparation of a clear plasma specimen. Significant cloudiness due to inadequate removal of platelets or in the presence of lipaemia can produce difficulty with optical end-point measurements. Appropriately prepared plasma samples have the advantages that they can be stored for future confirmatory testing and that they lend themselves to a variety of end-point detection methods. On the other hand, they have the substantial disadvantages of difficulty in effectively preparing a platelet-free specimen and the time required for preparation. As indicated below, some robotic devices can now prepare adequate plasma samples but most laboratories still use a separate centrifugation procedure and manual aliquoting.

Unanticoagulated whole blood, whether obtained by venepuncture or capillary collection, presents the problem of uncontrolled coagulation activation at the time of collection (Peterson and Gottfried, 1982). This adds a pre-analytical variable to the measurements made by devices using unanticoagulated whole blood. Hospital laboratory instruments using anti-coagulated whole blood methods have been described but are not widely used at the present time.

14.1.2 Specimen transport

Difficulties can arise in the preparation of anticoagulated specimens for transport to the hospital or reference laboratory. This delay, at times, can extend to many hours or even a day between the time of collection and the performance of the test. Most published data derive from anticoagulated specimens from which the plasma has been separated and in which testing has commenced within an hour or less of specimen collection. If it is necessary to analyse transported samples, it is clearly essential to demonstrate that transportation does not affect the result of the test and, therefore, its interpretation.

14.1.3 Sample and reagent pipetting

At points of care and in smaller hospital laboratories, sample and reagent pipetting are performed manually. Adjustable, hand-held pipettes and capillary tube techniques have reduced procedural imprecision and variation in both intra- and inter-operator performance. The creation of consolidated central laboratories results in sufficient test numbers being generated to justify, economically, robotic instruments with positive displacement automated pipetting. This development significantly improves reproducibility.

Some of the newer point-of-care, hand-held instruments used for the PT and (less commonly) the APTT use cuvettes with capillary channels coated with dry reagents (Oberhardt *et al.*, 1991; Rose *et al.*, 1993). The specimen can then be placed into a receiving well containing a cuvette directly from the fingerstick incision. This removes the need for pipetting both specimen and reagent. Precision studies of this method have not yet been reported.

14.1.4 Reaction temperatures

Coagulation testing must be performed at a constant temperature, preferably 37°C. A substantial difficulty with small, hand-held and large instruments alike is reliance on the instrument to maintain and/or detect any temperature fluctuation. Temperature fluctuation in the reaction chamber can lead to substantial error.

14.2 END-POINT DETECTION

14.2.1 Optical methods

Optical methods, particularly spectrophotometry and turbidity measurement, are time-honoured techniques for quantifying chemical analytes in the clinical chemistry laboratory (Davey *et al.*, 1972; Sibley and Singer, 1972; Bostick *et al.*, 1975; Weisbrot and Waldner, 1977; Klee *et al.*, 1978; Gogstad *et al.*, 1986). The development of optical methods for the detection of coagulation end-points was a natural extension. These methods were introduced in the 1970s and, since that time, have continued to develop in a variety of ways. The generation of fibrin following coagulation activation results in the conversion of the sample from liquid to solid, i.e. a change in optical density occurs. This forms the basis of different methods of clot detection.

In the classical turbidimetric method, the detector is placed opposite a light source shining through the specimen and the decrease in light transmittance resulting from fibrin-monomer polymer formation is measured as a function of time (Fig. 14.1). In the typical nephelometric or light-scattering methods, the detector is placed at an angle (90°–135°) from the line of the light being transmitted into the specimen. At such an angle, the light transmitted to the detector is minimal until fibrin-monomer polymer occurs leading to reflection of the light to the detector. Light scattering is then measured as a function of time with increasing scattered light being proportional to increasing particle formation. Both fluorometric and spectro-

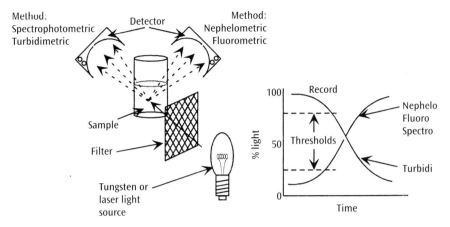

Fig. 14.1 *Optical methods for measuring the coagulation end-point. Spectrophotometric and turbidimetric methods measure light passing directly through the specimen, whereas nephelometric and fluorometric methods measure light at an angle to the light source. The amount of light passing through the sample decreases during the reaction in turbidometric and spectrophotometric methods, and increases during the reaction for nephelometric and fluorometric methods. (Modified with permission, Olson, J.D., 1995.)*

photometric methods have been used in the newer coagulation instruments. Although not common, thrombin or factor Xa-sensitive synthetic substrates can be used as detection reagents, even for high-volume tests like the PT and APTT, with the resulting generation of a colour (spectrophotometric) (Kapke *et al.*, 1981; Bartl *et al.*, 1983; Becker *et al.*, 1984; Berthier *et al.*, 1985; Mitchell *et al.*, 1985) or fluorescent (fluorometric) signal (Umlas *et al.*, 1984), the intensity of which increases as a function of time and is detected by appropriate sensors. Though not commonly used for the performance of routine coagulation procedures, these methods are becoming prominent in the assay of specific factors.

As mentioned above, optical methods require careful preparation of a plasma sample, and reagents used should not add to its opacity. Because of this, commonly used activators for the APTT used in the 1950 and 1960s (kaolin and celite) have been replaced with micronized silica and elagic acid.

14.2.2 Mechanical methods

CONDUCTIVITY

One of the oldest methodologies for the detection of the fibrin clot end-point is the use of conductivity (Fig. 14.2) (Barnett and Pinto, 1966). The principle of this method involves a moving hook rising and falling sequentially, at half-second intervals, breaking the surface of the sample. An electrical current is passed between the cycling and stationary probes, the latter remaining in the sample. When the clot forms, the hook will pick up the fibrin strand and fail to break the circuit, stopping the clock. The method has proved reliable. It is still commonly used in small laboratories and provides 'back-up' in larger laboratories. The procedure remains predominantly manual in all of its components except end-point detection. The instrument can be used with whole blood or plasma samples; however, the results generated from these two sample types are substantially different.

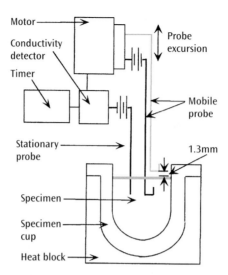

Fig. 14.2 *Mechanical measurement of coagulation using change in conductivity as the end-point. The cycling motion of the moving probe breaks the conductivity at 0.5-second intervals. When fibrin is formed, the fibrin strand prevents the interruption of conductivity, stopping the timer. (Modified with permission, Olson, J.D., 1995.)*

ELECTROMAGNETIC END-POINT METHODS

In the early 1970s a method was developed for performing a whole blood clotting time using kaolin or celite activation on a unanticoagulated specimen. The specimen tubes contain a stir bar set in motion within the instrument and whose loss of motion detects the end-point of coagulation (Bull *et al.*, 1975a,b; Doty *et al.*, 1979). This is one method for determining the activated coagulation time (ACT), a mainstay in the management of heparin therapy at points of care during cardiopulmonary bypass and dialysis. ACT tests generally use specimen collection tubes containing an activator (kaolin or celite), the collection tube serving as the 'cuvette' in the instrument.

The electromagnetic detection method has also extended to the detection of the motion of a metal ball in a test sample. This has been performed by two different techniques (Fig. 14.3) (van den Besselaar and Peters, 1996). The first uses an electromagnet(s) to set the ball in continuous oscillating motion, with end-point detection occurring when the viscosity of the specimen is sufficiently increased to stop the ball. Conversely, an electromagnet has been used to hold the metal ball in the sample at the wall of the cuvette with continuous rotation of the cuvette. When fibrin forms, the ball is forced from the electromagnet by the rotation of the tube, indicating the end-point. Both methods have been used successfully with plasma and whole blood.

VISCOMETRY

Piston and cylinder One of the earliest coagulation devices exploited changes in sample viscosity during fibrin monomer polymerization for end-point recognition (Anonymous, 1995; Traverso *et al.*, 1995a,b). This is the piston-cylinder viscometer in which a piston is located within a cylinder with whole blood or plasma acting as the interface between the two. The test is generally performed with an unanticoagulated specimen at point of care. The cylinder oscillates around the piston, the latter being attached to a strain gauge to measure its

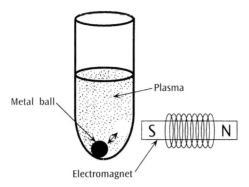

Fig. 14.3 *Mechanical measurement of coagulation using an electromagnetic end-point. The continuously rotating cuvette moves the metal ball away from the magnet when the ball is trapped by fibrin, stopping the timer, or the motion of the continuously moving (oscillating) ball is impeded by the fibrin formation. (Modified with permission, Olson, J.D., 1995.)*

motion. With a liquid sample, the energy created by the cylinder is not effectively transmitted and motion of the piston does not occur, but, as the viscosity of the sample increases with fibrin monomer polymerization, the piston is set in motion and the strain gauge sends a signal to the detector (Fig. 14.4). This method has the advantage of being able to examine not only the formation of the clot and platelet function, but also the subsequent stability or otherwise of the clot.

Sonar This technology has also been used in viscometry. A probe is placed in the sample and vibrates at a constant frequency (Fig. 14.5) (Sugiura *et al.*, 1982; Saleem *et al.*, 1983; Hett *et al.*, 1995). The instrument is designed to maintain this constant frequency of probe vibration, but in so doing uses more energy as the sample viscosity increases. This increase in energy is transduced to a chart recorder. This method has been used successfully both for clot detection and for the measurement of plasma, serum and whole blood viscosity. The sonar method also affords the opportunity to examine, over time, the formation (including platelet function), the stability and subsequent lysis of the clot.

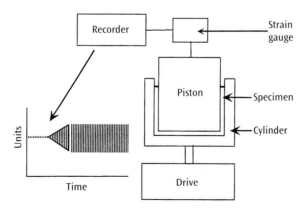

Fig. 14.4 *Mechanical (viscometric) measurement of coagulation with a piston and cylinder. Increased viscosity caused by fibrin formation increases energy transfer from cylinder to piston, and therefore the signal to the strain gauge. (Modified with permission, Olson, J.D., 1995.)*

Falling flag and rising bubble Two other methods have been used to measure the ACT, in addition to the electromagnetic method described previously. These are the 'falling flag' and 'rising bubble' methods, both of which depend on increasing viscosity (Fig. 14.6). In the falling flag method, a small, rigid plastic flag is continuously raised mechanically in the sample and allowed to fall back by gravity. As the sample viscosity increases, the rate at which the flag falls is reduced and the end-point detected. In the rising bubble method, a stream of air bubbles is passed from the bottom of a small-calibre cuvette through the sample. As the viscosity rises due to the fibrin formation, the clotted specimen is physically pushed into a light beam, thus detecting the end-point. These two devices have been developed primarily for use in monitoring heparin therapy, particularly the titration of heparinized specimens with protamine sulphate to assist in appropriate dosing for heparin neutralization.

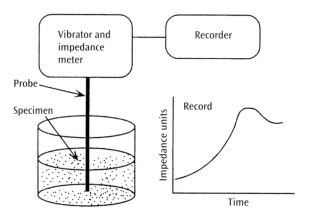

Fig. 14.5 *Mechanical (viscometric) measurement of coagulation by sonar. Increasing energy required to maintain a constant frequency of probe vibration during fibrin formation is measured. (Modified with permission, Olson, J.D., 1995.)*

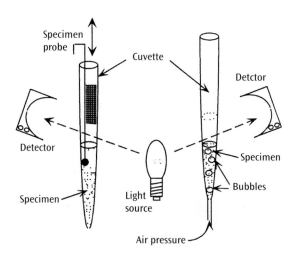

Fig. 14.6 *Mechanical (viscometric) measurement of coagulation by falling flag (left) and rising bubble (right).* Falling flag: *Change in the rate of probe movement by increased viscosity following fibrin formation is detected by the failure of the flag to interrupt light transmission to the detector.* Rising bubble: *Fibrin formation allows the bubbles to push the clotted specimen into the light path, blocking light transmission. (Modified with permission, Olson, J.D., 1995.)*

Capillary flow Instruments used at point of care and for home testing have exploited the natural flow of unanticoagulated whole blood through capillary tubes coated with PT or APTT reagent. Drops of blood are passed directly into the sample chamber of the cuvette, the latter being placed in the instrument and the capillary flow to a receiving chamber monitored. In the two methods described, capillary flow proceeds until fibrin-monomer polymerization increases the viscosity, which in turn eventually slows and stops the sample flow (Fig. 14.7) (Rose *et al.*, 1993; Carter *et al.*, 1996). One method uses laser light to assess flow, and when this slows and stops the end-point is reached. As an alternative approach, paramagnetic iron oxide particles (PIOPs) are present in the cuvette (Oberhardt *et al.*, 1991). In this method, capillary flow is detected by the movement of the paramagnetic particles in the blood. Magnetic techniques are employed to detect the cessation of flow of the particles. More recently, devices utilizing the movement of PIOPs for end-point detection have been modified to monitor the rate of fibrinolysis. As the clot dissolves, the iron particles begin to respond to magnetic forces again. The resumption corresponds to the lysis onset time (LOT), an indicator of fibrinolysis (Oberhardt *et al.*, 1997).

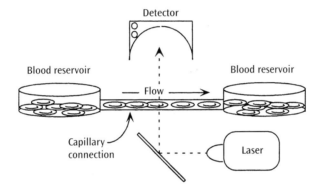

Fig. 14.7 *Mechanical (viscometric) measurement of coagulation in a whole blood specimen by capillary flow. Fibrin formation impedes the movement of erythrocytes, changing the rate of laser signal to the detector. A similar method detects the decreased motion of paramagnetic iron oxide particles. (Modified with permission, Olson, J.D., 1995.)*

14.3 HOSPITAL AND REFERENCE LABORATORY TESTING

As with the development of instrumentation in other areas of the laboratory, coagulation systems have evolved with a variety of approaches, ranging from manual tilt tube testing to high-volume, random access, robot systems.

In smaller laboratories where coagulation testing is performed on relatively few specimens each day, simple instruments, with any of the end-point detection methods described above, are used with manual methods for plasma separation and pipetting of the samples and reagents. In addition, results are manually transcribed from an instrument print-out into the laboratory's information system or a paper copy transported to the patient's record. The advantages of these simple, manual methods are as follows:

- reduced costs of instrumentation;
- added reliability of a uniform mechanism for end-point detection.

The disadvantages are:

- added labour costs to perform the sample preparation, pipetting and data transcription;
- increased possibility for error due to variation in pipetting technique;
- potential for clerical or transcription error.

As test numbers rise, either through centralized testing for multiple clinics and hospitals or because of the high volume in a single hospital/clinic system, the expense of the more advanced instrumentation can be distributed over a large number of specimens. The largest of these instruments are now capable of:

- automated pipetting of the sample;
- automated pipetting of the reagents (often many reagents, requiring automated timing between reagent additions);
- ability of end-point determination by more than one method (Pernod *et al.*, 1994; Aulesa *et al.*, 1996).

For some instruments, as many as three dozen different reagents can be loaded into the instrument in a single exercise with separate compartments for temperature control (refrigeration, room temperature or other temperatures). These instruments are capable of reading a previously generated bar code label for positive specimen identification. A bi-directional interface exists between the instrument computer and the laboratory information system. The latter can download patient demographics and test orders and subsequently pass the new data generated to the host system. Finally, there are large multi-functional laboratory systems which have successfully automated specimen labelling, centrifugation and robot-assisted placement of the samples in the analyser. Justifying the cost of these highly roboticized systems (particularly for coagulation) requires a substantial specimen workflow.

Advantages of these more highly automated instruments include:

- positive displacement pipetting of the patient sample and reagents;
- tightly controlled incubation times;
- positive specimen identification;
- bidirectional communication between instrument and host computer;
- reduced error rate both in technique and in transcription.

The disadvantage is their complexity and, therefore, difficulty in adequately controlling all aspects of function including pipetting volumes, temperature, timing, accuracy of data transmission, and others. The cost can be prohibitive depending on the setting.

14.4 COAGULATION TESTING AT THE POINT OF CARE

14.4.1 General considerations

The demand for rapid, reliable coagulation test results has driven the development of coagulation point-of-care instrumentation. Specifically, these tests have been advocated for monitoring procedures requiring heparinization (particularly haemodialysis, coronary artery bypass grafting [CABG] and percutaneous transluminal coronary angioplasty [PTCA]), fluid replacement during exsanguinating haemorrhage, and clinic or home monitoring of oral anti-coagulant therapy. The technologies involved in generating a coagulation test result at the point of care are varied; however, they share several common features.

All point-of-care technologies attain the goal of decreasing the turnaround time primarily by reducing the pre-analytical phase of testing. The location of the instrument at the bedside, nurse's station, operating room or in the home decreases the transport time to the test site, resulting in substantial time savings (15 minutes to as much as 24 hours or more for specimens mailed in from home for warfarin monitoring). Many instruments produce further time savings by performing the test on a single drop of unanticoagulated whole blood obtained by capillary (fingerstick) techniques rather than plasma obtained by venepuncture and centrifugation, thus eliminating the centrifugation step. These features also eliminate variability introduced by underfilling or overfilling tubes containing anticoagulant, effects of temperature and storage time on coagulation factor function, as well as the effect of centrifuge function on the ability to generate platelet poor plasma.

The use of unanticoagulated whole blood as the substrate for testing generates some problems that are not present when a venous specimen is drawn into a tube containing the appropriate amount of anticoagulant. Activation of coagulation factors by traumatic venepuncture has long been recognized as a source of falsely prolonged coagulation test results (Peterson and Gottfried, 1982), and the likelihood of a traumatic fingerstick is high if the operator is not experienced in the technique. If the finger must be squeezed to generate a drop of blood large enough to perform the test, the specimen may not provide accurate test results. Even a specimen obtained non-traumatically will eventually clot in the absence of anticoagulant, and thus testing performed on whole blood necessitates close proximity of patient and instrument. On the other hand, an anticoagulated specimen transported to a central laboratory for testing does not represent reality in the patient, even at the time the specimen was obtained, because of continuous loss of activity of clotting factors during transport (Palkuti, 1984); thus the specimen tested at the point of care may more closely represent the patient's clinical condition. Presently, most clinicians are used to correlating results from central laboratory testing with the patient's condition, and despite potentially more accurate representation by point-of-care testing, the algorithm for decision-making based on test results cannot be identical in these very different settings.

The location of point-of-care instrumentation also necessitates operation by individuals not formally trained in laboratory technology, such as physicians, nurses, perfusion technologists and, in the case of home testing, the patients themselves. Operation of the instrument is generally not complex, but training is still required to ensure proper technique in sample acquisition and instrument operation. Competency testing and/or proficiency testing are not usually part of routine nurse training and are certainly issues that need to be addressed for patients who use a coagulation testing instrument in their home. Additionally, the importance of maintaining the instrument in good working order and performance of quality control to ensure that the test results are valid may not be fully appreciated by these individuals. Some devices automatically prevent test performance if the quality control fails, until the instrument is serviced, which may prevent the inadvertent use of a malfunctioning device by an inexperienced operator. Appropriate controls are generally considered to be those that are physiologically identical to a patient specimen and contain the analyte in question at a known concentration. There are currently no commercially available controls that accurately mimic unanticoagulated whole blood samples. The product marketed as a whole blood control (Ciba Corning Diagnostics) is a mixture of plasma and stabilized blood cells, and does not contain platelets. To address this issue, manufacturers have recommended using plasma controls for instruments which are capable of analysing plasma specimens as well as whole blood specimens, or the use of electronic controls. There are no published data demonstrating that proper performance of a plasma control invariably indicates proper function of the whole blood channel of the instrument. Electronic controls send a signal through the instrument which simulates that sent by a patient specimen in order to assess the ability of the instrument to interpret the signal properly. Because they do not require placing a specimen into the instrument, they do not provide any information about the user's technique. Regardless of the nature of the controls used in point-of-care instrumentation, the fact that each test is performed in an independent cartridge means that the control is technically only valid for that cartridge and does not necessarily ensure proper performance of subsequent cartridges. The ability to detect a low failure rate in these systems is thus limited.

Data management also presents unique challenges in point-of-care instrumentation. Most instruments are not designed to interface directly to a laboratory or hospital information system. Thus, the data must be collected and transferred manually to the medical record. This provides an opportunity for transcription errors and adds to the workload of overburdened clerks or nurses. Some point-of-care instruments have the capability to store limited amounts of data for later retrieval, and some provide a print-out of the data. Both these features make data retrieval easier than with instruments that only display the data electronically and have no memory function. No point-of-care device to date allows wireless communication to a hospital information system.

14.4.2 Monitoring heparin therapy

ACTIVATED COAGULATION TIME

Several features of point-of-care coagulation instrumentation are specific to the clinical situation being monitored. One of the oldest coagulation tests in use at the point of care is the activated clotting time (ACT; described previously). This test was initially advocated for ensuring adequate anticoagulation during cardiopulmonary bypass (Bull *et al.*, 1975a,b) and has been used successfully in this setting for more than two decades. Since then, its utility has also been demonstrated for ensuring adequate heparinization during PTCA and following heparin clearance prior to sheath removal after the procedure (Ogilby *et al.*, 1989; Rath and Bennett, 1990). The therapeutic ranges may differ among instruments and thus direct comparison of test results between two systems is not appropriate (Uden *et al.*, 1991; Dougherty *et al.*, 1992; Ferguson, 1992). Because the APTT is not linear at the high levels of heparin needed for these procedures (Schriever *et al.*, 1973), it is not a useful test for following such patients. No central laboratory test is available that provides information equivalent to the ACT, and therefore correlation of ACT results with those obtained on a random access or batch analyser is not an issue.

ACTIVATED PARTIAL THROMBOPLASTIN TIME

Point-of-care monitoring of heparin anticoagulation at levels of 0.2–0.6 U/mL using the APTT or protamine titration has also been advocated. Such testing has potential utility rapidly to establish therapeutic levels of heparin in patients with recent thromboembolic events (Groce *et al.*, 1987; Becker *et al.*, 1994) or patients with microvascular bleeding following cardiac surgery (Despotis *et al.*, 1994a). However, APTT test results from whole blood and plasma specimens cannot be considered interchangeable. If APTT testing using identical reagents and instrumentation is performed on a heparinized whole blood specimen and the same specimen following the removal of erythrocytes, the results obtained will not be identical (Schlueter *et al.*, 1997). This is due in part to the neutralization of heparin by platelet factor IV in the whole blood specimen (van den Besselaar *et al.*, 1987). Despite the fact that the whole blood assay may provide the more physiologically relevant result, clinicians are used to monitoring heparin therapy by plasma APTT measurements. The manufacturers of whole blood assay systems have addressed this issue by mathematically converting the results obtained on a whole blood specimen to a plasma equivalent APTT (Macik, 1995).

Correction for specimen type does not ensure identical APTT results, however. It is well known from studies of APTT results generated by standard laboratory methods that differences in instrumentation and reagents have a large effect on the value obtained from a heparinized sample (Shapiro *et al.*, 1977; Barrowcliffe and Gray, 1981; Brandt and Triplett, 1981). There is presently no accepted method for standardizing APTT results generated with different instrumentation and reagents, as the international normalized ratio (INR) does for the PT. It is not surprising, therefore, that point-of-care instruments that generate APTT results are subject to this sort of variability. Most studies that compare central laboratory and point-of-care generated APTT results on the same specimen show that the variability is no more than would be expected between two standard laboratory instruments or two reagents (Ansell *et al.*, 1991; Despotis *et al.*, 1994b). However, this degree of variability may necessitate having two (or more) normal and therapeutic ranges for APTT results within a single institution, depending on how many different point-of-care instruments are in use within the facility. Direct comparison of point-of-care and central laboratory results remains a goal that will be difficult to attain. The current movement towards harmonization among different methods within health care systems will continue to exert pressure on improving these comparisons.

The effect of this degree of variability on clinical decision-making has been studied. In one study, if a three-way decision algorithm was used for adjusting heparin therapy (sub-therapeutic, therapeutic, supratherapeutic), the two test results differed in a clinically significant manner in 22% of the samples (Werner *et al.*, 1994). Another study of five whole blood point-of-care APTT monitors demonstrated that one instrument was unable to distinguish therapeutic from supratherapeutic heparin levels in 32% of the cases and another failed in 12% of cases (O'Neill *et al.*, 1991). Variability between identical instruments using the same lot of reagent does not appear to be a problem in the point-of-care setting, as would be expected from the experience of standard laboratory instruments (Ansell *et al.*, 1991).

Patients to be maintained on oral anticoagulation often continue to be monitored for therapeutic heparinization while attaining therapeutic warfarin levels. It has traditionally been assumed that the APTT will continue to reflect primarily heparin levels during this time period and the PT will reflect increasing warfarin levels without interference from heparin. While this is generally true for standard laboratory instrumentation, at least one point-of-care instrument shows excessive prolongation of the APTT in patients on warfarin in the presence or absence of heparin (Ray *et al.*, 1994). Similar changes have also been demonstrated for patients receiving aprotinin therapy (Despotis *et al.*, 1995).

14.4.3 Monitoring life-threatening haemorrhage

Over the past decade there has been considerable growth in liver transplantation. During the development of this technique, as surgeons were gaining expertise, exsanguinating haemorrhage was a frequent complication. Despite remarkable improvement in intra-operative management and improvement in surgical technique, there are still infrequently patients who undergo substantial blood loss. In the early days, a variety of methods evolved for monitoring coagulation in patients intraoperatively. At that time the Thromboelastograph, a piston-cylinder viscometer originally developed in the 1920s, resurfaced and gained considerable popularity in this clinical setting. In addition, the sonar device for whole blood coagulation testing was also found to be of some value. During liver transplantation, in the anhepatic phase, patients do undergo activation of fibrinolysis. Both technologies have, as an advantage, the ability not only to detect the rate of clot formation but also to detect accelerated fibrinolysis. Most patients undergoing liver transplantation or exsanguinating haemorrhage in other surgical settings can be managed successfully using more routine monitors of coagulation such as the PT and fibrinogen assay. Instruments using the principle of viscosity have also been used, less extensively, in many other clinical settings (Anonymous, 1995; Hett et al., 1995; Traverso et al., 1995a,b).

Comparison of point-of-care and standard PT test results is simplified by the use of the INR, but it should be stressed that the INR system of reporting is designed solely for oral anticoagulation. In studies at the point of care in patients with microvascular bleeding following cardiac surgery, the results correlated well with standard laboratory results (Despotis et al., 1994b). If the rapid turnaround time of point-of-care results facilitates the use of a transfusion algorithm based on coagulation studies, the transfusion requirements of patients undergoing these procedures may be decreased (Despotis et al., 1994a). Similar results might be expected in cases of massive transfusion following exsanguinating haemorrhage, although such a study has not been conducted to date.

14.4.4 Monitoring oral anticoagulation

In an outpatient setting, either clinic or home, monitoring of warfarin therapy by point-of-care PT has been advocated. Several studies have assessed the ability of patients to monitor their anticoagulation with a device in the home, and make necessary adjustments in their warfarin doses based on the results. These studies demonstrated that significantly more patients remain within the therapeutic range with home testing, presumably because of more frequent monitoring of their INR (White et al., 1989; Ansell et al., 1995). The ability to distinguish therapeutic from supratherapeutic levels of coumadin, based on point-of-care monitoring, appears to be fairly straightforward. When INR results on specimens from patients taking warfarin were compared in parallel on point-of-care and standard instrumentation, the results agreed well within the therapeutic range. Specimens with supratherapeutic warfarin levels gave high INR values in both tests, but the magnitude of the INR at high warfarin levels was less with the point-of-care devices than with standard laboratory instrumentation (Becker et al., 1993; Foulis et al., 1995; Kaatz et al., 1995; Douketis et al., 1998). If the likelihood of bleeding correlates with the degree to which the INR is elevated beyond the therapeutic range, point-of-care instrumentation may underestimate the risk of bleeding in patients with supratherapeutic anticoagulation levels.

Demand for more rapid turnaround time is driven by the hypothesis that more frequent monitoring (and dose modification) will lead to better patient care by responding to change in patient status more quickly, and ultimately decrease complications. As described above, some data demonstrate improvement in short-term patient outcome using point-of-care instrumentation. No studies are yet available which demonstrate influence on mortality, rethrombosis or bleeding.

Only a few studies have assessed the costs associated with point-of-care testing. Because of the disposable cartridge format of point-of-care instrumentation, the reagent cost per test is as much as 100 times higher than standard laboratory instrumentation (College of American Pathologists, 1997b). Savings in operator labour costs partially offset the increased reagent costs, but the point-of-care test is still more expensive to perform than the standard laboratory test, when a parallel standard test is available (White et al., 1989; Schlueter et al., 1997). Thus any cost savings generated by point-of-care testing must result from parameters such as decreased hospital stay, operating room time, complication rate or use of other medical resources. Such parameters are difficult to quantify. Despotis et al. (1994a) demonstrated significantly decreased operative times as well as red cell and platelet transfusions for patients monitored by point-of-care testing and a transfusion algorithm following cardiovascular surgery, but no direct cost comparison with standard laboratory monitoring and transfusion algorithm was performed. On the other hand, Nichols *et al.* (2000) were unable to generate an improvement in total time for preoperative work-up on the basis of point-of-care availability for coagulation testing. It is likely that point-of-care instrumentation will indeed prove to provide cost savings for certain groups of patients. To maximize benefit, it is important to use this modality only in situations where the results of testing will be acted upon as soon as they are available.

14.5 INSTRUMENT IMPACT ON RESULT VARIABILITY

Since the early 1980s there has been considerable interest in the degree of variability observed in interlaboratory comparisons of common coagulation tests. This variability was considered, at the time, to be somewhat surprising because the expectation was that the more uniform approaches to end-point measurement would actually decrease the amount of variability seen. Data generated confirm substantial contributions to this variability from reagents used in testing and the instruments in which those reagents are used. Table 14.1 depicts the number of reagents and instruments which were reported to the College of American Pathologists survey in the CG1 and CG2 participant summary of 1997 (College of American Pathologists, 1997a). These surveys have approximately 4300 and 850 participants, respectively. Because of substantial pressure to purchase capital equipment (instruments), consumables and reagents at the lowest possible cost, laboratories often elect to use reagents for routine testing based on cost. This leads to a substantial number of different instrument and reagent combinations. Hidden in the data presented in Table 14.1 is the additional contribution of different lot numbers of reagent. This number of different lots would cause an additional, substantial increase to the number of different instrument reagent combinations available.

Since the latter part of the 1980s, the development of an instrument-specific ISI (International Sensitivity Index) has been the subject of considerable investigation (Poggio *et al.*, 1989; Poller *et al.*, 1989, 1994; van Rijn *et al.*, 1989; D'Angelo *et al.*, 1990; Ray and Smith, 1990; Clarke *et al.*, 1992; Cunningham *et al.*, 1994; Cunningham and Olson, 1996). A recent report of the effect of instrument on ISI showed that not only was there an effect of instrument on sensitivity, but also that the same model of instrument from the same manufacturer had significant variation (Poller *et al.*, 1995). Other data have been reported indicating that 'same model' variation is minimal (Cunningham and Olson, 1996).

The surveys of the College of American Pathologists from 1994 and 1996 demonstrate the changes imparted by instrument/reagent combinations and those due to instrument alone (College of American Pathologists, 1994, 1996). In each case the same specimens are being

Table 14.1 *Data from the College of American Pathologists (1997) CG1 and CG2 (Survey Set B)*

	PT		APTT	
	1977 CG1B	1997 CG2B	1997 CG1B	1997 CG2B
Number of participants	4311	810	4140	850
Total number of instruments	51	34	47	32
Total number of reagents	34	27	33	22
Total number of reagent/instrument combinations	269	109	283	121

examined. The effect of the instrument/reagent combination is remarkable even within instrument type (Fig. 14.8). When both the thromboplastin and the specimen are supplied, the degree of variability is reduced, but it is still sufficient to produce a wide range of results in both the PT and the INR (Fig. 14.9).

Data such as these, and those described above, have led to efforts to provide ISI calibration reagent for use in each laboratory, with each instrument. Preliminary data indicate that such an approach can improve concordance among instruments, but the number of calibrators required may be impractical for widespread use (Poller *et al.*, 1995).

Information regarding the instrument effect on the APTT is available but not as comprehensive. Most information provided is for instrument/reagent combination, with limited data isolating the instrument effect (Marlar *et al.*, 1984; Hoffman and Verhappen, 1988; D'Angelo *et al.*, 1990). Attempts to develop an approach similar to the INR for monitoring heparin using the APTT have not been fruitful. Variability of drug, reagent, instrument

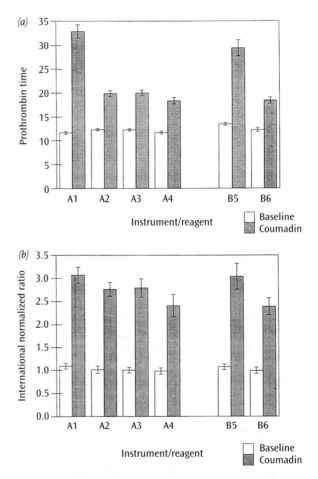

Fig. 14.8 *Variability of PT (a) and international normalized ratio (b) due to differences in both reagent and instrumentation. Normal and coumadinized plasma specimens were provided to the laboratories participating in the survey. Two instruments (A and B) were used with six different prothrombin reagents (1–6) as denoted on the x-axis. The number of laboratories using each of these instrument/reagent combinations is as follows: A1 = 42, A2 = 15, A3 = 132, A4 = 13, B5 = 27, B6 = 100 (College of American Pathologists Participant Summary, 1996).*

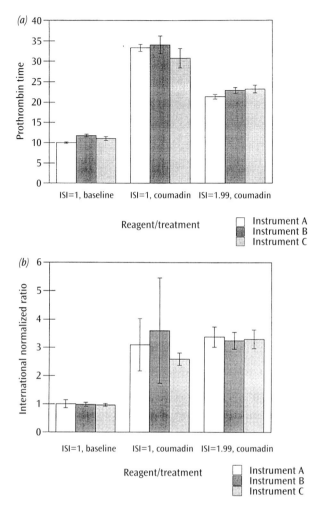

Fig. 14.9 *Variability of PT (a) and international normalized ratio (b) due to differences in instrumentation alone. Three reagent/specimen combinations were provided to the laboratories, as denoted on the x-axis. The specimens were either normal or coumadinized plasma, and the ISI of the reagents is indicated. One of three instruments (A, B or C) was used. The number of laboratories using each instrument is as follows: A = 135, B = 242, C = 16 (College of American Pathologists Participant Study, 1994, 1996).*

and patient responses have, to date, been too great for such standardization (Van der Velde and Poller, 1995).

It is interesting that instruments would have such a profound effect on the coagulation time. One would intuitively think that the reaction, and therefore its measurement, would be constant. There appear to be two major contributors to this variability. First, the variations among methods to measure end-point contribute to these differences. Optical methods reach the end-point faster than mechanical ones. Turbidimetric and nephelometric methods will also vary.

Second, within each instrument, small variations can occur in key components. These issues are more easily addressed with simpler testing methods. Larger, random access, robotic instruments in which the volume of pipetting, the timing of events, the temperature of reactions, the output of the light source and the functionality of the detectors are instrument-controlled present many areas of opportunity for variation in function. Validation of these functions becomes an interesting challenge for the instrument operator. Instrument manufacturers have developed internal checks that can be helpful, but instruments and their functions fail and instrument operators must assume that the instrument is malfunctioning when they begin a testing process. This requires that the instrument be validated on a regular basis in all its functional parameters and that appropriate controls for testing both within the reference range and in the relevant abnormal range be a part of all testing performed. These quality control and quality assurance issues are much less complex with the smaller, simpler instruments. As the instruments become more complex, the potential for one or more of these instrument-controlled events to malfunction and contribute to variability is significant.

14.6 SUMMARY

During the past three decades, a large variety of different methods have been developed to measure the coagulation end-point. Many continue to be used in instruments today. In addition, development of instrumentation is continuing to proceed at both ends of the size spectrum. In order to try to improve the management of oral anticoagulation, smaller devices designed for use by the patient at home are being actively studied. At the same time, hospital laboratories are using larger, highly automated, random access analysers capable of performing most tests of haemostasis in a single device. These widely disparate technologies present ever-changing challenges for both the laboratorian and the clinician, change that can be expected to continue.

REFERENCES

Aller, R. (1997) Coagulation analyzers: a new year, another look. *CAP Today* **11**, 50–67.

Anonymous (1995) Thromboelastography. Special issue dedicated to Professor Dr. Hellmut Hartert. *Sem. Thromb. Hemost.* **21**(Suppl. 4), 1–93.

Ansell, J.E., Tiarks, C., Hirsh, J. *et al.* (1991) Measurement of the activated partial thromboplastin time from a capillary (fingerstick) sample of whole blood. A new method for monitoring heparin therapy. *Am. J. Clin. Pathol.* **95**, 222–7.

Ansell, J.E., Patel, N., Ostrovsky, D. *et al.* (1995) Long-term patient self-management of oral anticoagulation. *Arch. Intern. Med.* **155**, 2185–9.

Aulesa, C., Petit, M., Sentis, M. *et al.* (1996) Initial evaluation of the ACL-Futura coagulation analyzer. *Sangre* **41**, 417–26.

Barnett, R.N. and Pinto, C.L. (1966) Reproducibility of prothrombin time determinations between technologists. Comparison of the fibrometer and tilt-tube methods. *Tech. Bull. Reg. Med. Technol.* **36**, 146–9.

Barrowcliffe, T.W. and Gray, E. (1981) Studies of phospholipid reagents used in coagulation II: factors influencing their sensitivity to heparin. *Thromb. Haemost.* **46**, 634–7.

Bartl, K., Becker, U. and Lill, H. (1983) Application of several chromogenic substrate assays to automated instrumentation for coagulation analysis. *Sem. Thromb. Hemost.* **9**, 301–8.

Becker, U., Jering, H., Bartl, K. *et al.* (1984) Automated prothrombin-time test with use of a chromogenic peptide substrate and a centrifugal analyzer. *Clin. Chem.* **30**, 524–8.

Becker, D.M., Humphries, J.E., Walker, F.B. *et al.* (1993) Standardizing the prothrombin time. Calibrating coagulation instruments as well as thromboplastin. *Arch. Pathol. Lab. Med.* **117**, 602–5.

Becker, R.C., Cyr, J., Corrao, J.M. *et al.* (1994) Bedside coagulation monitoring in heparin-treated patients with active thromboembolic disease: a coronary care unit experience. *Am. Heart J.* **128**, 719–23.

Berthier, A.M., Pommereuil, M., Scarabin, P.Y. *et al.* (1985) A multicenter study on amidolytic factor X evaluation in oral anticoagulant therapy. *Thromb. Haemost.* **53**, 433–6.

Bostick, W.D., Bauer, M.L., Morton, J.M. *et al.* (1975) Coagulation-time determination with automatic multivariable analysis, by use of a miniature centrifugal fast analyzer. *Clin. Chem.* **21**, 1288–93.

Brandt, J.T. and Triplett, D.A. (1981) Laboratory monitoring of heparin: effect of reagents and instruments on the activated partial thromboplastin time. *Am. J. Clin. Pathol.* **76**(suppl), 530–7.

Bull, B.S., Korpman, R.A., Huse, W.M. *et al.* (1975a) Heparin therapy during extracorporeal circulation: I. Problems inherent in existing heparin protocols. *J. Thorac. Cardiovasc. Surg.* **69**, 674–84.

Bull, B.S., Huse, W.M., Brauer, F.S. *et al.* (1975b) Heparin therapy during extracorporeal circulation: II. The use of a dose-response curve to individualize heparin and protamine dosage problems inherent in existing heparin protocols. *J. Thorac. Cardiovasc. Surg.* **69**, 674–84.

Carter, A.J., Hicks, K., Heldman, A.W. *et al.* (1996) Clinical evaluation of a microsample coagulation analyzer, and comparison with existing techniques. *Cathet. Cardiovasc. Diagn.* **39**, 97–102.

Clarke, K., Taberner, D.A., Thomson, J.M. *et al.* (1992) Assessment of value of calibrated lyophilised plasmas to determine International Sensitivity Index for coagulometers. *J. Clin. Pathol.* **45**, 58–60.

Cunningham, M.T. and Olson, J. D. (1996) Low inter-instrument variability of the international normalized ratio with the Coagamate X2/Simplastin excel system. *Am. J. Clin. Pathol.* **105**, 301–4.

Cunningham, M.T., Johnson, G.F., Pennell, B.J. *et al.* (1994) The reliability of manufacturer-determined, instrument-specific international sensitivity index values for calculating the international normalized ratio. *Am. J. Clin. Pathol.* **102**, 128–33.

D'Angelo, A., Seveso, M.P., D'Angelo, S.V. *et al.* (1990) Effect of clot-detection methods and reagents on activated partial thromboplastin time (APTT). Implications in heparin monitoring by APTT. *Am. J. Clin. Pathol.* **94**, 297–306.

Davey, F.R., Fiske, L. and Maltby, A. (1972) Evaluation of a photoelectric automatic prothrombin analyzer. *Am. J. Clin. Pathol.* **58**, 687–92.

Despotis, G.J., Santoro, S.A., Spitznagel, E. *et al.* (1994a) Prospective evaluation and clinical utility of on-site monitoring of coagulation in patients undergoing cardiac operation. *J. Thorac. Cardiovasc. Surg.* **107**, 271–9.

Despotis, G.J., Santoro, S.A., Spitznagel, E. *et al.* (1994b) On-site prothrombin time, activated partial thromboplastin time, and platelet count. *Anesthesiology* **80**, 33–51.

Despotis, G.J., Alsoufiev, A., Goodnough, L.T. *et al.* (1995) Aprotinin prolongs whole blood activated partial thromboplastin time but not whole blood prothrombin time in patients undergoing cardiac surgery. *Anesth. Analg.* **81**, 919–24.

Doty, D.B., Knott, H.W., Hoyt, J.L. *et al.* (1979) Heparin dose for accurate anticoagulation in cardiac surgery. *J. Cardiovasc. Surg.* **20**, 597–604.

Dougherty, K.G., Gaos, C.M., Bush, H.S. *et al.* (1992) Activated clotting times and activated partial thromboplastin times in patients undergoing coronary angioplasty who receive bolus doses of heparin. *Cathet. Cardiovasc. Diagn.* **26**, 260–3.

Douketis, J.D., Lane, A., Milne, J. *et al.* (1998) Accuracy of a portable international normalization ratio monitor in outpatients receiving long-term oral anticoagulant therapy: comparison with a laboratory reference standard using clinically relevant criteria for agreement. *Thromb. Res.* **92**, 11–17.

Ferguson, J. J. (1992) All ACTs are not created equal. *Texas Heart Inst. J.* **19**, 1–3.

Foulis, P.R., Wallach, P.M., Adelman, H.M. *et al.* (1995) Performance of the Coumatrak system in a large anticoagulation clinic. *Am. J. Clin. Pathol.* **103**, 98–102.

Gogstad, G.O., Dahl, K.H. and Christophersen, A. (1986) Turbidimetric determination of prothrombin time by clotting in a centrifugal analyzer. *Clin. Chem.* **32**, 1857–62.

Groce III, J.B., Gal, P., Douglas, J.B. *et al.* (1987) Heparin dosage adjustment in patients with deep-vein thrombosis using heparin concentrations rather than activated partial thromboplastin time. *Clin. Pharm.* **6**, 216–22.

Hett, D.A., Walker, D., Pilkington, S.N. *et al.* (1995) Sonoclot analysis (Review – 41 references). *Br. J. Anaesth.* **75**, 771–6.

Hoffmann, J.J. and Verhappen, M.A. (1988) Automated nephelometry of fibrinogen: analytical performance and observations during thrombolytic therapy. *Clin. Chem.* **34**, 2135–40.

Kaatz, S.S., White, R.H., Hill, J. *et al.* (1995) Accuracy of laboratory portable monitor International Normalization Ratio determinations: comparison with a criterion standard. *Arch. Intern. Med.* **155**, 1861–7.

Kapke, G.F., Feld, R.D., Witte, D.L. *et al.* (1981) Esterolytic method for determination of heparin in plasma. *Clin. Chem.* **27**, 526–9.

Klee, G.G., Didisheim, P., Johnson, R.J. *et al.* (1978) An evaluation of four automated coagulation instruments. *Am. J. Clin. Pathol.* **70**, 646–54.

Langdell, R.D., Wagner, R.H. and Brinkhous, K.M. (1953) Effect of antihemophilic factor on one-stage clotting tests: a presumptive test for hemophilia and a simple one-stage antihemophilic factor assay procedure. *J. Lab. Clin. Med.* **41**, 637–47.

Macik, B.G. (1995) Designing a point-of-care program for coagulation testing. *Arch. Pathol. Lab. Med.* **119**, 929–38.

Marlar, R.A., Bauer, P.J., Endres-Brooks, J.L. *et al.* (1984) Comparison of the sensitivity of commercial APTT reagents in the detection of mild coagulopathies. *Am. J. Clin. Pathol.* **82**, 436–9.

Mitchell, G.A., Solorzano, M.M., Riesgo, M.I. *et al.* (1985) Novel rhodamine tripeptide substrate for manual and automated colorimetric prothrombin time test. *Throm. Res.* **40**, 339–49.

Nichols, J.H., Kickler, T.S., Dyer, K.L. *et al.* (2000) Clinical outcomes of point-of-care testing in interventional radiology and cardiology setting. *Clin. Chem.* **46**, 453–550.

O'Neill, A.I., McAllister, C., Corke, C.F. *et al.* (1991) A comparison of five devices for the bedside monitoring of heparin therapy. *Anaesth. Intensive Care* **19**, 592–601.

Oberhardt, B.J., Dermott, S.C., Taylor, M. *et al.* (1991) Dry reagent technology for rapid, convenient measurement of blood coagulation and fibrinolysis. *Clin. Chem.* **37**, 520–6.

Oberhardt, B.J., Mize, P.D. and Pritchard, C.G. (1997) Point-of-care fibrinolytic tests: the other side of blood coagulation. *Clin. Chem.* **43**, 1697–702.

Ogilby, J.D., Kopelman, H.A., Klein, L.W. *et al.* (1989) Adequate heparinization during PTCA: assessment using activated clotting times. *Cathet. Cardiovasc. Diagn.* **18**, 206–9.

Palkuti, H. (1984) Deterioration of factor VIII:C in stored plasma for use in activity curves. *Lab. Med.* **15**, 840–2.

Pernod, G., Bouabana, B., Desrousseau, B. *et al.* (1994) A simultaneous evaluation of three multiparametric coagulation instruments: BFA, HEMOLAB and STA. *Nouv. Rev. Fr. Hematol.* **36**, 409–18.

Peterson, P. and Gottfried, E. (1982) The effects of inaccurate blood sample volume on prothrombin time and activated partial thromboplastin time. *Thromb. Haemost.* **47**, 101–3.

Poggio, M., van den Besselaar, A.M., van der Velde, E.A. *et al.* (1989) The effect of some instruments for prothrombin time testing on the International Sensitivity Index (ISI) of two rabbit tissue thromboplastin reagents. *Thromb. Haemost.* **62**, 868–74.

Poller, L., Thomson, J.M. and Taberner, D.A. (1989) Effect of automation on prothrombin time test in NEQAS surveys. *J. Clin. Pathol.* **42**, 97–100.

Poller, I., Thomson, J.M., Taberner, D.A. *et al.* (1994) The correction of coagulometer effects on international normalized ratios: a multicentre evaluation. *Br. J. Haematol.* **86**, 112–17.

Poller, L., Triplett, D.A., Hirsh, J. *et al.* (1995) The value of plasma calibrants in correcting coagulometer effects on International Normalized Ratios – An International Multicenter Study. *Am. J. Clin. Pathol.* **103**, 358–65.

Quick, A.J., Stanley-Brown, M. and Bancroft, F.W. (1935) A study of the coagulation defect in hemophilia and in jaundice. *Am. J. Med. Sci.* **190**, 501–11.

Rath, B. and Bennett, D.H. (1990) Monitoring the effect of heparin by measurement of activated clotting time during and after percutaneous transluminal coronary angioplasty. *Br. Heart. J.* **63**, 18–21.

Ray, M.J. and Smith, I.R. (1990) The dependence of the International Sensitivity Index on the coagulometer used to perform the prothrombin time. *Thromb. Haemost.* **63**, 424–9.

Ray, M.J., Carroll, P.A., Just, S.J.E. *et al.* (1994) The effect of oral anticoagulant therapy on APTT results from a bedside coagulation monitor. *J. Clin. Monit.* **10**, 97–100.

Rose, V.L., Dermott, S.C., Murray, B.F. *et al.* (1993) Decentralized testing for prothrombin time and activated partial thromboplastin time using a dry chemistry portable analyzer. *Arch. Pathol. Lab. Med.* **117**, 611–17.

Saleem, A., Blifeld, C., Saleh, S.A. *et al.* (1983) Viscoelastic measurement of clot formation: a new test of platelet function. *Ann. Clin. Lab. Sci.* **13**(2), 115–24.

Schlueter, A.J., Pennell, B.J. and Olson, J.D. (1997) Evaluation of a new protamine titration method to assay heparin in whole blood and plasma. *Am. J. Clin. Pathol.* **107**, 511–20.

Schriever, H.G., Epstein, S.E. and Mintz, M.D. (1973) Statistical correlation and heparin sensitivity of activated partial thromboplastin time, whole blood coagulation time, and an automated coagulation time. *Am. J. Clin. Pathol.* **60**, 323–9.

Shapiro, G., Huntzinger, S.W. and Wilson, J.E. (1977) Variation among commercial activated partial thromboplastin time reagents in response to heparin. *Am. J. Clin. Pathol.* **67**, 477–80.

Sibley, C. and Singer, J.W. (1972) Comparison of the Fibrometer System and the Bio-Data Coagulation Analyzer. *Am. J. Clin. Pathol.* **57**, 369–72.

Sugiura, K., Ikeda, Y., Ono, F. *et al.* (1982) Detection of hypercoagulability by the measurement of the dynamic loss modulus of clotting blood. *Thromb. Res.* **27**, 161–6.

Traverso, C.I., Caprini, J.A. and Arcelus, J.I. (1995a) The normal thromboelastogram and its interpretation. *Sem. Thromb. Hemost.* **21**(Suppl. 4), 7–13.

Traverso, C.I., Caprini, J.A. and Arcelus, J.I,. (1995b) Application of thromboelastography in other medical and surgical states. *Sem. Thromb. Hemost.* **21**(Suppl. 4), 50–2.

Uden, D.L., Seay, R.E., Kriesmer, P.J. *et al.* (1991) The effect of heparin on three whole blood activated clotting tests and thrombin time. *ASAIO Trans.* **37**, 88–91.

Umlas, J., Gauvin, G. and Taff, R. (1984) Heparin monitoring and neutralization during cardiopulmonary bypass using a rapid plasma separator and a fluorometric assay. *Ann. Thorac. Surg.* **37**, 301–3.

van den Besselaar, A.M. and Peters, R.H. (1996) Multicentre evaluation of the Thrombotest International Sensitivity Index used with a still ball coagulometer. *J. Clin. Pathol.* **49**, 414–17.

van den Besselaar, A.M.H.P., Meeuwisse-Braun, J., Jansen-Grüter, R. *et al.* (1987) Monitoring heparin therapy by the activated partial thromboplastin time: the effect of preanalytical conditions. *Thromb. Haemost.* **57**, 226–31.

Van der Velde, E.A. and Poller, L. (1995) The APTT monitoring of heparin – the ICTH/ICSH collaborative study. *Thromb. Haemost.* **73**, 73–81.

van Rijn, J.L.M.L., Schmidt, N.A. and Rutten, W. (1989) Correction of instrument and reagent based differences in determination of the international normalized ratio (INR) for monitoring anticoagulant therapy. *Clin. Chem.* **355**, 840–3.

Weisbrot, I.M. and Waldner, D.K. (1977) Evaluation of a single-channel photo-optical clot-timing instrument. *Am. J. Clin. Pathol.* **68**, 361–7.

Werner, M., Gallagher, J.V., Ballo, M.S. *et al.* (1994) Effect of analytic uncertainty of conventional and point-of-care assays of activated partial thromboplastin time on clinical decisions in heparin therapy. *Am. J. Clin. Pathol.* **102**, 237–41.

White, R.H., McCurdy, S.A., von Marensdorff, H. *et al.* (1989) Home prothrombin time monitoring after the initiation of warfarin therapy. *Ann. Intern. Med.* **111**, 730–7.

15

Reference ranges in haemostasis

ISOBEL D. WALKER

INTRODUCTION

Although molecular biology techniques are rapidly emerging as major tools in the confirmation of the diagnosis of haemostatic disorders, tests based on phenotype analysis remain fundamental to the initial screening procedures. Thus the repertoire of tests which haemostasis laboratories offer for diagnosis and research purposes continues to expand, with specific assays of coagulation factors, natural inhibitors and fibrinolytic system components.

Reference populations

Many factors influence the results which a laboratory will obtain for any particular test or assay and it is essential that each laboratory constructs its own comparator ranges for each of the assays it performs. In the past, many laboratories used samples obtained from patients to establish their comparator ranges. However, whilst these samples were easy to obtain, the ranges constructed were heavily influenced by the fact that, by definition, the population was 'diseased'. In recognition of the frequent inappropriateness of comparator ranges based on patient samples, laboratories moved to constructing ranges from results on samples drawn from healthy individuals. Unfortunately it became, and remains, widespread practice to use laboratory staff for this purpose. Whilst laboratory staff may in general be viewed as healthy, laboratory staff populations tend to be skewed towards younger age groups and may also have a gender bias.

Ideally, comparator ranges should be based on blood samples drawn from the population from which the eventual test samples will be drawn, paying due regard to the characteristics of that population which might affect the haemostatic variable in question.

Terminology

The term 'reference range' is preferable to the term 'normal range' since it accepts that normality is somewhat abstract and even healthy populations will contain individuals with many diverse attributes. Construction of reference ranges requires that clinical and laboratory staff understand the many factors, both pathological and physiological, which influence the level of the particular variable in which they are interested and construct their reference range (or reference ranges), taking into account all of the variables that are relevant to the population in whom the specific assay will subsequently be used for either diagnostic or epidemiological purposes.

The requirement for reference ranges

There is little necessity for elaborate sets of reference ranges in the initial laboratory diagnosis of severe coagulation factor deficiencies such as haemophilia which are characterized by zero (or virtually zero) levels of clotting factor. Difficulties in interpretation arise, however, in trying to distinguish between carrier states or mild haemophilia and genetically normal individuals who have clotting factor activity within the lower limits of normality. Particular problems occur with the laboratory diagnosis of some thrombophilic defects where there is overlap between levels of some coagulation inhibitors in genetically normal individuals and individuals who are heterozygous for a variant gene. It is this latter area of the detection of individuals with thrombophilic defects which is currently raising most diagnostic difficulty and has highlighted for routine diagnostic laboratories the importance of establishing references ranges.

Theory of reference values

An Expert Panel on the Theory of Reference Values was created in 1970 by the Committee on Standards (currently the Scientific Committee) of the International Federation of Clinical Chemistry (IFCC). The remit of this expert panel was to develop nomenclature and procedures for the production of reference values. A corresponding Standing Committee on Reference Values was established in 1977 by the then International Committee (now Council) for Standardization in Haematology (ICSH). This latter group has adopted for haematology recommendations produced by other scientific organizations, where appropriate, and has extended and developed them. A series of recommendations on the theory of reference values prepared by the IFCC and the ICSH was published in 1987 and remains useful background reading (Dybkaer and Solberg, 1987; PetitClerc and Solberg, 1987; Solberg, 1987a,b). The validity of any reference range is dependent on the appropriate selection of individuals to be sampled, the definition of sample collection and handling procedures, and the definition and control of the analytical process. The reference values obtained from the reference population provide a reference distribution from which reference limits may be calculated.

15.1 REFERENCE POPULATIONS

When collecting blood samples to determine reference ranges, it is important that the population from which the samples are collected is, as far as possible, similar to the population from which test samples will be drawn. Whilst this may seem obvious, it is often very difficult to match exactly the reference population with the patient or study population and compromises have to be made. What compromises are acceptable will depend, at least in part, on the purpose for which the reference range is being constructed – diagnostic, epidemiological or research. It is essential that clinicians and laboratory staff are conscious of the compromises that have been made in selecting donors for reference range samples and take them into account when using the reference values.

Many 'clinical' variables, some modifiable and others not, influence the concentration of haemostatic factors in the blood. The variables about which we have most information are those which are known (or have been suspected) to increase the risk of either arterial disease or venous thrombosis. Few studies have explored more broadly other variables which might influence components of coagulation or fibrinolysis. Furthermore, we lack information about the effect of even the most widely studied 'clinical' variables on the full range of components of haemostasis, since most attention has been directed to the possible associations between deviations in the concentrations of a limited range of clotting factors or fibrinolytic components and the incidence of coronary heart disease or other arterial disease; or on the potential association between plasma concentrations of natural anticoagulants and the incidence of venous thrombosis.

Any population is to some extent selected; blood donors, although they span a wide age range, are basically fit and healthy; industrial populations span roughly the same age range, but also tend to exclude those who are sick; studies examining risk factors for particular pathologies (e.g. coronary heart disease or venous thromboembolism) tend to be smaller studies with restrictions such as age or gender, and so on. Even where a whole community is studied, because of its specific geographical location, the community may not be entirely representative of other communities or groups. In any study, the participant response rate is inevitably less than 100% and this too introduces an element of bias. In some circumstances, population-based reference ranges may not be ideal and it is conceivable that for at least some variables, admission to hospital may in itself cause some changes which may make comparison of hospital patients with individuals in the community inappropriate.

15.2 NON-MODIFIABLE CLINICAL VARIABLES

The most obvious variables that may influence haemostatic components and which are not modifiable are gender, race and age, but it has also been shown that the levels of some coagulation factors are blood group-related.

15.2.1 Effect of age, gender and the menopause on haemostasis variables

In view of the known associations between increasing age and increasing risk of both arterial and venous thrombotic disease, numerous investigators have sought to examine the effects that the ageing process has on components of haemostasis and to establish relationships between these changes and the incidence of thrombotic disease. Most of these studies have included, for comparison, both males and females and many of them have also looked at the effect of the menopause in women. The relationships between gender, age or the menopause and components of haemostasis are extremely complex since each of these clinical variables is in itself related to a wide range of other clinical variables, including body mass indices, blood pressure, cholesterol and triglyceride levels. In assessing the ranges of haemostatic variables which occur in women between the ages of about 45 and 60, it may be virtually impossible to separate the changes that are due to age from those that are the effect of changing oestrogen levels at the time of the menopause.

Many studies have shown that fibrinogen is positively associated with age and is higher in females than in males (Meade *et al.*, 1983; Meade *et al.*, 1990; Lowe *et al.*, 1997). Even in adolescents aged 15–17 years, fibrinogen levels are significantly higher in women than in men (Prisco *et al.*, 1996). Most studies have also shown that postmenopausal women have significantly higher fibrinogen levels than premenopausal women and that this difference persists after standardization for other variables including age.

Factor VIII:C and von Willebrand factor are normally strongly correlated with each other and have similar associations with clinical variables. Mean levels of both factor VIII:C and von Willebrand factor increase with age (Conlan *et al.*, 1993a; Lowe *et al.*, 1997) and both factor VIII:C and von Willebrand factor are higher in females than in males of similar age. In particular, factor VIII:C levels are significantly higher in postmenopausal females than in men of the same age.

In a very small study, Notelovitz *et al.* (1981) recorded that both the activated partial thromboplastin time (APTT) and the thrombin clotting time were shorter in women following the natural menopause than in younger premenopausal women, but noted no difference in the prothrombin time. Since many studies have shown quite clearly that both fibrinogen and factor VIIIC are higher in women after the age of natural menopause than in younger women, it is perhaps not surprising that postmenopausal women have relatively shorter APTTs. The original APTT-based activated protein C:sensitivity ratio (APC:SR) is lower in females than in males, but menopausal status does not appear to influence the APC:SR significantly (Tosetto *et al.*, 1997).

Many laboratories have shown that factor VII:C, like factor VIII:C, is positively associated with age and is higher in females than in males, particularly following the menopause (Balleisen *et al.*, 1985; Lowe *et al.*, 1997). However, in teenagers no significant difference between factor VII antigen levels was noticed between males and females (Prisco *et al.*, 1996). Although no significant gender differences have been described in factor IX:C activity, Lowe *et al.* (1997) have demonstrated significant increasing factor IX:C levels with increasing age.

The increases in factor VIII:C and factor IX:C which occur with age may complicate the diagnosis of carriership of haemophilia A or B by phenotype analysis in older women – particularly following the menopause (Peake *et al.*, 1993). Similarly, the diagnosis of mild haemophilia A or B in older men may be difficult if plasma levels of factor VIII:C or IX:C increase with age in mild haemophiliacs as they do in the general population. If the original unmodified APTT-based APC:SR test is used to screen for the factor V Leiden mutation then it may be advisable to use separate reference ranges for females and males, otherwise an unnecessarily high number of women may be subjected to DNA testing and there may be an increased risk of failing to detect males who should be offered further investigation.

In the West of Scotland Blood Donor Study, premenopausal females had lower antithrombin activity compared with their male contemporaries until around 45 years, but postmenopausal females had higher mean antithrombin levels than both males of the same age and younger premenopausal females (Tait *et al.*, 1993a). These findings are broadly in keeping with those reported by many other groups (Meade *et al.*, 1977, 1983).

Tait *et al.* (1993b) reported that protein C activity displays a significant variation with age. This is most marked in young adult males. Premenopausal females have mean protein C activity below that of their male contemporaries and show a less marked rise with age until the menopause, when protein C activity in females is significantly higher than in men of the same age. These age- and sex-related changes in protein C activity are sufficiently striking for Tait *et al.* (1993b) to have recommended the use of age- and sex-restricted references ranges when interpreting protein C activity, a recommendation supported by Lowe *et al.* (1997). The gender- and age-related differences in protein C levels reported by Tait *et al.* (1993b) and Lowe *et al.* (1997) are different from those reported by Miletich *et al.* (1987), who reported no difference in protein C levels between men and women, but reported a 4% increase in protein C for each 10-year increase in age.

Many surveys have now shown quite clearly that protein C levels are strongly correlated to serum triglyceride and total cholesterol levels (Conlan *et al.*, 1993b; Rodeghiero and Tosetto, 1996; Woodward *et al.*, 1997) and some workers have demonstrated that once covariates including triglycerides and total cholesterol are taken into account age has a negligible effect on plasma protein C levels. However even in these studies, postmenopausal women had a higher mean protein C level than premenopausal women and premenopausal women had lower protein C levels than their male contemporaries.

There are very few reports of protein S levels in large population samples. Tait *et al.* (1997) have reported that females have lower median values of both total and free protein S antigen levels than males of a similar age. In women, both total and free protein S antigen levels rise slightly with increasing age, but in males total protein S antigen is unaffected by increasing age whilst free protein S antigen levels fall slightly. These results are in general agreement with reports that females have lower protein S activity than males and that protein S activity shows little change with age in men but a significant increase with age in women (Lowe *et al.*, 1997). These observations are consistent with a protein S-lowering effect of oestrogen and would suggest that the failure to employ carefully constructed age- and sex-specific ranges could lead to the false diagnosis of protein S deficiency in females.

Females have slightly lower mean plasminogen values compared with their male contemporaries in the age range between 25 and 55 years. After the menopause, plasminogen levels increase in women and the mean plasminogen activity in postmenopausal women is higher than the mean level in males of similar age (Tait *et al.*, 1992), but the differences are small and unlikely to be of clinical importance.

It must be re-emphasized that the interrelationships between components of haemostasis and clinical variables are extremely complex and correlations exist between the levels of the haemostatic components themselves. Lowe *et al.* (1997) have reported significant positive correlations between protein S, protein C, antithrombin, factors VII:C, VIII:C and IX:C and fibrinogen. It has been suggested that natural anticoagulant levels (antithrombin, protein C and protein S) may rise to compensate for increasing levels of procoagulants, fibrinogen and factor VII:C, or alternatively that these associations are a reflection of correlation of the synthesis of procoagulant and anticoagulant factors (Lowe *et al.*, 1997).

Whilst several authors have suggested that, for a variety of haemostatic variables, age- and gender-specific reference ranges should be constructed, for the majority of routine diagnostic laboratories this would not be feasible and it may be preferable to construct either a single or a strictly limited number of reference ranges. If this option is adopted, it is essential that clinicians using the laboratory service are aware of the clinical variables which affect the parameter in which they are interested and interpret the result taking into account the age, gender and menopause status of their patient. Undoubtedly many patients have already been incorrectly assigned a diagnosis of protein C or protein S deficiency, because either the laboratory performing the tests or the clinicians interpreting the results have not been adequately aware of the effects that age and gender (and their associated body mass and plasma lipid changes) bring to bear on the components of haemostasis.

15.2.2 Haemostasis variables in neonates and children

Not only do neonates have levels of many haemostatic variables which are quite different from those in adults, but the levels of some of these variables change rapidly within the first days, weeks and months of life. For many haemostatic variables, the levels found in term neonates are different from those found in preterm neonates. All of these facts produce particular problems for epidemiologists studying neonates and young infants and for neonatologists and paediatricians looking after them. It is usually impossible to produce local reference ranges for all haemostatic variables in neonates and children because of the many practical and ethical difficulties of obtaining sufficient numbers of blood samples.

15.2.3 Effect of race on haemostasis variables

In the ARIC (Atherosclerosis Risk in Communities) study, race was found to be a major determinant of factor VIII:C and von Willebrand factor levels (Conlan et al., 1993a). Blacks have significantly higher levels of factor VIII:C and von Willebrand factor than Whites.

The influence of race on antithrombin levels was found to be of greater magnitude than that of either age or gender: the antithrombin activity in Blacks in the ARIC Study was approximately 3.4% higher than in Whites regardless of gender (Conlan et al., 1994). The reverse was found for protein C antigen levels, protein C antigen being higher in Whites than in Blacks (Conlan et al., 1993b).

Global tests of overall fibrinolytic activity have shown that Africans, and Blacks in general, have greater fibrinolytic potential than Whites, and Blacks have been shown to have higher levels of cross-linked fibrin degradation products (D-dimers) than Whites (Currie et al., 1994).

There are many reasons why there may be racial differences in haemostatic variables. The genetic background differs from ethnic group to ethnic group and there is clear evidence that the level of some haemostatic variables, including fibrinogen and factor VII:C, is influenced by genotype (Kario et al., 1995). The distribution of ABO blood groups varies from race to race and there is evidence that the level of some haemostatic variables is associated with ABO blood groups. Furthermore, there may be major diet and lifestyle differences in different ethnic groups and there are relationships between haemostatic variable levels and diet and lifestyle.

In constructing reference ranges for haemostatic variables, it is important to take into account the racial mix of the reference group and to ensure that it is representative of the eventual test population.

15.2.4 Effect of ABO blood group on haemostasis variables

There is a well recognized relationship between ABO blood group and the level of von Willebrand factor antigen (Gill et al., 1987), von Willebrand factor antigen being significantly lower in individuals of blood group O than in those with non-O blood groups. Since the gene for von Willebrand factor is on chromosome 12 and the gene for ABO blood group determination is on chromosome 9, direct genetic linkage does not explain the significant variation in plasma von Willebrand factor concentrations amongst individuals of different ABO blood groups.

The relationship between von Willebrand factor antigen levels and ABO blood group has implications for the diagnosis of von Willebrand's disease. There may be a subset of type I von Willebrand's disease patients who have decreased concentrations of structurally normal von Willebrand factor antigen on the basis of blood group, rather than on specific inherited abnormalities of von Willebrand factor production or release (Gill et al., 1987).

In phenotype screening for von Willebrand's disease, it may be necessary to establish ABO blood group-related reference ranges for factor VIII:C and von Willebrand factor. If blood group-specific reference ranges are not used, von Willebrand factor gene defects may be over-looked in patients with non-O blood groups, because von Willebrand factor antigen levels in their blood are higher than expected.

Because of their higher levels of factor VIIIC, non-O blood group individuals have APC:SR levels lower than individuals with blood group O when the original unmodified APTT-based test is used (Tosetto *et al.*, 1997). In some circumstances, blood group specific reference ranges for APC:SR tests may be useful.

15.3 MODIFIABLE CLINICAL VARIABLES

15.3.1 Effect of plasma lipids and dietary fat intake on haemostasis variables

Woodward *et al.* (1997), in a survey of 746 men and 816 women aged 25–74 years, randomly sampled from a Glasgow population, found that serum total cholesterol and triglycerides were positively associated with factors VII:C and IX:C. The relationship of triglycerides to factor VIIC activity appears to be due partly to factor VII antigen (Carvalho de Sousa *et al.*, 1989; Lowe *et al.*, 1991) and partly to activation of factor VII by triglyceride-rich particles (Millar *et al.*, 1985; Silveira *et al.*, 1994). Factor VII:C has been shown to correlate directly not only with total plasma cholesterol and triglyceride levels but also with dietary fat intake in middle age (Vaisanen *et al.*, 1995). In men who reported avoidance of fatty foods in the month prior to blood sampling, the age-adjusted factor VII:C levels were found to be lower than in men who had not adjusted their diet and who had significantly higher serum cholesterol levels (Connelly *et al.*, 1993), suggesting that the effect of altering dietary fat intake on haemostasis variables is rapid.

There is little published epidemiological data on factor IX:C levels. However, in the Glasgow MONICA (WHO Multinational Monitoring of Trends in Cardiovascular Disease) study (Woodward *et al.*, 1997), factor IX:C activity was positively related to serum total cholesterol and triglyceride levels.

Fibrinogen levels correlate with cholesterol, blood pressure and body mass index more strongly in women than in men (Lee *et al.*, 1990; Woodward *et al.*, 1997). In the ARIC study, univariate analysis demonstrated that both factor VIII:C and von Willebrand factor are positively correlated with plasma triglyceride, body mass index, waist-to-hip ratio, serum insulin and diabetes, and both were negatively associated with HDL cholesterol (Conlan *et al.*, 1993a). Although there is no consistently described clear relationship between factor VIII:C levels and plasma cholesterol and triglyceride, the original APTT-based APC:SR is negatively associated with serum triglycerides and total cholesterol (Tosetto *et al.*, 1997).

Several studies have examined the relationships between plasma lipid levels and natural anticoagulant levels. The VITA (Vicenza Thrombophilia and Atherosclerosis) Project reported that both serum triglycerides and total cholesterol are positively related to plasma levels of antithrombin, protein C, heparin cofactor II and plasminogen. An increase in triglycerides or total cholesterol of 100 mg/dL increases the corresponding protein C activity level by 20.1 or 11.7 IU/dL, respectively (Rodeghiero and Tosetto, 1996). The effect on antithrombin activity is rather less – an increase of 100 mg/dL in serum cholesterol increasing the antithrombin level 4.3 IU/dL. The Glasgow MONICA survey confirmed the positive relationship of total cholesterol and triglyceride with antithrombin and protein C activity (Woodward *et al.*, 1997) and also reported a positive relationship between protein S activity and serum total cholesterol and triglyceride.

The vitamin K-dependent coagulation inhibitors (protein C and protein S) appear to be similarly positively related in both men and women with triglycerides, cholesterol, blood pressure and body mass index. These associations reflect those found for factors VII:C and IX:C, suggesting that the variables associated with insulin resistance may be related not only to increases in vitamin K-dependent clotting factors but also to the vitamin K-dependent natural anticoagulants.

These findings of strong correlations between plasma lipid levels and haemostasis variables have important implications for diagnostic laboratories. Some workers have suggested that, because of the apparent relationships between age and gender and haemostasis variables, for some variables age- and gender-specific reference ranges should be constructed. Other workers, however, have suggested that the construction of age- and gender-specific reference ranges may not be appropriate for diagnostic purposes since, once the effects of triglyceride and total cholesterol are taken into account, age has a negligible effect. It is not feasible for diagnostic laboratories to construct many separate reference ranges for increments in plasma lipid levels, but it is abundantly clear that in interpreting levels of haemostasis variables (including the natural anticoagulants) the patient's current plasma lipid status is important.

15.3.2 Effect of social class, education, smoking status and alcohol intake on haemostasis variables

In men, low social class or low education level has been shown to be positively associated with factor VIII:C, factor IX:C and fibrinogen levels (Conlan et al., 1993a; Woodward et al., 1997). One possible explanation for the higher factor VIII:C and fibrinogen levels in lower social groups may be an increased prevalence of infections (Khaw and Woodhouse, 1995). Increased antithrombin and protein C levels have also been shown to be associated with low social class or low education level (Conlan et al., 1994; Woodward et al., 1997).

Current cigarette smoking is strongly positively associated with fibrinogen level in both men and women (Woodward et al., 1997). Factor IX:C is also positively correlated with current smoking in both men and women but factor VII:C shows no correlation with smoking in men, although factor VII:C levels are higher in women who smoke than in non-smoking women (Woodward et al., 1997). According to some reports, factor VIII:C is negatively associated with smoking in both sexes (Conlan et al., 1993a). Others, however, have failed to find any association between smoking status and either factor VIII:C or von Willebrand factor (Woodward et al., 1997). It has been reported that current cigarette smokers have a higher mean APTT-based APC:SR than non-smokers (Tosetto et al., 1997).

Several studies have shown a positive relationship between antithrombin levels and cigarette smoking (Tait et al., 1993a; Conlan et al., 1994; Woodward et al., 1997), but no significant relationship between antithrombin activity and cigarette smoking was noted in the VITA Study (Rodeghiero and Tosetto, 1996). Cigarette smoking appears to have little or no effect on protein C levels (Tait et al., 1993b; Woodward et al., 1997), although some studies have suggested that protein C levels may be reduced slightly in cigarette smokers (Conlan et al., 1993; Rodeghiero and Tosetto, 1996). There is little reported data on the effect of smoking on protein S levels but Woodward et al. (1997) suggested that smokers may have slightly higher mean protein S activity levels than non-smokers. On the other hand, Tait et al. (1993c) found no significant difference in protein S antigen levels between smokers and non-smokers.

Alcohol intake has been shown to be positively related to protein S activity and inversely related to fibrinogen and antithrombin activity in males (Woodward et al., 1997).

These findings of relationships between levels of haemostasis variables and social class, education, smoking status and alcohol intake demand that, in constructing reference ranges, the reference population must be selected to be representative of these aspects of the eventual test population.

15.3.3 Effect of pregnancy on haemostasis variables

Pregnancy is normally associated with significant changes in many aspects of haemostasis. Towards the end of pregnancy, the overall 'balance' of the haemostatic system is shifted towards apparent hypercoagulability. All coagulation factors, with the exception of factor XI:C, increase during pregnancy (Clark *et al.*, 1998). The greatest changes occur in the factor VIII complex (factor VIII:C and von Willebrand factor), but factor VII:C also shows a substantial rise towards term.

Mean antithrombin activity increases slightly during pregnancy, but protein C activity does not change. However, following delivery there is a significant increase in protein C activity which, like the increase in factor VII:C activity, may be related to changes in plasma lipid levels. During pregnancy there is a significant decrease in both total and free protein S antigen levels and in protein S activity. In pregnancy, the APC:SR obtained using the original un-modified APC:SR test falls until, at term, almost 50% of women have APC:SRs which are beneath the 95th percentile of the reference range for non-pregnant women of similar age (Mathonnet *et al.*, 1996).

There are also major changes in the balance of the fibrinolytic system during pregnancy. The concentration of plasminogen increases significantly along with the antigen concentrations of tissue plasminogen activator and urinary-type plasminogen activator. At the same time, the concentration and activity of plasminogen activator inhibitor-1 increases almost fivefold and an additional plasminogen activator inhibitor (plasminogen activator inhibitor-2) not generally detectable in the blood of non-pregnant women is produced by the placenta and released into maternal plasma.

The changes in factor VIII:C and von Willebrand factor mean that, during pregnancy, phenotype diagnosis of carriership of haemophilia A or of von Willebrand's disease may be impossible. Similarly, because of the changes in protein S level, the phenotype diagnosis of protein S deficiency is very difficult (or impossible) in pregnant women. The original un-modified APC:SR test is not a useful screening test for factor V Leiden during pregnancy.

Most diagnostic laboratories do not consider it feasible to construct separate sets of reference ranges for haemostasis variables in pregnancy. However, because of the profound effect which pregnancy has on some variables, it is essential that, in interpreting test results, both the fact of pregnancy and the stage of gestation are taken into account.

15.3.4 Effect of oral contraceptives and hormone replacement therapy on haemostasis variables

Studies have consistently shown that the use of oral contraceptives affects the blood concentrations of many separate components of haemostasis. Many studies have shown that oral contraceptives increase plasma levels of fibrinogen, von Willebrand factor and factor VII:C (Meade *et al.*, 1976; Balleisen *et al.*, 1985). However, Lowe *et al.* (1997) reported that current users of oral contraceptive pills had higher levels of factor VIII:C and factor IX:C, but not of factor VII:C or fibrinogen, than non-pill users. The finding of no influence of contraceptive pill use on factor VII:C levels may reflect the lower oestrogen dose in current contraceptive pills. However, others have found that the effect of oral contraceptives on factor VII:C levels is strong even with the lowest oestrogen dose pills and to a significant extent is related to the newer types of progesterone (Bloemenkamp *et al.*, 1996). It has been suggested that in the study reported by Lowe *et al.* (1997) a 'low risk' population of women was inadvertently selected. Some authors have warned that oral contraceptives have larger effects on coagulation in smokers than in non-smokers (Fruzzetti *et al.*, 1994).

Older high-dose oral contraceptives were associated with reduction in antithrombin activity (Tait *et al.*, 1993a), but modern low oestrogen content pills are no longer associated with antithrombin activity reduction (Norris and Bonnar, 1996). In the West of Scotland Blood Donor study, contraceptive pill users had slightly higher mean protein C activity than non-pill users (Tait *et al.*, 1993b). Lowe *et al.* (1997) did not find this effect of oral contraceptive use on protein C levels. Oral contraceptive use results in a lowering of both total and free protein S antigen and also of protein S activity (Boerger *et al.*, 1987; Lowe *et al.*, 1997; Tait *et al.*, 1997). Women who use oestrogen-containing oral contraceptives have a reduced APTT-based APC:SR relative both to women not using oral contraceptives and to men (Tosetto *et al.*, 1997).

Rather similar results are reported with hormone replacement therapy. In the ARIC study, it was reported that hormone supplementation was associated with increased mean protein C levels and decreased antithrombin activity (Conlan *et al.*, 1993b, 1994), and Tait *et al.* (1993a) reported that hormone replacement use abrogates the rise in antithrombin activity associated with the menopause. Similarly, Lowe *et al.* (1997) have shown that hormone replacement use attenuates the rise in protein S activity which normally occurs in women following the menopause. It has been shown that current users of hormone replacement therapy have a non-significant trend towards lower fibrinogen levels than non-users (Lee *et al.*, 1993; Nabulsi *et al.*, 1993).

The effects of oral contraceptives on factor VIII:C and factor IX:C may be relevant in the context of the phenotype diagnosis of carriership of haemophilia A or B and the diagnosis of protein S deficiency may be difficult in women using oestrogen-containing contraceptives or hormone replacement therapy. Similarly, because the APC:SR is lower in women using oestrogens than in those not using oestrogens, the originally described APTT-based APC:SR may not be a suitable test for screening women using oestrogens for the FV Leiden mutation.

15.4 ANALYTICAL AND PRE-ANALYTICAL VARIABLES

15.4.1 Analytical variables

INSTRUMENTS AND REAGENTS

It is widely accepted that for reliable, accurate and reproducible results, laboratories must establish standardized analysis systems. Reference ranges are applicable only to specific machine and reagent combinations, and if either machine or reagent is changed new reference ranges should be established.

Some assays may not give valid results over the entire observable range of a particular variable. For example, it has been shown that fibrinogen results derived from prothrombin times may overestimate fibrinogen levels, particularly where the fibrinogen level is elevated (Chantarangkul *et al.*, 1994; Chitoli *et al.*, 1994). Thus in choosing assays and establishing reference ranges, care must be taken to select assays, the results of which will be valid over the entire range likely to be met subsequently in the test population. It is important that, wherever possible, assays are reported with reference to International Standards.

15.4.2 Pre-analytical variables

It is perhaps less widely recognized that in constructing reference ranges and subsequently using these ranges, not only analytical variables, but also pre-analytical variables, must be strictly controlled.

PATIENT PREPARATION

At least for some measures of haemostasis parameters, the circumstances and timing of blood sampling are important. It may be necessary to take into account such variables as the time of day at which blood samples are collected (e.g. for some measurements of fibrinolytic parameters which have a clear diurnal rhythm), and for some purposes the stage of the menstrual cycle or even the season of the year may be important.

Some haemostasis variables are affected by fat intake, and sampling of fasting individuals may be necessary. The same is also true of physical exertion or mental stress; some haemostasis variables are altered by exercise or stress and it may be essential to ensure that prior to blood collection the donors are resting and relaxed. Similarly, it may be necessary to define the donor's use of alcohol, caffeine or nicotine prior to blood sampling: how much is acceptable and, if abstention is necessary, the length of the period of abstinence. In some circumstances, a number of other variables may be relevant and have to be taken into account, e.g. the site of blood sampling, the avoidance of the use of a tourniquet, etc.

It is essential that as far as possible the sampling conditions applied to participants in the reference group are also applicable to the eventual test population. If the reference group population is sampled fasting and resting in the early morning after abstention from alcohol, nicotine and caffeine then it is essential that the same constraints are applied to patients when they are being sampled. Obviously, when reference ranges are being established for research or epidemiological purposes, where the subsequent test population may be expected to comply with instructions on how to prepare themselves for blood sampling, it is sensible and necessary to build into the sampling procedure as many patient or donor requirements as appropriate. On the other hand, where the reference range is being developed for diagnostic purposes, it is mandatory that the reference population is not subjected to sampling requirements which cannot be imposed on the subsequent patient population. This means that a laboratory which has both diagnostic and research interests may require to develop different reference ranges for its routine diagnostic service and for its research studies.

BLOOD SAMPLING AND SAMPLE TUBES

Laboratories should advise on the technique of sample collection. In general, evacuated tubes are suitable for collecting samples for most haemostasis tests and assays. Where they are not acceptable, advice to this effect should be given. Some clinicians prefer to use simple needles and syringes, and in some circumstances blood sampling using a butterfly and syringe might be clinically easiest. In establishing reference ranges, laboratories must consider the different possible methods of blood sample collection and must decide whether different collection techniques will influence specific tests and assays and take this into account in the blood sampling of their reference population.

The most widely used anticoagulant included in sample tubes for haemostasis tests is trisodium citrate. However, there is no international consensus on the optimal citrate concentration. The citrate concentration and sample tube additives, such as platelet stabilizers, may influence some assay results. It is important, therefore, that laboratories establish reference ranges using blood samples collected into the same type of sample tubes as those collected for test purposes.

SAMPLE HANDLING

Reference ranges must be constructed from samples handled in the same fashion as test samples, taking into account such variables as the time from sample collection until it is centrifuged and separated, the temperature at which the whole blood sample is held during transportation before it is centrifuged, centrifugation variables such as time, speed and temperature, whether or not the sample is subjected to a single spin or a double spin, the technique for aliquoting the plasma and the platelet count in the plasma following centrifugation.

SAMPLE STORAGE

Reference samples must be stored in the same fashion as test samples. Where samples will be tested fresh, it is important that reference ranges are established on fresh blood samples. Similarly, where patient samples will be tested after freezing, it is important that the reference ranges are established using frozen samples. If frozen samples are to be used then the conditions of frozen storage must be equivalent in terms of the volume of the aliquots stored, the method of freezing (slow freezing or snap freezing), the temperature at which the frozen aliquots are held and the duration for which samples are stored frozen prior to analysis. A standard protocol for thawing frozen samples must be adhered to for both reference and test samples.

15.5 DETERMINATION OF REFERENCE LIMITS

For clinical purposes, reference intervals defined by fractiles are most commonly used and by convention the reference interval contains the central 0.95 fraction or 95% of the reference distribution. The reference limits are thus estimated as the 0.025 and 0.975 fractiles and these limits cut off a fraction of 0.025 of the values in each tail of the reference distribution. The fractiles may be estimated by parametric or non-parametric methods. Parametric estimation techniques require that the data fit a specific distribution type or that such a distribution is gained by transforming the data (e.g. using logarithmic transformation). Non-parametric techniques make no assumptions about the type of distribution. Although in theory parametric estimation of fractiles is more precise with smaller sample sizes than non-parametric estimates, in practice there is little real difference in the precision between the two methods, and in general non-parametric methods are recommended because of their simplicity (Solberg, 1987b).

15.5.1 Number of reference values

In general, the number of reference values available is limited, but estimation of fractiles becomes increasingly more imprecise as the sample size decreases. The absolute minimum number of values necessary to determine the 0.025 and 0.975 fractiles is 40, but to obtain reasonably reliable estimates the number of values should preferably be at least 120 (Dybkaer and Solberg, 1987). However many samples are available, the confidence intervals of the fractiles must be computed to allow a conclusion to be drawn as to whether the precision of the reference limits is sufficient for their intended use.

In circumstances where a large set of values is not available (e.g. in paediatric practice) and precise estimates are impossible, the smaller number of values may still be useful as a guide.

15.5.2 Procedure for estimation of reference limits

The statistical procedures for the estimation of reference limits are described in the published series of recommendations of the theory of reference values (Solberg, 1987b).

15.6 CONCLUSIONS

Multiple demographic and laboratory variables exert strong effects on plasma levels of many or most haemostatic components. These influences may impact greatly on our ability to diagnose abnormalities. For epidemiological studies with large numbers of samples, co-variance analysis taking into account the effect of many different variables on the component being studied may be useful. For research purposes, the use of a carefully selected reference population which, as closely as possible, matches the test population in age, gender, weight, oestrogen use etc. is essential.

For clinical purposes, though, the problem is complex and greatest in the phenotype diagnosis of heterozygous bleeding or thrombotic disorders, including haemophilia carriers, mild von Willebrand's disease, protein C deficiency and protein S deficiency. Some authors have suggested the use of multiple separate reference ranges for particular haemostasis components, e.g. age- and sex-specific ranges for protein C and gender, and oestrogen use-specific ranges for protein S. In some circumstances, the use of separate reference ranges is evidently necessary, e.g. in the neonate and perhaps during pregnancy. In other circumstances, whilst it might be possible for large specialist laboratories to collect a number of separate reference ranges for specific age or gender groups, for most routine clinical laboratories the collection of multiple separate reference ranges may not be feasible. In these circumstances, clinical laboratories must ensure that they understand the variables that influence the test for which the reference range is being developed and that they include in their reference population an adequate number of individuals representative of all the influencing variables and ensure that no subgroup of individuals is over- or under-represented. In using the reference ranges so developed, clinicians must be aware of the factors which have the strongest influences on the parameter they are measuring and be aware of the presence or absence of these influencing factors in each patient whose blood sample is sent for diagnosis.

In short, for most clinical laboratories, the reference ranges which they develop will provide an indication of whether or not patients subsequently compared with these ranges are likely to have an abnormality. For the diagnosis of acquired abnormalities of haemostasis, these reference ranges may be adequate, but for the final diagnosis of heritable bleeding or thrombotic disorders, extended investigation, including DNA studies and family studies, are usually necessary.

REFERENCES

Balleisen, L., Bailey, J., Epping, P.H. *et al.* (1985) Epidemiological study on factor VII, factor VIII and fibrinogen in an industrial population: baseline data on the relation to age, gender, body weight, smoking, alcohol, pill using and menopause. *Thromb. Haemost.* **54**, 475–9.

Bloemenkamp, K.W.M., Gevers Leuven, J.A., Helmerhorst, F.M. *et al.* (1996) In low-dose oral contraceptives containing 20 μg or 30 μg ethinylestradiol, gestodene is associated with a lower increase in coagulant factor VII than is desogestrel. *Gynaecol. Endocrinol.* **10**(Suppl 2), 145–8.

Boerger, L.M., Morris, P.C., Thurnau, G.I. *et al.* (1987) Oral contraceptives and gender affect protein S status. *Blood* **69**, 692–4.

Carvalho de Sousa, J., Bruckert, A., Giral, P. *et al.* (1989) Coagulation factor VII and plasma triglycerides: decreased catabolism as a possible measure of factor VII hyper activity. *Haemostasis* **19**, 125–30.

Chantarengkul, V., Tripodi, A. and Mannucci, P.M. (1994) Results of a collaborative study for fibrinogen measurement: evidence that the use of a common calibrator improves inter laboratory agreement. *Blood Coag. Fibrinol.* **5**, 761–6.

Chitoli, A., Mackie, I.G., Grant, D. *et al.* (1994) Inaccuracy of the 'derived' fibrinogen measurement. *Blood Coag. Fibrinol.* **5**, 955–7.

Clark, P., Brennand, J., Conkie, J.A. *et al.* (1998) Activated protein C sensitivity, protein C, protein S and coagulation in normal pregnancy. *Thromb. Haemost.* **79**, 1166–70.

Conlan, M.G., Folsom, A.R. and Finch, A. *et al.* (1993a) Associations of factor VIII and von Willebrand factor with age, race, sex and risk factors for atherosclerosis. The Atherosclerosis Risk in Communities (ARIC) Study. *Thromb. Haemost.* **70**, 380–5.

Conlan, M.G., Folsom, A.R., Finch, A. *et al.* (1993b) Correlation of plasma protein C levels with cardiovascular risk factors in middle aged adults: the Atherosclerosis Risk in Communities (ARIC) Study. *Thromb. Haemost.* **70**, 762–7.

Conlan, M.G., Folsom, A.R., Finch, A. *et al.* (1994) Antithrombin III: associations with age, race, sex and cardiovascular disease risk factors: the Atherosclerosis Risk in Communities (ARIC) Study. *Thromb. Haemost.* **72**, 551–6.

Connelly, J.B., Roderick, P.J., Cooper, J.A. *et al.* (1993) Positive association between self reported fatty food consumption and factor VII coagulant activity, a risk factor for coronary heart disease in 4246 middle aged men. *Thromb. Haemost.* **70**, 250–2.

Currie, M.S., Rao, M.K., Blaser, D.G. and Cohen, H.G. (1994) Age and functional correlations of markers of coagulation and inflammation in the elderly: functional implications of elevated cross linked fibrin degradation products (D-dimers) *J. Am. Geriatr. Soc.* **42**, 738–42.

Dybkaer, R. and Solberg, H.E. (1987) Approved recommendation (1987) on the theory of reference values (part 6). Presentation of observed values related to reference values. *J. Clin. Chem. Clin. Biochem.* **25**, 657–62.

Fruzzetti, F., Ricci, C. and Fioretti, P. (1994) Haemostasis profile in smoking and non smoking women taking low-dose oral contraceptives. *Contraception* **49**, 579–92.

Gill, J.C., Enderes-Brooks, J., Bauer, P.J. *et al.* (1987) The effect of ABO blood group on the diagnosis of von Willebrand disease. *Blood* **69**, 1691–5.

Kario, K., Narita, N., Matsuo, T. *et al.* (1995) Genetic determinants of plasma factor VII in the Japanese. *Thromb. Haemost.* **73**, 617–22.

Khaw, K.T. and Woodhouse, P. (1995) Inter-relation of vitamin C, infection, haemostatic factors and cardiovascular disease. *Br. Med. J.* **310**, 1559–63.

Lee, A.J., Lowe, G.D.O., Smith, W.C.S. and Tunstall-Pedoe, H. (1993) Plasma fibrinogen in women: relationships with oral contraception, the menopause and hormone replacement therapy. *Br. J. Haematol.* **83**, 616–21.

Lowe, G.D.O., Wood, D.A., Douglas, J.T. *et al.* (1991) Relationships of plasma viscosity, coagulation and fibrinolysis to coronary risk factors and angina. *Thromb. Haemost.* **65**, 339–43.

Lowe, G.D.O., Rumley, A. and Woodward, M. (1997) Epidemiology of coagulation factors, inhibitors and activation markers: the third Glasgow MONICA Survey 1 illustrative reference ranges by age, sex and hormone use. *Br. J. Haematol.* **97**, 775–84.

Mathonnet, F., De Mazancourt, P., Bastenaire, B. *et al.* (1996) Activated protein C sensitivity ratio in pregnant women at delivery. *Br. J. Haematol.* **92**, 244–6.

Meade, T.W., North, W.R.S., Chakrabarti, R. *et al.* (1977) Population based distributions of haemostatic variables. *Br. Med. Bull.* **33**, 283–8.

Meade, T.W., Brozovic, M., Chakrabati, R. *et al.* (1976) An epidemiological study of the haemostatic effects of oral contraceptives. *Br. J. Haematol.* **34**, 353–64.

Meade, T.W., Brozovic, M., Chakrabati, R. *et al.* (1978) Ethnic group comparisons of variables associated with ischaemic heart disease. *Br. Heart J.* **40**, 789–95.

Meade, T.W., Haines, A.P., Imeson, J.D. *et al.* (1983) Menopausal status and haemostatic variables. *Lancet* **I**, 22–4.

Meade, T.W., Dyer, S., Howarth, D.J. *et al.* (1990) Antithrombin III and procoagulant activity: sex differences and effects of the menopause. *Br. J. Haematol.* **74**, 77–81.

Miletich, J., Sherman, L. and Broze, G., Jr (1987) Absence of thrombosis in subjects with heterozygous protein C deficiency. *N. Engl. J. Med.* **317**, 991–6.

Millar, G.J., Walter, S.J., Stirling, Y. *et al.* (1985) Assay of factor VII activity by two techniques: evidence for increased conversion of VII to alpha VIIa in hyperlipidaemia with possible implications for ischaemic heart disease. *Br. J. Haematol.* **59**, 249–58.

Nabulsi, A.A., Folsom, A.R., White, A. *et al.* (1993) Associations of hormone replacement therapy with various cardiovascular risk factors in post menopausal women. *N. Engl. J. Med.* **328**, 1069–75.

Norris, L.A. and Bonnar, J. (1996) The effect of oestrogen dose and progestogen type on haemostatic changes in women taking low dose oral contraceptive. *Br. J. Obstet. Gynaecol.* **103**, 261–7.

Notelovitz, M., Kitchens, C.S., Rapport, V. *et al.* (1981) Menopausal status associated with increased inhibition of blood coagulation. *Am. J. Obstet. Gynaecol.* **141**, 149–52.

Peake, I.R., Lillicrap, D.P.O., Boulyjenkof, V. *et al.* (1993) Report of a joint WHO/WFH meeting on the control of haemophilia: carrier detection and prenatal diagnosis. *Blood Coag. Fibrinol.* **4**, 313–44.

PetitClerc, C. and Solberg, H.E. (1987) Approved recommendation (1987) on the theory of reference values (part 2). Selection of individuals for the production of reference values. *J. Clin. Chem. Clin. Biochem.* **25**, 639–44.

Prisco, D., Fedi, S., Brunelli, T. *et al.* (1996) Fibrinogen and factor VII ag in healthy adolescents: the Floren-teen (Florence teenager) study. *Thromb. Haemost.* **75**, 778–81.

Rodeghiero, F. and Tosetto, A. (1996) The VITA Project: population based distributions of protein C, antithrombin III, heparin cofactor II and plasminogen – relationship with physiological variables and establishment of reference ranges. *Thromb. Haemost.* **76**, 226–33.

Silveira, A., Karpe, F., Blomback, M. *et al.* (1994) Activation of coagulation factor VII during alimentary lipemia. *Arterioscler. Thromb.* **4**, 60–9.

Solberg, H.E. (1987a) Approved recommendations (1986) on the theory of reference values (part 1). The concept of reference values. *J. Clin. Chem. Clin. Biochem.* **25**, 337–42.

Solberg, H.E. (1987b) Approved recommendation (1987) on the theory of reference values (part 5). Statistical treatment of collected reference values. Determination of reference limits. *J. Clin. Chem. Clin. Biochem.* **25**, 645–56.

Tait, R.C., Walker, I.D., Conkie, J.A. *et al.* (1992) Plasminogen levels in healthy volunteers – influence of age, sex, smoking and oral contraceptives. *Thromb. Haemost.* **68**, 506–10.

Tait, R.C., Walker, I.D., Islam, S.I.A.M. *et al.* (1993a) Influence of demographic factors on antithrombin III activity in a healthy population. *Br. J. Haematol.* **84**, 467–80.

Tait, R.C., Walker, I.D., Islam, S.I.A.M. *et al.* (1993b) Protein C activity in healthy volunteers: influence of age, sex, smoking and oral contraceptives. *Thromb. Haemost.* **70**, 281–4.

Tait, R.C., Walker, I.D. and Islam, S.I.A.M. (1993c) Natural anticoagulants in smokers (letter). *Am. Heart J.* **125**, 1806.

Tait, R.C., Wright, E.M. and Walker, I.D. (1997) Influence of age and sex on the diagnosis of protein S deficiency (abstract). *Thromb. Haemost.* (Suppl.).

Tosetto, A., Missiagila, E., Gatto, E. and Rodeghiero, F. (1997) The VITA Project: phenotypic resistance to activated protein C and factor V Leiden mutation in the general population. *Thromb. Haemost.* **78**, 859–63.

Vaisanen, S., Rankinen, T., Penttila, I. and Rauramaa, R. (1995) Factor VII coagulant activity in relation to serum lipoproteins and dietary fat in middle aged men. *Thromb. Haemost.* **73**, 435–8.

Woodward, M., Lowe, G.D.O., Rumley, A. *et al.* (1997) Epidemiology of coagulation factors, inhibitors and activation markers: The Third Glasgow MONICA Survey II. Relationships to cardiovascular risk factors and prevalent cardiovascular disease. *Br. J. Haematol.* **97**, 785–97.

16

Lupus anticoagulant testing

DOUGLAS A. TRIPLETT

INTRODUCTION

Lupus anticoagulants (LAs) belong to a family of antibodies designated as antiphospholipid antibodies (APAs) (Love and Santoro, 1990; Shapiro, 1995; Triplett, 1995). APAs were originally thought to be antibodies with specificity for phospholipids (PLs) (Moore and Mohr, 1952; Moore and Lutz, 1955; Frick, 1955). However, recent studies suggest that these anti-bodies recognize complexes of protein–phospholipid or perhaps proteins alone which expose neo-epitopes when binding to activated cellular membranes (*in vivo*) or negatively charged plastic surfaces in ELISA assays (*in vitro*) (Galli *et al.*, 1990; McNeil *et al.*, 1990; Bevers *et al.*, 1991; Oosting *et al.*, 1993; Triplett, 1995). This family of antibodies has been defined by laboratory tests. LA was first identified in patients with systemic lupus erythematosus (SLE) in 1952 (Conley and Hartmann, 1952). Circulating anticoagulants (synonym: inhibitors) are typically associated with clinical bleeding (e.g. factor VIII inhibitors); however, in the case of LA, the vast majority of patients have no evidence of clinical bleeding and, paradoxically, often present with venous or arterial thromboembolic events (Green and Lechner, 1981; Shapiro, 1995; Triplett, 1995). Also, the vast majority of LA patients do not have underlying SLE. LA may be encountered in a wide variety of clinical situations including post-infections (viral, bacterial, protozoal), autoimmune diseases (SLE, RA), lymphoproliferative disorders, and in association with the administration of certain drugs (Box 16.1). LAs may be defined as immunoglobulins (IgG, IgM, IgA, or mixtures) which prolong *in vitro* PL-dependent tests of coagulation (e.g. activated partial thromboplastin time [APTT], kaolin clotting time [KCT], dilute prothrombin time [dPT], dilute Russell viper venom time [dRVVT]).

Lupus anticoagulants may be seen in virtually any patient population. In large studies, there appear to be three distinct groups of patients with LAs: children, young adults and the geriatric population (Jude *et al.*, 1988). In children, LA is often seen in association with infections (e.g. chronic otitis media, tonsillitis). In this patient group, the distribution of males and females is essentially equal (Jude *et al.*, 1988). During the young adult years of life, females predominate and the presence of LA is indicative of an increased risk of thrombosis or recurrent spontaneous abortion (RSA) (Horellou *et al.*, 1987; Triplett, 1989). LA in the geriatric population is often seen in association with the use of various medications (e.g. procainamide, quinidine and quinine) and may also reflect a loss of regulation of the immune system (Table 16.1) (Manoussakis *et al.*, 1987). A few cases of familial APA with associated LA activity have been described (Mackie *et al.*, 1987; Ford *et al.*, 1990).

Both LA and anticardiolipin antibodies (ACAs) are associated with a number of clinical complications, including recurrent thrombosis involving either arteries or veins, RSA, thrombocytopenia and a variety of other clinical findings, e.g. livedo reticularis, skin necrosis, etc. (Shapiro, 1995; Triplett, 1995). In the early 1980s, the above associations between LA/ACA and clinical complications led to the concept of an antiphospholipid antibody syndrome (APS) (Harris, 1987; Hughes, 1993). APS is defined by both clinical and laboratory

Box 16.1   Antiphospholipid antibody (APA) classification

Autoimmune
- Primary
    Do not fulfil criteria for systemic lupus erythematosus
- Secondary
    Systemic lupus erythematosus
    Other connective tissue diseases
- Drug-induced
    Procainamide
    Quinine
    Quinidine
    Alpha-interferon

Alloimmune
- Infections
    Viral
    Bacterial
    Protozoal
    Fungal
- Malignancies
    Hairy cell leukaemia
    Lymphoproliferative

Table 16.1   *Lupus anticoagulant: demographics*

	Paediatric	Adult	Geriatric
Sex	M = F	F > M	F > M
Thrombosis	+	+++	−
Antigen			
II	++	++	+?
2 GPI	+	+	+
Asso.	Infections	Autoimmune	Imm; drugs

M, male; F, female; II, prothrombin; 2 GPI = glycoprotein I; Imm, decreased immune regulation; Asso., association with various clinical conditions.

findings (Table 16.2). Recent prospective studies have found the presence of LA to be a risk factor for both venous and arterial thrombosis (Ginsburg *et al.*, 1992; IR-APA, 1993). In series of patients with venous thromboembolic disease, LA has been identified in 8–14% of this group (Ginsburg *et al.*, 1995; Simioni *et al.*, 1996).

One of the most important aspects of LA is the marked variability between patients. Patients with LA have a marked heterogeneity of antibodies. For instance, it is possible to separate LA activity and ACA activity from individual patient plasmas (McNeil *et al.*, 1988). In fact, it appears that the mixture of antibodies within a given patient is unique. With such marked patient-to-patient variability, the diagnosis of LA in many cases can be difficult. Thus, it is necessary to use multiple tests when evaluating patients for possible LA (Brandt *et al.*, 1995a).

Table 16.2 *Criteria for antiphospholipid antibody syndrome (APS). (From Harris et al., 1987)*

Clinical	Laboratory
Venous thrombosis	IgG anticardiolipin antibody (> 10 GPL units)[a]
Arterial thrombosis	Positive lupus anticoagulant test
Recurrent fetal loss	IgM anticardiolipin antibody (> 10 MPL units)[a] and positive LA test
Thrombocytopenia	

[a]GPL and MPL refer to IgG and IgM phospholipid antibodies. The units refer to the standards proposed by Harris *et al.* (1987).
Patients with the APS syndrome should have at least one clinical and one laboratory finding during their disease. The APA test(s) should be positive on at least two occasions more than 8 weeks apart. The diagnosis of LA should be established using the criteria established by the SSC Subcommittee for Lupus Anticoagulant/Phospholipid-dependent Antibodies (Brandt *et al.*, 1995b).

16.1 LABORATORY DIAGNOSIS OF LUPUS ANTICOAGULANT

16.1.1 General

Historically, the diagnosis of LA was often made by serendipity through the diligence of the laboratory staff. A preoperative coagulation panel in many cases was ordered by the surgeon and the laboratory identified a prolonged APTT or KCT. This unexpected finding led to a series of tests ultimately establishing the presence of a circulating anticoagulant. With the realization of the important clinical associations seen with LA, many clinicians from a variety of specialities are now asking the question: 'Does my patient have a LA?' This question may be better phrased: 'Does my patient have an APA?' The latter question obligates the laboratory not only to evaluate the sample for the presence of LA but also to test for ACA. The recommended approach to testing for APA is outlined in Figure 16.1 (Brandt *et al.*, 1995a). It is imperative for the laboratory to have a well-developed scheme to establish the diagnosis of APA. Careful planning is necessary to optimize the evaluation which often requires multiple coagulation studies as well as ELISA assays for ACA and, more recently, antibodies to α-2 glycoprotein I [synonym: Apolipoprotein(H)] (Harris *et al.*, 1987; Roubey, 1996). The International Society of Thrombosis and Haemostasis/Scientific Subcommittees (SSC) are responsible for developing guidelines for testing in the field of haemostasis and thrombosis. The Subcommittee on Lupus Anticoagulants/Phospholipid-dependent Antibodies recently published an updated series of recommendations for the diagnosis of LA (Brandt *et al.*, 1995a). These recommendations incorporate four steps (Fig. 16.2):

1 Screening the plasma for prolongation of coagulation tests. Because of the marked heterogeneity of LA, it is necessary to employ two or more screening procedures. These screening procedures should evaluate different aspects of the coagulation system (i.e. final common pathway, intrinsic pathway and extrinsic pathway).

2 Mixing studies are used to identify the cause of the prolongation of the screening test. Procedures for mixing studies are widely variable between laboratories. Failure to correct a prolonged screening test suggests the presence of an inhibitor.

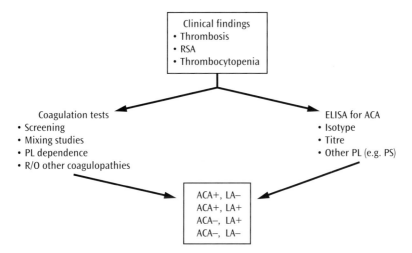

Fig. 16.1 *Antiphospholipid antibody (APA) laboratory evaluation. ELISA assays for antibodies to β_2 glycoprotein (β_2 GPI) are now commercially available. Antibodies to β_2 GPI appear to be more specific for clinical complications seen in patients with APA. PL, phospholipid; RSA, recurrent spontaneous abortion; ACA, anticardiolipin antibody; LA, lupus anticoagulant.*

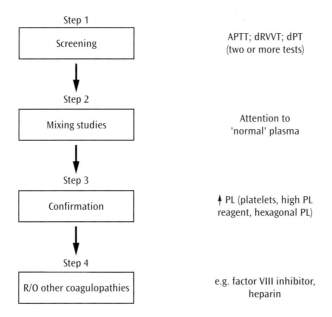

Fig. 16.2 *Lupus anticoagulant: identification. APTT, activated partial thromboplastin time; dRVVT, dilute Russell viper venom time; dPT, dilute prothrombin time; PL, phospholipid.*

3 Confirmatory studies are based on the addition of excess or reconfigured PLs to the patient sample to correct or significantly shorten the prolonged clotting time. This step is important in order to establish PL-dependence of the anticoagulant.
4 Rule out other coagulopathies. This step is critical in identifying other situations which may yield false-positive results if only the first three steps are employed. For instance, it is possible to misdiagnose a factor VIII inhibitor as a LA. Such a mistake may have catastrophic consequences (Ballard and Nyamuswa, 1993; Biron *et al.*, 1996).

The most common problem in the diagnosis of LA is failure to adhere to LA/APA Subcommittee guidelines. If laboratories rigidly follow the above recommendations, there will be very few false-positive or false-negative diagnoses.

16.1.2 Pre-analytical variables in the diagnosis

One of the more common confounding factors encountered in any coagulation laboratory relates to specimen collection and processing. Since many patients with LA present with thrombotic events, it is not uncommon for the laboratory to receive a sample which has been obtained through an indwelling venous or arterial line. Often, in the thrombotic patient, heparin is initiated and the attending physician then decides that studies for a thrombophilic work-up are needed. The heparinized sample not only compromises the potential diagnosis of LA but also other functional tests for physiological inhibitors (protein C, protein S, and AT III assays). There are now a number of commercially available products to neutralize heparin (e.g. Heparinase).

Care in venepuncture and specimen processing is important. Today, most laboratories employ evacuated collection tubes with 0.109 mol/L sodium citrate (3.2%). Patients who present with a thrombotic event or during pregnancy will have evidence of an 'acute-phase reaction'. The resulting increase in various plasma proteins, including fibrinogen, factor VIII, fibronectin, etc. tends to shorten baseline coagulation studies (e.g. APTT, KCT). The diagnosis of LA in pregnancy is often very difficult due to changes in coagulation proteins (Triplett, 1989).

Perhaps the most important aspect of processing a sample is preparing platelet-poor plasma (PPP). Ideally, the PPP should contain less than 5000 platelets/mL. Failure to prepare appropriate PPP may result in missing the diagnosis of LA. If the PPP is to be frozen and tested at a later time, it is recommended that the plasma be filtered through a 0.22 μm filter (Exner, 1985). If frozen plasmas have not been filtered, the freeze/thaw process may lead to false-negative results. Residual platelets in improperly prepared plasma may neutralize a LA upon thawing, with rupture of the platelets and exposure of PL.

16.1.3 Screening tests (step 1)

One of the major difficulties with LA relates to the marked intra- and interpatient hetero-geneity. The uniqueness of each individual's mix of antibodies presents a challenge. The SSC Subcommittee on Lupus Anticoagulant/Phospholipid-dependent Antibodies recommends at least two screening tests with documented sensitivity to LA (Brandt *et al.*, 1995a). However, many laboratories now employ at least three screening tests. The optimal combination includes tests which evaluate the three pathways of coagulation: intrinsic, extrinsic and final common pathway. An example of such a screening strategy would include APTT, dPT and dRVVT (Johns *et al.*, 1994; Brandt *et al.*, 1995b; Denis-Magdelaine *et al.*, 1995). This panel of tests will identify approximately 95% of LA-positive samples (Johns *et al.*, 1994). The subsequent steps in the diagnosis (mixing and confirmation) are based on the same test procedure which is prolonged in the screening studies. For instance, if an APTT is prolonged, the mixing and confirmatory steps are based on the APTT system (reagent/instrument combination) used in the screening procedure.

The choice of screening tests is dependent upon individual laboratory preference. An important point which was stressed above (pre-analytical) is the need to rule out heparin in the sample prior to initiating a full evaluation for the presence of LA. Often a thrombin time is helpful. If the thrombin time is prolonged, a normal reptilase time confirms the presence of heparin. Also, one can employ Heparinase or cationic resins to neutralize heparin.

16.1.4 Mixing studies (step 2)

Mixing studies are one of the most difficult areas in the coagulation laboratory (Kaczor et al., 1991). A variety of approaches have been utilized. Most laboratories employ a mixture of 1 part patient/1 part normal plasma. It is important to obtain an immediate result on the 1:1 mixture and also to incubate the mixture over a period of 60–120 minutes. Typically, LAs have an immediate effect (prolongation after the 1:1 patient/normal mix). Factor VIII inhibitors are usually time-dependent; consequently, the initial mixing study may suggest a factor deficiency (i.e. there is correction or shortening of the clotting time) (Kasper, 1996). However, with incubation of 1–2 hours, there is progressive prolongation of the clotting time. Studies have suggested that approximately 30% of LA samples will demonstrate a time-dependent effect (Clyne and White, 1988). Consequently, when evaluating a sample for LA, it is important to perform an immediate test followed by incubation of at least 1 hour.

One of the biggest variables in mixing studies is the choice of 'normal plasma' which is mixed with patient plasma. Various 'normal plasmas' are employed, including lyophilized control plasmas provided by commercial reagent manufacturers, aliquots of frozen normal plasma prepared by the laboratory, or fresh plasma obtained from laboratory personnel. The amount of PL present in commercial plasma samples is unknown. Therefore, laboratories should not use commercial plasma for mixing studies. In the case of frozen aliquoted normal plasma, it is important to filter the sample prior to freezing. If there are residual platelets in the sample, one may see a false-negative mixing study in a LA-positive sample (due to freeze/thaw rupture of platelet membranes and 'neutralization' of the LA in the patient sample).

16.1.5 Confirmatory testing (step 3)

In order to establish PL dependence of prolonged screening studies, it is necessary to demonstrate 'neutralization' or 'bypass' of the LA by adding a source of PL to the patient sample. A variety of different techniques have been employed, including the addition of freeze-thawed platelets (platelet neutralization procedure, PNP), excess bovine brain thromboplastin, platelet vesicles and hexagonal phase phosphatidylethanolamine (Triplett et al., 1983; Rosove et al., 1986; Arnout et al., 1992; Triplett et al., 1993). These various techniques will result in shortening the clotting times in LA-positive samples. Commercially available reagents for the PNP and the hexagonal phase PE are available (Blanco et al., 1997). Occasionally, a false-positive result may be seen in the presence of an underlying high titre factor VIII inhibitor (Blanco et al., 1997). In most cases, the clinical history (unexplained bleeding or bruising) will prevent an inappropriate diagnosis. Nevertheless, it is important for the laboratory to be vigilant in evaluating the entire sequence of test results on a patient being evaluated for a possible LA (Ballard and Nyamuswa, 1993; Biron et al., 1996).

16.1.6 Rule out other coagulopathies (step 4)

The most important coagulopathy which may lead to an incorrect diagnosis of LA is a factor VIII inhibitor. There are situations where patients may have both a factor VIII inhibitor and a LA. This is, for instance, not uncommonly found in the setting of haemophilia patients who have received replacement therapy utilizing commercial concentrates (Al-Saeed *et al.*, 1994; Blanco *et al.*, 1997). Many HIV-positive patients also have a demonstrable LA (Cohen *et al.*, 1986, 1989). Thus, a LA may be incorrectly diagnosed as a factor VIII inhibitor.

Recently, the association of LA with true or pseudofactor deficiencies has been documented. Not uncommonly, LA is associated with low levels of factor XII (Horellou *et al.*, 1987; Jaeger *et al.*, 1993; Halbmayer *et al.*, 1996; Jones *et al.*, 1996). In addition, factor XI activity in LA-positive patients may be decreased (Triplett and Barna, 1994; Dolan *et al.*, 1997). In these instances, despite progressive dilution of the patient sample, there is a failure to correct the factor activity. Table 16.3 summarizes the differences between true and pseudofactor deficiencies seen in patients with LA. The most common true factor deficiency seen in LA is hypoprothrombinaemia (Eberhard *et al.*, 1994). Virtually, all LA-positive patients have demonstrable antibodies to prothrombin (Galli *et al.*, 1997a; Fleck *et al.*, 1988). A small subset of these patients also have true hypoprothrombinaemia (Triplett, 1995). This is due to accelerated clearance of antiprothrombin complexes by the reticuloendothelial system (Bajaj *et al.*, 1985). Often, the hypoprothrombinaemia patients who bleed are children (Small, 1988). Typically, they respond well to prednisone.

Table 16.3 *Lupus anticoagulant: true and pseudofactor deficiencies*

	True factor deficiencies	Pseudofactor
Factor assay human substrate	Abnormal	Abnormal
Factor assay animal substrate	Abnormal	Normal
Parallelism of factor assay	Yes	No[a]
Antigenic factor assay	Decreased	Normal
Chromogenic factor assay	Decreased	Normal

[a]Apparent increase of factor activity and dilution of patient plasma.

16.2 THE CONCEPT OF INTEGRATED TEST SYSTEMS FOR LA

The sequential steps necessary to establish the diagnosis of LA present difficulties for many laboratories. The choice of test systems and maintaining consistency through the four steps of the diagnosis may be challenging and perhaps confusing in some cases. Recently, the concept of 'integrated systems' has been introduced by reagent manufacturers. These integrated systems allow one to perform the first three steps in the recommended diagnostic protocol by using matched reagents (e.g. screening dRVVT and dRVVT with an increased amount of PL). In designing this pairing of reagents, there is also a source of normal plasma and heparin neutralizing agent (polybrene) in the reagents. Testing can be performed if the patient is receiving heparin or oral anticoagulants. The StaClot LA system (Triplett *et al.*, 1993) also employs an integrated diagnostic approach (Fig. 16.3).

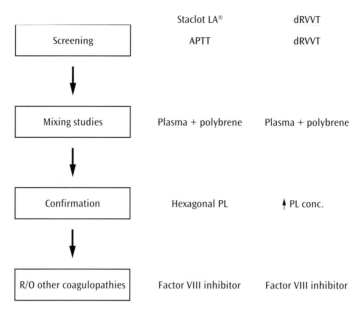

Fig. 16.3 *Lupus anticoagulant: integrated test systems. Occasionally, factor VIII inhibitors with relatively high titres (> 10 Bethesda units) will yield false-positive Staclot® and dRVVT (dilute Russell viper venom time) results. APTT, activated partial thromboplastin time; PL, phospholipid.*

16.3 CLINICAL RELEVANCE OF LA DIAGNOSIS

As noted earlier, LAs have been associated with a variety of thromboembolic complications involving the venous and arterial sites (Love and Santoro, 1990; Shapiro, 1995; Triplett, 1995). The diagnosis of LA must be interpreted in the context of the clinical setting. The presence of LA in children with infections does not carry the same implication as a LA diagnosed in a patient presenting with DVT. Optimally, a test system which identifies patients at increased risk for thromboembolic events would be extremely useful. Recent studies suggest that dRVVT may be more 'sensitive' in identifying LAs which predispose to thrombosis (Galli *et al.*, 1995, 1997b; Norbis *et al.*, 1997). There have also been attempts to quantitate LA (Speck, 1996); unfortunately, quantitation does not appear to have relevance in identifying patients at increased risk of thrombosis or RSA.

16.4 LABORATORY PERFORMANCE: QUALITY ASSURANCE/INTERNAL QUALITY CONTROL

Internal quality control requires careful adherence to the appropriate guidelines for preparing PPP and following the recommendations of the SSC Subcommittee on Lupus Anticoagulant/Phospholipid-dependent Antibodies. With each evaluation of patient plasma for the possibility of LA, it is necessary also to run a known LA-positive control. This will assure the laboratory that the tests being utilized are performing appropriately.

A variety of external quality assurance programmes have been utilized to evaluate laboratory performance. These include: International Survey for Lupus Anticoagulants (ISLA), College of American Pathologists surveys, UK National External Quality Assessment

Scheme, Société Française de Biologie Clinique, and a recent Belgian survey (Barna and Triplett, 1991; Haemostasis Committee of the 'Société Française de Biologie Clinique", 1992; Jennings *et al.*, 1997; Capel *et al.*, 1997). In these various schemes, 'unknown' samples are sent to laboratories with the request to evaluate the sample using local techniques. In most instances, 'strong' LA-positive samples are identified by the vast majority of laboratories (Jennings *et al.*, 1997). However, in many cases, weak LAs are not identified; alternatively, in some cases, a factor deficiency may be incorrectly identified as LA (Jennings *et al.*, 1997). With greater frequency of use of the SSC Guidelines for the Diagnosis of LA, the performance on external assessment programmes appears to be improving.

There is a need for commercial products which can be used to evaluate various tests and their relative sensitivity and specificity. Currently, appropriate reference materials are limited to frozen samples of known LA-positive plasma. Various surrogate plasmas have been proposed (Gempeier-Messina *et al.*, 1997).

16.5 CONCLUSIONS

The diagnosis of LA remains one of the more challenging areas in the laboratory. By adhering to the SSC Subcommittee on Lupus Anticoagulant/Phospholipid-dependent Antibody diagnostic guidelines, there has been significant improvement. Nevertheless, there remain a number of areas which need further refinement, including the ability to identify LA-positive samples which may be linked to a higher incidence of clinical complications. Also, the ready availability of reference materials and control samples for use in day-to-day laboratory operations is necessary.

REFERENCES

Al-Saeed, A., Makris, M., Malia, R.G. *et al.* (1994) The development of antiphospholipid antibodies in haemophilia is linked to infection with hepatitis C. *Br. J. Haematol.* **88**, 845–8.

Arnout, J., Huybrechts, E., Vanrusselt, E. and Vermylen, J. (1992) A new lupus anticoagulant neutralization test based on platelet-derived vesicles. *Br. J. Haematol.* **80**, 341–6.

Bajaj, S.P., Rapaport, S.I., Barclay, S. *et al.* (1985) Acquired hypoprothrombinemia due to nonneutralizing antibodies to prothrombin, mechanism and management. *Blood* **65**, 1538–43.

Ballard, H.S. and Nyamuswa, G. (1993) Life-threatening haemorrhage in a patient with rheumatoid arthritis and a lupus anticoagulant coexisting with acquired autoantibodies against factor VIII. *Br. J. Rheumatol.* **32**, 515–17.

Barna, L.K. and Triplett, D.A. (1991) A report on the First International Workshop for Lupus Anticoagulant Identification. *Clin. Exp. Rheumatol.* **9**, 557–67.

Bevers, E.M., Galli, M., Barbui, T. *et al.* (1991) Lupus anticoagulant IgG's (LA) are not directed to phospholipids only but to a complex of lipid bound prothrombin. *Thromb. Haemost.* **66**, 629–32.

Biron, C., Durand, L., Lemkecher, T. *et al.* (1996) Simultaneous occurrence of lupus anticoagulant, factor VIII inhibitor and localized pemphigoid. *Am. J. Hematol.* **51**, 250–1.

Blanco, A.N., Cardozo, M.A., Candela, M. *et al.* (1997) Anti-factor VIII inhibitors and lupus anticoagulants in haemophilia A patients. *Thromb. Haemost.* **77**, 656–9.

Brandt, J.T., Barna, L.K. and Triplett, D.A. (1995a) Laboratory identification of lupus anticoagulants: results of the second international workshop for identification of lupus anticoagulants. *Thromb. Haemost.* **74**, 1597–603.

Brandt, J.T., Triplett, D.A., Alving, B. and Scharrer, I. (1995b) Criteria for the diagnosis of lupus anticoagulants: an update. *Thromb. Haemost.* **74**, 1185–90.

Capel, P., Arnout, J., Cauchie, P. *et al.* (1997) Comparative study of antiphospholipid antibody detection in eleven Belgian laboratories. *Acta Clinica Belgica* **52**, 84–91.

Clyne, L.P. and White, P.F. (1988) Time dependency of lupus-like anticoagulants. *Arch. Int. Med.* **148**, 1060–3.

Cohen, A.J., Philips, T.M. and Keffler, C.M. (1986) Circulating coagulation inhibitors in the acquired immunodeficiency syndrome. *Ann. Int. Med.* **104**, 175–80.

Cohen, H., Mackie, I.J., Anagnostopoulos, N. *et al.* (1989) Lupus anticoagulant, anticardiolipin antibodies and human immunodeficiency virus in haemophilia. *J. Clin. Pathol.* **42**, 629–33.

Conley, C.L. and Hartmann, R.C. (1952) A hemorrhagic disorder caused by circulating anticoagulant in patients with disseminated lupus erythematosus. *J. Clin. Invest.* **31**, 621–2.

Denis-Magdelaine, A., Flahaut, A. and Verdy, E. (1995) Sensitivity of sixteen APTT reagents for the presence of lupus anticoagulants. *Haemostasis* **25**, 98–105.

Dolan, G., Kirby, R., Vong, S.T. *et al.* (1997) Interference on factor XI: measurement by antiphospholipid antibodies: potential source of error in diagnosis of factor XI deficiency. *Br. J. Haemost.* **97**, 85.

Eberhard, A., Sparling, C., Sudbury, S. *et al.* (1994) Hypoprothrombinemia in childhood systemic lupus erythematosus. *Sem. Arth. Rheum.* **24**, 12–8.

Exner, T. (1985) Comparison of two simple tests for the lupus anticoagulant. *Am. J. Clin. Pathol.* **83**, 215–18.

Fleck, R.A., Rapaport, S.I. and Rao, L.V.M. (1988) Antiprothrombin antibodies and the lupus anticoagulant. *Blood* **72**, 512–19.

Ford, P.M., Brunet, D., Lillicrap, D.P. and Ford, S.E. (1990) Premature stroke in a family with lupus anticoagulant and antiphospholipid antibodies. *Stroke* **21**, 66–71.

Frick, P. (1955) Acquired circulating anticoagulant in systemic 'collagen disease'. Autoimmune thromboplastin deficiency. *Blood* **10**, 691–706.

Galli, M., Comfurius, P., Maassen, C. *et al.* (1990) Anticardiolipin antibodies (ACA) directed not to cardiolipin but to a plasma cofactor. *Lancet* **335**, 1544–7.

Galli, M., Finazzi, G., Bevers, E.M. and Barbui, T. (1995) Kaolin clotting time and dilute Russell's viper venom time distinguish between prothrombin-dependent and α2 glycoprotein I-dependent antiphospholipid antibodies. *Blood* **86**, 617–23.

Galli, M., Beretta, G., Daldossi, M. *et al.* (1997a) Different anticoagulant and immunological properties of anti-prothrombin antibodies in patients with antiphospholipid antibodies. *Thromb. Haemost.* **77**, 486–91.

Galli, M., Finazzi, G. and Barbui, T. (1997b) Antiphospholipid antibodies: predictive value of laboratory tests. *Thromb. Haemost.* **78**, 75–8.

Gempeier-Messina, P.M., Muller, C., Triplett, D.A. and Stocker, K.F. (1997) Artificial positive control plasma for lupus anticoagulant assays. *Ann. Hematol.* **74**, A94.

Ginsburg, K.S., Liang, M.H., Newcomer, L. *et al.* (1992) Anticardiolipin antibodies and the risk for ischemic stroke and venous thrombosis. *Ann. Intern. Med.* **117**, 997–1002.

Ginsberg, J.S., Wells, P.S., Brill-Edwards, P. *et al.* (1995) Antiphospholipid antibodies and venous thromboembolism. *Blood* **86**, 3685–91.

Green, D. and Lechner, K. (1981) A study of 215 non-hemophilic patients with inhibitors to factor VIII. *Thromb. Haemost.* **45**, 200–3.

Haemostasis Committee of the "Société Francaise de Biologie Clinique" (1992) Laboratory heterogeneity of the lupus anticoagulant: a multicentre study using differing clotting assays on a panel of 78 samples. *Thromb. Res.* **66**, 349–64.

Halbmayer, W.M., Haushofer, A., Angerer, V. and Fischer, M. (1996) The discrimination of factor XII deficiency and lupus anticoagulant. *Thromb. Haemost.* **75**, 698–9.

Harris, E.N. (1987) Syndrome of the black swan. *Br. J. Rheumatol.* **26**, 324.

Harris, E.N., Gharavi, A.E., Patel, S.P. and Hughes, G.R.V. (1987) Evaluation of the anti-cardiolipin test: report of an international workshop held 4 April 1986. *Clin. Exp. Immunol.* **68**, 215–22.

Horellou, M.H., Aurousseau, M.H., Boffa, M.C. *et al.* (1987) Biological and clinical heterogeneity of lupus and lupus-like anticoagulants in fifty-seven patients. *J. Med.* **18**, 199–217.

Hughes, G.R.V. (1993) The antiphospholipid syndrome: ten years on. *Lancet* **342**, 341–4.

Italian Registry of Antiphospholipid Antibodies (IR-APA) (1993) Thrombosis and thrombocytopenia in antiphospholipid syndrome (idiopathic and secondary to SLE) first report from the Italian Registry. *Haematologica* **78**, 313–18.

Jaeger, U., Kapiotis, S., Pabinger, I. *et al.* (1993) Transient lupus anticoagulant associated with hypoprothrombinemia and factor XII deficiency following adenovirus infection. *Ann. Haematol.* **67**, 95–9.

Jennings, I., Kitchen, S., Woods, T.A.L. *et al.* (1997) Potentially clinically important inaccuracies in testing for the lupus anticoagulant, an analysis of results from three surveys of the UK National External Quality Assessment Scheme (NEQAS) for blood coagulation. *Thromb. Haemost.* **77**, 934–7.

Johns, A.S., Chamley, L., Ockelford, P.A. *et al.* (1994) Comparison of tests for the lupus anticoagulant and antiphospholipid antibodies in systemic lupus erythematosus. *Clin. Exp. Rheumatol.* **12**, 523–6.

Jones, D.W., Gallimore, M.J. and Winter, M. (1996) Pseudo factor XII deficiency and phospholipid antibodies. *Thromb. Haemost.* **75**, 696–7.

Jude, B., Goudemand, J., Dolle, I. *et al.* (1988) Lupus anticoagulant: a clinical and laboratory study of 100 cases. *Clin. Lab. Haematol.* **10**, 41–51.

Kaczor, D.A., Bickford, N.M. and Triplett, D.A. (1991) Evaluation of different mixing study reagents and dilution effect in lupus anticoagulant testing. *Am. J. Clin. Pathol.* **95**, 408–11.

Kasper, C.K. (1996) Laboratory tests for factor VIII inhibition, their variation, significance and interpretation. *Blood Coagul. Fibrinolysis* **2**, 7–10.

Love, P.E. and Santoro, S.A. (1990) Antiphospholipid antibodies: anticardiolipin and the lupus anticoagulant in systemic lupus erythematosus (SLE) and in non-SLE disorders. *Ann. Int. Med.* **112**, 692–8.

Mackie, I.J., Colaco, C.B. and Machin, S.J. (1987) Familial lupus anticoagulants. *Br. J. Haematol.* **67**, 359–63.

McNeil, H.P., Krilis, S.A. and Chesterman, C.N. (1988) Purification of anti-phospholipid antibodies using a new affinity method. *Thromb. Res.* **52**, 641–8.

McNeil, H.P., Simpson, R.J., Chesterman, C.N. and Krilis, S.A. (1990) Antiphospholipid antibodies are directed against a complex antigen that includes a lipid binding inhibitor of coagulation, B_2 Glycoprotein I (apolipoprotein H). *Proc. Natl Acad. Sci. USA* **87**, 4120–4.

Manoussakis, M.N., Tziousfas, A.G., Silis, M.P. *et al.* (1987) High prevalence of anticardiolipin and other autoantibodies in a healthy elderly population. *Clin. Exp. Immunol.* **69**, 557–65.

Moore, J.E. and Lutz, W.B. (1955) The natural history of systemic lupus erythematosus: an approach to its study through chronic biologic false positive reactors. *J. Chronic. Dis.* **1**, 297–316.

Moore, J.E. and Mohr, C.F. (1952) Biologically false positive serologic tests for syphilis. *J. Am. Med. Assoc.* **150**, 467–73.

Norbis, F., Barbui, T. and Galli, M. (1997) Diluted Russell's viper venom time and colloidal silica clotting time for the identification of the phospholipid dependent inhibitors of coagulation. *Thromb. Res.* **85**, 427–31.

Oosting, J.D., Derksen, R.H.W.M., Bobbink, I.W.G. *et al.* (1993) Antiphospholipid antibodies directed against a combination of phospholipids with prothrombin, protein C or protein S: an explanation for their pathogenic mechanism? *Blood* **81**, 2618–25.

Rosove, M.H., Ismail, M., Kozoil, B.J. *et al.* (1986) Lupus anticoagulants: improved diagnosis with a kaolin clotting time using rabbit brain phospholipid in standard and high concentrations. *Blood* **68**, 472–8.

Roubey, R.A.S. (1996) Antigenic specificities of antiphospholipid autoantibodies: implications for clinical laboratory testing and diagnosis of the antiphospholipid syndrome. *Lupus* **5**, 425–30.

Shapiro, S.S. (1995) The lupus anticoagulant/antiphospholipid syndrome. *Ann. Rev. Med.* **47**, 533–53.

Simioni, P., Prandoni, P., Zanon, E. *et al.* (1996) Deep venous thrombosis and lupus anticoagulant. A case control study. *Thromb. Haemost.* **76**, 187–9.

Small, P. (1988) Severe hemorrhage in a patient with circulating anticoagulant acquired hypoprothrombinemia and systemic lupus erythematosus. *Arth. Rheum.* **31**, 1210–1.

Speck, R. (1996) New method for quantifying lupus anticoagulant. *Clin. Appl. Thromb. Haemost.* **2**, 237–40.

Triplett, D.A. (1989) Antiphospholipid antibodies and recurrent pregnancy loss. *Am. J. Reprod. Immunol.* **20**, 52–67.

Triplett, D.A. (1995) Antiphospholipid-protein antibodies: laboratory detection and clinical relevance. *Thromb. Res.* **78**, 1–31.

Triplett, D.A. and Barna, L.K. (1994) Use of a factor XI assay to screen for α2 GPI dependent or prothrombin dependent lupus anticoagulants. *Lupus* **3**, 354.

Triplett, D.A., Brandt, J.T., Kaczor, D. and Schaeffer, J. (1983) Laboratory diagnosis of lupus inhibition: a comparison of the tissue thromboplastin inhibition procedure with a new platelet neutralization procedure. *Am. J. Clin. Pathol.* **79**, 678–82.

Triplett, D.A., Barna, L.K. and Unger, G.A. (1993) A hexagonal (II) phase phospholipid neutralization assay for lupus anticoagulant identification. *Thromb. Haemost.* **70**, 787–93.

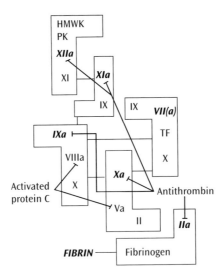

Fig. 17.1 *Illustration of sites of regulatory function of antithrombin and activated protein C. The clotting cascade is represented by an integrated set of individual complexes. Enzymes in each complex are indicated in bold.*

17.2.2 The protein C pathway

In the protein C pathway, the key enzyme is APC, which functions by proteolytically inhibiting factors Va and VIIIa in the prothrombinase and tenase complexes, respectively (Fig. 17.1). APC derives from limited proteolysis of protein C by thrombin complexed to an endothelial cofactor, the integral membrane protein thrombomodulin. Protein S functions as a cofactor to APC presumably by anchoring it to negatively charged membranes (Fig. 17.2). Both protein C and protein S are synthesized by the liver and both undergo post-translational modifications, one of which is γ-carboxylation in glutamic acid residues at the N-terminal end of the protein (gla-domain) (Furie and Furie, 1990). This modification occurs in the liver and is blocked by warfarin or acenocoumarol. This has important implications in testing for these anticoagulant proteins, since partially carboxylated or decarboxylated molecules do not bind phospholipids and are not adsorbed by barium citrate or aluminium hydroxide, employed in some functional tests. The plasma concentrations of protein C and protein S are 80 and 260 nmol/L, respectively (Esmon, 1992).

Protein S is not an enzyme: the amino-terminal half of the molecule has a modular structure similar to that of other coagulation proteins, while the carboxy-terminal half does not contain a serine-protease-like active site but is homologous to sex hormone-binding globulin. Protein S is also physiologically bound to C4b-binding protein (a complement regulator) at equimolar concentration. Only the β, but not the α, chain arm of the spider-like C4b-binding protein molecule can bind protein S and only free protein S is the cofactor of APC (Dahlbäck, 1991). It has been shown that even though C4b-binding protein is an acute-phase reactant, the equilibrium in synthesis and assembly of the different chains by which it is composed is maintained, so that little or no increase in protein S-binding (no increase in β-chain) is observed during acute reaction, in contrast to what was previously believed (Garcia de Frutos *et al.*, 1994). It follows that the measurement of C4b-binding protein concentration when evaluating protein S deficiency is of little importance.

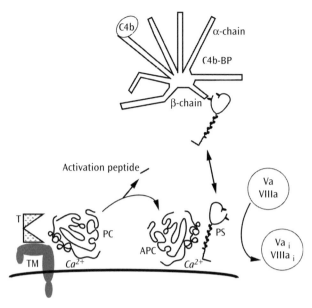

Fig. 17.2 *Schematic representation of the components of the protein C pathway. Protein C (PC) is activated at the cell surface by thrombin (T) complexed to thrombomodulin (TM) by cleavage of a small peptide (activation peptide). The enzyme-activated protein C (APC) then inhibits, by limited proteolysis, activated factors V and VIII. Its cofactor, protein S (PS), is in equilibrium with the complement regulator C4b-binding protein (C4b-BP). Calcium-mediated binding of the gla-domain regions of proteins C and S is also illustrated. The figure aims to give an overall view of the components of the protein C anticoagulant pathway and it does not purport to represent reciprocal molecular interactions or sizes of the various components.*

Thrombomodulin participates in protein C activation by binding thrombin with high affinity and modifying its prothrombotic functions (Esmon, 1987). Thrombomodulin expression at the endothelial surface is regulated by inflammatory mediators and therefore represents a good example of integration between haemostatic and inflammatory mechanisms (Esmon, 1987).

A recently described molecule, the endothelial protein C receptor, is a high-affinity membrane receptor for protein C and APC. It also is regulated by inflammatory mediators, and recent evidence indicates that one of its functions is enhancement of protein C activation by the thrombin–thrombomodulin complex (Regan *et al.*, 1996; Stearns-Kurosawa *et al.*, 1996). Its DNA and protein sequence have been resolved and structure–function studies are under way.

17.3 DEFECTS ASSOCIATED WITH THROMBOPHILIA

17.3.1 Defects of the anticoagulant pathways and thrombophilia

There is convincing clinical and epidemiological evidence of an association between deficiency of antithrombin and protein C and venous thromboembolism (Koster *et al.*, 1995a; De Stefano *et al.*, 1996; Lane *et al.*, 1996a,b). The association between protein S deficiency and venous thromboembolism, however, is less well documented, the reason possibly being related to the difficulty of measuring the concentration and function of protein S and of defining good reference ranges (Koster *et al.*, 1995a; Faioni *et al.*, 1997). Protein S deficiency might be a mild risk factor and a rare disease and therefore very large and selected studies are needed to pinpoint the association. Recently, a large family study of a kindred of 122 members showed that protein S deficiency associated with a Gly295Val substitution confers an approximately 11-fold risk of venous thromboembolism (Simmonds *et al.*, 1998). Another large study of several different families established a risk of approximately 5 for carriership of a genetic alteration in the protein S gene (Makris *et al.*, 2000). So, when analysed genetically, protein S does in fact seem to confer an increased risk of venous thromboembolism.

The structure and sequence of antithrombin, as well as that of its gene, are known (Olds *et al.*, 1993). A database of mutations and single publications report over 80 different mutations in the antithrombin gene (Lane *et al.*, 1993; Aiach *et al.*, 1995). Inherited deficiency of antithrombin can be detected by both antigenic and functional tests. According to the more recently proposed classification, deficiencies of antithrombin are subdivided in type I, characterized by parallel reduction in functional antithrombin and its antigen, and type II, characterized by derangement of function and normal antigenic concentration. A subdivision of type II antithrombin deficiency is based on mutation site: in one group, mutations affect the reactive site (II RS); in a second group, mutations affect the heparin binding site (IIHBS); and in a third group, mutations determine multiple functional defects (pleiotropic effect, II PE) (Lane *et al.*, 1993).

The structure and sequence of protein C, and those of its gene, are also known (Plutzky *et al.*, 1986). Over 160 different mutations have been reported for protein C deficiency (Aiach *et al.*, 1995; Reitsma *et al.*, 1995). The classification is still based on the combination of functional and immunological assays. In type I deficiency, characterized by low levels of functional protein C measured by clotting and chromogenic assays and by a parallel decrease in concentration, the most frequent genetic defects are missense mutations. In type II deficiency, characterized by normal or elevated concentration and decrease in function measured by one or more functional assays (chromogenic and/or clotting), the underlying genetic defects are missense mutations, nonsense mutations, small deletions and insertions.

Two genes for protein S have been identified, one being a pseudogene (Ploos van Amstel *et al.*, 1990). This, together with the complexity of the protein S active gene, has somewhat delayed the analysis of genetic defects underlying protein S deficiency. Furthermore, classification of protein S deficiency has been rather confusing. However, two main types of deficiency can be recognized: a type I deficiency with a parallel decrease in function and concentration, and a type II deficiency with reduced function and normal concentration of free and total protein S. Normal levels of total protein S and reduced free protein S levels and function can be considered a phenotypic variant of type I deficiency (Zoller *et al.*, 1995; Simmonds *et al.*, 1997). Different mutations and a polymorphism (PS Heerlen) which shows a high frequency in the general population and in thrombophilic patients have been reported (Bertina *et al.*, 1990; Aiach *et al.*, 1995) and are summarized in a database of protein S mutations (Gandrille *et al.*, 1997). Two novel polymorphisms which affect protein S levels (free and total) have been identified lately (Leroy-Matherton *et al.*, 1999; Leroy-Matherton *et al.*, 2000).

Since thrombomodulin is an integral membrane protein, its measurement by traditional assays is not possible. Circulating fragments in plasma, which are the product of cleavage by cellular proteases, have been measured in various diseases but their exact meaning remains to be fully clarified (Takano *et al.*, 1990). Since the DNA sequence of the thrombomodulin gene is known (Jackman *et al.*, 1987), molecular approaches to study mutations associated with thrombosis are currently employed. A polymorphism (van der Velden *et al.*, 1991) was shown to be equally distributed in healthy individuals and thrombophilic patients. Possibly this polymorphism is associated with myocardial infarction in the young (Norlund *et al.*, 1997), while another missense mutation was found in men with myocardial infarction in a large study (Doggen *et al.*, 1998). Several point mutations in the gene of thrombomodulin have been found in patients with venous thromboembolism, and three different mutations in the promoter of thrombomodulin in patients with myocardial infarction (Ohlin and Marler, 1995, 1997; Ireland *et al.*, 1997). Even though all these reports suggest a role for thrombo-modulin gene mutations in thrombophilia, further evidence that specific mutations are associated with a thrombotic risk is required before introducing tests for thrombomodulin defects in routine screening for inherited thrombophilia.

17.3.2 Procoagulant molecules and thrombophilia

The biochemical pathways of the coagulation cascade are complex, and various mechanisms may operate to produce a thrombophilic state. Alterations of procoagulant proteins that are cofactors in the haemostatic mechanism (such as factor V) or that participate in procoagulant complexes regulated by the naturally occurring anticoagulants (such as factor II in the prothrombinase complex) have been shown to be associated with an increased risk of venous thromboembolism.

17.3.3 Resistance to activated protein C

The enzyme APC inactivates factor Va and factor VIIIa by sequential lysis of three Arg bonds (Kalafatis *et al.*, 1994). Substitution of Arg 506 in factor V for Gln (factor V R506Q, 1691G→A) is the molecular basis of resistance to activated protein C (Bertina *et al.*, 1994). This amino acid substitution slows inactivation of factor Va and consequently impairs rapid inhibition of thrombin production (Kalafatis *et al.*, 1996). This may not be the only mechanism by which thrombin inhibition is dampened in resistance to APC. It has been shown that factor V functions as a cofactor to APC in the inactivation of factor VIII/VIIIa (Shen and Dahlback, 1994) and this cofactor activity appears diminished in factor V R506Q (Tans *et al.*, 1997).

Resistance to APC is the phenotypic expression of factor V R506Q in most cases. In a small percentage of patients, however, resistance to APC measured by some clotting-based functional assays is not due to factor V R506Q. Although this finding was initially attributed to a lack of specificity of these assays, it has been shown recently that in selected cases a polymorphism different from the mutation underlying factor V R506Q can contribute to this phenotype (Bernardi *et al.*, 1997). Furthermore, resistance to APC in the absence of factor V R506Q has been clearly shown to be an independent risk factor for venous thromboembolism (de Visser *et al.*, 1999; Rodeghiero and Tosetto, 1999).

17.3.4 Prothrombin mutation 20210G→A

A point mutation in the 3′ untranslated region of the gene for prothrombin (20210G→A) is the latest identified inherited risk factor for venous thrombosis (Poort *et al.*, 1996). Reports indicate that the 20210G→A mutation is frequent in the general population and more frequent in patients with venous thrombosis (Poort *et al.*, 1996; Cooper *et al.*, 1997; Cumming *et al.*, 1997; Ferraresi *et al.*, 1997; Hillarp *et al.*, 1997). The association of the prothrombin variant with cardiovascular disease is less well defined (Franco *et al.*, 1997; Rosendaal *et al.*, 1997). The mechanism whereby a mutation in the 3′ untranslated region of this gene is a risk factor for venous thrombosis has not yet been elucidated. In more than 80% of cases, the mutation is associated with elevated plasma prothrombin (above the 75th percentile), which is a risk factor for venous thrombosis in itself, so that the 20210A allele might act through the elevated prothrombin levels (Poort *et al.*, 1996). Whether the elevation of prothrombin is a consequence of an altered function of prothrombin or thrombin is at present unknown. The possibility exists that the prothrombin 20210A allele is in linkage disequilibrium with another sequence variation which is directly connected to the increased risk of thrombosis.

17.3.5 Metabolic defects and thrombophilia

Mild or moderate hyperhomocysteinaemia [reviewed by Cattaneo (1997) and D'Angelo and Selhub (1997)] is associated with both venous and arterial thromboembolism. It can be an acquired or a genetic defect; in the first case it is associated with nutritional deficiencies of essential cofactors of homocysteine metabolism such as cobalamin, folate and pyridoxine, and chronic renal insufficiency. Common genetic defects are heterozygous cystathionine-β-synthase deficiency and the presence in the homozygous state of a thermolabile mutant of methylene-tetrahydrofolate reductase. Both enzymes participate in the metabolic pathways that convert homocysteine to methionine or cysteine. These genetic defects are not invariably associated with elevated homocysteine levels, and other factors, such as the above-mentioned nutritional deficiencies, are likely to contribute to the hyperhomocysteinaemia phenotype. The mechanisms by which hyperhomocysteinaemia is thrombogenic are not completely understood, although several experimental data point to direct or mediated vascular and endothelial cell injury or perturbation.

17.3.6 Others

Other genetic defects have been reported in families with thrombophilia. Segregation of the phenotype with the genotype and the thrombotic symptoms has not always been demonstrated and most reports are anecdotal. In some instances, as with hereditary dysfibrinogenaemia, the disease is so rare in patients with thrombosis that studies of causal relationship and risk are very difficult to perform. In other cases, although biochemical and experimental studies are very promising, no clear-cut clinical evidence or formal studies of risk are as yet available; this is the case for defects in fibrinolysis, tissue factor pathway inhibitor, heparin cofactor II and factor XII deficiency. An exception is the report of an approximately twofold risk of venous thromboembolism associated with elevated levels of factor VIII (Koster *et al.*, 1995b), factor IX (van Hylckama *et al.*, 2000) and factor XI (Meijers *et al.*, 2000). The inherited nature of these defects is yet to be demonstrated. Some evidence exists so far only for factor VIII (Kamphuisen *et al.*, 1998).

17.3.7 Epidemiological notes

Table 17.1 illustrates the prevalence in the general population, in unselected patients and in familial thrombophilia, of the defects so far described (De Stefano *et al.*, 1996; Lane *et al.*, 1996a,b; Poort *et al.*, 1996). As previously stated, in more than 50% of the cases of familial thrombophilia, one or more defects can be identified, while the percentage is much lower in unselected patients. Some defects are more frequent than others in patients and in healthy individuals and there are differences in the prevalence of some defects in different ethnic groups. This is the case, for example, in resistance to APC (Rees, 1996).

Table 17.1   *Defects in thrombophilia: prevalence in the general population, in unselected and selected patients with thrombosis*

Type of defect	Prevalence (%)		
	In general population	In unselected patients	In thrombophilia
Antithrombin deficiency	0.02	1	1–7
Protein C deficiency	0.2–0.4	3	1–9
Protein S deficiency	–	1–3	1–13
Factor V R506Q[a]	3–7	12–20	52
Prothrombin 20210G→A[a]	2.3	6.2	18
Hyperhomocysteinemia	–	10	19

[a]Heterozygous

17.4 WHAT DO WE MEASURE AND HOW?

17.4.1 General considerations

The coagulation molecules which we seek to measure are mostly glycoproteins. We can therefore measure their concentration in a medium (plasma, serum, cell extract, depending on where they are prevalently stored) or their function. How we measure their function strictly depends on what we know of the biochemistry and physiology of the molecule. Let us take protein S as an example to illustrate this concept. Protein S, as discussed above, circulates in both a complexed and a free form, the latter only expressing cofactor activity to APC. Most functional assays of protein S have been set up with the aim of separating the free from the complexed form and of measuring the cofactor activity of protein S in a system where excess amounts of activated protein C are present and where free protein S is the limiting step. However, at present, little is known about the role of complexed protein S: it is not known, for instance, if protein S has a role in complement regulation, and if this does or does not influence its anticoagulant activity during inflammation. Similarly, though, some evidence indicates that hormonal status might modify protein S concentration (and consequently, function); the extent and importance of this aspect have not been fully investigated. If more information were available, completely different functional assays might be set up. An example is a new type of functional assay for protein S (van Wijnen *et al.*, 1997) which reflects its APC-independent role (Heeb *et al.*, 1994). Thus, to summarize, all functional assays must be viewed as incomplete answers to the question we are asking when we perform them, i.e. is the protein that is being measured functional? Functional assays that measure newly established functions may become available as scientific knowledge accumulates.

When tests that measure concentration and function are both available, their combined use permits classification into two main categories: a deficiency where both the concentration and the function of the protein are equally reduced (often termed type I deficiency) and a deficiency where the concentration is normal (or slightly above normal) and the function is strongly reduced (often termed type II or dysfunctional deficiency). This type of classification has proved unimportant from a clinical standpoint since there is no difference in the site and severity of the thrombotic events between the two groups. One notable exception is a particular subtype of a heparin binding site defect of antithrombin, the heterozygous form of which is associated with a low prevalence of thrombotic episodes (Finazzi *et al.*, 1987). However, this type of classification, which now, in some cases, has been replaced by more complex ones based on molecular defects, has been very useful for two main reasons. The first is to illustrate the point that functional tests are more useful screening tools than tests which determine concentration in that they detect both types of deficiency. The second is that detection of type II deficiencies has fostered a number of biochemical and molecular studies that have provided useful insight into structure–function relationships.

Before describing details of the tests available for each single analyte, some considerations concerning general laboratory procedures and good laboratory practice are necessary. In coagulation testing, as in other laboratory assays, pre-analytical variables must be controlled. These include venepuncture technique, type of anticoagulant, transportation and storage requirements, and centrifugation procedure. All are essential issues. Each laboratory should have well-standardized written protocols that need to be verified periodically and rigorously followed. In general, evaluation of the anticoagulant pathway is carried out using plasma. Blood is drawn from the antecubital vein without stasis, rapidly mixed with trisodium citrate (105 mmol/L) and then centrifuged within 2 hours at $3000 \times g$ and 4°C for 20 minutes. Plasma is separated and either tested directly or divided into aliquots for storage and later use. Optimal storage conditions are required due to the lability of most of the proteins. Snap freezing (ethanol and dried ice or liquid nitrogen) and storage at –80°C for up to 1 year are suggested procedures. Rapid thawing at 37°C and mixing before testing is also recommended. If the freezers are kept in optimal condition and seldom opened, storage for longer periods can be accomplished, but functionality of the proteins should be periodically assessed. Some measurements may require different anticoagulants or particular processing of plasma before storage or other special treatment. Genetic analysis is generally carried out on DNA that must be extracted from the white cells. DNA extraction procedures have been amply described and each laboratory should choose its own, depending on the workload, the storage space and the possibility of storing DNA for a long time (DNA banking). It has been reported that the levels of some haemostatic variables are modified when tested soon after a thrombotic episode (Reiter *et al.*, 1995). The recommended time between the event and blood sampling is at least 1 month.

Method reproducibility and expression of results are other critical features of laboratory tests. In general, each laboratory should have a reference plasma which optimally should be a pool of at least 40 different plasmas derived from healthy donors. To this plasma pool, 100% of activity and antigen of the substance that is to be measured is arbitrarily assigned. To make results comparable in different laboratories and within the same laboratory at different times, pooled plasma should be calibrated against an international standard. The measured protein can then be expressed either as a percentage or in absolute units. International standards are available for antithrombin, protein C and protein S (Hubbard, 1988). Daily quality control can be accomplished by running one or two samples of known concentration in each assay. Such samples can be prepared within the laboratory and stored frozen; however, most commercial assay kits contain control plasmas which are also available separately. Coefficients of variation are widely different in the different assays. In general they are lower for chromogenic functional or immunoenzymatic assays, and higher for traditional, clotting-based functional assays, even if automation has improved assay performance greatly. Reference values for each measurement must be calculated by each laboratory because ethnic differences are common in haemostatic variables. Variability due to local assay performance (operator, instrumentation, reference pooled plasma) must be added to this. The best, though not always practicable, way to generate reference ranges, is to measure the variable in at least 100 subjects not affected by the disease to which the variable is associated. The reference population should, if possible, be balanced for sex and age to the population usually referred for thrombophilia screening to that centre. Normalization of measurements must be verified and obtained by appropriate mathematical transformation if necessary (usually logarithmic transformation suffices). Outliers should be eliminated when found outside the mean ± 3 standard deviations. The normal range can then be established by calculating the mean ± 1.96 standard deviations. In some instances, the levels of the variable to be measured change with age or differ by gender or some other demographic factor. In this case, different reference ranges should be chosen. This is the case, for example, with protein S and homocysteine, which show gender differences, protein C which shows age differences, and resistance to APC which shows age and gender differences.

17.4.2 The global tests

In contrast to the development of tests for the detection of haemostatic defects where the use of global tests preceded that of specific assays, the investigation of venous thrombotic disease was initially through specific assays and only recently through global tests. The prothrombin time (PT) and the activated partial thromboplastin time (APTT) used for the initial screening of haemorrhagic diseases are global, easy to perform and rather inexpensive tests. The average screening for thrombophilia, on the other hand, is costly and time-consuming and prospectively bound to become even more cumbersome and expensive as other risk factors are detected. The need for a global screening test, therefore, is evident. Recently, PT-based and APTT-based global tests have been proposed by different groups: all of these assess the functional integrity of the protein C pathway and are unaffected by antithrombin deficiency or the 20210G→A mutation in prothrombin (Kraus *et al.*, 1995; Preda *et al.*, 1996; Engelhardt *et al.*, 1997). The principle of these assays is that endogenous protein C is activated by the addition of a snake activator, and its global activity (which requires integrity of protein C, protein S and the natural substrates factor V and factor VIII) is tested by measuring prolongation of the clotting time. The performance of these tests is still to be fully evaluated prospectively in large clinical cohorts. However, some data are available from pilot studies indicating that APTT-based tests are sensitive to factor V R506Q (100%), less so to protein C deficiency (91%) and even less so to protein S deficiency (84%) (Engelhardt *et al.*, 1997). On the other hand, a PT-based global test seems to perform better, having sensitivity and specificity both above 90% (Preda *et al.*, 1996). What is not clear yet is if the low sensitivity of the APTT-based global test for protein S deficiency is in fact due to previous misdiagnosis of protein S deficiency. Moreover, specificity less than 100% is determined by false-positive results in thrombophilic patients who have no known defect associated with thrombosis. This suggests that these individuals might have a defect that is detected by the global tests, but that at present we cannot identify. There is currently little evidence that global tests at this stage of development represent any kind of advantage over more traditional assays.

17.4.3 Antithrombin

Functional assays of antithrombin explore three of the known properties of antithrombin: inhibition of thrombin, inhibition of Xa and heparin binding. Antithrombin activity is measured by adding appropriate dilutions of the sample plasma or reference to a solution containing excess thrombin and heparin, and then measuring residual thrombin by lysis of a specific chromogenic substrate. Colour development is proportional to the amount of thrombin present in the sample, and therefore inversely related to the amount of anti-thrombin (Mannucci and Tripodi, 1987; De Stefano *et al.*, 1996; Lane *et al.*, 1996b).

Quantitation is performed using an appropriate standard curve. A problem with this assay is that heparin cofactor II, when present in the plasma sample at high concentration, can participate in thrombin inhibition and therefore lead to overestimation of antithrombin activity (Tran *et al.*, 1985). This problem is bypassed when the anti-Xa function is measured instead by the same assay principle. Both tests are run in the presence of heparin. A modification of the method (also called progressive antithrombin and anti-Xa activity assays) allows measurement of the functional inhibitory activity of antithrombin in the absence of heparin, i.e. depending only on integrity of the reactive site and substrate binding capacity and independent of heparin binding capacity. A comparison of the results of these two assays suggests a heparin binding or a reactive site defect. For the purpose of screening a large number of patients, the test of choice should be the anti-Xa in the presence of heparin. The only drawback is that one might miss the few cases in which antithrombin capacity is altered and anti-Xa capacity is preserved. One should be aware that, although extremely rare, these cases do exist.

Concentration of antithrombin can be measured by different immunoassays: radial immunodiffusion, ELISA, rocket immunoelectrophoresis. Each one presents the same advantages or disadvantages that these immunological methods have in general. A good compromise between costs and precision is the radial immunodiffusion with precast gels.

Crossed immunoelectrophoresis of antithrombin in the presence and absence of heparin is a diagnostic tool to detect a dysfunctional antithrombin that does not bind heparin (Mannucci and Tripodi, 1987). The availability of molecular studies has replaced the necessity for in depth diagnostic studies of dysfunctional defects. However, in most cases, integration of biochemical and molecular analyses allows better understanding of protein function. Table 17.2 summarizes the diagnostic approach to antithrombin deficiency.

Table 17.2   *Diagnostic approach to antithrombin deficiency*

Suggested screening test	Anti-Xa with heparin
Additional tests	Anti-IIa with heparin
	Anti-IIa without heparin
	Measurement of concentration
	Crossed immunoelectrophoresis
	Genetic analysis

17.4.4 Protein C

Functional assays of protein C can be divided into two main groups: amidolytic assays that test the functional integrity of the active site of protein C after its activation, and clotting assays that test the global anticoagulant activity of protein C after activation. The principle of the first type of test is that protein C is activated and then added to a solution containing a specific chromogenic substrate. Colour development is proportional to APC concentration. This assay is dependent on the capacity of protein C to be activated and on the integrity of the serine protease catalytic triad. Amidolytic activity is not dependent on gla-domain-related phospholipid binding or protein S binding. On the other hand, clotting assays explore the proteolytic activity of protein C after activation against the natural substrates factor Va and factor VIIIa, resulting in an increased plasma clotting time. This type of assay depends on the susceptibility of protein C to activation, on the integrity of the active site, and on phospholipid and protein S binding capacity. Thus, in some instances, amidolytic activity may be preserved while clotting tests are altered. This is the case with mutations leading to amino acid substitutions in the gla-domain or propeptide region. More often, amidolytic and clotting tests are concomitantly altered. The variables in the different proposed assays for protein C are the activator and whether and how protein C is extracted from plasma before testing. In the older assays, the activator was α-thrombin (Francis and Patch, 1983; Bertina et al., 1984). However α-thrombin activates protein C very slowly; more recent assays employ either the thrombin–thrombomodulin complex or a venom derived from *Agkistrodon contortrix contortrix*, the copperhead snake (Comp et al., 1984a; Francis, 1986; Martinoli and Stocker, 1986; Francis and Seyfert, 1987). Most commercial assays activate protein C directly in plasma, which is then diluted in protein C-deficient plasma to standardize clotting factor concentration, and the clotting time evaluated in a coagulometer (Martinoli and Stocker, 1986; Francis and Seyfert, 1987). In previous tests protein C was first extracted from plasma by different methods: immunoaffinity to a monoclonal antibody (Vigano-D'Angelo et al., 1986), barium citrate or aluminium hydroxide adsorption and elution (Francis and Patch, 1983; Bertina et al., 1984; Sala et al., 1984). Obviously, the ideal test for protein C is one where protein C is extracted from plasma (to avoid interference from other plasma components in the test) by a highly specific and harmless method such as immunoaffinity, is activated by the physiological complex thrombin–thrombomodulin and is then tested against its natural substrates, factor Va and factor VIIIa (Vigano-D'Angelo et al., 1986). However, the best is rarely the most practicable. Monoclonal antibodies are costly when not produced locally, so is thrombomodulin, and this type of assay is difficult to automate. A feasible alternative is a clotting-type test in which protein C is activated in plasma by the snake venom. This type of test can be automated, is commercially available and fairly cost-effective. The limits of this test are that, being plasma-based, it is subject to interferences (Ireland et al., 1995; Faioni et al., 1996). The suggested alternative is the amidolytic equivalent of this test, which will not detect all types of dysfunctional defect but affords many advantages in screening large numbers of samples (Lane et al., 1996b). Several comparisons of functional and immunological tests for protein C have been performed (Tripodi et al., 1985; Mannucci et al., 1987; Vinazzer and Pangraz, 1987; Franchi et al., 1988).

Concentration of protein C in plasma can be measured by any of the different immunological methods available (Boyer et al., 1984; Epstein et al., 1984; Mannucci and Tripodi, 1987; Mannucci et al., 1987). As for antithrombin, measurement of concentration is not a recommended screening procedure since dysfunctional deficiencies would go undetected. It should, rather, be used as an additional diagnostic tool to indicate the subtype of deficiency and the probable site of molecular derangement. In general, ELISA is the most sensitive and reproducible method, but the most costly. Home-made ELISAs employing commercially available antibodies are an option. In this case, attention should be paid to the choice of antibodies. A double monoclonal antibody sandwich ELISA using Fab fragments can easily be set up, but caution should be exercised in selecting antibodies that have different and distant epitopes.

Crossed immunoelectrophoresis of protein C in the absence and presence of calcium has been successfully employed to detect protein C molecules with defective calcium binding (Barbui et al., 1984). The same arguments discussed for antithrombin apply. Table 17.3 summarizes the diagnostic approach to protein C deficiency.

17.4.5 Protein S

Functional assays of protein S explore the cofactor function of protein S to APC. These assays are based on clotting tests in the presence of excess amounts of APC and limiting amounts of protein S derived from the sample plasma at appropriate dilutions. Protein S to be tested is

Table 17.3 *Diagnostic approach to protein C deficiency*

Suggested screening test	Amydolytic test with venom activator
Additional tests	Measurement of concentration
	Crossed immunoelectrophoresis
	Genetic analysis

either supplied with the whole plasma of the patient (Comp *et al.*, 1984b; Suzuki and Nishioka, 1988; Wolf *et al.*, 1989; Preda *et al.*, 1990) or extracted from the plasma by immunoaffinity to a monoclonal antibody (D'Angelo *et al.*, 1988). Functional assays of protein S have not been very successful. The reasons are many and can be summarized as follows:

- Protein S circulates in a free form (which expresses cofactor activity to APC) and a complexed form (which does not express cofactor activity). Only the assay which extracts protein S from plasma with a free protein S-specific monoclonal antibody separates the two forms. In the other assays, a dilution of test plasma in protein S-deficient plasma is required. The latter often contains residual protein S and invariably C4b-binding protein, which determine unknown and unpredictable redistribution of protein S in the sample between the bound and complexed forms.
- Protein S-dependent anticoagulant activity of activated protein C is not reproducible. It depends in part on APC concentration, an often uncontrollable variable in most of the proposed assays.
- Protein S is more labile than other coagulation proteins: repeated freezing and thawing of samples, traces of thrombin and low concentration all limit its activity.
- The 'cleanest' method proposed, that based on the antibody-mediated extraction of free protein S and its test in a Xa-based clotting assay (D'Angelo *et al.*, 1988), is costly, requires a specific monoclonal antibody, is time-consuming and not applicable for routine screening. The commercially available functional assays, on the other hand, are all, to a different extent, subject to various interferences. Resistance to APC and antiphospholipid antibodies can both interfere with these assays (Faioni *et al.*, 1993; Cooper *et al.*, 1994; Simioni *et al.*, 1995; Lawrie *et al.*, 1995).

The need for a reliable, easy-to-perform and inexpensive functional test for protein S is obvious. A multicentre comparison of protein S functional tests has been performed (Boyer-Neumann *et al.*, 1993). So far, the problem remains unsolved. We suggest, however, that with due caution, a functional assay for protein S be used in parallel with an assay to measure its concentration. This, at present, is the only way that a dysfunctional defect can be detected.

As is the case for antithrombin and protein C, all common immunological methods can be employed to measure the concentration of protein S. The issue, however, is complicated by the necessity to separate the free from the bound form, or at least to consider the different reactivity of free versus bound protein S. Total protein S (free plus complexed) can be measured after separation of bound protein S from C4b-binding protein. This can be achieved by using EDTA-containing buffers, long incubation times, high dilutions or antibody binding, all of which shift the equilibrium between free and complexed protein S (Schwarz *et al.*, 1984; Bertina *et al.*, 1985; Boyer-Neumann *et al.*, 1988; Krachmalnicoff *et al.*, 1990; Tripodi *et al.*, 1992). Free protein S needs to be measured after it is separated from complexed protein S. This can be achieved by physical methods, such as polyethylene glycol (PEG) precipitation (Comp *et al.*, 1986; Malm *et al.*, 1988), or by immunoaffinity to monoclonal antibodies, as described for the functional test based on the same principle (D'Angelo *et al.*, 1988). The first is a commonly used method that allows precipitation of the protein S-C4b-binding protein complex by the addition to plasma of PEG: free protein S remains in the supernatant where it can be measured by commonly employed immunological methods. The limitations of this method are mainly related to its great variability, especially between laboratories. Within a single laboratory, if standard conditions are carefully maintained, the between-assay co-efficient of variation can be kept at reasonable levels. Another drawback is that plasma samples that have marked physical alterations cannot be handled appropriately: examples are plasmas derived from myeloma or strongly hyperlipidaemic patients. Advantages of this method are its very low cost and relatively low technical requirement. Recently, monoclonal antibodies that recognize only the free form of protein S have been successfully employed in a double antibody ELISA, which is commercially available (Amiral *et al.*, 1994). The clinical performance of this assay has been assessed, though no multicentre evaluation has yet been performed (Aillaud *et al.*, 1996). Table 17.4 summarizes the diagnostic approach to protein S deficiency.

Table 17.4 *Diagnostic approach to protein S deficiency*

Suggested screening test	Measurement of free protein S concentration (measurement of function)
Additional tests	Measurement of total protein S concentration

17.4.6 Resistance to APC

The phenotype originally described associated with factor V R506Q is a lack of prolongation of plasma clotting time on addition of exogenous APC in an APTT. This is the basis for the originally proposed functional test for resistance to APC (Dahlbäck *et al.*, 1993). Several other tests have been proposed; some are modifications of the original that in addition require pre-dilution of the test plasma in factor V-deficient plasma, while others explore the coagulation cascade downstream from factor Xa, and still others are PT-based. A comparison of the diagnostic efficacy of some of these methods (Tripodi *et al.*, 1997) using the presence of factor V R506Q as reference has established that the APTT-based methods have highly variable discriminating capacity between carriers and non-carriers of the mutation. The best discriminatory capacity belongs to those methods that promote clotting by Xa addition or Russell's viper venom (RVV). Also, pre-dilution in factor V-deficient plasma elevates the sensitivity and specificity considerably. In the choice of the method to use for screening, one should consider the goal. If large populations are to be screened, and the aim is to detect APC resistance associated with factor V R506Q, good alternatives to genetic studies, which are expensive and not widely available, are the Xa or RVV methods that are rather inexpensive and which discriminate well also between heterozygotes and homozygotes. In settings where molecular diagnosis is largely applied, the cost-effectiveness of genetic analysis should be evaluated against these tests. As discussed earlier, a polymorphism different from the 1691G→A mutation can contribute to the phenotype APC resistance. Moreover, as mentioned earlier, resistance to APC in the absence of factor V R506Q is an independent risk factor for venous thromboembolism, so that one might want to choose a method which is not at all specific for the mutation, such as the originally proposed functional test for resistance to APC (Dahlbäck *et al.*, 1993).

Detection of the point mutation in factor V responsible for the majority of the phenotype resistance to APC has been made mostly by restriction enzyme cleavage after DNA extraction and amplification of the nucleotide region enclosing G 1691 (de Ronde and Bertina, 1994). Different approaches have also been proposed to enable the handling of larger sample numbers (Corral *et al.*, 1996; De Lucia *et al.*, 1996; Ripoll *et al.*, 1997). Table 17.5 summarizes the diagnostic approach to resistance to APC-factor V R506Q.

Table 17.5 *Diagnostic approach to resistance to APC*

Suggested screening test alternatively	Xa-based or RVV-based clotting tests APTT-based with factor V-deficient plasma
Additional tests	Genetic analysis

17.4.7 Prothrombin 20210G→A

Measurement of prothrombin levels is a rather easy and well-established diagnostic procedure. However, the functional tests have low sensitivity and specificity. Moreover, it is not only elevated levels of prothrombin that are a risk factor, but the association of elevated levels with the 20210G→A mutation (Poort *et al.*, 1996). Approximately 20% of patients with the mutation, however, do not have elevated prothrombin levels (Poort *et al.*, 1996), and thus screening is best performed by genetic analysis.

Prothrombin function can be measured by clotting or chromogenic assays. The underlying principle in both is the activation of prothrombin to thrombin. Different activators can be used, generally derived from snake venom, or physiological activation via the extrinsic pathway can be exploited. Prothrombin concentration can be measured by classical immunological methods (Bertina *et al.*, 1979).

The genetic defect is a point mutation which does not create or abolish a restriction site. Such a site can be created by introducing a nucleotide substitution during amplification, designing an appropriately mutated oligonucleotide (Poort *et al.*, 1996). Other methods have also been proposed (Ferraresi *et al.*, 1997; Ripoll *et al.*, 1997; Poort *et al.*, 1997). Table 17.6 summarizes the diagnostic approach to prothrombin 20210 G→A.

17.4.8 Homocysteine

Homocysteine is a sulphydryl amino acid derived from metabolic conversion of methionine (Ueland *et al.*, 1993). Determination of total homocysteine in plasma or serum requires the reduction of the disulphide bond between homocysteine and other thiols or albumin. Hyperhomocysteinaemia is diagnosed by measuring, after an overnight fast, plasma levels of total homocysteine by radioenzymatic assays, gas chromatography-mass spectrometry, or high-performance liquid chromatography with electrochemical or fluorescent detection (Ueland *et al.*, 1993). In heterozygotes for defects of cystathionine-β-synthase, plasma levels of homocysteine may overlap with those found in normals; measurement of homocysteine levels after a methionine load improves discrimination (Boers *et al.*, 1985; Rees and Rodgers, 1993). Table 17.7 summarizes the diagnostic approach to hyperhomocysteinaemia.

Table 17.6 *Diagnostic approach to prothrombin 20210G/ÆA*

Suggested screening test	Genetic analysis
Additional tests	Measurement of levels of prothrombin with functional clotting, amidolytic and concentration tests

Table 17.7 *Diagnostic approach to hyperhomocysteinemia*

Suggested screening test	Measurement of total plasma homocysteine before and after methionine load

17.4.9 A note of caution

The result of a laboratory test is just a 'number'. Its interpretation, once we are reasonably sure that the number is correct, rests with the acquisition of as much additional information as possible. First we must be sure that all acquired causes of deficiency are excluded. For example, we must be sure the patient is not on oral anticoagulants. This, which may seem an obvious statement, is certainly one of the most frequent situations of differential diagnosis after the test is done, and leads to the performance of a number of useless tests. Considering the half-lives of the vitamin K-dependent proteins we measure and the clearance of oral anticoagulants, it is safe to consider that oral anticoagulants should have been withheld for at least 10 days before testing. A good relationship between the attending clinicians and the laboratory is mandatory to avoid misinterpretation of test results or costly and useless testing. Table 17.8 illustrates some of the more frequent causes of acquired deficiency. Attention should be always paid to anamnesis related to drug use and to associated diseases.

When acquired deficiency can reasonably be ruled out, an inherited deficiency can be identified by establishing that relatives have the same phenotypic and/or genotypic defect. The number of relatives to be tested is a subject of never-ending debate. In fact, one tests the relatives that are available for screening, and who are willing to come to be tested even from far away, and whom one can afford to test. The actual testing must be accompanied by accurate collection of documented family history of thrombosis. In the end, one should have a fairly complete picture of a family, possibly extending through two or more generations, with phenotypes and genotypes and thromboembolic events. This constitutes the basis for good family counselling and of correct interpretation of laboratory results.

Table 17.8   *Frequent acquired causes of defects associated with thrombophilia*

Pregnancy
Oral contraceptive use
Disseminated intravascular coagulation
Renal disease
Liver disease
Nutritional deficiencies
Specific antibodies to naturally occurring anticoagulants
Antiphospholipid antibodies
Malignancy

17.4.10 Pitfalls

Even when all the correct procedures are followed, and no major or minor mistakes have been made, a test result can be wrong. The reason often lies with interference in the test by concomitant defects. This obviously is more frequent the less specific the test. Plasma-based clotting tests are more subject to interference. Thus, as mentioned, resistance to APC can interfere with some protein S and protein C functional clotting tests, leading to misdiagnosis of protein S or protein C deficiency (see specific subchapters). Elevated levels of factor VIII can interfere with APTT-based assays of resistance to APC (Henkens *et al.*, 1995). It must be remembered that thrombophilic patients may have more than one defect associated with thrombosis so that interferences are not uncommon. Caution in the interpretation of results must be exercised in these cases. Moreover, an unknown number of defects is still to be uncovered and may yet interfere with functional assays. This is possibly the explanation for a number of pathological results that are confirmed at second testing and are not associated with a molecular inherited defect. In these cases, additional explanations are the occurrence of a spontaneous mutation or parental uncertainty.

17.5 FUTURE PROSPECTS

In line with a modern concept of thrombophilia that considers the interaction of multiple genetic (and acquired) traits in determining the individual risk of a thrombotic event, it is safe to assume that new risk factors will be sought, and found, in the near future. Candidate genes are to be looked for in the area of haemostatic proteins, but also in those molecules that participate in inflammatory processes and in cellular interactions. From the point of view of the laboratory, this means a rapid increase of workload and expenditure. Social health issues such as cost–benefit of extended screening procedures and the ethical issue of giving better care to more people underline the need for more rapid, inexpensive and technically easy-to-perform automated techniques. This, together with continuous scientific progress, should be a goal for the near future.

REFERENCES

Aiach, M., Gandrille, S. and Emmerich, J. (1995) A review of mutations causing deficiencies of antithrombin, protein C and protein S. *Thromb. Haemost.* **74**, 81–9.

Aillaud, M.F., Pouymayou, K., Brunet, D. *et al.* (1996) New direct assay of free protein S antigen applied to diagnosis of protein S deficiency. *Thromb. Haemost.* **75**, 283–5.

Amiral, J., Grosley, M., Boyer-Neumann, C. *et al.* (1994) New direct assay of free protein S antigen using two distinct monoclonal antibodies specific for the free form. *Blood Coag. Fibrinol.* **5**, 179–86.

Barbui, T., Finazzi, G., Mussoni, L. *et al.* (1984) Hereditary dysfunctional protein C (protein C Bergamo) and thrombosis. *Lancet* **239**, 819.

Bernardi, F., Faioni, E.M., Castoldi, E. *et al.* (1997) A factor V genetic component differing from factor V R506Q contributes to the APC resistance phenotype. *Blood* **90**, 1522–57.

Bertina, R.M., van der Marel-van Nieuwkoop, W. and Loeliger, E.A. (1979) Spectrophotometric assays of prothrombin in plasma of patients using oral anticoagulants. *Thromb. Haemost.* **42**, 1296–305.

Bertina, R.M., Broekmans, A.W., Krommenhoek-van Es, C. and van Wijngaarden, A. (1984) The use of a functional and immunologic assay for plasma protein C in the study of the heterogeneity of congenital protein C deficiency. *Thromb. Haemost.* **51**, 1–5.

Bertina, R.M., Reinalda-Poot, J., van Wijngaarden, A. *et al.* (1985) Determination of plasma protein S, the protein cofactor of activated protein C. *Thromb. Haemost.* **53**, 268–72.

Bertina, R.M., Ploos van Amstel, H.K., van Wijngaarden, A. *et al.* (1990) Heerlen polymorphism of protein S, an immunologic polymorphism due to dimorphism of residue 460. *Blood* **76**, 538–48.

Bertina, R.M., Koeleman, B.P.C., Koster, T. *et al.* (1994) Mutation in blood coagulation factor V associated with resistance to activated protein C. *Nature* **369**, 64–7.

Boers, G.H.J., Fowler, B., Smals, A.G.H. *et al.* (1985) Improved identification of heterozygotes for homocystinuria due to cystathionine synthase deficiency by the combination of methionine loading and enzyme determination in cultured fibroblasts. *Hum. Genet.* **69**, 164–9.

Boyer, C., Rothschild, C., Wolf, M. *et al.* (1984) A new method for the estimation of protein C by ELISA. *Thromb. Res.* **36**, 579–89.

Boyer-Neumann, C., Wolf, M., Amiral, J. *et al.* (1988) Familial type I protein S deficiency associated with severe thrombosis. A study of five cases. *Thromb. Haemost.* **60**, 128.

Boyer-Neumann, C., Bertina, R.M., Tripodi, A. *et al*. (1993) Comparison of functional assays for protein S: European collaborative study of patients with congenital and acquired deficiency. *Thromb. Haemost.* **70**, 946–50.

Cattaneo, M. (1997) Hyperhomocysteinaemia. *Vessels* **3**, 16–21.

Comp, P.C., Nixon, R.R. and Esmon, C.T. (1984a) Determination of functional levels of protein C, an antithrombotic protein, using thrombin-thrombomodulin complex. *Blood* **63**, 15–21.

Comp, P.C., Nixon, R.R., Cooper, M.R. and Esmon, C.T. (1984b) Familial protein S deficiency is associated with recurrent thrombosis. *J. Clin. Invest.* **74**, 2082–8.

Comp, P.C., Doray, D., Patton, D. and Esmon, C.T. (1986) An abnormal plasma distribution of protein S occurs in functional protein S deficiency. *Blood* **67**, 504–8.

Cooper, P.C., Hampton, K.K., Makris, M. *et al*. (1994) Further evidence that activated protein C resistance can be misdiagnosed as inherited functional protein S deficiency. *Br. J. Haematol.* **88**, 201–3.

Cooper, P.C., Beauchamp, N.J., Daly, M.E. *et al*. (1997) The prothrombin 20210 G→A variant is associated with increased levels of prothrombin and increased incidence of venous thrombosis (abstr. # OC-1546). *Thromb. Haemost.* **78**(Suppl.), 378.

Corral, J., Iniesta, J.A., Gonzalez-Conejero, R. and Vicente, V. (1996) Detection of factor V Leiden from a drop of blood by PCR-SSCP. *Thromb. Haemost.* **76**, 735–7.

Cumming, A.M., Keeney, S., Salden, A. *et al*. (1997) The prothrombin gene G20210A variant: prevalence in a U.K. anticoagulant clinic population. *Br. J. Haematol.* **98**, 353–5.

D'Angelo, A. and Selhub, J. (1997) Homocysteine and thrombotic disease. *Blood* **90**, 1–11.

D'Angelo, A., Vigano-D'Angelo, S., Esmon, C.T. and Comp, P.C. (1988) Acquired deficiencies of protein S. *J. Clin. Invest.* **81**, 1445–54.

Dahlback, B. (1991) Protein S and C4b-binding protein: components involved in the regulation of the protein C anticoagulant system. *Thromb. Haemost.* **66**, 49–61.

Dahlback, B., Carlsson, M. and Svensson, P.J.(1993) Familial thrombophilia due to a previously unrecognized mechanism characterized by poor anticoagulant response to activated protein C: prediction of a cofactor to activated protein C. *Proc. Natl Acad. Sci. USA* **90**, 1004–8.

De Lucia, D., Cerbone, A.M., Belli, A. *et al*. (1996) Resistance to APC in adults with a history of juvenile transient ischemic attacks. *Thromb. Haemost.* **76**, 627–8.

de Ronde, H. and Bertina, R.M. (1994) Laboratory diagnosis of APC-resistance: a critical evaluation of the test and the development of diagnostic criteria. *Thromb. Haemost.* **72**, 860–86.

De Stefano, V., Finazzi, G. and Mannucci, P.M. (1996) Inherited thrombophilia: pathogenesis, clinical syndromes, and management. *Blood* **87**, 3531–44.

De Visser, M.C., Rosendaal, F.R. and Bertina, R.M. (1999) A reduced sensitivity for activated protein C in the absence of factor V Leiden increases the risk of venous thrombosis. *Blood* **93**, 1271–6.

Doggen, C.J.M., Kunz, G., Rosendaal, F.R. *et al*. (1998) A mutation in the thrombomodulin gene, 127G to A coding for Ala25Thr, and the risk of myocardial infarction in men. *Thromb. Haemost.* **80**, 743–8.

Engelhardt, W., Girolami, A., Kraus, M. *et al*. (1997) Multicenter evaluation of new assays for determination of total function of the protein C system and of APC sensitivity (abstr. # PS-114). *Thromb. Haemost.* **78**(Suppl.), 378.

Epstein, D.J., Bergum, P.W., Bajaj, S.P. and Rapaport, S.I. (1984) Radioimmunoassays for protein C and factor X. *Am. J. Clin. Pathol.* **82**, 573–81.

Esmon, N.L. (1987) Thrombomodulin. *Semin. Thromb. Hemost.* **13**, 454–63.

Esmon, C.T. (1992) The protein C anticoagulant pathway. *Arterioscler. Thromb.* **12**, 135–45.

Faioni, E.M., Franchi, F., Asti, D. *et al*. (1993) Resistance to activated protein C in nine thrombophilic families: interference in a protein S functional assay. *Thromb. Haemost.* **70**, 1067–71.

Faioni, E.M., Franchi, F., Asti, A. and Mannucci, P.M. (1996) Resistance to activated protein C mimicking dysfunctional protein C: diagnostic approach. *Blood Coag. Fibrinol.* **7**, 349–52.

Faioni, E.M., Valsecchi, C., Palla, A. *et al*. (1997) Free protein S deficiency is a risk factor for venous thrombosis. *Thromb. Haemost.* **78**, 1343–6.

Ferraresi, P., Legnani, C., Quaglio, S. *et al.* (1997) Study of a G/A variation in the 3´ untranslated region of prothrombin mRNA in Italian patient with venous thrombosis (abstr. # OC-1547). *Thromb. Haemost.* **78**(Suppl.), 378.

Finazzi, G., Caccia, R. and Barbui, T. (1987) Different prevalence of thromboembolism in the subtypes of congenital antithrombin III deficiency: review of 404 cases. *Thromb. Haemost.* **58**, 1094.

Franchi, F., Tripodi, A., Valsecchi, C. *et al.* (1988) Functional assay for protein C: comparison of two snake-venom assays with two thrombin assays. *Thromb. Haemost.* **60**, 145–7.

Francis, R.B. Jr (1986) A simplified PTT-based protein C activity assay using the thrombin-thrombomodulin complex. *Thromb. Res.* **37**, 337–44.

Francis, R.B. and Patch, M.J. (1983) A functional assay for protein C in human plasma. *Thromb. Res.* **32**, 605–13.

Francis, R.B. and Seyfert, U. (1987) Rapid amidolytic assay of protein C in whole plasma using an activator from the venom of Agkistrodon Contortrix. *Am. J. Clin. Pathol.* **87**, 619–25.

Franco, F.R., Trip, M.D., ten Cate, H. *et al.* (1997) The prevalence of the 20210 G→A mutation in the 3´-untranslated region of the prothrombin gene in patients with premature coronary artery disease (abstr. # HI-12). *Thromb. Haemost.*, **78**(Suppl.), 769.

Furie, B. and Furie, B.C. (1990) Molecular basis of vitamin K-dependent γ-carboxylation. *Blood* **75**,1753–62.

Gandrille, S., Borgel, D., Ireland, H. *et al.* (1997) Protein S deficiency: a database of mutations. For the plasma coagulation inhibitors subcommittee of the Scientific and Standardization Committee of the International Society on Thrombosis and Haemostasis. *Thromb. Haemost.* **77**, 1201–14.

Garcia de Frutos, P., Alim, R.I.M., Hardig, Y. *et al.* (1994) Differential regulation of α and β chains of C4b-binding protein during acute-phase response resulting in stable plasma levels of free anticoagulant protein S. *Blood* **84**, 815–22.

Heeb, M.J., Rosing, J., Bakker, H.M. *et al.* (1994) Protein S binds to and inhibits factor Xa. *Proc. Natl Acad. Sci. USA* **91**, 2728–32.

Henkens, C.M.A., Bom, V.V.J. and van der Meer, J. (1995) Lowered APC-sensitivity ratio related to increased factor VIII clotting activity. *Thromb. Haemost.* **74**, 1198–9.

Hillarp, A., Zeller, B., Svensson, P. and Dahlback, B. (1997) The 20210 A allele of the prothrombin gene is a common risk factor among Swedish outpatients with verified deep venous thrombosis. *Thromb. Haemost.* **78**, 990–2.

Hubbard, A.R. (1988) Standardization of protein C in plasma: establishment of an international standard. *Thromb. Haemost.* **59**, 464–7.

Ireland, H., Bayston, T., Thompson, E. *et al.* (1995) Apparent heterozygous type II deficiency caused by the factor V 506 Arg to Gln mutation. *Thromb. Haemost.* **73**, 731–2.

Ireland, H., Kunz, G., Kyriakoulis, K. *et al.* (1997) Thrombomodulin gene mutations associated with myocardial infarction. *Circulation* **96**, 15–18.

Jackman, R.W., Beeler, D.L., Fritze, L. *et al.* (1987) Human thrombomodulin gene is intron depleted: nucleic acid sequences of the cDNA and gene predict protein structure and suggest sites of regulatory control. *Proc. Natl Acad. Sci. USA* **84**, 6425–9.

Kalafatis, M., Rand, M.D. and Mann, K.G. (1994) The mechanism of inactivation of human factor V and human factor Va by activated protein C. *J. Biol. Chem.* **269**, 31869–80.

Kalafatis, M., Haley, P.E., Lu, D. *et al.* (1996) Proteolytic events that regulate factor V activity in whole plasma from normal and activated protein C (APC)-resistant individuals during clotting: an insight into the APC-resistance assay. *Blood* **87**, 4695–707.

Kamphuisen, P.W., Houwing-Duistermaat, J.J., van Houwelingen, H.C. *et al.* (1998) Familial clustering of factor VIII and von Willebrand factor levels. *Thromb. Haemost.* **79**, 323–7.

Koster, T., Rosendaal, F.R., Briet, E. *et al.* (1995a) Protein C deficiency in a controlled series of unselected outpatients: an infrequent but clear risk factor for venous thrombosis (Leiden Thrombophilia Study) *Blood* **85**, 2756–61.

Koster, T., Blann, A.D., Briet, E. *et al.* (1995b) Role of clotting factor VIII in effect of von Willebrand factor on occurrence of deep vein thrombosis. *Lancet* **345**, 152–5.

Krachmalnicoff, A., Valsecchi, C., Tombesi, S. *et al.* (1990) A monoclonal antibody to human protein S used as the capture antibody for measuring total protein S by enzyme immunoassay. *Clin. Chem.* **36**, 43–7.

Kraus, M., Noah, M. and Fickenscher, K. (1995) The PCAT – a simple screening assay for assessing the functionality of the protein C anticoagulant pathway. *Thromb. Res.* **79**, 217–22.

Lane, D.A. and Caso, R. (1989) Antithrombin: structure, genomic organization, function and inherited deficiency. In: Tuddenham, E.G.D. (ed.), *The Molecular Biology of Coagulation*. London: Baillière Tindall, 961–88.

Lane, D.A., Olds, R.J., Boisclair, M. *et al.* (1993) Antithrombin III mutation database: first update. *Thromb. Haemost.* **70**, 361–9.

Lane, D.A., Mannucci, P.M., Bauer, K.A. *et al.* (1996a) Inherited thrombophilia: Part 1. *Thromb. Haemost.* **76**, 651–62.

Lane, D.A., Mannucci, P.M., Bauer, K.A. *et al.* (1996b) Inherited thrombophilia: Part 2. *Thromb. Haemost.* **76**, 824–34.

Lawrie, A.S., Lloyd, M.E., Mohamed, F. *et al.* (1995) Assay of protein S in systemic lupus erythematosus. *Blood Coag. Fibrinol.* **6**, 322–4.

Leroy-Matheron, C., Duchemin, J., Levant, M. *et al.* (1999) Genetic modulation of plasma PS levels by two frequent dimorphisms in the PROS1 gene. *Thromb. Haemost.* **82**, 1088–92.

Leroy-Matheron, C., Duchemin, J., Levant, M. *et al.* (2000) Influence of the nt 2148 A to G substitution (Pro 626 dimorphism) in the PROS1 gene on circulating free protein S levels in healthy volunteers – reappraisal of protein S normal ranges. *Thromb. Haemost.* **83**, 798–9.

Makris, M., Leach, M., Beauchamp, N.J. *et al.* (2000) Genetic analysis, phenotypic diagnosis, and risk of venous thrombosis in families with inherited deficiencies of protein S. *Blood* **95**, 1935–41.

Malm, J., Laurell, M. and Dahlback, B. (1988) Changes in the plasma levels of vitamin K-dependent protein C and S and of C4b-binding protein during pregnancy and oral contraception. *Br. J. Haematol.* **68**, 437–48.

Mannucci, P.M. and Tripodi, A. (1987) Laboratory screening of inherited thrombotic syndromes. *Thromb. Haemost.* **57**, 247–51.

Mannucci, P.M., Boyer, C., Tripodi, A. *et al.* (1987) Multicenter comparison of five functional and two immunologic assays for protein C. *Thromb. Haemost.* **57**, 44–8.

Martinoli, J.L. and Stocker, K. (1986) Functional protein C assay using Protac®, a novel protein C activator. *Thromb. Res.* **43**, 253–64.

Meijers, J.C.M., Tekelenburg, W.L.H., Bouma, B.N. *et al.* (2000) High levels of factor XI as a risk factor for venous thrombosis. *N. Engl. J. Med.* **342**, 696–701.

Norlund, L., Holm, J., Zoller, B. and Ohlin, A-K. (1997) A common thrombomodulin amino acid dimorphism is associated with myocardial infarction. *Thromb. Haemost.* **77**, 248–51.

Ohlin, A.K. and Marlar, R.A. (1995) The first mutation identified in the thrombomodulin gene in a 45 year old man presenting with thromboembolic disease. *Blood* **85**, 330–6.

Ohlin, A.K. and Marlar, R.A. (1997) Thrombomodulin gene variations and thromboembolic disease. *Thromb. Haemost.* **78**, 396–400.

Olds, R.J., Lane, D.A., Chowdhury, V. *et al.* (1993) Complete nucleotide sequence of the antithrombin gene: evidence for homologous recombination causing thrombophilia. *Biochemistry* **32**, 4216–24.

Ploos van Amstel, H.K., Reitsma, P.H., van der Logt, C.P.E. and Bertina, R.M. (1990) Intron-exon organization of the active human protein S gene PSα and its pseudogene PSβ: duplication and silencing during primate evolution. *Biochemistry* **29**, 7853–61.

Plutzky, J., Hoskins, J.A., Long, G.L. and Crabtree, G.R. (1986) Evolution and organization of the human protein C gene. *Proc. Natl Acad. Sci. USA* **83**, 546–50.

Poort, S.R., Rosendaal, F.R., Reitsma, P.H. and Bertina, R.M. (1996) A common genetic variation in the 3'-untranslated region of the prothrombin gene is associated with elevated plasma prothrombin levels and an increase in venous thrombosis. *Blood* **88**, 3698–703.

Poort, S.R., Bertina, R.M. and Vos, H.L. (1997) Rapid detection of the prothrombin 20210 A variation by allele specific PCR. *Thromb. Haemost.* **78**, 1157–8.

Preda, L., Tripodi, A., Valsecchi, C. *et al.* (1990) A prothrombin time-based functional assay of protein S. *Thromb. Res.* **60**, 19–32.

Preda, L., Simioni, P., Legnani, C. *et al.* (1996) A new global test for the evaluation of the protein C-protein S system. *Blood Coag. Fibrinol.* **7**, 465–9.

Rees, D.C. (1996) The population genetics of factor V Leiden (Arg 506 Gln). *Br. J. Haematol.* **95**, 579–86.

Rees, M.W. and Rodgers, G.M. (1993) Homocysteinemia: association of a metabolic disorder with vascular disease and thrombosis. *Thromb. Res.* **71**, 337–59.

Regan, L.M., Stearns-Kurosawa, D.J., Kurosawa, S. *et al.* (1996) The endothelial cell protein C receptor. *J. Biol. Chem.* **271**, 17499–503.

Reiter, W., Ehrensberger, H., Steinbruckner, B. and Keller, F. (1995) Parameters of haemostasis during acute venous thrombosis. *Thromb. Haemost.* **74**, 596–601.

Reitsma, P.H., Bernardi, F., Doig, R.G. *et al.* (1995) Protein C deficiency: a database of mutations, 1995 update. *Thromb. Haemost.* **73**, 876–89.

Ridker, P.M., Hennekens, C.H., Lindpaintner, K. *et al.* (1995) Mutation in the gene coding for coagulation factor V and the risk of myocardial infarction, stroke and venous thrombosis in apparently healthy men. *N. Engl. J. Med.* **332**, 912–17.

Ripoll, L., Paulin, D., Thomas, S. and Drouet, L.O. (1997) Multiplex PCR-mediated site-directed mutagenesis for one-step determination of factor V Leiden and G20210A transition of the prothrombin gene. *Thromb. Haemost.* **78**, 960–1.

Rodeghiero, F. and Tosetto, A. (1999) Activated protein C resistance and factor V Leiden mutation are independent risk factors for venous thromboembolism. *Ann. Intern. Med.* **130**, 643–50.

Rosendaal, F.R., Siscovick, D.S., Schwartz, S.M. *et al.* (1997) A common prothrombin variant (20210 G→A) increases the risk of myocardial infarction in young women (abstr. # HI-11). *Thromb. Haemost.* **78**(Suppl.), 769.

Sala, N., Owen, W.G. and Collen, D. (1984) A functional assay of protein C in human plasma. *Blood* **63**, 671–5.

Schwarz, H.P., Fisher, M., Hopmeier, P. *et al.* (1984) Plasma protein S deficiency in familial thrombotic disease. *Blood* **64**, 1297–300.

Shen, L. and Dahlback, B. (1994) Factor V and protein S as synergistic cofactors to activated protein C in degradation of factor VIIIa. *J. Biol. Chem.* **269**, 18735–8.

Simioni, P., Gavasso, S., Luni, S. *et al.* (1995) A protein S functional assay yields unsatisfactory results in patients with activated protein C resistance. *Blood Coag. Fibrinol.* **6**, 286–7.

Simmonds, R.E., Zoller, B., Ireland, H. *et al.* (1997) Genetic and phenotypic analysis of a large (122) member protein S-deficient kindred provides an explanation for the familial coexistence of type I and type III plasma phenotypes. *Blood* **89**, 4364–70.

Simmonds, R.E., Ireland, H., Lane, D. *et al.* (1998) Clarification of the risk for venous thrombosis associated with hereditary protein S deficiency by investigation of a large kindred with a characterized gene defect. *Ann. Intern. Med.* **128**, 8–14.

Stearns-Kurosawa, D.J., Kurosawa, S., Mollica, J.S. *et al.* (1996) The endothelial cell protein C receptor augments protein C activation by the thrombin-thrombomodulin complex. *Proc. Natl Acad. Sci. USA* **93**, 10212–6.

Suzuki, K. and Nishioka, J. (1988) Plasma protein S activity measured using Protac, a snake venom derived activator of protein C. *Thromb. Res.* **49**, 241–51.

Takano, S., Kimura, S., Ohdama, S. and Aoki, N. (1990) Plasma thrombomodulin in health and diseases. *Blood* **76**, 2024–29.

Tans, G., Nicolaes, G.A. and Rosing, J. (1997) Regulation of thrombin formation by activated protein C: effect of the factor V Leiden mutation. *Semin. Haematol.* **34**, 244–55.

Tran, T.H. and Duckert, F. (1985) Influence of heparin cofactor II (HCL II) on the determination of antithrombin (AT). *Thromb. Res.* **40**, 571–6.

Tripodi, A., Valsecchi, C., Bottasso, M. *et al.* (1985) Comparison of a functional assay for protein C with two immunoassays. *Thromb. Res.* **40**, 243–8.

Tripodi, A., Bertina, R.M., Conard, J. *et al.* (1992) Multicenter evaluation of three commercial methods for measuring protein S antigen. *Thromb. Haemost.* **68**, 149–54.

Tripodi, A., Negri, B., Bertina, R.M. and Mannucci, P.M. (1997) Screening for the FV:Q^{506} mutation – evaluation of thirteen plasma-based methods for their diagnostic efficacy in comparison with DNA analysis. *Thromb. Haemost.* **77**, 436–9.

Ueland, P.M., Refsum, H., Stabler, S.P. *et al.* (1993) Total homocysteine in plasma or serum: methods and clinical applications. *Clin. Chem.* **39**, 1764–79.

van der Velden, P.A., Krommenhoek-Van Es, T., Allaart, C.F. *et al.* (1991) A frequent thrombomodulin amino acid dimorphism is not associated with thrombophilia. *Thromb. Haemost.* **65**, 511–13.

Van Hylckama, V.A., van der Linden, I.K., Bertina, R.M. *et al.* (2000) High levels of factor IX increase the risk of venous thrombosis. *Blood* **95**, 3678–82.

van Wijnen, M., van't Veer, C., Meijers, J.C.M. *et al.* (1997) A plasma coagulation assay to determine the activated protein C independent anticoagulant activity of protein S (abstr. # OC-756). *Thromb. Haemost.* **78**(Suppl.), 187.

Vigano-D'Angelo, S., Comp, P.C., Esmon, C.T. and D'Angelo, A. (1986) Relationship between protein C antigen and anticoagulant activity during oral anticoagulation and in selected disease states. *J. Clin. Invest.* **77**, 416–25.

Vinazzer, H. and Pangraz, U. (1987) Protein C: comparison of different assays in normal and abnormal plasma samples. *Thromb. Res.* **46**, 1–8.

Wolf, M., Boyer-Neumann, C., Martinoli, J.L. *et al.* (1989) A new functional assay for human protein S activity using activated factor V as substrate. *Thromb. Haemost.* **62**, 1144–5.

Zoller, B., Garcia de Frutos, P. and Dahlback, B. (1995) Evaluation of the relationship between protein S and C4b-binding protein isoforms in hereditary protein S deficiency demonstrating type I and type III deficiencies to be phenotypic variants of the same genetic disease. *Blood* **85**, 3524–31.

18

Standardization and control of oral anticoagulant therapy[1,2]

ANTON M.H.P. VAN DEN BESSELAAR

INTRODUCTION

The prothrombin time (PT) is the primary laboratory test for monitoring oral anticoagulant treatment. Different drugs are used (e.g. warfarin, acenocoumarin and phenprocoumon), but can be monitored by the same laboratory methods. It is now generally accepted that laboratory monitoring of oral anticoagulant treatment should be reported using the international normalized ratio (INR). The concept of INR was introduced in the early 1980s (Loeliger and Lewis, 1982; Kirkwood, 1983) and was adopted by the World Health Organization Expert Committee on Biological Standardization (ECBS) (WHO, 1983). After more than 10 years of experience with the INR system, it was felt that several improvements were required, with regard to definitions and methods. Although revised guidelines were adopted by the ECBS in October 1997 (WHO, 1999), a few issues remain to be resolved. The use of lyophilized plasmas for calibration is still problematic. This chapter includes the revised definitions and methods for determination of the INR. The uncertainty of the INR will be assessed, including pre-analytical, analytical and biological variations. The importance and limitations of external quality assessment schemes will be highlighted.

[1]The author would like to thank the following for fruitful collaboration in many studies: R.M. Bertina, J. Meeuwisse-Braun, H. Schaefer-van Mansfeld, E. Witteveen, C. van Rijn, F.J.M. van der Meer and E.A. van der Velde.
[2]Results of the Netherlands EQAS were kindly provided by the 'Federatie van Nederlandse Thrombosediensten' and the 'Stichting Subcommissie Stolling van de CCKL'. Immuno AG (Vienna, Austria) kindly provided samples of frozen and lyophilized coumarin plasmas for analysis. Dr A. Tripodi kindly provided Figure 18.2. Mrs. E. van Duijn provided secretarial assistance.

18.1 DEFINITIONS

TISSUE FACTOR

Tissue factor is an integral transmembrane protein functioning as a cofactor of factor VIIa towards factors IX and X in the blood. Tissue factor needs to be associated with phospholipids for full expression of its cofactor function.

THROMBOPLASTIN

Thromboplastin is a reagent containing tissue factor and phospholipids. Many thromboplastins are crude extracts prepared from mammalian tissues in which tissue factor is only a minor component on a weight basis and which also contains phospholipids. A preparation of a thromboplastin consisting of a tissue extract alone, either with or without added calcium chloride, is termed 'plain'. When the preparation contains adsorbed plasma as a source of additional factor V and fibrinogen, it is termed 'combined'. Thromboplastins may also be grouped into types according to the tissue source from which they are derived, e.g. human brain, bovine brain, rabbit brain or lung, or human placenta. The tissue factor component of recombinant thromboplastin reagents is produced by recombinant DNA techniques and then lipidated *in vitro*.

PROTHROMBIN TIME (PT)

The prothrombin time (PT) or tissue factor-induced coagulation time (Blombäck *et al.*, 1994) is the clotting time of a plasma or whole blood sample in the presence of thromboplastin and the appropriate amount of calcium ions. The PT is reported in seconds.

PROTHROMBIN-TIME SYSTEM

A prothrombin-time system is defined as a procedure by which the prothrombin time is determined using a specific thromboplastin reagent and a particular method which may be manual, e.g. a tilt-tube method, or involve the use of an instrument which records the end-point automatically. The description of the method should include all procedures and equipment used, e.g. the pipettes and test tubes.

MEAN NORMAL PROTHROMBIN TIME (MNPT)

Although it is difficult to define normality, plasma obtained from a healthy adult person is considered to be normal and can be used for calibration of prothrombin-time systems. There are no *a priori* exclusion criteria for normal donors. The mean normal prothrombin time (MNPT) is defined as the geometric mean of prothrombin times of the healthy adult population. For practical purposes, the geometric mean of the prothrombin time calculated from at least 20 fresh samples from healthy individuals (including both sexes) is a reliable approximation of the MNPT (Van den Besselaar *et al.*, 1993). The geometric mean is the antilogarithm of the arithmetic mean of the logarithms of the individual PT values (Kirkwood, 1983).

It is not necessary to collect and test all the individual samples in one session. It is recommended that each laboratory should determine the MNPT using its own prothrombin-time system.

The MNPT as defined above should be distinguished from the prothrombin time of pooled normal plasma. The latter may be shorter than the MNPT of the individual plasmas used to prepare the pool (Burgess-Wilson *et al.*, 1993). This observation might be explained by minor partial deficiencies of single coagulation factors in individual plasmas which are compensated by one another in the pool.

PROTHROMBIN-TIME RATIO

The prothrombin-time ratio is the prothrombin time obtained with a test plasma or blood sample divided by the MNPT, all times having been determined using the same prothrombin-time system.

INTERNATIONAL SENSITIVITY INDEX (ISI)

The international sensitivity index is a quantitative measure in terms of the first primary international reference preparation (coded 67/40) of the responsiveness of a prothrombin-time system to the defect induced by oral anticoagulants. The ISI of the first primary international reference preparation (coded 67/40) is 1.0 by definition.

INTERNATIONAL NORMALIZED RATIO (INR)

The INR is defined for a given plasma or blood specimen from a patient on long-term oral anticoagulant therapy. The INR is calculated from the prothrombin-time ratio using a prothrombin-time system with a known ISI according to the formula:

$$INR = (PT/MNPT)^{ISI}$$

The INR can be interpreted as the prothrombin-time ratio that would have been obtained, if the first primary international reference preparation (coded 67/40) had been used.

18.2 INTERNATIONAL STANDARDIZATION

International standardization of the PT can be achieved by relating any given test system to an established primary reference system. In 1977, a research standard prepared by the International Committee on Thrombosis and Haemostasis in collaboration with the National Institute of Biological Standards and Control, London, UK, was established by the WHO as the primary international reference preparation (IRP) for thromboplastin (WHO, 1977). This material, coded 67/40, was prepared from human brain supplemented with adsorbed bovine plasma (combined reagent), to be used according to meticulously defined instructions (Bangham *et al.*, 1973).

18.3 WHO CALIBRATION MODEL

Kirkwood (1983) proposed a model for the calibration of any PT system in terms of the primary IRP. In this model, a linear relationship is hypothesized between the logarithms of PTs obtained with the primary IRP method and the logarithms of PTs obtained with the test system (Fig. 18.1). Furthermore, the model requires that a single relationship be valid for fresh plasma specimens of normal individuals and fresh specimens of patients stabilized on oral anticoagulant therapy. The relation can be described by the following formula:

$$\log PT_{67/40} = a + b \log PT_{test}$$

in which *a* and *b* are the intercept and slope of the calibration line, respectively. The model leads to a simple formula to transform a PT ratio obtained with the test system (R_{test}) into one which would have been obtained had the primary IRP 67/40 been used:

$$R_{67/40} = (R_{test})^{ISI}$$

$R_{67/40}$ is also called the international normalized ratio (INR) and the slope *b* is equal to the international sensitivity index (ISI). This calibration model was tested successfully in an international collaborative exercise organized by the European Community Bureau of Reference (BCR) and the International Committee for Standardization in Haematology (Hermans *et al.*, 1983). The model was then adopted by the WHO (1983). It is the thromboplastin manufacturers' responsibility to provide calibration data for each lot of their reagents (Loeliger, 1985).

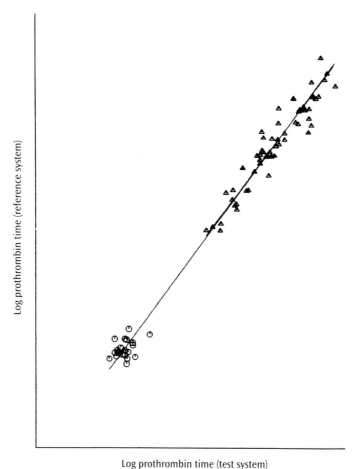

Fig. 18.1 *Calibration of a working thromboplastin system ('test' system) against the primary international reference preparation (IRP) method (reference system). The logarithms of prothrombin times determined with the test system are plotted along the horizontal axis, and the logarithms of prothrombin times with the reference system along the vertical axis. Samples of normal individuals are represented by circles; and samples of patients on long-term oral anticoagulant treatment by triangles. The calibration line is calculated by orthogonal regression analysis. The slope of the line is the designated ISI of the test system.*

18.4 SECONDARY INTERNATIONAL REFERENCE PREPARATIONS FOR THROMBOPLASTINS

18.4.1 The family of secondary international reference preparations for thromboplastins

For the determination of ISI and INR, prothrombin-time systems must be calibrated using international reference preparations (IRPs) of thromboplastins. Each calibration involves the determination of the relation between the prothrombin times of the new prothrombin-time system and those of the reference system. The first primary IRP (coded 67/40) was prepared from human brain thromboplastin supplemented with adsorbed bovine plasma as a source of fibrinogen and factor V. It was available in limited supply only. It was evident that IRP 67/40 could not be used for direct calibration of local PT systems. For calibration of local working thromboplastins, the production of secondary IRPs was required. These secondary IRPs were calibrated against IRP 67/40 in multicentre collaborative studies and each secondary IRP was characterized with a mean ISI value resulting from the collaborative studies. Before a reference preparation was consumed completely, it had to be replaced by a new material and the replacement preparation calibrated against the former. The hierarchy of IRP is shown in Figure 18.2. At present, there are three IRPs available from the WHO. Each represents a different species of thromboplastin, i.e. human, rabbit and bovine. The second human IRP (coded BCT/253) has been replaced by a human recombinant thromboplastin, coded rTF/95 (Tripodi et al., 1998). The current human and rabbit IRP are 'plain' thromboplastins, i.e. without addition of adsorbed plasma as a source of fibrinogen and factor V. The third WHO IRP, coded OBT/79, is a bovine thromboplastin combined with adsorbed bovine plasma.

All three WHO IRPs are in the custody of the Central Laboratory of the Netherlands Red Cross Blood Transfusion Service, Amsterdam. An example of thromboplastin calibration and

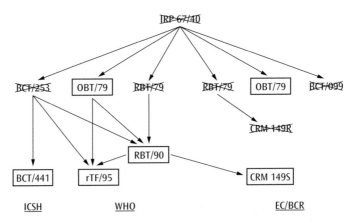

Fig. 18.2 *Hierarchy of international reference preparations (IRPs). Preparation coded 67/40 was the primary WHO standard with an ISI = 1.0 by definition. Each arrow represents a historical multicentre calibration study, relating a new preparation to the previous. Currently available preparations are boxed. Discontinued preparations are crossed out. BCT/441 is available from the International Council for Standardization in Haematology (ICSH), OBT/79, RBT/90 and rTF/95 from the World Health Organization (WHO), and CRM 149S and OBT/79 from the European Commission's Institute for Reference Materials and Measurements (formerly Community Bureau of Reference, BCR).*

the statistical methods for calculation of the ISI are given in Appendix A.18.1. The calibration of a thromboplastin is, in general, more precise when comparisons are made between similar preparations from the same species (Tomenson, 1984; Van den Besselaar and Bertina, 1993). The current IRPs represent different species and types of reagents. It is recommended that laboratories and manufacturers use the secondary IRP of the same species for the calibration of their materials. It is also recommended that 'combined' thromboplastins be calibrated against OBT/79, which is the only 'combined' IRP currently available. In addition to the WHO IRPs, several other secondary reference preparations have been provided by other organizations, i.e. the European Community Bureau of Reference (BCR, now succeeded by the Institute for Reference Materials and Measurements, IRMM) and the International Council for Standardization in Haematology (ICSH). These reference preparations have also been calibrated against the WHO IRPs. Since all secondary IRPs have been calibrated, directly or indirectly, against the first primary IRP (coded 67/40), it is expected that ISI values obtained with any IRP will be independent of the route of calibration. In contrast, it became evident that there is a systematic difference between ISI values obtained with BCT/253 and with RBT/79 (Poller et al., 1993; Van den Besselaar, 1993; Tripodi et al., 1994). ISI values obtained with OBT/79 were in good agreement with those of RBT/79 (Van den Besselaar, 1993). To resolve this problem, it was recommended that all future IRPs be calibrated against all current IRPs (Tripodi et al., 1995a). In this way, discrepancies between routes of calibration will become smaller after each multi-centre IRP calibration study. Thus, RBT/90 and rTF/95 have been calibrated against all three IRPs and their assigned ISI values were the mean of the three separate calibrations.

18.4.2 Between-laboratory variation of ISI

It should be realized that all multicentre IRP calibration studies have been performed with the manual technique for prothrombin time determination. There is a compelling reason for using the manual technique. All participant laboratories should use the same technique and this technique should be available in all parts of the world. Furthermore, this technique should be available during the period that the IRP is being provided by the custodian. There is no 'instrument' complying with these requirements but the human being. Although each participant laboratory used the manual technique, considerable interlaboratory variation of the ISI was observed. The coefficient of variation (CV) of the ISI ranged from 1.7 to 6.8% (Van den Besselaar, 1996a). The lower CV values were obtained when very similar thromboplastins were compared, in agreement with the requirement for like-versus-like calibrations.

Part of the interlaboratory variation may be caused by differences in manual technique, e.g. the frequency of tilting the tube. Another source of error may be pre-analytical conditions (see below). The within-laboratory variation of the ISI is usually smaller than the between-laboratory variation (Van den Besselaar, 1996a), suggesting that the latter has an important systematic component. The within-laboratory precision of the ISI may be excellent but this does not guarantee that the value determined by one laboratory is as accurate when used by other laboratories. This is one of the central problems of prothrombin time standardization. In view of the interlaboratory variation observed in multicentre calibration studies, it is recommended by the WHO ECBS (1999) that calibration of national reference preparations or manufacturers' working standards should be performed by at least two laboratories.

18.4.3 Effects of instruments

The thromboplastin IRPs issued by the WHO and BCR have been calibrated by means of manual techniques, and the ISI values of the IRPs relate to the manual technique. Presently, clinical laboratories rely largely on automated instruments for PT determination (coagulo-meters), while laboratories involved in calibration studies use the manual technique almost exclusively. For reliable INR determination, it is important to know the effect of coagulo-meters on the ISI of commercial reagents. Recent studies have shown that instruments may have a significant effect on the PT ratio and hence on the ISI (D'Angelo, et al., 1989; Peters et al., 1989; Poggio et al., 1989; Ray and Smith, 1990; Chantarangkul et al., 1992; Van den Besselaar et al., 1999). The difference in ISI observed between two photo-optical instruments could amount to approximately 10% (Poggio et al., 1989). The relative effect of an instrument may not be the same for various reagents. It is therefore difficult to predict the effect.

18.4.4 Uncertainty of the INR

The analytical errors of the ISI and MNPT are propagated to the INR. The effect of analytical errors can be evaluated by external quality assessment schemes for the prothrombin time and INR. In addition to pre-analytical and analytical errors, there is another source of uncertainty which has been described as residual variation. This type of uncertainty is caused by the prothrombin time's lack of specificity. The prothrombin time is influenced by many different factors in each individual's plasma. Thus, there is an interaction between the prothrombin-time system and the patient's sample. It is not easy to assess the magnitude of the isolated interaction effect on the INR because it is compounded by analytical errors. Some authors have attempted to calculate the total variation of the INR, including analytical variation and interaction effects (Tomenson, 1984; Loeliger et al., 1985; Van den Besselaar, 1996a). Tomenson (1984) showed that the total uncertainty of the INR, expressed as the approximate 95% confidence interval, depends on the similarity between the thromboplastin used to estimate the INR and the reference thromboplastin defining the INR. The secondary IRP for bovine thromboplastin (OBT/79) is relatively similar to the primary IRP 67/40, because both are 'combined' reagents. The secondary IRP for rabbit thromboplastin (RBT/79) is not similar to IRP 67/40 because of species difference and the fact that RBT/79 is 'plain' (i.e. not combined with adsorbed plasma). The confidence interval of INR predicted from clotting times determined with OBT/79 is smaller than the interval of INR predicted from clotting times determined with RBT/79 (Tomenson, 1984). Currently recommended therapeutic target ranges are 2–3 INR and 3–4.5 INR for various clinical states (British Society for Haematology, 1990; Hirsh et al., 1995). The widths of these target ranges are similar to the 95% confidence intervals calculated for a single patient's INR (Fig. 18.3). It is clear that some patients whose INR is well within the recommended target range with one reagent system could appear to be underdosed or overdosed when evaluated with another system. Clinical studies suggest that the inherent uncertainty of the INR does not impair the efficacy and safety of anticoagulant therapy (Boekhout-Mussert et al., 1981; Brophy et al., 1994; Finazzi et al., 1994; Barcellona et al., 1996).

18.5 CALIBRATION OF PROTHROMBIN-TIME SYSTEMS

18.5.1 Types of calibration

Four types of calibration should be distinguished:

1 calibration of IRPs;
2 calibration of national reference preparations and manufacturers' working standards ('house' standards);

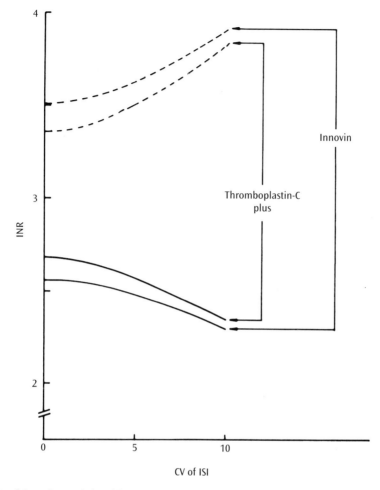

Fig. 18.3 *Confidence intervals (95%) for predicted international normalized ratios (INRs) about a target value of 3 as a function of the coefficient of variation (CV) of the international sensitivity index (ISI). The confidence intervals were estimated according to the method proposed by Tomenson (1984). In this method, the residual standard deviation about the orthogonal regression line is used. These were estimated for two working thromboplastin systems, i.e. Thromboplastin-C Plus and Innovin, calibrated against RBT/90. The lower limits of the 95% confidence intervals are represented by continuous curves, and the upper limits by interrupted curves. (Reprinted from Van den Besselaar (1996a) by permission of S. Karger AG, Basel, Switzerland.)*

3 calibration of manufacturers' commercial preparations against the corresponding working standard ('lot-to-lot' calibration);
4 local system calibration.

In general, the results of type 1, 2 or 3 calibrations are used by laboratories other than the calibrating laboratories. The user laboratories should therefore be aware of the interlaboratory variation in ISI values. The possibility of correcting for local thromboplastin/instrument combination effects by means of type 4 calibration is presently under study by several groups, e.g. the European Concerted Action on Anticoagulation (Poller, 1996). Type 4 calibration involves the use of deep-frozen or lyophilized plasmas with assigned INR or prothrombin-time values. Type 1 and 2 calibrations must be carried out with a large number of fresh plasma or whole blood samples. Several studies suggest that, under certain circumstances, fresh plasmas for type 3 calibrations can be replaced reliably by frozen, lyophilized, pooled or artificially depleted plasmas (Van den Besselaar *et al.*, 1980; Denson, 1986; Tripodi *et al.*, 1996).

Prothrombin-time systems must be calibrated in terms of the appropriate IRP of thromboplastin and the response to the coagulation defect induced by oral anticoagulants must be defined by the ISI obtained in the calibration procedure. Supplies of IRPs are limited and it is not possible to use these materials to calibrate each lot of the many thromboplastins produced by different manufacturers. Calibration of individual lots of thromboplastin must be carried out by comparison with a secondary 'house' standard, which must be a lot of the same or very similar thromboplastin calibrated against the appropriate IRP.

The basis of the thromboplastin calibration model (Kirkwood, 1983) is necessarily an empirical one. While there is good evidence that the calibration relationship defined in a double-logarithmic plot of prothrombin times is usually linear and that the same line represents data points for both anticoagulated patients and normal, healthy subjects, the possibility of departure from these assumptions cannot be ruled out. Statistical methods to test deviations from the latter assumption have been described (Tomenson, 1984; Van der Velde, 1984). In the case of marked deviation, the assignment of an ISI would not be meaningful, and a modified model may be appropriate (Tomenson, 1984; Gogstad *et al.*, 1986). For practical purposes, the assignment of an ISI is acceptable if INRs calculated with the ISI derived from the overall regression line (i.e. determined from data from anticoagulated patients plus normal subjects) do not differ from INRs calculated with the regression line for patients only by more than 10% in the 2–4.5 INR range.

18.5.2 Calibration of international reference preparations

The calibration of IRPs of thromboplastins and their replacements must be carried out in international multicentre collaborative studies using fresh plasma samples from normal individuals and patients under stable oral anticoagulant treatment. Prothrombin times must be determined by manual techniques. Each collaborative study for replacement of an IRP must include the testing of all existing WHO IRPs. The ISI assigned to the replacement material shall be the mean of the ISIs obtained by calibration with all existing WHO IRPs (Tripodi *et al.*, 1995a).

18.5.3 Calibration of secondary standards

National reference preparations or manufacturers' 'house' standards of human origin must be calibrated against the current international standard for thromboplastin, human, recombinant, plain (coded rTF/95); plain thromboplastins of rabbit brain or rabbit lung must be calibrated against the current international reference reagent of thromboplastin, rabbit, plain (coded RBT/90); and thromboplastins of bovine origin must be calibrated against the current international reference preparation of thromboplastin, bovine, combined (coded OBT/79). Thromboplastins of rabbit tissue combined with adsorbed bovine plasma must also be calibrated against OBT/79.

In view of the interlaboratory variation observed in multicentre calibration studies, it is recommended that calibration of national reference preparations or manufacturers' 'house' standards be performed by at least two laboratories, and the mean ISI be used for further calibrations.

18.5.4 Calibration of individual lots of thromboplastins

The precision of calibration is greatest when similar materials and methods are compared. For this reason, a national reference preparation or manufacturer's 'house' standard used for the calibration of individual lots of thromboplastin must be a thromboplastin derived from the same tissue of the same species, using a similar manufacturing process. Lot-to-lot calibration must be performed by the manufacturer before release of the thromboplastin.

18.6 CALIBRATION PROCEDURES

18.6.1 Application

Each calibration procedure entails the determination of a series of prothrombin times, using normal and abnormal plasmas or whole blood samples, with both the reference and the test thromboplastin. The tests are performed with either fresh samples from individual subjects (procedure 1) or frozen or lyophilized plasmas (procedure 2). Abnormal plasmas for procedure 1 are obtained from patients undergoing long-term oral anticoagulant treatment. Frozen or lyophilized plasmas for procedure 2 may be pooled plasmas from normal subjects and from patients undergoing long-term oral anticoagulant treatment.

Procedure 1 is recommended for the calibration of secondary standards (e.g. manu-facturers' house standards) against the appropriate IRP and for the calibration of whole blood coagulometers. Procedure 1 can also be used for the calibration of individual batches of thromboplastin against the corresponding secondary standard (i.e. lot-to-lot calibration), but may be replaced by procedure 2 if the same results are obtained.

The precision of the calibration relationship depends on the number of plasmas and on a balanced distribution of normal and abnormal plasmas over the therapeutic range of INR values. The recommended number of abnormal plasmas is three times the number of normal plasmas.

18.6.2 Procedure 1: Calibration of a secondary standard using individual fresh plasma or whole blood samples

This procedure consists of a set of tests using freshly opened or reconstituted thromboplastins and different individual samples of fresh plasma or whole blood. The procedure must be repeated on at least five separate occasions using fresh reagents on each occasion. The procedure need not be repeated on consecutive days but should be completed as soon as possible. The tests in any one laboratory on any one day should be performed by the same person. The order in which the thromboplastins are tested must be changed from day to day (Hermans *et al.*, 1983) to avoid a bias induced by plasma instability. Traditionally, the total numbers of abnormal and normal samples for procedure 1 have been 60 and 20, respectively (Hermans *et al.*, 1983; Thomson *et al.*, 1984).

BLOOD SAMPLES

Blood samples from healthy subjects and patients who have been on oral anticoagulants for at least 6 weeks should be selected. Samples from patients treated with heparin should not be used. It is recommended that patients' samples with INR values in the range 1.5–4.5 are selected. Selection of samples with the reference system may induce a small bias of the calibration line (Van den Besselaar and Van der Velde, 1984; Van den Besselaar *et al.*, 1999). Selection of patient samples may well be performed using the clinic's routine system for monitoring the patients. Once selected, the samples should be used for the calibration even if the INRs determined with the reference system appear to be outside the 1.5–4.5 INR range.

Blood should be obtained by venepuncture, avoiding haemolysis and contamination with tissue fluids, and be drawn either with a plastic syringe and transferred to a plastic tube, or with other non-contact activation equipment. Nine volumes of blood are decalcified with one volume of 0.109 mol/L trisodium citrate solution (Ingram and Hills, 1976). A mixture of trisodium citrate and citric acid is also acceptable if the total citrate plus citric acid concentration is 0.109 mol/L and the pH is no lower than 5. The same procedure and materials must be used for all the samples in a given calibration study.

If evacuated tubes are used for blood collection, their lot number should be noted, as there may be lot-to-lot variation. If evacuated tubes are made of glass, they must be properly siliconized internally and the pH of the trisodium citrate plus citric acid solution must be in the range 5–6 (Van den Besselaar *et al.*, 1983). The sample is centrifuged as soon as it is received, but no later than 2 hours after blood collection. The centrifugation is such that the plasma is rendered poor in platelets. The plasma should be taken off the red cell layer with a plastic pipette, stored undisturbed in a narrow, stoppered, non-contact tube at room temperature and tested within 5 hours after blood collection.

Some techniques or instruments require the use of capillary non-citrated blood (Tripodi *et al.*, 1993). Capillary blood can be obtained by finger or heel puncture. The capillary blood must be obtained without squeezing and should be tested immediately with the technique or instrument to be calibrated. Venous blood is obtained from the same subjects (normals and patients) within 5 minutes for comparative measurements.

THE PROTHROMBIN-TIME TEST

The classical prothrombin-time test is performed by mixing equal volumes of citrated plasma, thromboplastin and calcium chloride solution (0.025 mol/L) (Ingram and Hills, 1976). Alternatively, reagents are available in which thromboplastin and calcium chloride are pre-mixed. The time taken for the mixture to clot when maintained at a temperature of between 36.5 and 37.5°C is recorded. Specific instructions for the test with commercial thromboplastins shall be provided by the manufacturers. Specific instructions for use of IRPs shall be supplied by the custodian of these materials.

The coagulation end-point for IRPs of thromboplastin is detected by the manual (tilt-tube) technique. The coagulation end-point for other thromboplastins is detected by a manual technique or with the aid of an automatic end-point recorder. The same technique must be used throughout the series of tests with a given thromboplastin.

Each laboratory must have a system for internal quality control. Records are maintained of the lot number of all reagents and disposable equipment used. Periodic checks of the temperature of incubation baths or heating blocks and of the volumes of pipettes or pumps are made and recorded (Van den Besselaar *et al.*, 1997).

STATISTICAL EVALUATION

An orthogonal regression line is calculated on the basis of the logarithm of the prothrombin time (log PT) of 20 normal subjects plus 60 patients stabilized on long-term therapy (Van der Velde, 1984). Log PT for the IRP is plotted on the vertical axis and log PT for the test system on the horizontal (Kirkwood, 1983). Orthogonal regression analysis provides an estimate of the standard deviation about the regression line ('residual standard deviation'). Any samples with a perpendicular distance greater than three residual standard deviations from the line are excluded. After removal of the latter samples, the final orthogonal regression line is calculated. The suggested procedure for reporting and calculation of the ISI is given in Appendix A.18.1. To define the ISI of the test system, a sufficient number of separate tests must be carried out to obtain a within-laboratory coefficient of variation of the slope of the orthogonal regression line of 3% or less.

CALIBRATION OF NEAR-PATIENT TESTING DEVICES

A simple bedside prothrombin-time test was described many years ago (Ziffren *et al.*, 1940) as an alternative to the classical prothrombin-time test. In this bedside test, freshly drawn blood without sodium citrate anticoagulant was added immediately to a thromboplastin reagent in a test tube and the clotting time determined by a manual technique. However, the bedside test was never used as widely as the classical prothrombin-time test.

In recent years, portable devices for near-patient coagulation testing have been developed and are now being introduced on the market. These devices are called whole blood analysers or coagulation monitors. In some types, whole blood (either venous or capillary) without sodium citrate anticoagulant is used (Lucas *et al.*, 1987); in other types, citrated whole blood can be used (Oberhardt *et al.*, 1991). All devices consist of a portable instrument or analyser and disposable test cards or cuvettes. The test cards or cuvettes contain a sample application zone connected to a reaction chamber. The reaction chamber contains dried thromboplastin and other particles if required. The test cards or cuvettes are placed in the analyser and the sample is dropped into the sample well and is drawn via capillary action into the reaction chamber, which is maintained in a temperature-controlled 37°C environment. The sample entering the reaction chamber dissolves the thromboplastin reagent and signals the beginning of the timing sequence. In some systems, a laser photometer detects the cessation of blood flow (clotting) by sensing variation in light scatter caused by the movement of red blood cells. Other systems contain paramagnetic iron oxide particles which begin to oscillate in response to an applied oscillating magnetic field. This movement is monitored optically by the analyser. With the onset of fibrin polymerization, a significant restriction in the movement of the paramagnetic iron oxide particles occurs and is detected. The time elapsed between application of blood and cessation of flow or restricted particle movement is measured by the monitor and is converted mathematically to a plasma equivalent prothrombin time or INR. After a prothrombin time or INR is displayed, a new test card may be inserted for the next test.

Several studies have been published comparing INRs read from near-patient coagulation monitors and INRs determined with conventional prothrombin-time systems using commercial reagents (McCurdy and White, 1992; Kapiotis *et al.*, 1995; Gosselin *et al.*, 1997; Ruzicka *et al.*, 1997). Systematic differences in INR have been reported which are probably caused by inaccurate calibration of either the near-patient device or the conventional system, or both.

There are a few publications in which near-patient devices have been calibrated with an IRP according to the WHO guidelines (Tripodi *et al.*, 1993; Kaatz *et al.*, 1995; Kitchen and Preston, 1997; Tripodi *et al.*, 1997). Systematic differences in INR between near-patient device and international reference system have been reported. In one case the INR bias was attributed to erroneous ISI determination by the monitor's manufacturer (Tripodi *et al.*, 1993). In other studies, the manufacturer's MNPT value appeared to be the cause of INR differences between monitor and international reference system (Tripodi *et al.*, 1997; Kitchen and Preston, 1997). ISI and MNPT values determined by the manufacturer are encoded in the test cards and cannot be changed by the user. It has been suggested (Tripodi *et al.*, 1997) that the option for the user to change ISI and MNPT encoded in the test card should be offered by the manufacturers of near-patient devices.

18.6.3 Procedure 2: Calibration of individual lots of thromboplastin

Calibration of individual lots of thromboplastin may be carried out with pooled normal plasmas and pooled coumarin plasmas or plasmas artificially depleted of vitamin K-dependent coagulation factors (Van den Besselaar *et al.*, 1980; Denson, 1986). The number of plasma pools required for precise calibration is, in general, much smaller than the number of fresh individual plasma samples required for procedure 1. The scatter of data points about the line of relationship is relatively small because the test lot is very similar to the secondary standard and/or because the biological variation caused by individual samples is reduced by the pooling of plasmas. It has been reported that lot-to-lot calibration of bovine and rabbit thromboplastins could be performed with as few as three plasma pools (Van den Besselaar *et al.*, 1980; Denson, 1986), but the accuracy of such a simplified procedure may depend on the quality of the pooled plasmas and the thromboplastins being compared. At least three plasma pools are required to permit the testing of linearity. When one normal plasma pool is used, at least two different abnormal plasma pools are necessary with an INR of between 1.5 and 4.5 and a difference of at least 1.0 in their INRs. It is recommended that any procedure using pooled or artificially depleted plasmas is validated against the fresh plasma procedure (procedure 1).

The requirements for pooled plasmas are detailed in the revised guidelines issued by WHO (1999). The citrate concentration for pooled plasmas must be the same as the concentration for fresh individual plasmas (see procedure 1). For deep-frozen and lyophilized plasmas, the pH must be within the 7.3–7.9 interval and the factor V content within 60–140 U/dL to avoid INR discrepancies (Tripodi *et al.*, 1995b). To obtain an acceptable degree of precision, the prothrombin-time testing procedure is repeated on at least four separate occasions (Tripodi *et al.*, 1996).

STATISTICAL EVALUATION

An orthogonal regression line is calculated on the basis of log PT of the pooled plasmas. Individual determinations are entered when multiple determinations for each plasma pool are available. Log PT for the reference system (house standard) is plotted on the vertical axis, and log PT for the test batch of thromboplastin on the horizontal. Determinations at a perpendicular distance greater than three residual standard deviations from the line are removed before the final orthogonal regression line is calculated.

To define the ISI of a batch of thromboplastin, a sufficient number of tests is carried out to obtain a within-laboratory coefficient of variation of the slope of the orthogonal regression line of 3% or less. The recommended procedure for calculation of the ISI is given in Appendix A.18.2.

Manufacturers of commercial reagents should state on the package insert the ISI of the relevant batch of thromboplastin together with the IRP against which it has been determined and the instrument for which it is valid.

18.7 LOCAL SYSTEM CALIBRATION

One approach to correcting for instrument and reagent effects is for each laboratory to determine its own 'local system ISI' with lyophilized plasmas calibrated centrally using an international reference thromboplastin and the manual technique (Poller *et al.*, 1994, 1995a,b). In this way the local laboratory avoids using an international reference thromboplastin and the manual technique for prothrombin-time testing. However, this approach still requires the determination of the MNPT, which involves measuring the prothrombin time of at least 20 normal subjects. Determination of local system ISI and MNPT is a time-consuming process and ideally should be repeated with each batch of reagent. Many laboratories are unable to undertake this extra workload and so tend to use the ISI and MNPT values provided by the manufacturers of the thromboplastins.

Several studies have been performed to test whether a reduction in the number of calibrant plasmas is possible without compromising the reliability of the calibration. The minimum number of samples needed for reliable local system ISI calibration using a manual technique and a low ISI thromboplastin is 20 abnormal lyophilized plasma samples and seven lyophilized normal plasma samples (Poller *et al.*, 1998). Other studies have shown that plasma selection becomes critical when less than 12 samples are used (Dufty *et al.*, 1997). These observations were based on the use of individual plasmas from single sources. It is possible, however, that plasma pools from multiple donors may reduce the biological variation and permit the use of fewer calibrant plasmas. In fact, it has been shown that accurate and precise ISI values could be obtained for two rabbit thromboplastins using a set of two lyophilized plasma pools from normal donors and six lyophilized pools from patients on long-term oral anticoagulant treatment (Tripodi *et al.*, 1996). Three days of repeated testing were required to achieve acceptable precision of the slope of the regression line.

Since adsorbed plasma calibrants do not completely mimic plasmas from patients stabilized on oral anticoagulant therapy, there is an expectation that the use of coumarin plasmas may be more appropriate. Poller *et al.* (1995b) concluded that the agreement between adsorbed and coumarin plasma calibrants in calculation of system ISI was reassuring. In contrast, Stevenson *et al.* (1997) demonstrated that lyophilized coumarin plasma calibrants are superior in system ISI calibration.

An alternative approach to INR estimation is the use of INR calibrated reference plasmas, which does not require the determination of a local system ISI or MNPT (Van den Besselaar, 1994a; Houbouyan and Goguel, 1997; Hubbard *et al.*, 1997). This method uses at least three calibrated reference plasmas to construct a calibration curve by plotting the local PT against the assigned INR. The INR value of test plasma samples can then be directly interpolated from the local PT (Fig. 18.4). This method has been found to give major improvements in inter-laboratory variability (Houbouyan and Goguel, 1997).

Standard lyophilized plasmas with INR values assigned against RBT/90 have been used for local verification of the accuracy of the INR (Critchfield *et al.*, 1996). To perform reliable calibration verification, the assigned INR values of the plasma standards must be accurate. Manufacturers must assign INR values by techniques that are independent of the working prothrombin time method used in a laboratory, to ensure a more absolute standard of INR 'truth'. Manufacturers of plasma standards must warrant that their INRs have been assigned properly so that laboratories can be confident of the accuracy of INR assignment.

Differential performance of standard plasmas across different reagent/instrument systems ('matrix effects') can be a problem. Truly 'universal' plasma standards would ideally behave like real patient specimens across different analytical systems. This may be difficult to achieve (Van den Besselaar, 1996b, 1997). When it is not possible to assign a single INR value to a given lyophilized plasma, it may be useful to assign reagent-specific INR-equivalent values (Van den Besselaar, 1997). It will be important for manufacturers to specify clearly the set of reagent/instrument combinations for which their plasma standards may be reliably used (Critchfield *et al.*, 1996).

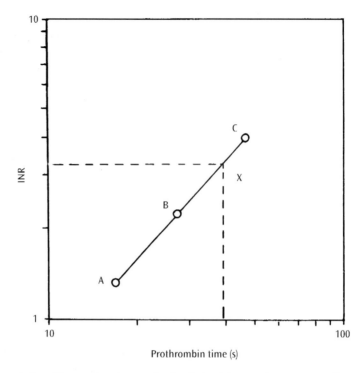

Fig. 18.4 *Interpolation of international normalized ratio (INR) for test plasma X, according to Hubbard* et al. *(1997). The calibration curve is constructed by plotting local prothrombin time against assigned INR value for reference plasmas A, B and C. (Reprinted by permission of Blackwell Science Ltd, Oxford, UK.)*

18.8 PRE-ANALYTICAL CONDITIONS

18.8.1 Blood sampling

Many pre-analytical conditions may affect the results of routine coagulation assays. NCCLS (the National Committee for Clinical Laboratory Standards) recommends that coagulation testing, including prothrombin time, is not performed on plasma from the first blood tube drawn from a patient, but on plasma from a second or subsequent tube drawn during the same phlebotomy (NCCLS, 1991). This guideline is based on the assumption that tissue factor is likely to contaminate the first tube and produce erroneous test results. Several studies have shown that no statistically or clinically significant difference was found in the prothrombin times measured on the first or second tube (Yawn *et al.*, 1996; Brigden *et al.*, 1997; Gottfried and Adachi, 1997). Thus, under the real-life working conditions of a busy hospital or out-patient clinic, in which experienced phlebotomists draw blood specimens, the first tube yields accurate results for the prothrombin time and protocols that call for discarding the first tube drawn are unnecessary.

18.8.2 Sodium citrate concentration

Sodium citrate is the recommended anticoagulant for routine blood coagulation assays. Nine volumes of blood should be mixed with one volume of sodium citrate solution. The prothrombin-time ratio is influenced by the calcium chloride concentration for recalcification (Van den Besselaar, 1994b) and it can be inferred that the ionized calcium rather than total calcium concentration determines the clotting times. Since the citrate concentration influences the ionized calcium concentration, it can be inferred that the prothrombin-time ratio can be influenced by the sodium citrate concentration. Different sodium citrate concentrations are being used by clinical laboratories for anticoagulation of blood specimens. Many laboratories use 3.8% trisodium citrate (i.e. 0.129 mol/L), but others favour 3.2% (i.e. 0.109 mol/L). Recent studies have shown that results of routine coagulation tests may depend on the concentration of citrate used (Adcock et al., 1997). Duncan et al. (1994) reported that the citrate concentration can affect the calculation of the INR and the ISI-calibration of certain thromboplastins. Since a concentration of 0.109 mol/L trisodium citrate ($C_6H_5Na_3O_7.2H_2O$) has been used in major studies to calibrate IRPs, it is the recommended anticoagulant for coagulation testing and should be adopted worldwide.

18.8.3 Centrifugation

It is recommended that the blood sample be centrifuged as soon as received by the laboratory. The centrifugation shall be such that the plasma is rendered platelet-poor, i.e. at least $2500 \times g$ for 10 minutes, at a controlled room temperature (18–24°C).

18.8.4 Storage of blood

The stability of blood specimens for prothrombin time testing has been investigated in various studies. Both shortening and prolongation of clotting times have been observed depending on the conditions of storage. Temperature, pH, type of container, time of storage and thromboplastin are important parameters. Prothrombin time shortening occurs when whole blood is stored in borosilicate or siliconized borosilicate tubes at 4°C (Palmer et al., 1982). Subsequent studies have demonstrated the pivotal roles of the contact phase of coagulation in initiating activation of the prothrombin time (Palmer and Gralnick, 1982, 1984). Prothrombin time shortening also occurs when whole blood is stored at room temperature, even in siliconized tubes (Palmer et al., 1982; Thomson et al., 1983; Van den Besselaar et al., 1983). Shortening of the prothrombin time occurs also in plasmas when separated immediately after centrifugation and stored at room temperature (Ho and Wu, 1991). Shortening of the prothrombin time occurs predominantly in the first 4 hours after blood collection. Prolongation of the prothrombin time is observed mostly after 24 hours or longer (Baglin and Luddington, 1997; Brigden et al., 1997). The magnitude of the change of the INR depends on the reagent used (Baglin and Luddington, 1997). These authors concluded that there is no clinically significant change in the INR when analysis is delayed for up to 3 days with any thromboplastin. This contrasts with the requirement of testing plasmas for calibration within 5 hours after blood collection.

18.8.5 Influence of containers

Both the needle/syringe method and evacuated blood collection systems are in widespread use by clinical laboratories. Glass syringes and evacuated tubes should be properly siliconized to avoid contact activation (Van den Besselaar et al., 1983). It should be realized that the silicone layer on the interior glass tube wall becomes unstable when it is in contact with non-buffered trisodium citrate solution (pH > 8). Such systems eventually induced contact activation when the silicone layer had deteriorated under the influence of the citrate solution (Van den Besselaar and Loeliger, 1982). Silicone layers in contact with mixtures of sodium citrate and citric acid (pH 5–6) are much more stable.

The reduced pressure in the evacuated tubes should be such that the volume ratio of blood drawn to citrate solution is 9:1. Evacuated blood collection tubes can influence the prothrombin-time ratio and hence the ISI (Table 18.1). These effects may be caused by contact with different tube surfaces or by different composition of the anticoagulant (citrate) solutions in these tubes. Untoward effects of blood collection systems should be eliminated by rigorous standardization of these systems (Van den Besselaar *et al.*, 1998).

Table 18.1 *Mean prothrombin time (PT), prothrombin time ratio and international sensitivity index (ISI). Blood specimens were collected by venepuncture using three evacuated systems: Vacuette (Greiner Labortechnik, Kremsmunster, Austria) (lot 099710), Vacutainer (Becton Dickinson, Franklin Lakes, New Jersey, USA) (lot 6K883), and Venoject (Terumo Europe, Leuven, Belgium) (lot 97F26L1). PT was determined with Recombiplastin (Ortho Clinical Diagnostics) (lot RTF-159) on an MLA Electra-1800, and with Recombiplastin lot RTF-167 on a KC-10 steel ball coagulometer. The ISI of the latter system had been determined previously with plasma samples collected in Vacutainer tubes and was used as a reference system for calculation of the ISI of the other systems. The coefficients of variation (CVs) of the slopes of the orthogonal regression lines (log PT of the reference system plotted against log PT with the other system) are given as percentages. Differences between PT ratios obtained with Vacutainer tubes and either Vacuette or Venoject were tested with Student's t-test on paired observations. A significant difference (P < 0.01) is indicated by an asterisk*

Instrument	Blood collection tube	Mean PT (s) Normals (*n* = 21)	Patients (*n* = 80)	Mean PT ratio	ISI	CV of slope
MLA 1800	Vacuette	11.6	37.9	3.26*	0.95	0.8
MLA1800	Vacutainer	11.2	32.9	2.94	1.04	0.8
MLA1800	Venoject	10.9	31.7	2.92	1.05	0.8
KC10	Vacuette	10.7	39.3	3.66*	0.87	0.7
KC10	Vacutainer	10.3	36.1	3.50	0.90	–
KC10	Venoject	10.0	33.8	3.38*	0.92	0.6

18.9 LYOPHILIZED PLASMAS

18.9.1 General

Lyophilized plasmas are used for internal and external quality assessment (Preston, 1995) and have been investigated for local ISI and INR calibration (Houbouyan and Goguel, 1997; Hubbard *et al.*, 1997; Poller *et al.*, 1997). The advantage of lyophilized plasmas is their good stability. They can be stored for years at 4°C and be shipped at ambient temperatures without loss of activity. Lyophilized materials have been prepared, not only from individual donations but also by pooling donations from many individuals or patients treated with oral anticoagulants. In addition, lyophilized materials have been prepared from pooled normal plasma by artificial depletion of coagulation factors. Artificial depletion may be performed by adsorption onto aluminium hydroxide or barium sulphate.

18.9.2 Effects of buffering and freeze-drying

Prior to lyophilization, a buffer must be added to plasma to stabilize the pH and the pro-thrombin time (Zucker *et al.*, 1970). Many manufacturers use N-2-hydroxyethyl-piperazinc-N′-2-ethanesulphonic acid (HEPES) because it provides excellent pH and coagulation factor stability. Addition of HEPES prolongs the PT and INR in a dose-dependent way, caused by a decrease of the pH. After lyophilization, the pH is increased due to loss of carbon dioxide and the INR is reduced (Table 18.2). Hubbard *et al.* (1997) suggested using an optimal HEPES concentration of 20 mmol/L. After lyophilization, the turbidity of plasma is increased, which may influence the clotting times determined by photo-optical instruments (Hirst and Poller, 1992). The residual moisture content of the lyophilized product is critical for stability, and secondary desiccation with P_2O_5 resulted in improved stability (Lang and Kleindel, 1984). It has been reported that the effect of freeze-drying on the PT ratio may depend on the type of thromboplastin reagent (Poller *et al.*, 1999).

Table 18.2   *International normalized ratio (INR) equivalent values for pooled coumarin plasma. Samples were tested in different stages of processing this plasma towards a lyophilized product. HEPES/glycine (1% w/v) was added before dispensing in siliconized glass vials. INRs were assessed with Thrombotest (bovine brain thromboplastin, combined), Diagen (rabbit brain thromboplastin, plain), British Comparative Thromboplastin (BCT, a human brain thromboplastin, plain) and Simplastin (rabbit brain/lung thromboplastin, plain)*

Stage of processing	INR (Thrombotest)	INR (Diagen)	INR (BCT)	INR (Simplastin)
Plasma without addition	2.2	2.5	2.8	2.9
Plus HEPES and glycine	2.7	3.0	3.0	3.3
Beginning of filling vials	2.7	3.0	3.0	3.3
End of filling vials	2.7	3.1	2.9	3.1
Lyophilized product	2.5	2.5	2.7	2.7

18.10 EXTERNAL QUALITY ASSESSMENT

18.10.1 External quality assessment schemes

External quality assessment schemes (EQASs) in chemistry and haematology have been established in a number of countries (Preston, 1995). These vary considerably in respect of the number of analytes offered, the number of participants, the source and composition of samples, and the frequency of distribution. In this chapter, only EQASs of INR determinations will be considered. Participants are requested to determine the INR using their routine method and thromboplastin. The results are returned to the scheme organizer for analysis, and individual participant's results are then related using various statistical methods to produce either overall or group mean or median values.

The primary function of EQAS is optimal patient care through improved laboratory performance. This is largely achieved through the analysis of individual laboratory results and the identification of those laboratories which are performing poorly. EQASs with large numbers of participants have considerable advantage over smaller schemes in that the large volume of data generated by participants also permits an analysis of reagent and instrument performance. This is of considerable value to scheme participants, manufacturers and purchasers. The advantage of the INR system is that for any given patient sample, approximately the same INR will be obtained irrespective of the thromboplastin and method used. However, the EQA schemes in both the UK (Kitchen *et al.*, 1994) and the Netherlands (Van den Besselaar, 1994a, 1997) have demonstrated thromboplastin-related differences in results of INR determination. One possible explanation for these discrepancies is the preparation and/or lyophilization process of the survey samples.

It should be realized that variability caused by pre-analytical conditions is not adequately reflected by EQAS. The survey samples are the same for all participants, but the local MNPT and ISI are influenced by pre-analytical conditions such as blood collection tubes (Van den Besselaar *et al.*, 1998). Thus, when two laboratories obtain the same prothrombin time for a survey sample using the same reagent and instrument, their INRs calculated for the sample may be different because of different local MNPT values (Peters *et al.*, 1991).

In the Netherlands, two EQA schemes have been established which include the INR. The first EQA scheme is organized by the Federation of Netherlands Thrombosis Centres and was originally devised for the member laboratories using the Thrombotest® method for whole blood samples (Van Dijk-Wierda *et al.*, 1980). The Thrombotest® reagent is composed of bovine brain thromboplastin and adsorbed bovine plasma ('combined' reagent) and has an ISI close to 1.0. The survey samples for this scheme consist of artificial blood prepared by combining various pooled plasmas with red cells. The artificial blood samples are mailed to the participants at ambient temperatures. In general, participants receive the samples within 24 hours. Ambient temperature differences between various parts of the Netherlands are small because of the influence of the Gulf Stream and the small distances in this flat country. The blood samples deteriorate slowly but this process is the same for samples mailed to different parts of the country. It is essential that all participants store the samples at room temperature and perform the determinations on the same day, i.e. 4 days after preparation. In the 1990s many participants of this scheme replaced their routine Thrombotest method with plain thromboplastin systems. These participants can use the same survey specimens, after centrifugation.

In Figures 18.5 and 18.6, the between-laboratory variation of the INR is plotted as a function of the mean INR calculated for each survey sample. For the Thrombotest users, a different pattern was observed when compared with the pattern for the users of a plain rabbit thromboplastin (PT-HS, Instrumentation Laboratory) with an ISI of approximately 1.4. For the rabbit thromboplastin, the CV of the INRs tended to increase with increasing mean INR values (Fig. 18.5). In contrast, the CV of the INRs determined by Thrombotest users did not show such a trend, but appeared to be more or less constant for mean INRs between 2 and 4 (Fig. 18.6). One should be cautious in the interpretation of these results, and three points should be considered. First, Thrombotest determinations were performed with whole blood as provided by the scheme, whereas the plain thromboplastins were used with plasma obtained after centrifugation. Variability in the centrifugation step might increase the CV of the INR. Second, different types of instrument are used for Thrombotest and the plain thromboplastin reagents. Instruments are an integral part of the prothrombin time system and may influence the CV. Third, outlier values were excluded for calculation of the CV, but the exclusion limits depend on the number of participants (Reijnierse *et al.*, 1989). There were approximately 70 participants using Thrombotest in 1996, but only 22 participants using the plain rabbit thromboplastin PT-HS in the same period. The variability of the CV is greater for small groups of participants than for large groups. Thus, it cannot be excluded that differences in CV are related to different numbers of participants.

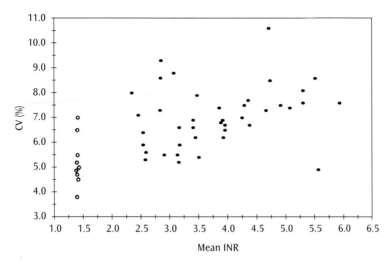

Fig. 18.5 *Between-laboratory variation of the international normalized ratio (INR) expressed as coefficient of variation (CV) in the external quality assessment scheme organized by the Federation of Netherlands Thrombosis Centres. Results were obtained by participants using reagent PT-HS (Instrumentation Laboratory) in 10 surveys in 1996. The mean INR of each sample calculated for these participants is plotted on the horizontal axis. Open symbols, samples prepared from pooled normal plasmas; filled symbols, samples prepared from pooled coumarin plasmas.*

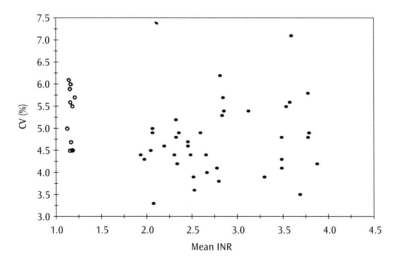

Fig. 18.6 *Between-laboratory variation of the international normalized ratio (INR) for EQAS participants using the Thrombotest (Nycomed) reagent. For further information, see Figure 18.5 caption.*

The second national (Netherlands) EQA scheme in blood coagulation is based on lyophilized plasma samples, as in most other countries. Survey samples are prepared by pooling large numbers of individual coumarin patients' samples. The advantage of lyophilized samples is their long-term stability and their possible use in multiple surveys. Typical results obtained through the two schemes are shown in Table 18.3. INR values reported by PT-HS

Table 18.3 *Results of international normalized ratio (INR) external quality assessment schemes in the Netherlands. Artificial blood samples are used in scheme I, lyophilized plasma samples in scheme II. Results are analysed according to reagent used by participants. n, number of participants; CV, coefficient of between-laboratory variation*

Reagent	Scheme I (Dec. 1997)			Scheme II (Sept. 1997)		
	n	Mean INR	CV (%)	*n*	Mean INR	CV (%)
Thrombotest	45	4.1	7.0	6	3.4	7.5
Recombiplastin	18	4.8	6.1	12	4.5	9.5
PT-HS (Instr. Lab.)	24	5.3	6.0	30	4.8	5.4
Thromborel-S	9	4.9	6.4	13	4.1	3.0
HepatoQuick	15	4.1	5.0	13	4.1	8.0
Innovin	–	–	–	11	4.1	8.7

users are systematically higher than INRs reported by Thrombotest, Innovin, Thromborel-S, and HepatoQuick users. However, the order of the mean INR values is not the same for the lyophilized plasma and artificial blood samples. In scheme II, mean INR values for Thromborel-S and HepatoQuick are practically the same, but in scheme I, mean INRs for Thromborel-S are always greater than those for HepatoQuick. It is unlikely that these differences are caused by calibration errors because participants of both schemes obtain their information from the same sources. Furthermore, there is considerable overlap of participants in the two schemes. These and other results from the author's laboratory (Van den Besselaar, 1997) demonstrate that there is an important interaction between the prothrombin-time system and the sample. It is not possible to determine a single INR value for a survey sample which is valid for all reagents (Van den Besselaar, 1997).

18.10.2 Performance criteria for EQAS participants

In the UK EQAS, individual participant's results are compared with the median value for the thromboplastin group to which the participants belong (Preston, 1995). Where there are less than 10 users of any thromboplastin, the individual's result is compared with the overall median value. If the participant's result is more than 15% removed from the median value to which it is compared, it is classed as an unsatisfactory performance.

In the EQAS organized by the Federation of Netherlands Thrombosis Centres, performance is assessed in terms of the deviation index (DI) (Lewis, 1988):

$$DI = (x - x_m)/SD$$

where x is the participant's result, x_m is the mean, and SD is the interlaboratory standard deviation of the INR values for the thromboplastin group to which the participants belong. When there are less than six users of any thromboplastin, the performance of the individual's result is not assessed in terms of the DI. The overall mean or median INR values may not be appropriate to assess the performance of minority thromboplastin users when there are important INR differences between thromboplastin groups as in Table 18.3. An alternative and more acceptable method is to assess the performance of the individual participant's result by comparison to a value determined by an established reference laboratory or group of reference laboratories using the same or similar prothrombin-time system.

REFERENCES

Adcock, D.M., Kressin, D.C. and Marlar, R.A. (1997) Effect of 3.2% vs 3.8% sodium citrate concentration on routine coagulation testing. *Am. J. Clin. Pathol.* **107**, 105–10.

Baglin, T. and Luddington, R. (1997) Reliability of delayed INR determination: implication for decentralized anticoagulant care with off-site blood sampling. *Br. J. Haematol.* **96**, 431–4.

Bangham, D.R., Biggs, R., Brozovic, M. and Denson, K.W.E. (1973) Calibration of five different thromboplastins, using fresh and freeze-dried plasma. *Thrombos. Diathes. Haemorrh.* **29**, 228–39.

Barcellona, D., Biondi, G., Vannini, M.L. and Marongiu, F. (1996) Comparison between recombinant and rabbit thromboplastin in the management of patients on oral anticoagulant therapy. *Thromb. Haemost.* **75**, 488–90.

Blombäck, M., Abildgaard, U., Van den Besselaar, A.M.H.P. *et al.* (1994) Nomenclature of quantities and units in thrombosis and haemostasis (Recommendations 1993). *Thromb. Haemost.* **71**, 375–94.

Boekhout-Mussert, M.J., Van der Kolk-Schaap, P.J., Hermans, J. and Loeliger, E.A. (1981) Prospective double-blind clinical trial of bovine, human, and rabbit thromboplastins in monitoring long-term oral anticoagulation. *Am. J. Clin. Pathol.* **75**, 297–303.

Brigden, M.L., Graydon, C., McLeod, B. and Lesperance, M. (1997) Prothrombin time determination. The lack of need for a discard tube and 24-hour stability. *Am. J. Clin. Pathol.* **108**, 422–6.

British Society for Haematology (1990) Guidelines on oral anticoagulant: second edition. *J. Clin. Pathol.* **43**, 177–83.

Brophy, M.T., Fiore, L.D., Lau, J. *et al.* (1994) Comparison of a standard and a sensitive thromboplastin in monitoring low intensity oral anticoagulant therapy. *Am. J. Clin. Pathol.* **102**, 134–7.

Burgess-Wilson, M.E., Burri, R. and Woodhaus, B.J. (1993) Important differences encountered in the normal plasma pools used for the control of oral anticoagulation. *Thromb. Haemost.* **69**, 1124.

Chantarangkul, V., Tripodi, A. and Mannucci, P.M. (1992) The effect of instrumentation on thromboplastin calibration. *Thromb. Haemost.* **67**, 588–9.

Craig, S., Stevenson, K.J., Dufty, J.M.K. and Taberner, D.A. (1997) Local INR correction: justification for a simplified approach. *J. Clin. Pathol.* **50**, 783–9.

Creasy, M.A. (1956) Confidence limits for the gradient in the linear functional relationship. *J. R. Stat. Soc. B.* **18**, 65–9.

Critchfield, G.C., Bennett, S.T. and Swaim, W.R. (1996) Calibration verification of the international normalized ratio. *Am. J. Clin. Pathol.* **106,** 786–94.

D'Angelo, A., Seveso, M.P., D'Angelo, S.V. *et al.* (1989) Comparison of two automated coagulometers and the manual tilt-tube method for the determination of prothrombin time. *Am. J. Clin. Pathol.* **92**, 321–8.

Denson, K.W.E. (1986) Artificially depleted plasma for manufacturers international calibration of thromboplastin. *Clin. Lab. Haematol.* **8**, 55–60.

Dufty, J.M.K., Craig, S., Stevenson, K.J. and Taberner, D.A. (1997) Calculation of system international sensitivity index: how many calibrant plasmas are required? *J. Clin. Pathol.* **50**, 40–4.

Duncan, E.M., Casey, C.R., Duncan, B.M. and Lloyd, J.V. (1994) Effect of concentration of trisodium citrate anticoagulant on calculation of the international normalised ratio and the international sensitivity index of thromboplastin. *Thromb. Haemost.* **72**, 84–8.

Finazzi, G., Falanga, A., Galli, M. *et al.* (1994) Recombinant versus high-sensitivity conventional thromboplastin: a randomized clinical study in patients on oral anticoagulation. *Thromb. Haemost.* **75**, 804–7.

Finney, D.J. (1995) Calibration of thromboplastins. *Proc. R. Soc. Lond. B.* **262**, 71–5.

Gogstad, G.O., Wadt, J., Smith, P. and Brynildsrud, T. (1986) Utility of a modified calibration model for reliable conversion of thromboplastin times to international normalized ratios. *Thromb. Haemost.* **56**, 178–82.

Gosselin, R.C., Owings, J.T., Lankin, E. *et al.* (1997) Monitoring oral anticoagulant therapy with point-of-care devices: correlations and caveats. *Clin. Chem.* **43**, 1785–6.

Gottfried, E.L. and Adachi, M.M. (1997) Prothrombin time and activated partial thromboplastin time can be performed on the first tube. *Am. J. Clin. Pathol.* **107**, 681–3.

Hermans, J., Van den Besselaar, A.M.H.P., Loeliger, E.A. and Van der Velde, E.A. (1983) A collaborative calibration study of reference materials for thromboplastins. *Thromb. Haemost.* **50**, 712–17.

Hirsh, J., Dalen, J.E., Deykin, D. *et al.* (1995) Oral anticoagulants. Mechanism of action, clinical effectiveness, and optimal therapeutic range. *Chest* **108**(supplement), 231–46S.

Hirst, C.F. and Poller, L. (1992) The cause of turbidity in lyophilised plasmas and its effects on coagulation tests. *J. Clin. Pathol.* **45**, 701–3.

Ho, C.-H. and Wu, S.-Y. (1991) The influence of time, temperature and packed cells on activated partial thromboplastin time and prothrombin time. *Thromb. Res.* **62**, 625–33.

Houbouyan, L.L. and Goguel, A.F. (1997) Long-term French experience in INR standardization by a procedure using plasma calibrants. *Am. J. Clin. Pathol.* **108**, 83–9.

Hubbard, A.R., Margetts, S.M.L. and Barrowcliffe, T.W. (1997) International normalized ratio determination using calibrated reference plasmas. *Br. J. Haematol.* **98**, 74–8.

Ingram, G.I.C. and Hills, M. (1976) Reference method for the one-stage prothrombin time test on human blood. *Thromb. Haemost.* **36**, 237–8.

Kaatz, S.S., White, R.H., Hill, J. *et al.* (1995) Accuracy of laboratory and portable monitor international normalized ratio determinations. *Arch. Intern. Med.* **155**, 1861–7.

Kapiotis, S., Quehenberger, P. and Speiser, W. (1995) Evaluation of the new method Coaguchek for the determination of prothrombin time from capillary blood: comparison with Thrombotest on KC-1. *Thromb. Res.* **77**, 563–7.

Kirkwood, T.B.L. (1983) Calibration of reference thromboplastins and standardisation of the prothrombin time ratio. *Thromb. Haemost.* **49**, 238.

Kitchen, S. and Preston, F.E. (1997) Monitoring oral anticoagulant treatment with the TAS near-patient test system: comparison with conventional thromboplastins. *J. Clin. Pathol.* **50**, 951–6.

Kitchen, S., Walker, I.D., Woods, T.A.L. and Preston, F.E. (1994) Thromboplastin related differences in the determination of international normalised ratio: a cause for concern? *Thromb. Haemost.* **72**, 426–9.

Lang, H. and Kleindel, M. (1984) Prüfung der Lagerstabilität von lyophilisiertem AK-Plasma durch beschleunigte Degradation. *Berichte der ÖGKC* **7,** 93–6.

Lewis, S.M. (1988) External quality assessment. In: Lewis, S.M., Verwilghen, R.L. (eds), *Quality Assurance in Haematology*. London: Baillière Tindall, 151–75.

Loeliger, E.A. (1985) ICSH/ICTH Recommendations for reporting prothrombin time in oral anticoagulant control. *Thromb. Haemost.* **53,** 155–6.

Loeliger, E.A. and Lewis, S.M. (1982) Progress in laboratory control of oral anticoagulants. *Lancet* **ii**, 318–20.

Loeliger, E.A., Van den Besselaar, A.M.H.P. and Lewis, S.M. (1985) Reliability and clinical impact of the normalization of the prothrombin times in oral anticoagulant control. *Thromb. Haemost.* **53**, 148–54.

Lucas, F.V., Duncan, A., Jay, R. *et al.* (1987) A novel whole blood capillary technic for measuring the prothrombin time. *Am. J. Clin. Pathol.* **88**, 442–6.

McCurdy, S.A. and White, R.H. (1992) Accuracy and precision of a portable anticoagulation monitor in a clinical setting. *Arch. Intern. Med.* **152**, 589–92.

National Committee for Clinical Laboratory Standards (NCCLS) (1991) Collection, transport and preparation of blood specimens for coagulation testing and performance of coagulation assays. *NCCLS document, H21-A2*. Villanova, PA: NCCLS.

Oberhardt, B.J., Dermott, S.C., Taylor, M. *et al.* (1991) Dry reagents technology for rapid, convenient measurements of blood coagulation and fibrinolysis. *Clin. Chem.* **37**, 520–6.

Palmer, R.N. and Gralnick, H.R. (1982) Cold-induced contact surface activation of the prothrombin time in whole blood. *Blood* **59**, 38–42.

Palmer, R.N. and Gralnick, H.R. (1984) Inhibition of the cold activation of factor VII and the prothrombin time. *Am. J. Clin. Pathol.* **81**, 618–22.

Palmer, R.N., Kessler, C.M. and Gralnick, H.R. (1982) Warfarin coagulation; difficulties in interpretation of the prothrombin time. *Thromb. Res.* **25**, 125–30.

Peters, R.H.M., Van den Besselaar, A.M.H.P. and Olthuis, F.M.F.G. (1989) A multi-centre study to evaluate method dependency of the international sensitivity index of bovine thromboplastin. *Thromb. Haemost.* **61**, 166–9.

Peters, R.H.M., Van den Besselaar, A.M.H.P. and Olthuis, F.M.F.G. (1991) Determination of the mean normal prothrombin time for assessment of international normalized ratios. *Thromb. Haemost.* **66**, 442–5.

Poggio, M., Van den Besselaar, A.M.H.P., Van der Velde, E.A. and Bertina, R.M. (1989) The effect of some instruments for prothrombin time testing on the International Sensitivity Index (ISI) of two rabbit tissue thromboplastin reagents. *Thromb. Haemost.* **62**, 868–74.

Poller, L. (1996) European concerted action on anticoagulation (ECAA). *Haemostasis* **26**(supplement 4), 266–8.

Poller, L., Taberner, D.A., Thomson, J.M. *et al.* (1993) Effect of the choice of WHO International Reference Preparation for thromboplastin on International Normalized Ratios. *J. Clin. Pathol.* **46**, 64–6.

Poller, L., Thomson, J.M., Taberner, D.A. and Clarke, D.K. (1994) The correction of coagulometer effects on international normalized ratios: a multicentre evaluation. *Br. J. Haematol.* **86**, 112–17.

Poller, L., Triplett, D.A., Hirsh, J. *et al.* (1995a). The value of plasma calibrants in correcting coagulometer effects on international normalised ratios: an international multicentre study. *Am. J. Clin. Pathol.* **103**, 358–65.

Poller, L., Triplett, D.A., Hirsh, J. *et al.* (1995b). A comparison of lyophilised artificially depleted plasmas and lyophilised plasmas from patients receiving warfarin in correcting for coagulometer effects on International Normalised Ratios. *Am. J. Clin. Pathol.* **103**, 366–71.

Poller, L., Barrowcliffe, T.W., Van den Besselaar, A.M.H.P. *et al.* (1996) European concerted action on anticoagulation (ECAA) – the multicentre calibration of rabbit and human ECAA reference thromboplastins. *Thromb. Haemost.* **76**, 977–82.

Poller, L., Barrowcliffe, T.W., Van den Besselaar, A.M.H.P. *et al.* (1997) A simplified statistical method for local INR using linear regression. *Br. J. Haematol.* **98**, 640–7.

Poller, L., Barrowcliffe, T.W., Van den Besselaar, A.M.H.P. *et al.* (1998) Minimum lyophilized plasma requirement for ISI calibration. *Am. J. Clin. Pathol.* **109**, 196–204.

Poller, L., Keown, M., Shepherd, S.A. *et al.* (1999) The effects of freeze drying and freeze drying additives on the prothrombin time and the international sensitivity index. *J. Clin. Pathol.* **52**, 744–8.

Preston, F.E. (1995) Quality control and oral anticoagualation. *Thromb. Haemost.* **74**, 515–20.

Ray, M.J. and Smith, I.R. (1990) The dependence of the international sensitivity index on the coagulometer used to perform the prothrombin time. *Thromb. Haemost.* **63**, 424–9.

Reijnierse, G.L.A., Van den Besselaar, A.M.H.P. and Hermans, J. (1989) Een nieuw verwerkingsprogramma van ingezonden uitslagen in het kader van externe kwaliteitsbewaking. Ervaringen in 1988. *Tijdschr NVKC* **14**, 122–7.

Ruzicka, K., Kapiotis, S., Quehenberger, P. *et al.* (1997) Evaluation of bedside prothrombin time and activated partial thromboplastin time measurement by coagulation analyzer. Coaguchek Plus in various clinical settings. *Thromb. Res.* **87**, 431–40.

Stevenson, K.J., Craig, S., Dufty, J.M.K. and Taberner, D.A. (1997) System ISI calibration: a universally applicable scheme is possible only when coumarin plasma calibrants are used. *Br. J. Haematol.* **96**, 435–41.

Thomson, J.M., Easton, A.C. and Faragher, E.B. (1983) The use of vacutainer tubes for collection and storage of blood for coagulation testing. *Clin. Lab. Haematol.* **5**, 413–21.

Thomson, J.M., Tomenson, J.A. and Poller, L. (1984) The calibration of the second primary international reference preparation for thromboplastin (thromboplastin, human, plain, coded BCT/253). *Thromb. Haemost.* **52**, 336–42.

Tomenson, J.A. (1984) A statistician's independent evaluation. In: van den Besselaar, A.M.H.P., Gralnick, H.R., Lewis, S.M. (eds), *Thromboplastin Calibration and Oral Anticoagulant Control*. Boston: Martinus Nijhoff, 87–108.

Tripodi, A., Arbini, A.A., Chantarangkul, V. *et al.* (1993) Are capillary whole blood coagulation monitors suitable for the control of oral anticoagulant treatment by the international normalized ratio? *Thromb. Haemost.* **70**, 921–4.

Tripodi, A., Chantarangkul, V., Braga, M. *et al.* (1994) Results of a multicenter study assessing the status of standardization of a recombinant thromboplastin for the control of oral anticoagulant therapy. *Thromb. Haemost.* **72**, 261–7.

Tripodi, A., Poller, L., Van den Besselaar, A.M.H.P. and Mannucci, P.M. (1995a) A proposed scheme for calibration of international reference preparations of thromboplastin for the prothrombin time. *Thromb. Haemost.* **74**, 1368–9.

Tripodi, A., Chantarangkul, V., Akkawat, B. *et al.* (1995b) A partial factor V deficiency in anticoagulated lyophilized plasmas has been identified as a cause of the international normalized ratio discrepancy in the external quality assessment scheme. *Thromb. Res.* **78**, 283–92.

Tripodi, A., Chantarangkul, V., Manotti, C. *et al.* (1996) A simplified procedure for thromboplastin calibration – the usefulness of lyophilized plasmas assessed in a collaborative study. *Thromb. Haemost.* **75**, 309–12.

Tripodi, A., Chantarangkul, V., Clerici, M. *et al.* (1997) Determination of the international sensitivity index of a near-patient testing device to monitor oral anticoagulant therapy. *Thromb. Haemost.* **78**, 855–8.

Tripodi, A., Chantarangkul, V., Negri, B. *et al.* (1998) International collaborative study for the calibration of a proposed reference preparation of thromboplastin, human recombinant, plain. *Thromb. Haemost.* **79**, 439–43.

Van den Besselaar, A.M.H.P. (1993) Multi-center study of replacement of the international reference preparation for thromboplastin, rabbit, plain. *Thromb. Haemost.* **70**, 794–9.

Van den Besselaar, A.M.H.P. (1994a) Use of lyophilized calibration plasmas and control blood for international normalized ratio calculation in external quality assessment of the prothrombin time. *Am. J. Clin. Pathol.* **102**, 123–7.

Van den Besselaar, A.M.H.P. (1994b) The response of Quick's prothrombin time test to oral anticoagulation. Influence of thromboplastin source and calcium chloride concentration. *Arch. Pathol. Lab. Med.* **118**, 145–9.

Van den Besselaar, A.M.H.P. (1996a) Precision and accuracy of the international normalized ratio in oral anticoagulant control. *Haemostasis* **26**(suppl 4), 248–65.

Van den Besselaar, A.M.H.P. (1996b) Comparison of lyophilized plasmas with fresh plasmas for calibration of thromboplastin reagents in oral anticoagulant control. *Br. J. Haematol.* **93**, 437–44.

Van den Besselaar, A.M.H.P. (1997) Field study of lyophilised plasmas for local prothrombin time calibration in The Netherlands. *J. Clin. Pathol.* **50**, 371–4.

Van den Besselaar, A.M.H.P. and Bertina, R.M. (1993) Multi-centre study of thromboplastin calibration precision – influence of reagent species, composition, and international sensitivity index (ISI). *Thromb. Haemost.* **69**, 35–40.

Van den Besselaar, A.M.H.P. and Loeliger, E.A. (1982) The effect of contact activation on the prothrombin time with special reference to the use of evacuated tubes. In: Triplett, D.A. (ed.), *Standardization of Coagulation Assays: an Overview*. Skokie: College of American Pathologists, 95–102.

Van den Besselaar, A.M.H.P.and Van der Velde, E.A. (1984) The manufacturers' calibration study. In: van den Besselaar, A.M.H.P., Gralnick, H.R., Lewis, S.M. (eds), *Thromboplastin Calibration and Oral Anticoagulant Control*. Boston: Martinus Nijhoff, 127–49.

Van den Besselaar, A.M.H.P., Van Halem-Visser, L.P., Hoekstra-Schuman, M. *et al.* (1980) Simplified thromboplastin calibration. Further experience of the Dutch reference laboratory for anticoagulant control. *Thromb. Haemost.* **43**, 53–7.

Van den Besselaar, A.M.H.P., Van Halem-Visser, L.P. and Loeliger, E.A. (1983) The use of evacuated tubes for blood collection in oral anticoagulant control. *Thromb. Haemost.* **50**, 676–7.

Van den Besselaar, A.M.H.P., Lewis, S.M., Mannucci, P.M. and Poller, L. (1993) Status of present and candidate international reference preparations (IRP) of thromboplastin for the prothrombin time. *Thromb. Haemost.* **69**, 85.

Van den Besselaar, A.M.H.P., Meeuwisse-Braun, J., Schaefer-Van Mansfeld, H. *et al.* (1997) Influence of plasma volumetric errors on the prothrombin time ratio and international sensitivity index. *Blood Coag. Fibrinol.* **8**, 431–5.

Van den Besselaar, A.M.H.P., Meeuwisse-Braun, J., Witteveen, E., and Van Meegen, E. (1998) Effect of evacuated blood collection tubes on thromboplastin calibration. *Thromb. Haemost.* **79**, 1062–3.

Van den Besselaar, A.M.H.P., Houbouyan, L.L., Aillaud, M.F. *et al.* (1999) Influence of three types of automated coagulometers on the international sensitivity index (ISI) of rabbit, human, and recombinant human tissue factor preparations. *Thromb. Haemost.* **81**, 66–70.

Van der Velde, E.A. (1984) Orthogonal regression equation. In: van den Besselaar, A.M.H.P., Gralnick, H.R., Lewis, S.M. (eds), *Thromboplastin Calibration and Oral Anticoagulant Control*. Martinus Nijhoff, 25–39.

Van Dijk-Wierda, C.A., Van den Besselaar, A.M.H.P. and Loeliger, E.A. (1980) Quality control of prothrombin time determinations in The Netherlands. *Scand. J. Haematol.* **25**(suppl. 37), 153–5.

WHO ECBS (Expert Committee on Biological Standardization) (1977) *Blood Products and Related Substances. Thromboplastins.* WHO Technical Report Series. Twenty-eighth report. Geneva: WHO, 14–15.

WHO ECBS (Expert Committee on Biological Standardization) (1983) Requirements for thromboplastins and plasma used to control oral anticoagulant therapy. WHO Technical Report Series. Thirty-third report. Geneva: WHO, 81–105.

WHO ECBS (Expert Committee on Biological Standardization) (1999) Guidelines for thromboplastins and plasma used to control oral anticoagulant therapy. WHO Technical Report Series. Forty-eighth report. Geneva: WHO, 64–93.

Yawn, B.P., Loge C. and Dale, J. (1996) Prothrombin time: one tube or two. *Am. J. Clin. Pathol.* **105**, 794–7.

Ziffren, S.E., Owen, C.A., Hoffman, G.R. and Smith, H.P. (1940) A simple bedside test for control of vitamin K therapy. *Am. J. Clin. Pathol.* **10**, 13–16.

Zucker, S., Cathey, M.H. and West, B. (1970) Preparation of quality control specimens for coagulation. *Am. J. Clin. Pathol.* **53**, 924–7.

APPENDICES

Appendix A.18.1: EXAMPLE OF USE OF SUGGESTED METHOD FOR REPORTING THE DATA FOR THE CALIBRATION OF A HOUSE STANDARD OF THROMBOPLASTIN AGAINST AN INTERNATIONAL REFERENCE PREPARATION

THROMBOPLASTINS

- Rabbit brain thromboplastin house standard;
- International reference preparation of thromboplastin, rabbit, plain, RBT/90.

END-POINT RECORDING TECHNIQUES

- Automated photoelectric coagulometer for house standard;
- Manual (tilt tube) technique for RBT/90.

The tests were conducted on 10 days. On each day, two fresh normal and six fresh patient samples were tested. On each day, different subjects were used. The automated coagulometer and manual determinations were performed more or less simultaneously.

CALCULATIONS

The international sensitivity index of the house standard (ISI_w) is obtained by plotting the prothrombin times using the two thromboplastins on logarithmic axes as shown in Figure A.18.1, fitting a straight line of the form:

$$Y = A + BX \tag{A.1}$$

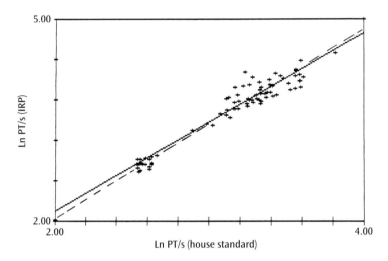

Fig. A.18.1 *Double-logarithmic plot of prothrombin times for determination of the international sensitivity index (ISI): ln (PT/s) with the secondary standard (horizontal axis) against ln$_e$ PT/s with the international reference preparation RBT/90 (vertical axis). The interrupted line represents the structural relation (orthogonal regression line) based on both normal and patient samples. The continuous line represents the relation based on the patients' samples alone.*

and estimating the slope B. The recommended method involves estimation of a linear structural relation (also called 'orthogonal regression equation'). With this technique, the slope (B) can be estimated as follows. Consider analysis for a set of N independent observations (x_i, y_i) where $i = 1, 2, 3, \ldots, N$; these symbols represent logarithms of the measured prothrombin times for N paired tests of the IRP (y) and the house standard (x). Write x_0, y_0, for the arithmetic means of the N values of x_i, y_i respectively. Write also Q_1, Q_2 for the sums of squares of ($x_i - x_0$) and ($y_i - y_0$), respectively, and P for the sum of their products. These quantities include all that is necessary for computing a and b, the least squares estimators for the parameters A and B of equation (A.1) Now define:

$$E = (Q_2 - Q_1)^2 + 4P^2 \tag{A.2}$$

Then

$$b = [Q_2 - Q_1 + E^{1/2}]/2P \tag{A.3}$$

and

$$a = y_0 - bx_0 \tag{A.4}$$

are the estimators that minimize the sum of squares of the perpendicular distances of the N points from the line (A.1).

The variance of b is given by:

$$\text{Var}(b) = \{[(1+b^2)P + NbV]bV\}/P^2 \tag{A.5}$$

where

$$V = (Q_2 - bP)/(N - 2) \tag{A.6}$$

The standard error of b (s_b) is the square root of $\text{Var}(b)$. If t is a deviate from the t-distribution, with $(N - 2)$ degrees of freedom and at a chosen probability, approximate confidence limits to B can now be obtained by setting an interval t^*s_b on either side of b.

The residual standard deviation is the square root of V. Outlying points should be rejected if their vertical distance from the calibration line is greater than three residual standard deviations.

The ISI for the house standard is calculated as follows:

$$\text{ISI}_w = \text{ISI}_{IRP} \times b \tag{A.7}$$

The coefficient of variation (%) of b is $100s_b/b$.

Creasy (1956) has suggested an ingenious alternative for the confidence limits for the slope, appropriate here if one can assume the frequency distribution of the random errors of the x_i and the y_i to be approximately normal. Creasy's result then determines confidence limits for B that rest upon rigorous theory; in practice, these limits are likely to be trustworthy unless N is so small as to introduce trouble from non-normality (Finney, 1995). With t as above, define:

$$D = 4t^2(Q_1Q_2 - P^2)/[E(N - 2)] \tag{A.8}$$

and form

$$b_0 = \tan^{-1}(b) \tag{A.9}$$

$$d_0 = \tan^{-1}\{[D/(1 - D)]^{1/2}\}/2 \tag{A.10}$$

Then the confidence limits are:

$$\tan(b_0 - d_0) \text{ and } \tan(b_0 + d_0) \tag{A.11}$$

In most cases at probability 0.95, $D < 1.0$. However, at higher probabilities an unusual conjunction of data can make the calculation of the confidence limits impossible because D exceeds 1.0 and the square root of a negative number is not defined (see equation A.10). There is no simple way of detecting this trouble until D has been calculated.

EXAMPLE

Using the data from Table A.18.1, the calculated MNPT values for RBT/90 and the rabbit thromboplastin are 17.16 and 13.12 seconds, respectively. The ISI of RBT/90 is 1.0. There was one outlier observation (patient no. 18) whose perpendicular distance to the orthogonal regression line was greater than 3 residual standard deviations. The data of this specimen were rejected. The calculated value for b based on the remaining 79 samples is 1.3753. Thus, the ISI for the house standard PT system is estimated as $1.0 \times 1.3753 = 1.3753$.

The standard error for b is calculated as 0.0372. The coefficient of variation for b is $100 \times 0.0372/1.3753 = 2.7\%$. The confidence limits for b are calculated according to Creasy's method, at probability 0.95: 1.3037 (lower limit) and 1.4522 (upper limit).

Table A.18.1 *Prothrombin times for the calibration of a house standard of rabbit thromboplastin*

Day (date)	Plasma	International reference preparation RBT/90	House standard
24.4.1996	Normal 1	16.9	12.5
	Patient 1	60.1	29.6
	Patient 2	48.1	24.1
	Patient 3	38.3	22.5
	Patient 4	55.2	26.0
	Patient 5	49.5	29.2
	Patient 6	36.2	21.5
	Normal 2	18.5	12.8
25.4.1996	Normal 3	15.9	13.6
	Patient 7	79.8	36.3
	Patient 8	55.4	29.7
	Patient 9	42.3	23.6
	Patient 10	54.2	30.2
	Patient 11	30.5	20.5
	Patient 12	49.5	29.8
	Normal 4	17.0	13.8
29.4.1996	Normal 5	17.1	12.7
	Patient 13	54.1	25.0
	Patient 14	31.3	19.7
	Patient 15	44.9	22.4
	Patient 16	46.4	22.8
	Patient 17	53.0	23.7
	Patient 18	67.3	25.3
	Normal 6	19.1	13.8
30.4.1996	Normal 7	18.6	13.3
	Patient 19	49.0	27.9
	Patient 20	35.2	22.4
	Patient 21	65.2	30.7
	Patient 22	61.5	26.5
	Patient 23	67.7	35.1
	Patient 24	28.3	18.0
	Normal 8	18.2	12.6
2.5.1996	Normal 9	17.0	13.0
	Patient 25	43.8	24.3
	Patient 26	44.5	26.4
	Patient 27	53.0	28.1
	Patient 28	51.0	27.8
	Patient 29	63.3	31.8
	Patient 30	60.7	32.4
	Normal 10	17.3	13.8
3.5.1996	Normal 11	18.2	13.6
	Patient 31	48.0	31.0
	Patient 32	45.5	27.3
	Patient 33	45.0	25.8
	Patient 34	38.5	23.7
	Patient 35	56.3	33.5
	Patient 36	69.1	35.1
	Normal 12	16.9	12.5

Day (date)	Plasma	International reference preparation RBT/90	House standard
6.5.1996	Normal 13	16.9	13.2
	Patient 37	43.3	28.1
	Patient 38	59.2	36.0
	Patient 39	46.9	30.3
	Patient 40	41.6	25.6
	Patient 41	64.3	35.9
	Patient 42	53.7	36.2
	Normal 14	19.3	14.3
7.5.1996	Normal 15	17.2	12.9
	Patient 43	52.7	34.9
	Patient 44	42.6	26.6
	Patient 45	41.8	27.9
	Patient 46	44.2	26.0
	Patient 47	39.1	24.2
	Patient 48	62.9	35.0
	Normal 16	16.9	12.6
8.5.1996	Normal 17	16.3	13.6
	Patient 49	34.1	23.0
	Patient 50	51.9	33.9
	Patient 51	48.8	28.7
	Patient 52	62.3	36.8
	Patient 53	48.1	27.2
	Patient 54	45.6	29.0
	Normal 18	16.0	12.6
13.5.1996	Normal 19	15.1	12.7
	Patient 55	58.7	36.1
	Patient 56	88.4	45.3
	Patient 57	44.1	27.7
	Patient 58	38.7	23.5
	Patient 59	40.1	25.7
	Patient 60	57.6	27.7
	Normal 20	15.6	12.8

In this example, there was a deviation from linearity. This can be shown by calculating the structural relation for the patients' samples only. The latter does not pass through the mean of the normals (see Fig. A.18.1). In this example, the assignment of an ISI based on all samples is acceptable because INRs calculated with the ISI do not differ by more than 10% from INRs calculated with the patients-only relation.

Appendix A.18.2: EXAMPLE OF USE OF SUGGESTED METHOD FOR REPORTING THE DATA ON THE CALIBRATION OF INDIVIDUAL BATCHES OF THROMBOPLASTIN

THROMBOPLASTINS

- Rabbit brain thromboplastin house standard;
- Batch of rabbit brain thromboplastin.

END-POINT RECORDING: AUTOMATED PHOTOELECTRIC COAGULOMETER

- Pooled coumarin plasmas, lots 960606, 1 through 5 (deep-frozen);
- Pooled normal plasma: lot 900423 (deep-frozen).

The ISI and MNPT of the rabbit brain thromboplastin house standard used with this particular automated photoelectric coagulometer are 1.31 and 12.7 seconds, respectively.

The tests were conducted in four separate runs. In each run, thromboplastins were reconstituted freshly and deep-frozen plasmas were thawed freshly. Since the house standard and the test batch were both used on the same photoelectric coagulometer, the order in which the two preparations were tested was alternated from one run to the next. This was done to avoid any bias due to possible instability of the thromboplastins and pooled plasmas.

CALCULATION

The International sensitivity index of the batch (ISI_b) is calculated as $ISI_b = ISI_w \times b$, where b is the slope of the straight line fitted to a double-logarithmic plot of the prothrombin times in Table A.18.2, with the prothrombin times for the house standard and the batch being shown on the vertical and horizontal axes, respectively (see Fig. A.18.2). The structural relation

Table A.18.2   *Prothrombin times for the calibration of an individual batch of rabbit thromboplastin*

Run no.	Plasma lot no.	House standard Order of testing (within-run)	Prothrombin time	Rabbit brain thromboplastin Order of testing (within-run)	Prothrombin time
1	900423	1	14.0	7	15.1
	960606-1	2	20.5	8	21.5
	960606-2	3	29.1	9	31.5
	960606-3	4	32.9	10	36.4
	960606-4	5	36.2	11	41.0
	960606-5	6	39.7	12	44.6
2	900423	7	14.1	1	15.4
	960606-1	8	20.3	2	22.6
	960606-2	9	29.5	3	31.2
	960606-3	10	32.8	4	37.6
	960606-4	11	37.3	5	40.8
	960606-5	12	39.8	6	44.5
3	900423	1	14.0	7	15.0
	960606-1	2	20.0	8	21.5
	960606-2	3	28.1	9	32.1
	960606-3	4	31.8	10	34.2
	960606-4	5	35.9	11	40.7
	960606-5	6	37.2	12	44.7
4	900423	7	13.9	1	15.0
	960606-1	8	20.0	2	21.9
	960606-2	9	27.9	3	30.9
	960606-3	10	31.5	4	35
	960606-4	11	34.6	5	39.2
	960606-5	12	37.6	6	44.4

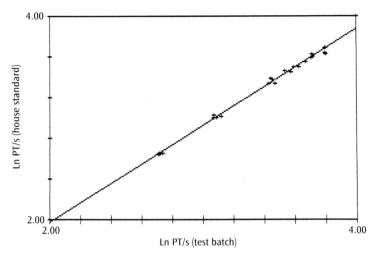

Fig. A.18.2 *Double-logarithmic plot of prothrombin times for determination of the international sensitivity index (ISI): ln (PT/s) with the test batch (horizontal axis) against ln (PT/s) with the secondary standard (vertical axis). The line represents the structural relation (orthogonal regression line) based on six deep-frozen pooled plasmas tested in four sessions.*

formula for b is, the necessary changes having been made, given by equation (A.3) above. The standard error of b is obtained from equation (A.5). The coefficient of variation (%) of b is $100 \times s_b/b$.

EXAMPLE

Using the data from Table A.18.2, the calculated value for b is 0.9466. The ISI for the house standard is given as 1.31. Thus, the ISI for the batch is estimated as $1.31 \times 0.9466 = 1.24$.

The standard error for b is calculated as 0.0142. The coefficient of variation for b is $100 \times 0.0142/0.9466 = 1.5\%$. The confidence limits for b at probability 0.95: 0.9175 and 0.9765 (Creasy's method).

Index

Note: page numbers in **bold** refer to tables